DIAGNOSTIC ULTRASOUND

Seventh Edition

DIAGNOSTIC ULTRASOUND

Principles and Instruments

Frederick W. Kremkau, PhD

Professor and Director
Center for Medical Ultrasound
Wake Forest University
School of Medicine
Winston-Salem, North Carolina

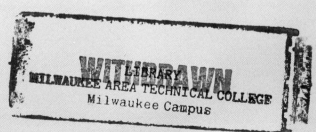
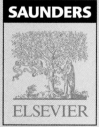

SAUNDERS

ELSEVIER

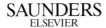
SAUNDERS
ELSEVIER

11830 Westline Industrial Drive
St. Louis, Missouri 63146

Notice

International Standard Book Number 0-7216-3192-4

Executive Editor: Jeanne Wilke
Senior Developmental Editor: Linda Woodard
Publishing Services Manager: Patricia Tannian
Project Manager: Kristine Feeherty
Designer: Jyotika Shroff

Printed in the United States of America

Working together to grow
libraries in developing countries

www.elsevier.com | www.bookaid.org | www.sabre.org

ELSEVIER   BOOK AID International   Sabre Foundation

Last digit is the print number: 9 8 7 6 5 4 3 2 1

To colleagues with whom I've been privileged to collaborate and publish:

Edwin Carstensen, PhD — *University of Rochester*
Barry Goldberg, MD — *Thomas Jefferson University*
Lennard Greenbaum, MD — *Orlando Regional Healthcare*
John Hobbins, MD — *Yale University (now at the University of Colorado)*
Dalane Kitzman, MD — *Wake Forest University*
Christopher Merritt, MD — *Thomas Jefferson University*
Lewis Nelson, MD — *Wake Forest University*
Charles Tegeler, MD — *Wake Forest University*
Larry Waldroup, BS, RDMS — *Thomas Jefferson University*

To the memory of former academic colleagues and coauthors:

Robert Apfel, PhD — *Yale University*
Hugh Flynn, PhD — *University of Rochester*
Raymond Gramiak, MD — *University of Rochester*
William McKinney, MD — *Wake Forest University*
Charles L. Spurr, MD — *Wake Forest University*
Kenneth Taylor, MD, PhD — *Yale University*

And to Lil, who for 38 years has walked with me down …

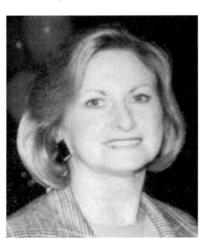
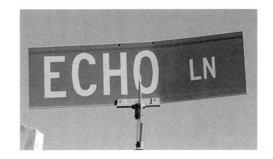

Reviewers

Joan M. Clasby, BvE, RDMS, RT
Sonography Program Director
Orange Coast College
Costa Mesa, California

Ana Maria P. De Jesus, MS, RDMS
MCDMS Clinical Coordinator and Assistant Professor
Montgomery College
Takoma Park, Maryland

Janice Dolk, MA, RT(R), RDMS
Director of Allied Health Education
University of Maryland, Baltimore County
Baltimore, Maryland

Stephanie Ellingson, BA, RDMS, RDCS, RVT, RTR
Program Director, Diagnostic Medical Sonography
University of Iowa Hospitals and Clinics
Iowa City, Iowa

Thomas J. Gervaise, BS, RT, RDMS
Ultrasound Division Director
Modern Technology School
Anaheim, California

Ecaterina Mariana Hdeib, MA, RDMS
Clinical Instructor, Diagnostic Medical Ultrasound
    Program
University of Missouri-Columbia
Columbia, Missouri

Felicia Jones, MSEd, RDMS, RVT
Director
Tidewater Community College
Virginia Beach, Virginia

Joseph Morton, MBA, RT(R), RDMS
Sonographer and Clinical Instructor
St. Mary's Hospital
Milwaukee, Wisconsin

Susanna L. Ovel, RT, RDMS, RVT
Senior Sonographer and Trainer
Radiological Associates of Sacramento
Sacramento, California

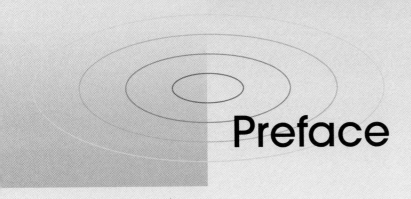

Preface

This book is intended for students, allied-health personnel, and physicians who need fundamental knowledge of the physical principles and instrumentation of diagnostic ultrasound. Understanding and applying these underlying principles of physics and electronics improves the quality of medical care involving diagnostic ultrasound. The best sonographers and image interpreters are those who understand these principles and apply them in their practice.

The purpose of this book is to explain how contemporary diagnostic ultrasound works. It serves as a principles textbook in sonography educational programs and helps readers handle artifacts properly, scan safely, evaluate instrument performance, and prepare for registry and board examinations. The content of the book, however, is not driven by published exam content outlines, but rather by the author's assessment of contemporary technology in the field and his approach to teaching this material in the classroom and at conferences and seminars. The book does not describe how to perform diagnostic examinations or how to interpret the results except, in a limited way, in the consideration of Doppler displays in Chapters 6 and 7, artifacts in Chapter 8, and safety in Chapter 9. Other books are available that concentrate on scanning techniques and interpretation of images.

Although the book is up to date regarding newer developments in the field, the emphasis is on the fundamentals. For the sake of beginners, the text is simplified while at the same time maintaining its integrity and usefulness for more experienced users. To provide broader coverage of the material for advanced readers while avoiding overwhelming beginners, some advanced concepts and topics are included in shaded boxes separated from the main text and also compiled in Appendix H. Beginners and those not interested in advanced concepts can skip these boxes. Advanced books with broad coverage, appropriate primarily for physicists, medical physicists, and engineers, are available.[1,2] A basic understanding of some mathematics and physics is assumed. These concepts are reviewed in Appendixes E and F. Although the book is intended for readers who lack a physics or engineering background, digestion of the material *will* require significant effort. Admittedly, for such readers, the material *is* difficult. It cannot be made easy and still maintain the necessary understanding for appropriate application in practice. However, 30 years of lecturing and publication experience has convinced the author that the material *can* be understandable with reasonable preparation and effort on the part of the student. For the sake of brevity and comprehension, many statements made in this book are simplifications of the actual situation. No attempt is made to present the history of the development of diagnostic ultrasound. This has been summarized in a series of articles in the *Journal of Ultrasound in Medicine* (Vol. 22-24, 2003-2005) and in other references.

DIFFERENCES WITH EARLIER EDITIONS AND WITH NATIONAL EXAMINATIONS

There are several differences between each new edition compared with earlier editions and compared with the content of ARDMS and board examinations. This is because this text is up to date with current technology, while exams change more slowly because of the necessarily thorough and time-consuming process requiring practice surveys, committee decisions, and item generation, review, and approval. For example, the receiver block in the instrument diagram and discussion of receiver functions (in editions 1 through 5) are now outmoded carry-overs from the analog electronics era. Four of these former functions are now accomplished in the beam former or the signal processor, and one has disappeared. Mechanical transducers, including annular arrays, have been largely phased out and are no longer included in Chapter 3. Static scanners and analog image memories have been gone for years. Outmoded descriptions of technology and instrument features that are no longer largely present in the field are eliminated with each new edition. Thus the book tends to change more rapidly than the exams. For exam preparation this is a disadvantage, but the philosophy of the book is to be, with each edition, as consistent as possible with contemporary technology, rather than to tailor material to current exam content outlines. Also, some topics that may appear in exams are, in the author's opinion, irrelevant or inappropriately in-depth for the nonphysicist/nonengineer readership of this book. Examples include wave interference, Huygens' principle, and diffraction. The material that *is* covered is broad and complicated as it is, without adding undue breadth or depth. Topics that in the author's opinion are superfluous or outmoded but are included in published exam outlines are treated briefly in Appendix G. In this way the integrity and relevance of the text are maintained while also covering other terms and topics the student may encounter in principles lectures, articles, courses, and examinations.

FEATURES

- Comprehensive coverage of all aspects of diagnostic ultrasound
- Latest developments in sonographic technology
- Two presentations of Doppler principles (broad and condensed)
- More than 1,000 images, several in color
- Learning objectives lists
- Review and practice exercises with answers
- Key points listings and compilation
- Descriptive subheadings
- Highlighted key terms
- Helpful boxes and tables
- Math and physics reviews
- National exam preparation material
- Advanced topics insertions and compilation
- Glossary

NEW TO THIS EDITION

The recent introduction of flat-panel displays in sonographic instruments prompted their inclusion. Discussions of coded excitation, 3D imaging, and contrast agents have been expanded. Mathematics and physics reviews, exam preparation material, advanced topics, and a condensed treatment of Doppler ultrasound (Appendix I) are new features. The advanced topics appear in shaded boxes at appropriate locations within the text and are compiled in Appendix H.

USING THIS TEXT

This book covers, in three parts, the principles of how diagnostic ultrasound works:

1. Sonographic Principles (Chapters 1-4)
2. Doppler Principles (Chapters 5-7)
3. Miscellaneous Topics (Chapter 8-10)

It is intended that the book be read in sequential chapter order, as each chapter builds on previously presented material. One exception to this is that Appendix I can be substituted for Chapters 5-7 for readers who need less depth and breadth of coverage on Doppler topics. The complete coverage in Chapters 5-7 is recommended for those working in echocardiography and vascular ultrasound. Key terms are boldface at first appearance in the text and are listed at the beginning of each chapter and defined in the Glossary. Exercises, numbering more than a thousand (including a comprehensive multiple-choice examination in Chapter 10), are provided to evaluate progress, strengthen concepts, and provide practice for registry and specialty board examinations. Answers are given at the back of the book. Also included are nine appendixes: Appendix A is a compilation of key points from each chapter, and Appendixes B, C, and D are compilations of the symbols, equations, and tables that appear throughout the book. Appendixes E and F provide mathematics and physics reviews for material relevant to diagnostic ultrasound. Appendix G treats additional material that may appear on board and registry exams. Appendix G and Chapter 10 provide review material for the student and those studying for registry and specialty board exams. Appendix H is a compilation of advanced material appearing throughout the book that is beyond that appropriate for beginners. Appendix I is a condensed version of the material on Doppler ultrasound in Chapters 5-7.

After studying this book, the student should be able to:

- Describe what ultrasound is.
- Explain how ultrasound detects and locates anatomic structures.
- Explain how ultrasound is sent into the body.
- Discuss how echoes are received from the body and processed in the instrument.
- Describe how anatomic information is presented on the display.
- Explain how ultrasound detects and measures tissue motion and blood flow.
- List the ways motion and flow information is presented.
- Explain how flow detection is localized to a specific site in tissue.
- List the common artifacts that can occur with diagnostic ultrasound.

- Discuss how performance of sonographic instruments is tested.
- Describe the risk and safety issues associated with diagnostic ultrasound.

FOR THE INSTRUCTOR

Several additions and modifications to the book are in response to reviews from 11 sonography educational program directors. Not all of their recommendations could be implemented because of differences of opinion with the author and even with each other. In the author's judgment, the best and most practical improvements have been incorporated into this edition.

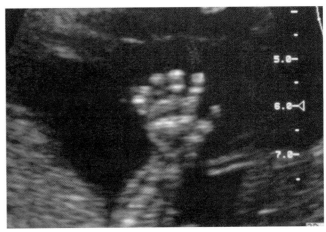

Any questions?

Acknowledgments

The author gratefully acknowledges helpful comments and suggestions from students and instructors who have used previous editions of the book. For contributions to text development and illustration acquisition, he thanks:

Gene Adamowski
Dick Begin
Jim Brown
Pam Burgess
Cindy Burnham
Peter Burns
Sandy Frazier Byrne
Marge Cappuccio
Jackie Carlson
Jackie Challender
George Cook
Ken Craig
Larry Crum
Diane Davis
Lou Davis
Tom Dew
Bob Dockendorff
Jean Ellison
Rob Entrekin
Karen Fowle
Sherry Francis
Rob Gill
Richard Hackel
Sharon Hardin
Tracey Heriot
Sharon Hughes
Clarence Hynes
Jim Jago
Teresa Jones
Marie King
Dalane Kitzman
Clay Larsen
Jill Leighton
Kathy Lewis

Anne Mansfield
Kristin Martin
Doug Maxwell
Dana Meads
Steve Meads
Chris Merritt
Don Milburn
Heather Miller
Mort Miller
Terry Needham
Lew Nelson
Mohsen Nomeir
Leif Penrose
Valerie Perry
Cam Pollock
Jeff Powers
Roy Preston
Delores Pretorius
Paul Ramsey
Scott Reavis
Joe Roselli
Helen Routh
Pam Rowland
Lars Shaw
John Sheldon
Jackie Sledge
Jacques Souquet
David Taylor
Chuck Tegeler
Paul Tesh
Kai Thomenius
Barbara Weinstein
Neil Wolfman

with special recognition to John Seksay for generating many images for a teaching and publication file.

For their cooperation and assistance he also thanks the American Institute of Ultrasound in Medicine (AIUM), the American Registry for Diagnostic Medical Sonography (ARDMS), and the following companies (with special appreciation to the engineers of Philips Ultrasound for on-site, enlightening, and in-depth discussions):

Aloka
ATS Laboratories
Computerized Imaging Reference Systems (CIRS)
Gammex RMI
GE Medical Systems
Medison
Medisonics
Nuclear Associates
Nuclear Enterprises
Philips Ultrasound
Siemens Ultrasound
Sonosite
Terason
Toshiba Medical Systems

He acknowledges, with appreciation, Jeanne Wilke for developmental assistance, Linda Woodard for editorial assistance, and Kristine Feeherty for production management.

Contents

DIAGNOSTIC ULTRASOUND

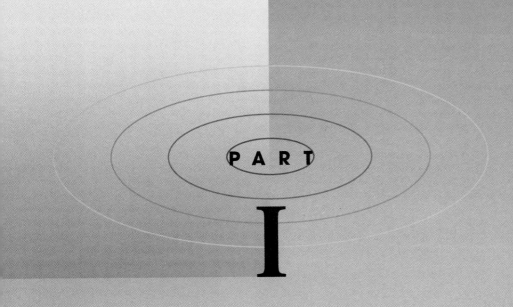

Sonographic Principles

1 Introduction

LEARNING OBJECTIVES

After reading this chapter, the student should be able to do the following:

- Explain how the pulse-echo principle is used in sonography.
- Describe the image formats used in sonography.
- Explain how the Doppler effect is applied in Doppler ultrasound.
- List the ways in which Doppler information is presented by Doppler instruments.

KEY TERMS

The following terms are introduced in this chapter:

Color Doppler display
Doppler effect
Gray-scale
Image
Instrument

Linear image
Pulse-echo technique
Scan line
Sector image
Sonography

Spectral displays
Transducer
Ultrasound

Bats, dolphins, and other animals used **ultrasound** long before human beings applied it to their needs. These animals use ultrasound to detect, locate, determine motion of, and capture prey; to avoid obstacles; to detect and avoid predators; and in the courtship of mates. Among other uses, human beings have applied ultrasound techniques, in the form of diagnostic ultrasound, to the challenges of diagnostic medicine. Diagnostic ultrasound encompasses **sonography** and Doppler ultrasound. Sonography is medical anatomic imaging using a **pulse-echo technique.** Doppler ultrasound includes detection, quantitation, and evaluation of tissue motion and blood flow using the **Doppler effect** with ultrasound.

SONOGRAPHY

The word *sonography* comes from the Latin *sonus* (sound) and the Greek *graphein* (to write). Diagnostic

sonography is medical two-dimensional and three-dimensional anatomic and flow imaging using ultrasound. Ultrasound imaging is not a passive push-button activity but rather an interactive process involving the sonographer, patient, **transducer, instrument,** and sonologist. Understanding the underlying physical and electronic principles presented in this book improves the quality of medical care involving diagnostic sonography.

Medical imaging with ultrasound is called sonography.

An **image** (from the Latin term for "imitate") is a reproduction, representation, or imitation of the physical form of a person or thing. An ultrasound image is the visible counterpart of an invisible object, produced by an electronic instrument. Ultrasound provides a noninvasive way of looking inside the human body (Figure 1-1)

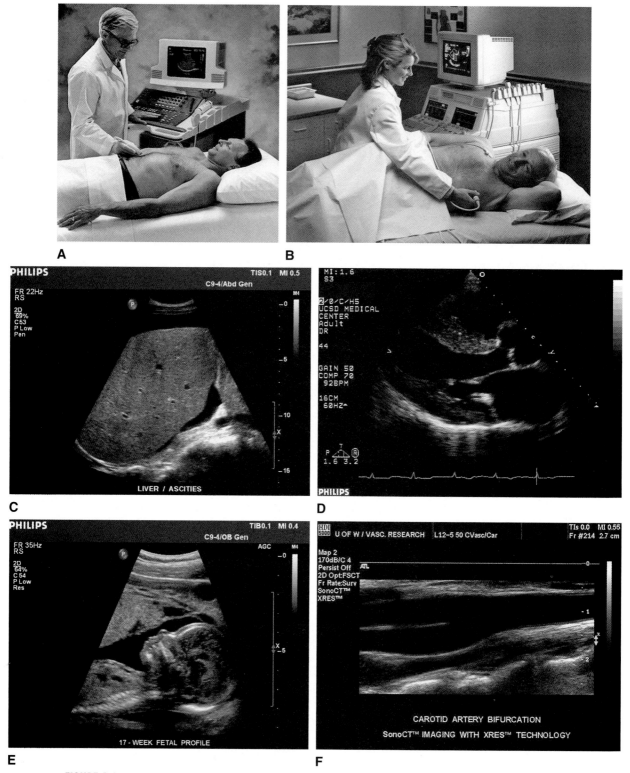

■ **FIGURE 1-1**   (**A** and **B**) Ultrasound provides a window into the human body, allowing us to see what we otherwise would not see: abdominal (**C**), cardiac (**D**), obstetric (**E**), and vascular (**F**) images.

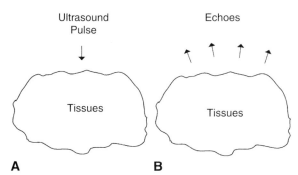

■ **FIGURE 1-2**   Pulse-echo technique. **A,** In diagnostic ultrasound, ultrasound pulses are sent into the tissues to interact with them and to obtain information about them. **B,** Echoes return from the tissues, providing information that is useful for anatomic imaging, flow measurement, and diagnosis.

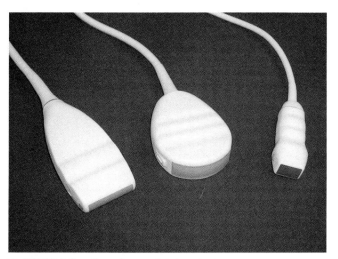

■ **FIGURE 1-3**   Transducers of various types.

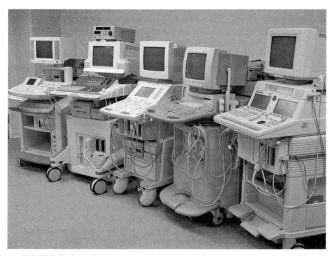

■ **FIGURE 1-4**   Sonographic instruments from various manufacturers.

to image otherwise unseen anatomy. Anatomic imaging with ultrasound is accomplished with a pulse-echo technique. Pulses of ultrasound are generated by a transducer and are sent into the patient (Figure 1-2), where they produce echoes at organ boundaries and within tissues. These echoes then return to the transducer, where they are detected and then presented on the display of a sonographic instrument. The transducer (Figure 1-3) generates the ultrasound pulses and receives the returning echoes. Sonography requires knowledge of the location of origin and the strength of the echoes returning from the patient. The ultrasound instrument (Figure 1-4) processes the echoes and presents them as visible dots, which form the anatomic image on the display. The brightness of each dot corresponds to the echo strength, producing what then is known as a **gray-scale** image. The location of each dot corresponds to the anatomic location of the echo-generating structure. Positional information is determined by knowing the direction of the pulse when it enters the patient and measuring the time it takes for its echo to return to the transducer. From a starting point on the display (usually at the top), the proper location for presenting the echo then can be determined. With knowledge of the sound speed, the echo arrival time is used to determine the depth of the structure that produced the echo.

Sonography is accomplished with a pulse-echo technique.

Echoes from anatomic structures represent these structures in a sonographic image.

If one pulse of ultrasound is sent into tissue, a series of dots (one line of echo information or one **scan line**) is displayed (Figure 1-5). Not all of the ultrasound pulse is reflected back from any interface. Rather, most of the original pulse continues to be reflected back from deeper interfaces. The echoes from one pulse appear as one scan line (Figure 1-5, *E* and *F*). If the process is repeated, but with different starting points for each subsequent pulse, a cross-sectional image of the anatomy is built up (Figure 1-6). Each pulse travels in the same direction but starts from a different point, yielding vertical parallel scan lines and a rectangular image as shown in Figure 1-7. These cross-sectional images are produced with vertical parallel scan lines that are so close together that they cannot be identified individually. The rectangular display resulting from this procedure often is called a linear scan or **linear image,** referring to the linear-array transducer used to produce it. A second approach to sending ultrasound pulses through the anatomy to be imaged is shown in Figure 1-8. With this method, each pulse originates from the same starting point, but subsequent pulses go out in slightly different directions. This results in a sector scan (**sector image**), which is shaped like a slice of pie (Figure 1-9). Figure 1-10 shows a format that is a combination of the two just described; that is, pulses (and scan lines) originate from different starting points (as in a linear image), but each pulse (and scan line) travels in a slightly different direction than the previous one (as in a sector image). In this example, the starting points form a curved line across the top of the scan rather than a straight line, as in the linear scans shown in Figure 1-7.

Sonographic images are composed of many scan lines.

Sonographic scan formats commonly are limited to these three types: linear, sector, and their combination. Other formats may be used occasionally, but in any case, what is required is that ultrasound pulses be sent through all portions of the anatomic cross section that is to be imaged. Each pulse generates a series of echoes, resulting in a series of dots (a scan line) on the display. The resulting cross-sectional image is composed of many (typically 96 to 256) of these scan lines. The scan format determines the starting points and paths for the individual scan lines according to the starting point and path for each pulse used in generating each scan line. The clinical cross-sectional gray-scale sonographic images produced sometimes are called B scans, indicating that the images are produced by *scanning* the ultrasound through the imaged cross section (i.e., sending pulses through all regions of the cross section) and converting the echo strength into the *brightness* of each represented echo on the display (hence, B scan or brightness scan). B scan and gray-scale scan mean the same thing.

Sonographic images are presented in linear and sector forms.

For many years, sonography was limited to two-dimensional (2D) cross-sectional scans (or "cuts") through anatomy. Now 2D imaging has been extended into three-dimensional (3D) scanning and imaging. This requires scanning the ultrasound through many adjacent tissue cross sections to build up a 3D volume of echo information (Figure 1-11). This 3D volume of echoes then can be processed and interrogated to present 2D or 3D images of the anatomy.

Sonographic images are of 2D and 3D types.

DOPPLER ULTRASOUND

Echoes produced by moving objects have frequencies different from the pulses sent into the body. This is called the Doppler effect, which is put to use in detecting and measuring tissue motion and blood flow. Animals sometimes apply the Doppler effect in their use of ultrasound. Human applications include the Doppler effect observed in light received from stars that indicates that the universe is expanding. The use of Doppler radar in weather forecasting, aviation safety, and vehicle speed detection with police radar has made the term a household word. In addition to experiencing the acoustic Doppler effect in everyday life (as demonstrated by the changing pitch of a siren or vehicle horn as the vehicle passes by), the Doppler effect has been applied to automatic door openers in public buildings and to burglar alarms (Figure 1-12). The Doppler effect is named after Christian Andreas Doppler, who conducted an extensive investigation into its nature.[5]

The Doppler effect is a change in frequency caused by moving objects.

Like sonography, Doppler ultrasound has been used in medicine for many years. Long-standing applications include monitoring the fetal heart rate during labor and delivery and evaluating blood flow in the heart and carotid arteries. Like sonography, Doppler ultrasound has been used in virtually all medical specialties. In addition to detecting tissue motion, Doppler ultrasound can determine the presence or absence of blood flow and its direction, speed, and character. Rapid scanning and processing of Doppler data allow color-coded presentations of Doppler information (**color Doppler displays**) to be superimposed on gray-scale anatomic images (Figure 1-13 and Color Plate 1). Doppler information is applied to loudspeakers for audible evaluation and to chart recorders and **spectral displays** for quantitative analysis (Figure 1-14 and Color Plate 2). Doppler instruments include sonographic imaging to determine the anatomic locations from which the Doppler information is acquired (Figure 1-15).

Doppler information is presented in audible, color display, strip-chart, and spectral display forms.

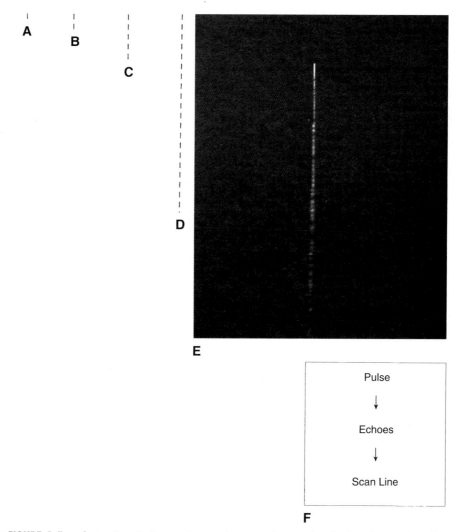

■ **FIGURE 1-5**   One pulse of ultrasound generates a single scan line (series of echoes) as it travels through tissue. Echoes are presented in sequence on a scan line as they return from tissue during pulse travel. **A,** The first echo is displayed. **B,** The second echo is added. **C,** Three more echoes are added. **D,** All the echoes from a single pulse have been received and displayed as a completed scan line. **E,** A complete scan line resulting from one emitted pulse. In practice, this is accomplished in less than one-thousandth of a second. **F,** According to the pulse-echo imaging principle, one pulse traveling through tissues produces a stream of echoes that become one scan line on the display.

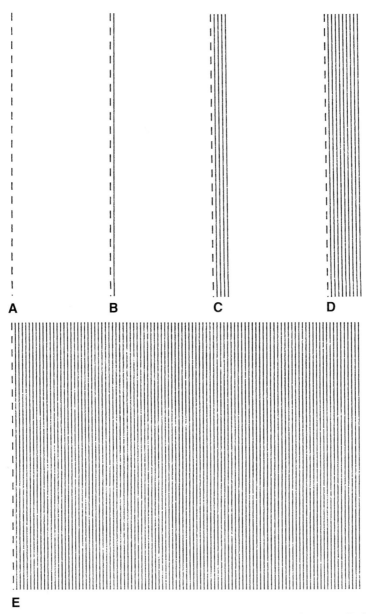

■ **FIGURE 1-6**   A single rectangular image or scan (frame) is composed of many vertical parallel scan lines. Each scan line represents a series of echoes returning from a pulse traveling through the tissues. **A,** One scan line from one pulse, as generated in Figure 1-5. **B,** A second scan line is added. **C** and **D,** Five and 10 scan lines, respectively. **E,** A complete frame consisting of (in this example) 100 scan lines.

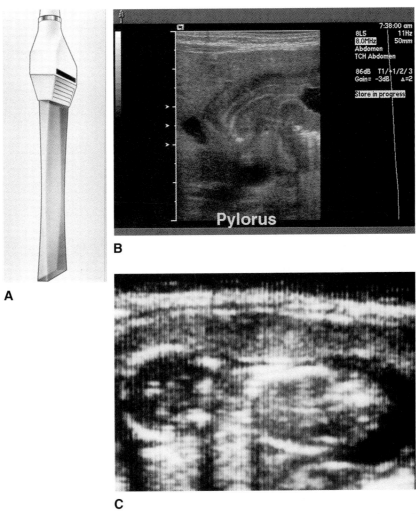

A

B

C

■ **FIGURE 1-7** **A,** Ultrasound is sent through a rectangular volume of tissue to produce rectangular images that commonly are called linear images or linear scans. **B,** Linear abdominal scan. **C,** Poor-quality (by current standards) fetal image from the late 1970s reveals the 120 vertical parallel scan lines of which it is composed.

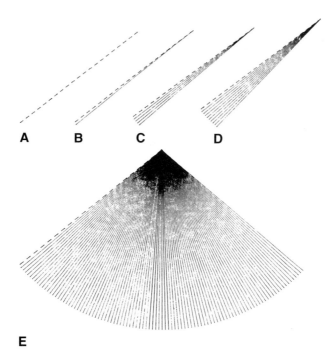

A   **B**   **C**   **D**

E

■ **FIGURE 1-8**   A single sector frame is progressively built up with 1 **(A)**, 2 **(B)**, 5 **(C)**, 10 **(D)**, and 100 **(E)** scan lines in sequence. All originate from a common origin and travel out in different directions.

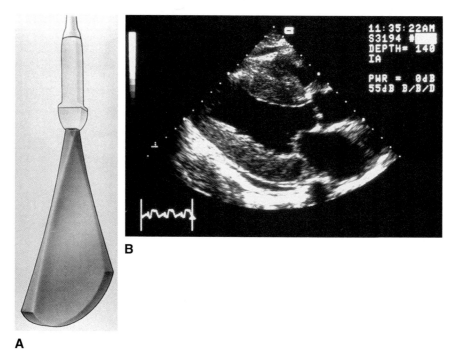

B

A

■ **FIGURE 1-9**   **A,** Ultrasound is sent through a pie slice–shaped volume of tissue to produce images that commonly are called sector images or sector scans. **B,** Sector scan of adult heart.

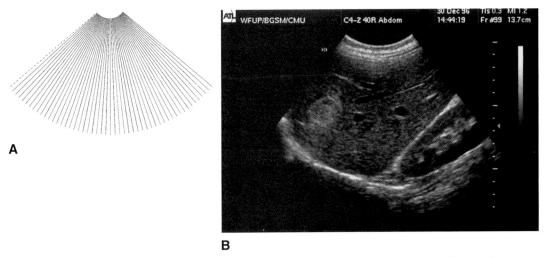

■ **FIGURE 1-10** **A,** A modified form of sector scan is produced when pulses and scan lines originate from different points across the top of a sector display. **B,** Abdominal scan of the liver and kidney using the scan format shown in **A.**

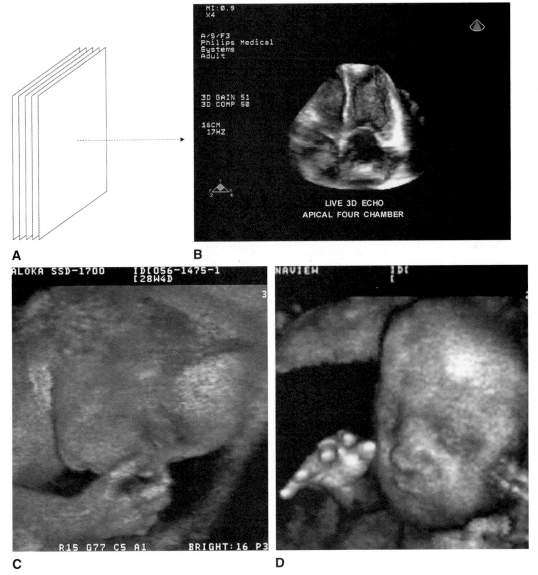

■ **FIGURE 1-11** Three-dimensional sonographic images. **A,** Three-dimensional echo data are acquired by obtaining many two-dimensional sections of echo information from the imaged anatomy. **B,** Cardiac four-chamber view. **C,** Fetus holding nose. **D,** Fetal head and hands.

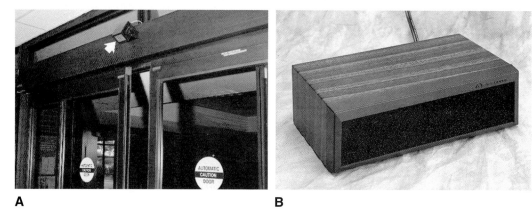

■ FIGURE 1-12   Ultrasonic devices that use the Doppler effect. **A,** An automatic door opener *(arrow).*
B, A motion-detection (burglar) alarm.

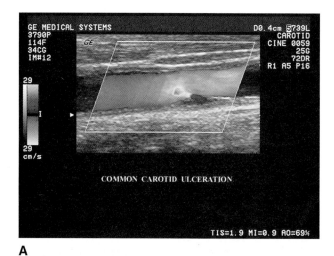

A

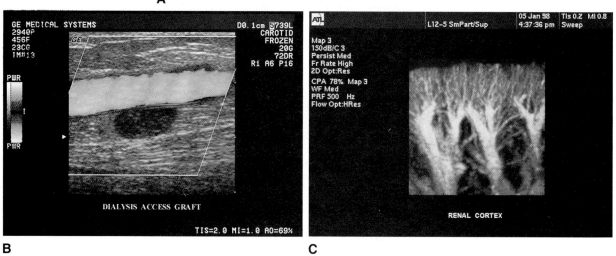

B   **C**

■ FIGURE 1-13   Color Doppler displays of blood flow presented in forms called **(A)** color Doppler-shift,
(B) color Doppler-power, and **(C)** 3D color Doppler-power displays. See Color Plate 1.

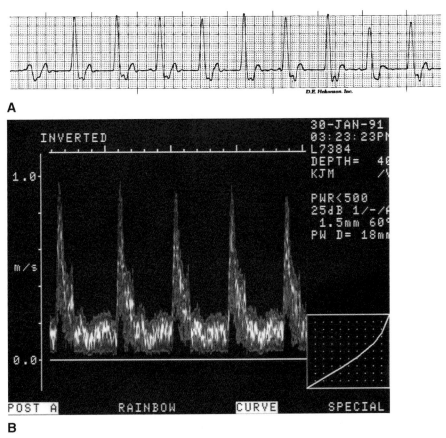

■ **FIGURE 1-14**   **A,** Strip-chart recording of Doppler information. **B,** Display of Doppler information (in a form called a spectral display) from common carotid arterial blood flow. See Color Plate 2 for **B.**

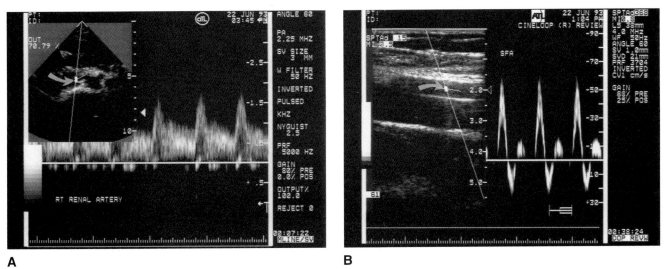

■ **FIGURE 1-15**   Spectral Doppler displays of blood flow in the right renal artery **(A)** and superficial femoral artery **(B),** with anatomic images showing the locations *(curved arrows)* from which the Doppler information was acquired.

REVIEW

The key points presented in this chapter are the following:
- Medical imaging with ultrasound is called sonography.
- Sonography is accomplished with a pulse-echo technique.
- Echoes from anatomic structures represent these structures in a sonographic image.
- Sonographic images are composed of many scan lines.
- Sonographic images are presented in linear and sector forms.
- Sonographic images are of 2D and 3D types.
- The Doppler effect is a change in frequency caused by moving objects.
- Doppler information is presented in audible, color display, strip-chart, and spectral display forms.

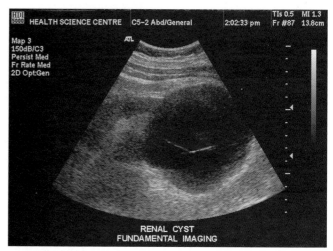

■ **FIGURE 1-16**   Illustration to accompany Exercise 9.

EXERCISES

1. The diagnostic ultrasound imaging (sonography) method has two parts:
   a. Sending _____ of _____ into the body.
   b. Using _____ received from the anatomy to produce an _____ of that anatomy.
2. Ultrasound gray-scale scans are _____-_____ images of tissue cross sections.
3. The brightness of an echo, as presented on the display, represents the _____ of the echo.
4. A linear scan is composed of many _____-_____ scan lines.
5. A sector scan is composed of many scan lines with a common _____.
6. A linear scan has a _____ shape.
7. A sector scan is shaped like a _____ of _____.
8. A sector scan can have a _____ or a _____ top.
9. Figure 1-16 is an example of an image in which the scan lines do *not* originate at a common _____.
10. Sonography is accomplished by using a _____-_____ technique. The information of importance in doing this includes the _____ from which each echo originated and the _____ of each echo. From this information, one can determine the echo _____ and _____ on the display.
11. The _____ is the interface between the patient and the instrument.
12. Transducers generate _____ _____ and receive returning _____.
13. Three-dimensional echo information is presented on _____ displays.
14. Acquisition of a 3D echo data volume requires scanning the ultrasound through several tissue _____ _____.

15. The Doppler effect is a change in echo
    a. amplitude.
    b. intensity.
    c. impedance.
    d. frequency.
    e. arrival time.
16. The change in Exercise 15 is a result of _____.
17. The motion that produces the Doppler effect is that of the
    a. transducer.
    b. sound beam.
    c. display.
    d. reflector.
18. In medical applications, the flow of _____ is commonly the source of the Doppler effect. Doppler information is applied to _____ for audible evaluation and to a _____ for visual analysis.
19. The visual display of Doppler information can be in the form of a _____-_____ recording, a _____ display, or a _____ display.
20. Color Doppler displays can present Doppler-_____ and Doppler-_____ information in color.
21. Figure 1-17 shows a
    a. 2D linear image.
    b. 2D sector image.
    c. modified sector image.
    d. 3D gray-scale image.
    e. spectral display.
22. Figure 1-18 shows a
    a. 2D linear image.
    b. 2D sector image.
    c. modified sector image.
    d. 3D gray-scale image.
    e. spectral display.

23. Figure 1-19 shows a
   a. 2D linear image.
   b. 2D sector image.
   c. modified sector image.
   d. 3D gray-scale image.
   e. spectral display.
24. Figure 1-20 shows a
   a. 2D linear image.
   b. 2D sector image.
   c. modified sector image.
   d. 3D gray-scale image.
   e. spectral display.
25. Figure 1-21 shows a
   a. 2D linear image.
   b. 2D sector image.
   c. modified sector image.
   d. 3D gray-scale image.
   e. spectral display.

Answers to the exercises begin on p. 361.

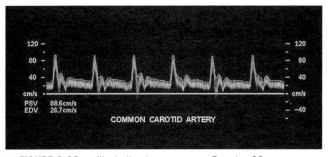

■ **FIGURE 1-19** Illustration to accompany Exercise 23.

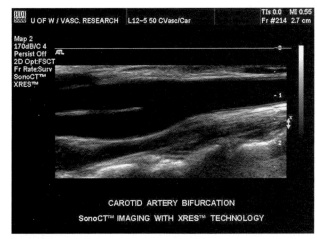

■ **FIGURE 1-17** Illustration to accompany Exercise 21.

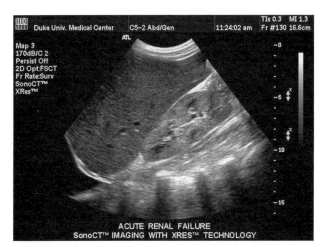

■ **FIGURE 1-20** Illustration to accompany Exercise 24.

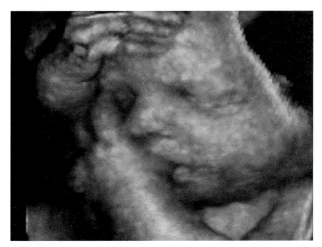

■ **FIGURE 1-18** Illustration to accompany Exercise 22.

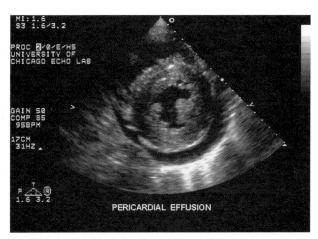

■ **FIGURE 1-21** Illustration to accompany Exercise 25.

LEARNING OBJECTIVES

After reading this chapter, the student should be able to do the following:

- Explain what frequency is and why it is important in diagnostic ultrasound.
- Define ultrasound and describe how it behaves.
- Discuss how harmonics are generated.
- Compare continuous and pulsed ultrasound.
- Describe the weakening of ultrasound as it travels through tissue.
- Discuss the generation of echoes in tissue.

KEY TERMS

The following terms are introduced in this chapter:

Absorption	Hertz	Pulse repetition period
Acoustic	Impedance	Pulsed ultrasound
Acoustic variables	Incidence angle	Range equation
Amplitude	Intensity	Rarefaction
Attenuation	Intensity reflection coefficient	Rayl
Attenuation coefficient	Intensity transmission coefficient	Reflection
Backscatter	Interference	Reflection angle
Bandwidth	Kilohertz	Reflector
Compression	Longitudinal wave	Refraction
Constructive interference	Medium	Scatterer
Continuous wave	Megahertz	Scattering
Contrast agent	Nonlinear propagation	Sound
Coupling medium	Oblique incidence	Spatial pulse length
Cycle	Penetration	Speckle
Decibel	Period	Specular reflection
Density	Perpendicular	Stiffness
Destructive interference	Perpendicular incidence	Strength
Duty factor	Power	Transmission angle
Echo	Pressure	Ultrasound
Energy	Propagation	Wave
Fractional bandwidth	Propagation speed	Wavelength
Frequency	Pulse	Work
Fundamental frequency	Pulse duration	
Harmonics	Pulse repetition frequency	

Ultrasound is like the ordinary **sound** that we hear except that it has a **frequency** higher than what human beings can hear. As **ultrasound** travels through the human body, it interacts with anatomy in ways that allow us to use it for diagnostic imaging. In this chapter we consider what ultrasound is, how it is described, and how it travels through and interacts with tissue.

SOUND

Waves

Diagnostic sonography uses ultrasound to produce images of anatomy and flow. Ultrasound is a form of sound. Through our sense of hearing we experience sound daily. But what is sound? In spoken communication, sound is produced by a speaker and is heard by a listener. Sound travels from the speaker to the listener, so it is something that travels (i.e., propagates) through a **medium** such as air. But what *is* this sound that is traveling through air? Sound is a traveling variation in **pressure** (Figure 2-1, *A*). When the speaker speaks, variations in pressure are produced in the throat and mouth. These pressure variations travel through the air to the listener, where they stimulate the auditory response in the ear and brain.

More generally, we can say that sound is a **wave**. A wave is a traveling variation in one or more quantities, such as pressure. For example, a water wave is a traveling variation in water surface height. Dropping a pebble into a pond disturbs the surface of the water, causing it to move up and down. These up-and-down movements then travel across the surface of the pond so that, at the far shore, motion eventually occurs that is similar to what was generated where the pebble entered the water. Like water waves, sound involves mechanical motion in the medium through which it travels. The pressure variations in the sound wave cause particles of the medium to vibrate back and forth.

A wave is a traveling variation of some quantity or quantities.

Associated with the pressure variations in a sound wave, there are **density** variations also. Density is the concentration of matter (mass per unit volume). Pressure, density, and particle vibration are called **acoustic variables** because they are quantities that vary in a sound wave (**acoustic** being derived from the Greek word for hearing). As sound travels through a medium, pressure and density go through **cycles** of increase and decrease, and particles of the medium oscillate back and forth. At any point in the medium, pressure and density increase and decrease in repetitive cycles as the sound wave travels past. Regions of low pressure and density are called **rarefactions**. Regions of high pressure and density are called **compressions**. Compressions and rarefactions travel through a medium with a sound

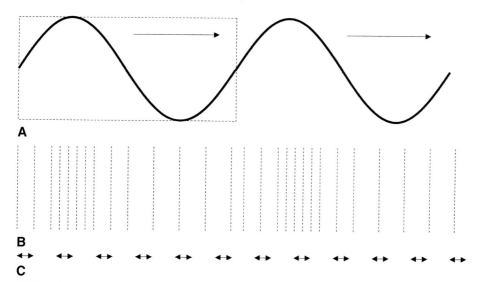

■ **FIGURE 2-1** **A,** Sound is a traveling pressure variation. The box encloses one cycle of pressure variation. The pressure wave in this example is traveling to the right as indicated by the arrows. **B,** Sound is also a traveling density variation. Regions of compression (high density) and rarefaction (low density) travel along with the high- and low-pressure regions of the wave. **C,** Particles vibrate back and forth in a sound wave. This vibratory motion is parallel to the direction of travel of the wave. Such a wave is called a longitudinal wave. Thus sound is a longitudinal, compressional pressure wave.

wave (Figure 2-1, *B*). Sound requires a medium through which to travel; that is, it cannot pass through a vacuum. Sound is a mechanical compressional wave in which back-and-forth particle motion is parallel to the direction of wave travel (Figure 2-1, *C*). Such a wave is called a **longitudinal wave**.

> *Sound is a traveling variation of acoustic variables.*

> *Acoustic variables include pressure, density, and particle motion.*

Sound is described by terms that are used to describe all waves. These terms include frequency, **period, wavelength, propagation speed, amplitude,** and **intensity.** Amplitude and intensity are covered in the later section on **attenuation.**

Frequency

Frequency is a count of how many complete variations (cycles) pressure (or any other acoustic variable) goes through in 1 second of time. In other words, frequency is how many cycles occur in a second. As shown in Figure 2-1, *A*, pressure starts at its normal (undisturbed) value. This would be the pressure in the medium if no sound were propagating through it. As a sound wave travels through a medium, the pressure at any point in the medium increases to a maximum value, returns to normal, decreases to a minimum value, and returns to normal. This describes a complete cycle of variation in pressure as an acoustic variable.

> *A cycle is one complete variation in pressure or other acoustic variable.*

The positive and negative halves of a pressure cycle correspond to compression and rarefaction, respectively. In other words, when the pressure is higher, the medium is more dense (more tightly packed), and when the pressure is lower, the medium is less dense. As a sound wave travels past some point in the medium, this cycle of increasing and decreasing pressure and density is repeated over and over. The number of times it is repeated in 1 second is called the frequency (Figure 2-2). Thus frequency is the number of cycles that occur per second. Frequency units include **hertz** (Hz), **kilohertz** (kHz), and **megahertz** (MHz). One hertz is one cycle per second. One kilohertz is 1000 Hz. One megahertz is 1,000,000 Hz.

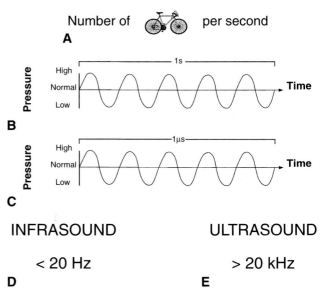

Frequency

■ **FIGURE 2-2**   **A,** Frequency is the number of complete variations (cycles) that an acoustic variable (pressure, in this case) goes through in 1 second. **B,** Five cycles occur in 1 second; thus the frequency is five cycles per second, or 5 Hz. **C,** If five cycles occur within one millionth of a second, also known as a microsecond (1 μs) (i.e., 5 million cycles occurring in 1 second), the frequency is 5 MHz. **D,** Infrasound is sound that human beings cannot hear because the frequencies are too low (less than 20 Hz). **E,** Ultrasound is sound that human beings cannot hear because the frequencies are too high (greater than 20 kHz).

> *Frequency is the number of cycles in a wave that occur in 1 second.*

> *One hertz is one cycle per second. The abbreviation for hertz is Hz.*

> *One kilohertz is 1000 cycles per second. The abbreviation for kilohertz is kHz.*

> *One megahertz is 1 million cycles per second. The abbreviation for megahertz is MHz.*

Human hearing operates over a frequency range of about 20 to 20,000 Hz, although there is great variation on the upper frequency limit in individuals. Sound having a frequency of less than 20 Hz is called infrasound because its frequency is too low for human hearing (*infra* is from the Latin meaning "below"). Sound with a frequency of 20,000 Hz or higher is called ultrasound (*ultra* is from the Latin meaning "beyond") because its frequency is too high for human hearing. Frequency is important in diagnostic ultrasound because of its impact on the resolution and **penetration** of sonographic images.

Infrasound is sound of frequency too low for human hearing.

Ultrasound is sound of frequency too high for human hearing.

Period

Period *(T)* is the time that it takes for one cycle to occur (Figure 2-3). In ultrasound the common unit for period is the microsecond (μs). One microsecond is one millionth of a second (0.000001 second). For example, the period for 5 MHz ultrasound is 0.2 μs. This is because 5 MHz ultrasound contains 5 million cycles in a second, so that each cycle has only one fifth of a millionth of a second (0.2 μs) to occur. The importance of period will become

apparent when **pulsed ultrasound** is considered in the next section. Table 2-1 lists common periods. Period decreases as frequency increases because, as more cycles are packed into 1 second, there is less time for each one. Indeed, period equals 1 divided by the frequency (*f*).

$$T \, (\mu s) = \frac{1}{f \, (MHz)}$$

Period is the time that it takes for one cycle to occur.

If frequency increases, period decreases.

TABLE 2-1   Common Ultrasound Periods and Wavelengths in Tissue

Frequency (MHz)	Period (μs)	Wavelength (mm)*
2.0	0.50	0.77
3.5	0.29	0.44
5.0	0.20	0.31
7.5	0.13	0.21
10.0	0.10	0.15
15.0	0.07	0.10

*Assuming a (soft tissue) propagation speed of 1.54 mm/μs (1540 m/s).

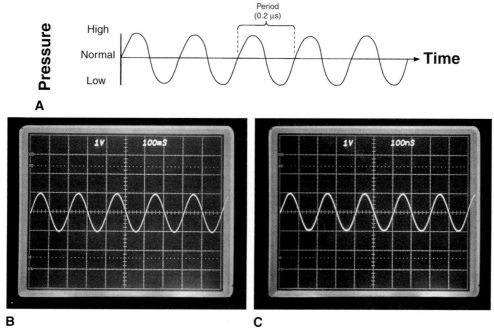

■ **FIGURE 2-3**   Period is the time it takes for one cycle to occur. **A,** Each cycle occurs in 0.2 μs, so the period is 0.2 μs. If one cycle takes 0.2 (or ⅕) millionths of a second to occur, then 5 million cycles occur in 1 second, so the frequency is 5 MHz. **B,** Photograph of a tracing of a 5-Hz electric voltage. The total screen width represents 1 second of time. One can see that five cycles occur in 1 second and each cycle takes one fifth (0.2) of a second to occur (period). If this were a pressure wave, it would be an example of infrasound (frequency is 5 Hz less than 20 Hz). **C,** In this tracing, the total screen width is 1 μs. If five cycles occur in 1 μs, the period is 0.2 μs and the frequency is 5 MHz, as in **A.** If this were a pressure wave, it would be an example of ultrasound (frequency greater than 20 kHz).

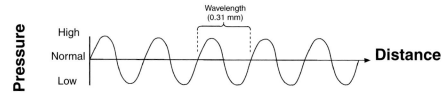

■ FIGURE 2-4   Wavelength is the length of space over which one cycle occurs. In this figure, each cycle covers 0.31 mm. Thus the wavelength is 0.31 mm. This figure differs from Figures 2-2 and 2-3 in that the horizontal axis represents distance rather than time. For a propagation speed of 1.54 mm/µs and a frequency of 5 MHz, the wavelength is 0.31 mm.

Wavelength

Wavelength is the length of space over which one cycle occurs (Figure 2-4). If we could stop the sound wave, visualize it, and measure the distance from the beginning to the end of one cycle, the measured distance would be the wavelength. The wavelength is the length of a cycle from "front" to "back." More precisely, it could be called the cycle length, but traditionally it has been called the wavelength. For ultrasound, wavelength commonly is expressed in millimeters. One millimeter (1 mm) is one thousandth of a meter (0.001 m). The importance of wavelength will be evident when detail resolution of images is considered. Table 2-1 lists common wavelengths used in ultrasonography of soft tissue.

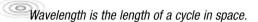

Wavelength is the length of a cycle in space.

Propagation Speed

Propagation speed is the speed with which a wave moves through a medium. For sound, propagation speed is the speed at which a particular value of an acoustic variable moves (Figure 2-5), at which a cycle moves, and at which the entire wave moves. All of these are the same speed. Propagation speed units include meters per second (m/s) and millimeters per microsecond (mm/µs).

ADVANCED CONCEPTS

Speed is the rate of change of position of an object. Speed sometimes is called velocity, although, strictly speaking, *velocity* is defined as speed *with* direction of motion specified. An example of wind speed might be 25 miles per hour (mph), but its velocity would be 25 mph out of the northwest.

Propagation speed is the speed at which a wave moves through a medium.

Wavelength (λ) depends on the frequency and propagation speed. The relationship between the three is that wavelength is equal to propagation speed (*c*) divided by frequency.

$$\lambda \text{ (mm)} = \frac{c \text{ (mm/µs)}}{f \text{ (MHz)}}$$

This equation predicts that wavelength decreases as frequency increases. This is confirmed in Table 2-1.

If frequency increases, wavelength decreases.

An example of this relationship between frequency, wavelength, and propagation speed is seen by comparing Figures 2-3, *C*; 2-4; and 2-5. In these figures, frequency is 5 MHz, wavelength is 0.31 mm, and propagation speed is 1.54 mm/µs. These values apply to the same wave because they are a compatible set according to the foregoing equation:

$$\lambda \text{ (mm)} = \frac{c \text{ (mm/µs)}}{f \text{ (MHz)}} = \frac{1.54 \text{ mm/µs}}{5 \text{ MHz}} = 0.31 \text{ mm}$$

Propagation speed is determined by the medium, primarily its **stiffness** (hardness). Stiffness is the resistance of a material to compression. Stiffness is the inverse of compressibility; that is, a compressible material such as a sponge has low stiffness, and a stiff (hard) material such as a rock has low compressibility. Stiffer media have higher sound speeds. Thus propagation speeds are lower in gases (which are highly compressible), higher in liquids, and highest in solids (which are nearly incompressible). The average propagation speed in soft tissues is 1540 m/s, or (in more relevant units for our purposes) 1.54 mm/µs. Values for soft tissues range from 1.44 to 1.64 mm/µs.[6] Not surprisingly, because soft tissue is mostly water, these values are similar to those for liquids like water.

Propagation speeds are highest in solids and lowest in gases.

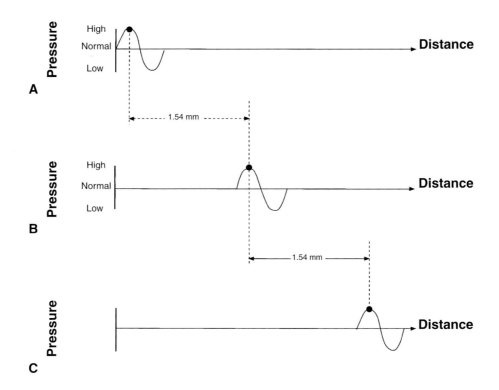

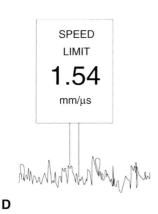

■ FIGURE 2-5 Propagation speed is the speed with which a particular value of an acoustic variable (also the rest of the cycle and indeed the entire wave) travels through a medium. The movement of a maximum (identified by the dot) is shown in this figure. **B** is 1 μs after **A. C** is 1 μs after **B** and 2 μs after **A.** The maximum (dot) moves 1.54 mm in 1 μs and 3.08 mm in 2 μs. The propagation speed is 1.54 mm/μs. The propagation speed in this figure (1.54 mm/μs), when divided by the frequency in Figure 2-3, *C* (5 MHz), equals the wavelength in Figure 2-4 (0.31 mm). **D,** Propagation speeds in soft tissue average 1540 m/s, or 1.54 mm/μs.

The average propagation speed of sound in tissues is 1.54 mm/μs.

In lung tissue, because it contains gas, the propagation speed of sound is much lower than in other soft tissues. However, this difference is not important because ultrasound does not penetrate air-filled lung well enough for imaging. In bone, because it is a solid, propagation speeds are higher (3.0 to 5.0 mm/μs) than in soft tissues. Soft tissue propagation speeds are within a few percent of the average, so that the average can be assumed for all soft tissues with little error. Fat is farthest from the average, about 6% lower. Propagation speed is important because sonographic instruments use it to locate echoes correctly on the display.

Harmonics

The dependence of propagation speed on pressure causes strong sound (pressure) waves to change shape as they travel (Figure 2-6). The reason for this is that the higher-pressure portions of the wave travel faster than the lower-pressure portions. This causes a wave that originally is shaped in a smooth curve form (called sinusoidal; illustrated in Figure 2-6, A) to progress toward a nonsinusoidal shape (Figure 2-6, C). **Propagation** in which speed depends on pressure and the wave shape changes is called **nonlinear propagation.** A sinusoidal waveform is characterized by a single frequency (equal to the number of cycles per second). Any other wave shape contains additional frequencies that are even and odd multiples of the original frequency. The original frequency is called the **fundamental frequency.** The even and odd multiples are called even and odd **harmonics,** respectively. A frequency analysis of the wave in Figure 2-6, A, would yield a single (fundamental) frequency such as 2 MHz. Parts B and C would reveal, in addition to the fundamental frequency, harmonics such as 4, 6, and 8 MHz. As the shape becomes less sinusoidal, the harmonics become stronger. Therefore they are stronger in part C than in part B. Using harmonic frequency echoes improves the quality of sonographic images.

> *Harmonics are even and odd multiples of the fundamental frequency.*

PULSED ULTRASOUND

Thus far we have discussed terms (frequency, period, wavelength, and propagation speed) that are sufficient to describe **continuous wave** (or CW) ultrasound where cycles repeat indefinitely. For sonography and much of Doppler ultrasound, pulsed ultrasound is used rather than continuous wave. An ultrasound **pulse** is a few cycles of ultrasound. Pulses are separated in time with gaps of no ultrasound. Ultrasound pulses are described by some additional parameters that we will discuss now.

> *With continuous wave ultrasound, cycles repeat indefinitely. Pulsed ultrasound consists of pulses separated by gaps in time. A pulse is a few cycles of ultrasound.*

Pulse Repetition Frequency and Period

Pulse repetition frequency *(PRF)* is the number of pulses occurring in 1 second (Figure 2-7). Diagnostic ultrasound involves a few thousand pulses per second, so that pulse repetition frequency commonly is expressed in kilohertz (kHz). One kilohertz is 1000 Hz. **Pulse repetition period** *(PRP)* is the time from the beginning of one pulse to the beginning of the next (Figure 2-8). Its common units are milliseconds (ms). One millisecond is one thousandth of a second. Pulse repetition period is the reciprocal of pulse repetition frequency. Pulse repetition period decreases as pulse repetition frequency increases because, as more pulses occur in a second, there is less time from one to the next.

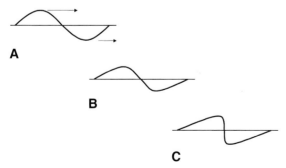

■ FIGURE 2-6 In nonlinear propagation, propagation speed depends on pressure. **A,** Higher-pressure portions of the wave travel faster than the lower-pressure portions. **B** and **C,** Thus the wave changes shape as it travels. This change from the initial sinusoidal shape introduces harmonics that are even and odd multiples of the fundamental frequency.

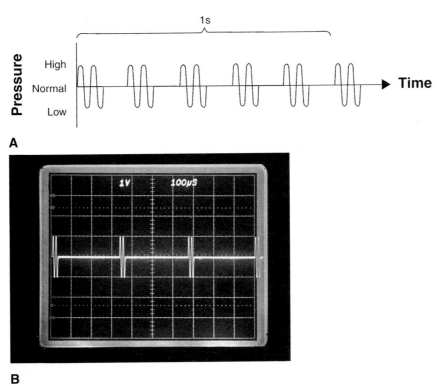

■ FIGURE 2-7   Pulse repetition frequency is the number of pulses occurring in 1 second. **A,** Five pulses (containing two cycles each) occur in 1 second; thus the pulse repetition frequency is 5 Hz. **B,** In this photograph, three pulses occur in 1 millisecond (or one thousandth of a second); thus the pulse repetition frequency is 3 kHz. The total screen width is 1 ms.

$$PRP\ (ms) = \frac{1}{PRF\ (kHz)}$$

The pulse repetition frequency is controlled automatically by sonographic instruments to satisfy requirements that are discussed later. With Doppler techniques, the operator controls pulse repetition frequency as described in later chapters.

Pulse repetition frequency is the number of pulses occurring in a second.

Pulse repetition period is the time from the beginning of one pulse to the beginning of the next one.

If pulse repetition frequency increases, pulse repetition period decreases.

Pulse Duration

Pulse duration *(PD)* is the time that it takes for one pulse to occur (Figure 2-8). Pulse duration is equal to the period (the time for one cycle) times the number of cycles in the pulse *(n)* and is expressed in microseconds. Sonographic pulses are typically 2 or 3 cycles long. Shorter pulses, compared with longer ones, improve the quality of sonographic images. Doppler ultrasound pulses are typically 5 to 30 cycles long.

$$PD\ (\mu s) = n \times T\ (\mu s)$$

Sonographic pulses are typically 2 or 3 cycles long. Doppler pulses are typically 5 to 30 cycles long.

Pulse duration decreases if the number of cycles in a pulse is decreased or if the frequency is increased (reducing the period). The instrument operator chooses the frequency.

Pulse duration is the time for a pulse to occur.

If frequency is increased, period is decreased, reducing the pulse duration. If the number of cycles in a pulse is reduced, pulse duration is decreased. Shorter pulses improve the quality of sonographic images.

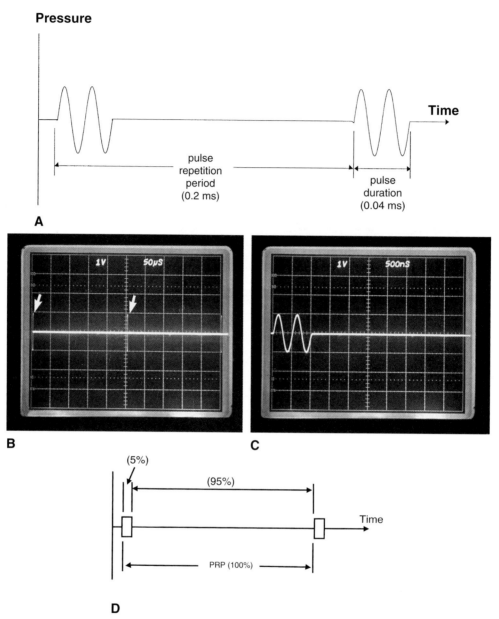

■ **FIGURE 2-8** Pulse repetition period is the time from the beginning of one pulse to the beginning of the next. **A,** The pulse repetition period is 0.2 ms (200 μs). Therefore the pulse repetition frequency is 5 kHz. Pulse duration is the time that it takes for one pulse to occur. Pulse duration is equal to the period multiplied by the number of cycles in the pulse. The pulse duration is 40 μs. The duty factor is the fraction of time that the sound is on. The duty factor is 40/200, which equals 0.2, or 20%. **B,** Photograph shows that the pulse repetition period is 0.25 ms. (The pulse repetition frequency is 4 kHz.) The period is 0.5 μs, as shown expanded in **C,** and the pulse duration is 1 μs. From one pulse to the next (pulse repetition period of 0.25 ms, or 250 μs), the sound is on (pulse duration) for 1 μs. The duty factor is, in this example, 0.004, or 0.4%. The screen width is 0.5 ms in **B** and 5 μs in **C. D,** The duty factor is the fraction of time that pulsed ultrasound is actually on. In this example the pulse repetition period *(PRP)* represents 100% of the time from the start of one pulse to the start of the next one. Of this time, the sound is on 5% of the time (the pulse duration divided by the pulse repetition period) and off 95% of the time.

Duty Factor

Duty factor *(DF)* is the fraction of time that pulsed ultrasound is on (Figure 2-8, *D*). Continuous wave ultrasound is on 100% of the time. Pulsed ultrasound, by definition, is not on all of the time. The duty factor indicates how much of the time the ultrasound *is* on. Longer pulses increase the duty factor because the sound is on more of the time.

> *Duty factor is the fraction of time that pulsed ultrasound is on.*

Higher pulse repetition frequencies increase duty factor because there is less "dead" time between pulses. Thus the duty factor increases with increasing pulse duration or pulse repetition frequency. Duty factor has no units because it is a fraction. Thus duty factor simply is expressed as a decimal, such as 0.10 or 0.25, or as a percentage, such as 10% or 25%. The importance of duty factor will become evident when intensities and safety issues are discussed later. The duty factor is equal to pulse duration divided by pulse repetition period. The reason for this is that pulse duration represents the amount of time that the sound is on, and pulse repetition period is the time from one pulse to the next. Thus the ratio of the two represents the *fraction* of time that pulsed ultrasound is on.

$$DF = \frac{PD\ (\mu s)}{PRP\ (\mu s)} = \frac{PD\ (\mu s) \times PRF\ (kHz)}{1000\ (kHz/MHz)}$$

The factor of 1000 converts kilohertz to megahertz to be consistent with microseconds of pulse duration. Multiplying the duty factor by 100 expresses it as a percentage. For example, if the pulse duration is 2 μs and the pulse repetition period is 250 μs, then

$$DF = \frac{2}{250} = 0.008 = \text{or } 0.8\%$$

A range of duty factors is encountered in diagnostic ultrasound because of various conditions chosen by the instrument and the operator. Typical duty factors for sonography are in the range of 0.1% to 1.0%. For Doppler ultrasound, because of longer pulse durations, the range of typical duty factors is 0.5% to 5.0%.

> *If pulse duration increases, the duty factor increases.*

> *If pulse repetition frequency increases, pulse repetition period decreases and the duty factor increases.*

Spatial Pulse Length

If we could stop a pulse, visualize it, and measure the distance from its beginning to its end, the measured distance would be the **spatial pulse length** *(SPL)*. Spatial pulse length is the length of a pulse from front to back (Figure 2-9, *A*). Spatial pulse length is equal to the length of each cycle times the number of cycles in the pulse. The length of each cycle is the wavelength. Thus the spatial pulse length increases with wavelength and increases with the number of cycles in the pulse.

$$SPL\ (mm) = n \times \lambda\ (mm)$$

> *Spatial pulse length is the length of space that a pulse takes up.*

Because wavelength decreases with increasing frequency, spatial pulse length decreases with increasing frequency (Figure 2-9, *B* and *C*). Units for spatial pulse length are millimeters. Spatial pulse length is an important quantity when considering image resolution. Shorter pulse lengths improve resolution.

> *If the number of cycles in a pulse increases, spatial pulse length increases. If frequency increases, wavelength and spatial pulse length decrease.*

> *Shorter pulses improve sonographic image resolution.*

Frequency

Recall that frequency expresses the number of cycles in a wave that occur in a second of time. This is fine for continuous wave ultrasound, but in pulsed ultrasound there are gaps between pulses so that some of the cycles are missing compared with continuous wave operation. For example, 5-MHz frequency continuous wave ultrasound has 5 million cycles occurring in a second. But what about 5-MHz pulsed ultrasound? The frequency, 5 MHz, gives the number of cycles per second, as if the wave were continuous wave, even though it is not. The actual number of cycles occurring in a second for pulsed ultrasound depends on the duty factor. For example, if the duty factor is 0.01, or 1%, the ultrasound is on only one hundredth of the time, and the actual number of cycles per second is 50,000, or 50 kHz. The quiet time between pulses eliminates 99% of the cycles in this example, even though the frequency implies that there are 5 million cycles per second. However, the frequency

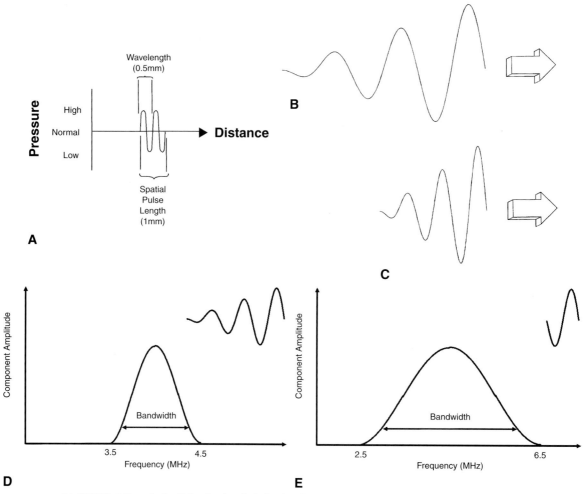

■ **FIGURE 2-9** **A,** Spatial pulse length is the length of space over which a pulse occurs. Spatial pulse length is equal to wavelength multiplied by the number of cycles in the pulse. In this figure, wavelength is 0.5 mm, there are two cycles in each pulse, and spatial pulse length is 0.5 × 2, or 1 mm. This figure differs from Figures 2-7, *A,* and 2-8, *A,* in that the horizontal axis represents distance rather than time. **B** and **C** show three-cycle damped (decreasing in amplitude) pulses of ultrasound traveling to the right. **B,** Lower-frequency pulse with longer wavelength and spatial pulse length. **C,** Higher-frequency pulse with shorter wavelength and spatial pulse length. **D** and **E,** Plots of the frequencies present in two ultrasound pulses. Component amplitude is the amplitude of each frequency component present. Bandwidth is the frequency range within which the amplitudes exceed some reference value. Compare the frequency spectrum for a narrowband, longer pulse **(D)** with the frequency spectrum for a broadband, shorter pulse **(E).**

for pulsed ultrasound is still given as 5 MHz because the behavior of the pulses (regarding period, wavelength, propagation speed, and other characteristics such as attenuation) is like that of 5-MHz continuous wave ultrasound.

Bandwidth

In contrast to continuous wave ultrasound, which can be described by a single frequency, ultrasound pulses contain a *range* of frequencies called the **bandwidth** (Figure 2-9, *D* and *E*). The shorter the pulse (the fewer the number of cycles), the more frequencies present in

it (broader bandwidth). **Fractional bandwidth** is the bandwidth divided by the operating frequency. Fractional bandwidth is unitless. It describes how large the bandwidth is compared with the operating frequency.

Bandwidth is the range of frequencies contained in a pulse.

Shorter pulses have broader bandwidths and fractional bandwidths.

Bandwidth is specified by some definition of where in the frequency range it starts and stops. For example, a 6-decibel (dB) bandwidth refers to the range of frequencies that includes those that have half or greater the amplitude (one fourth or greater the power) of the strongest one, which is the operating frequency. A 20-dB bandwidth includes amplitudes that are one tenth or greater of the strongest (one hundredth or greater the power). Clearly, a 20-dB bandwidth is greater that a 6-dB bandwidth.

The reciprocal of fractional bandwidth is called quality factor (Q). The quality factor is operating frequency divided by bandwidth. Shorter pulses (with their broader bandwidths) have lower Q's. This may seem like a contradiction because we stated previously that shorter pulses produce better resolution. So how could this be a lower quality? One does best to forget that Q originally stood for "quality" and simply to think of it as "Q." In the early days of electronics, for example, in radio, narrow bandwidth was good (for example, in radio to tune in one station and, at the same time, to tune out another station that is nearby on the frequency dial). In much of

modern electronics (including, for example, the Internet) broad bandwidth is good, being associated with, for example, high-fidelity sound and video and high information transmission rates. Thus in many cases, including sonography, low Q is good Q.

Shorter pulses have broader bandwidth and lower Q's. For short pulses (those having three cycles or fewer), the Q is approximately equal to the number of cycles in the pulse. Figure 2-10 gives two examples.

Bandwidth is an oft-mentioned term regarding connections to the Internet. Broader bandwidth connections permit faster information transfer and thus cost more. To achieve higher information transmission rates, a higher bit rate is required. Bits (and gaps) must be shorter in temporal length to be transmitted at a higher bit rate. Shorter bits have broader bandwidth just as shorter ultrasound pulses do. Thus higher bit rates require broader bandwidth connections to accomplish.

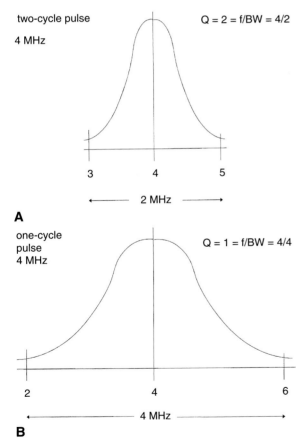

A

B

■ **FIGURE 2-10** **A,** A 4-MHz, two-cycle pulse has a Q factor of approximately 2, and therefore a bandwidth of approximately 2 MHz (from 3 to 5 MHz). **B,** A 4-MHz one-cycle pulse has a Q factor of approximately 1, and therefore a bandwidth of approximately 4 MHz (from 2 to 6 MHz). Shorter pulses have broader bandwidths and lower Q's.

ATTENUATION

We now consider the magnitude of the cyclic variations in a continuous or pulsed ultrasound wave. Amplitude and intensity are indicators of the **strength** of the sound. They are related to how loud the sound would be if it could be heard. Ultrasound, however, cannot be heard, and so loudness is irrelevant. Nevertheless, amplitude and intensity are important indicators of how strong or "intense" the ultrasound is.

Amplitude

Amplitude is the maximum variation that occurs in an acoustic variable. Amplitude is an indicator of how far a variable gets away from its normal, undisturbed value (its value if there were no sound present). Amplitude is the maximum value minus the normal (undisturbed or no-sound) value (Figure 2-11, *A*). Amplitude is expressed in units that are appropriate for the acoustic variable considered. Megapascals (MPa) are the units for pressure.

Intensity

Intensity *(I)* is the rate at which **energy** passes through a unit area. Intensity is equal to the power *(P)* in a wave divided by the area *(A)* over which the power is spread (Figure 2-11, *B* and *C*). Ultrasound is generated by transducers in the form of beams, somewhat like laser beams, but as sound instead of light. The average intensity of a sound beam is the total power in the beam divided by the cross-sectional area of the beam.

$$I \text{ (mW/cm}^2) = \frac{P \text{ (mW)}}{A \text{ (cm}^2)}$$

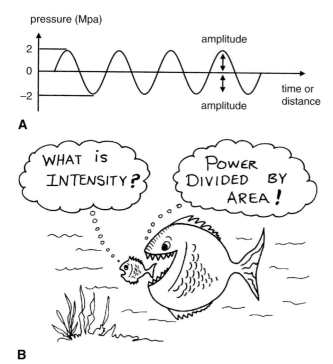

A

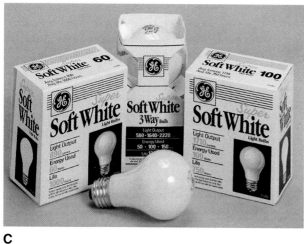

B

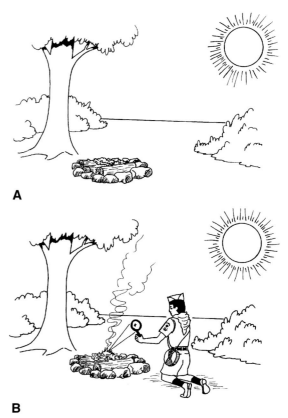

C

■ **FIGURE 2-11** **A,** Amplitude is the maximum amount of variation that occurs in an acoustic variable (pressure, in this case). In this figure the amplitude is 2 MPa. **B,** Intensity is the power in a sound wave divided by the area over which the power is spread (the beam area). **C,** A watt is the unit of power for a light bulb.

Increasing the power increases the intensity. Increasing the area decreases the intensity. Decreasing the area (focusing) increases the intensity because the power is more concentrated.

If beam power increases, intensity increases. If beam area decreases (focusing), intensity increases.

Energy is the capability of doing **work.** Sound, heat, light, and mechanical motion are forms of energy. Power

is the rate at which energy is transferred from one part of a system to another (e.g., a lamp plugged into a wall outlet) or from one location to another (e.g., traveling down a laser or ultrasound beam). Power is the energy transferred divided by the time required to transfer the energy, that is, the transfer rate. Power units include watts (W) and milliwatts (mW). One milliwatt is one thousandth of a watt. Beam area is expressed in centimeters squared (cm^2). Intensity units include milliwatts per centimeter squared (mW/cm^2) and watts per centimeter squared (W/cm^2). Intensity is an important quantity in describing the sound that is sent into the body by a transducer and in discussing bioeffects and safety. An analogy may be made to the effect of sunlight on dry kindling (Figure 2-12). Sunlight normally will not ignite the kindling, but if the same light power from the sun is concentrated into a small area (increased intensity) by focusing it with a magnifying glass, the kindling can be ignited. In this example, increasing the intensity produces an effect, even though the power remains the same. The beam area is determined by the transducer, in particular, how it focuses the beam. Intensity is proportional to amplitude squared. Thus if amplitude is doubled, intensity is quadrupled. If amplitude is halved, intensity is quartered.

A

B

■ **FIGURE 2-12** **A,** Sunlight does not normally ignite a fire. **B,** However, when the sunlight is focused, intensity increases, and ignition can occur.

ADVANCED CONCEPTS

Several intensities are encountered in diagnostic ultrasound. Reasons for this are as follows:

1. Like a flashlight beam, intensity is not constant across a sound beam but is usually highest in the center and falls off near the periphery (Figure 2-13).
2. In the case of pulsed ultrasound, intensity varies with time (Figure 2-14); that is, the intensity is some value during each pulse but is zero between pulses.
3. Intensity is not constant within pulses (Figure 2-15) but rather starts out high and then decreases toward the end of the pulse.

For spatial considerations, the spatial peak (SP) and spatial average (SA) values are used. Spatial peak is the greatest intensity found across the beam, usually at the center. Spatial average is the average for all values found across the beam, including the larger values found near the center and the small values near the periphery.

For temporal (time) considerations, temporal average (TA), pulse average (PA), and temporal peak (TP) values are used. Temporal peak is the greatest intensity found in the pulse as it passes by. Pulse average is the average for all values found in a pulse, including the larger values found at its beginning and the small values found near the end. Temporal average includes the "dead" time between pulses where there is zero intensity. Thus temporal average is the lowest value, temporal peak is the highest, and pulse average is in between for a given pulsed beam. Pulse average and temporal average values are related by the duty factor. Temporal average intensity (I_{TA}) is equal to the pulse average intensity (I_{PA}) multiplied by the duty factor.

$$I_{TA} = I_{PA} \times DF$$

Thus if the duty factor is 0.01 (the sound is on 1% of the time), the temporal average intensity will be one hundredth the pulse average intensity. The greater the duty factor, the greater the temporal average intensity will be. If the sound is continuous instead of pulsed, the duty factor is equal to 1, and the pulse average intensity and temporal average intensity are equal to each other.

The pulses shown in Figures 2-7 and 2-14 have constant amplitude and intensity within each pulse. Pulses used in sonography, however, are similar to those shown in Figure 2-15. The peak intensity occurring within each pulse is called the temporal peak intensity. The intensity averaged over the pulse duration is called the pulse average intensity. For constant amplitude pulses, temporal peak intensity and pulse average intensity are equal. Six intensities result from these spatial and temporal considerations:

1. Spatial average–temporal average (I_{SATA})
2. Spatial peak–temporal average (I_{SPTA})

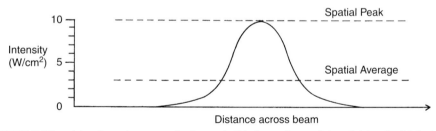

■ **FIGURE 2-13**   Intensity varies across the beam. In this figure, the spatial peak intensity (at the beam center) is 10 W/cm² and the spatial average is 3 W/cm². In addition to varying across the beam, intensity varies along the direction of beam travel because of focusing and attenuation.

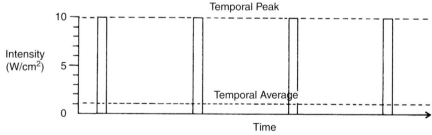

■ **FIGURE 2-14**   Intensity versus time for pulsed ultrasound. Temporal peak intensity (10 W/cm²) is the intensity when the sound is actually on. Temporal average intensity (1 W/cm²) is the intensity that is averaged over time. In this figure the duty factor is 0.1. This figure assumes constant intensity within pulses. Sonographic pulses are depicted more accurately in Figure 2-9, *B* and *C*, and in Figure 2-15.

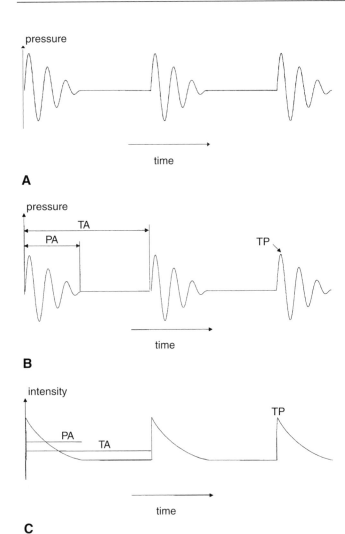

pressure

time

A

pressure

TA

PA

TP

time

B

intensity

TP

PA

TA

time

C

■ **FIGURE 2-15** **A,** The ultrasound pulses used in sonography have cycles of differing pressure amplitudes within each pulse. They are called damped pulses. **B,** The relevant times for three intensities are shown. Temporal average *(TA)* intensity is averaged over the pulse-repetition period; pulse average *(PA)* intensity is averaged over the pulse duration; and temporal peak *(TP)* intensity is not averaged over time. **C,** Intensity versus time for the pressure waveforms of **A** and **B.** The values for TP, PA, and TA intensities are shown. Temporal peak is the largest value (no averaging). Pulse average is smaller because it is averaged over pulse duration (including the portions with lower intensities). Temporal average is smallest because it is averaged over the pulse repetition period (including the time with no intensity).

3. Spatial average–pulse average (I_{SAPA})
4. Spatial peak–pulse average (I_{SPPA})
5. Spatial average–temporal peak (I_{SATP})
6. Spatial peak–temporal peak (I_{SPTP})
   Spatial average–temporal average averages spatially across the beam and temporally, yielding the lowest value for a given beam. Spatial peak–temporal peak is averaged neither spatially nor temporally, so it is the highest value.

Example 2-1

The spatial peak–pulse average intensity is 500 mW/cm², and the duty factor is 2% (0.02). Calculate spatial peak–temporal average.

$$I_{SPTA} = I_{SPPA} \times DF = 500 \times 0.02 = 10 \text{ mW/cm}^2$$

Example 2-2

The spatial peak–temporal peak and spatial peak–pulse average intensities are 6 and 2 W/cm², respectively. Calculate spatial peak–temporal average if the duty factor is 1%.

$$I_{SPTA} = I_{SPPA} \times DF = 2 \times 0.01 = 0.020 \text{ W/cm}^2 = 20 \text{ mW/cm}^2$$

Attenuation

Attenuation *(a)* is the weakening of sound as it propagates (Figure 2-16). One must understand attenuation because (1) it limits imaging depth and (2) its weakening effect on the image must be compensated by the diagnostic instrument. With an unfocused beam in any medium, such as tissue, amplitude and intensity will decrease as the sound travels through the medium. This reduction in amplitude and intensity as sound travels is called attenuation (Figure 2-17). Attenuation encompasses the **absorption** (conversion of sound to heat) of sound as it travels and the **reflection** and **scattering** of the sound as it encounters tissue interfaces and heterogeneous tissues. Absorption is the dominant factor contributing to attenuation of ultrasound in soft tissues. The generation of echoes by the reflection and scattering of sound is crucial to sonographic imaging but contributes little to attenuation in most cases. **Decibels** are the units used to quantify attenuation. The **attenuation coefficient** *(a_c)* is the attenuation that occurs with each centimeter the sound wave travels. Its units are decibels per centimeter (dB/cm). The farther the sound travels, the greater the attenuation is.

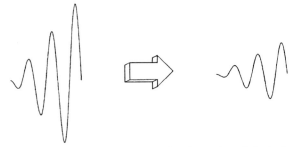

■ **FIGURE 2-16** An ultrasound pulse is weakened (reduction of amplitude) as it travels through a medium (in this case from left to right). This weakening is called attenuation.

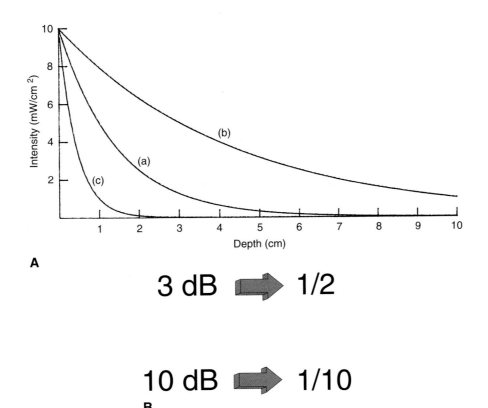

B

■ **FIGURE 2-17**   Attenuation of sound as it travels through a medium. **A,** In example (a), the intensity decreases by 50% for each 1 cm of travel. This corresponds to an attenuation coefficient of 3 dB/cm. In example (b), the attenuation coefficient is 1 dB/cm, whereas in (c), the attenuation coefficient is 10 dB/cm. **B,** Two easy-to-remember values for decibels and their corresponding intensity reduction are (1) a 3-dB attenuation corresponds to an intensity reduction (50%) to one half the original value, and (2) a 10-dB attenuation corresponds to an intensity reduction (90%) to one tenth the original value.

Decibels are good units for making comparisons. For example, they describe the relationships between various measured sound levels (Figure 2-18) and the threshold of human hearing (the weakest sound we can hear). Table 2-2 gives examples of various values. Decibels involve the logarithm of the ratio of two powers or intensities. In the case of attenuation, they are the intensities before and after the attenuation has occurred. Two decibel values have particular usefulness: 3 dB corresponds to an intensity ratio of one half, that is, an intensity reduction of 50%; and 10 dB corresponds to an intensity ratio of one tenth, that is, an intensity reduction of 90% (Figures 2-17 and 2-19). Logarithms and decibels are discussed in more detail in Appendix E.

Example 2-3

Compare the following two intensities in decibels: $I_1 = 20$ mW/cm^2, $I_2 = 10$ mW/cm^2.

I_2 is one half of I_1. Therefore I_2 is 3 dB less than I_1.

Example 2-4

Compare (in decibels) I_2 with I_1, where $I_1 = 10$ mW/cm^2 and $I_2 = 0.01$ mW/cm^2.

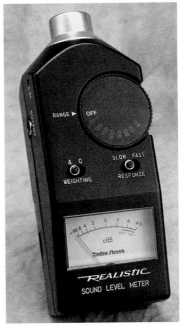

■ **FIGURE 2-18**   A sound level meter based on decibels.

Each factor of 10 is equivalent to 10 dB. I_1 is 1000 times I_2 so that I_2 is 30 dB less than I_1.

Example 2-5

As sound passes through tissue, its intensity at one point is 1 mW/cm^2; at a point 10 cm farther along, it is 0.1 mW/cm^2. What are the attenuation and attenuation coefficient values?

Because the intensity is reduced to one tenth from the first point to the second, the attenuation is 10 dB. The attenuation coefficient is the attenuation divided by the separation between the two points. In this case,

TABLE 2-2 Sound Levels

Sound	Level (dB)
Pain threshold	130
Rock concert	115
Chain saw	100
Lawn mower	90
Vacuum cleaner	75
Normal conversation	60
Whisper	30
Hearing threshold	0

$$a_c = \frac{10\ dB}{10\ cm} = 1\ dB/cm$$

Table 2-3 lists various values of intensity ratio and percent values with corresponding decibel values of attenuation. To determine the attenuation in decibels, multiply the attenuation coefficient by the sound path length (L) (how far the sound has traveled) in centimeters.

$$a\ (dB) = a_c\ (dB/cm) \times L\ (cm)$$

If attenuation coefficient increases, attenuation increases.

If path length increases, attenuation increases.

Attenuation increases with increasing frequency. Persons who live in apartments or dormitories experience this fact when they hear mostly the bass notes through the wall from a neighbor's sound system. For soft tissues, there is approximately (values of 0.3 to 0.7 are commonly used by various authors for various purposes) 0.5 dB of

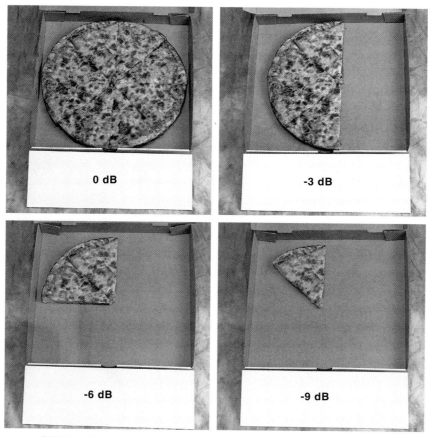

■ **FIGURE 2-19** Each reduction of 3 dB corresponds to removing half the pizza.

attenuation per centimeter for each megahertz of frequency (Table 2-4). In other words, the average attenuation coefficient in decibels per centimeter for soft tissues is approximately equal to one half the frequency in megahertz. To calculate the attenuation in decibels, multiply one half the frequency in megahertz by the path length in centimeters.

$$a \ (dB) = \tfrac{1}{2} \ (dB/cm\text{-}MHz) \times f \ (MHz) \times L \ (cm)$$

As frequency increases, attenuation increases.

TABLE 2-3   Attenuation for Various Intensity Ratios*

Attenuation (dB)	Intensity Ratio	Percent Intensity Ratio
0	1.00	100
1	0.79	79
2	0.63	63
3	0.50	50
4	0.40	40
5	0.32	32
6	0.25	25
7	0.20	20
8	0.16	16
9	0.13	13
10	0.10	10
15	0.032	3.2
20	0.010	1.0
25	0.003	0.3
30	0.001	0.1
35	0.0003	0.03
40	0.0001	0.01
45	0.00003	0.003
50	0.00001	0.001
60	0.000001	0.0001
70	0.0000001	0.00001
80	0.00000001	0.000001
90	0.000000001	0.0000001
100	0.0000000001	0.00000001

*The intensity ratio is the fraction of the original intensity remaining after attenuation.

The intensity ratio corresponding to that number of decibels may be obtained from Table 2-3. This ratio is equal to the fraction of the intensity (at the beginning of the path) that remains at the end of the path. If the intensity at the beginning is known, the intensity at the end may be found by multiplying the beginning intensity by the intensity ratio. *A summary of this four-step process follows:*

1. Multiplying the frequency by one half yields the approximate attenuation coefficient.
2. Multiplying the attenuation coefficient by the path length yields the attenuation.
3. The intensity ratio then is determined for the decibel value calculated in step 2 (using Table 2-3). This is the *fraction* of the original intensity remaining at the end of the path.
4. Multiplying the intensity ratio by the intensity at the start of the path yields the intensity at the end of the path.

Example 2-6

If 4-MHz ultrasound with 10 mW/cm^2 intensity is applied to a soft tissue surface, what is the intensity 1.5 cm into the tissue?

Step 1: Multiply the frequency by one half to yield an attenuation coefficient of 2 dB/cm.

Step 2: Multiply the attenuation coefficient (2 dB/cm) by the path length (1.5 cm) to yield an attenuation of 3 dB.

Step 3: From Table 2-3, an attenuation of 3 dB corresponds to an intensity ratio of 0.5. Thus 50% of the intensity remains after the sound travels through this path.

Step 4: Multiply the intensity ratio (0.5) by the intensity at the beginning of the path (10 mW/cm^2) to yield the intensity at the end of the path. The result is 5 mW/cm^2.

Attenuation is higher in lung than in other soft tissues because of the air present in the organ. Attenuation is higher in bone than in soft tissues.

TABLE 2-4   Average Attenuation Coefficients in Tissue

Frequency (MHz)	Average Attenuation Coefficient for Soft Tissue (dB/cm)	Intensity Reduction in 1-cm Path (%)	Intensity Reduction in 10-cm Path (%)
2.0	1.0	21	90
3.5	1.8	34	98
5.0	2.5	44	99.7
7.5	3.8	58	99.98
10.0	5.0	68	99.999

A practical consequence of attenuation is that it limits the depths of images (penetration) obtained. The penetration decreases as frequency increases (Figures 2-20 to 2-22). Table 2-5 lists attenuation coefficients and typical imaging depths for various frequencies in soft tissue.

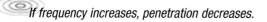

If frequency increases, penetration decreases.

The depths needed to reach human anatomy determine the frequencies used in diagnostic ultrasound, which range from 2 to 15 MHz for most applications. Within this range, the lower frequencies are used for deeper penetration and the higher frequencies for superficial applications and invasive transducers (rectal, vaginal, and esophageal). Even higher frequencies (up to 50 MHz) are used for some specialized applications, including ophthalmologic imaging and intravascular

imaging with catheter-mounted transducers. Frequencies less than 2 MHz are used in large-animal applications.

ECHOES

Ultrasound is useful as an imaging tool because of the reflection and scattering of sound waves at organ and tissue interfaces and scattering within heterogeneous tissues. The reflected and scattered sound waves produce the pattern of echoes that is necessary for diagnostic pulse-echo imaging with ultrasound. These phenomena are considered in this section.

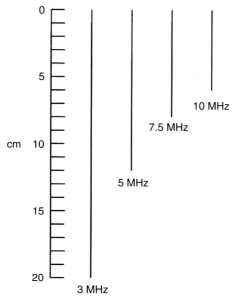

■ **FIGURE 2-21**   Typical imaging depths (penetrations) for several frequencies in soft tissues. Penetration decreases as frequency increases because attenuation increases.

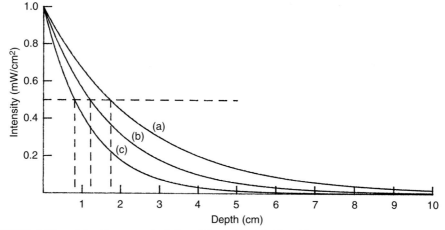

■ **FIGURE 2-20**   Intensity versus depth in soft tissue for 3.5 MHz (*a*), 5.0 MHz (*b*), and 7.5 MHz (*c*). The depth at which half-intensity (3-dB attenuation) occurs (1.7, 1.2, and 0.8 cm, respectively) is indicated for each.

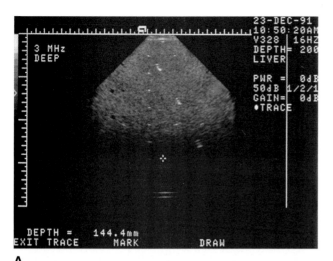

A

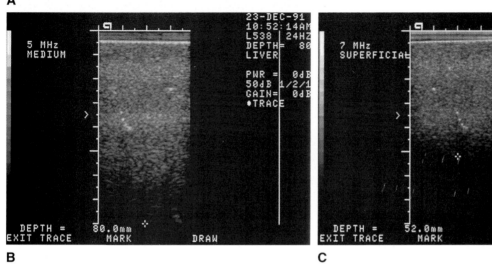

B   C

■ **FIGURE 2-22**   Examples of penetration in a tissue-equivalent phantom at 3 MHz **(A)**, 5 MHz **(B)**, and 7 MHz **(C)**. Penetration decreases as frequency increases.

TABLE 2-5   Common Values for Attenuation Coefficient and Penetration

Frequency (MHz)	Attenuation Coefficient (dB/cm)	Penetration (cm)
2.0	1.0	30
3.5	1.8	17
5.0	2.5	12
7.5	3.8	8
10.0	5.0	6
15.0	7.5	4

Perpendicular Incidence

Perpendicular incidence denotes a direction of travel of the ultrasound wave **perpendicular** to the boundary between two media (Figure 2-23). The incident sound may be reflected back into the first medium or transmitted into the second medium; most often, both

occur. When there is perpendicular incidence, reflected sound travels back through the first medium in a direction opposite to the incident sound (i.e., the reflected sound returns to the sound source). In the case of perpendicular incidence, the transmitted sound does not change direction; it moves through the second medium in the same direction as the incident sound did in the first. The intensities of the reflected sound (the **echo**) and the transmitted sound depend on the incident intensity at the boundary and the impedances of the media on either side of the boundary.

Impedance

Impedance *(z)* determines how much of an incident sound wave is reflected back through the first medium and how much is transmitted into the second medium. Impedance is equal to the density (ρ) of a medium multiplied by its propagation speed. Impedance units are

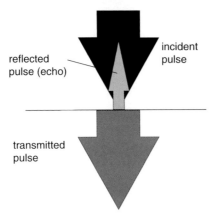

reflected
pulse (echo)

incident
pulse

transmitted
pulse

■ **FIGURE 2-23**   Reflection and transmission at a boundary with perpendicular incidence. The incident pulse is partially reflected (echo) with the remainder (transmitted pulse) continuing into the second medium. The strengths of the reflected and transmitted pulses are determined by the impedances of the two media at the boundary.

rayls. Impedance increases if the density is increased or if the propagation speed is increased. Average soft tissue impedance is 1,630,000 rayls.

$$z \text{ (rayls)} = \rho \text{ (kg/m}^3) \times c \text{ (m/s)}$$

If density increases, impedance increases. If propagation speed increases, impedance increases.

ADVANCED CONCEPTS

This impedance $(z = \rho c)$ is called the characteristic impedance. The characteristic impedance is the impedance for a propagating plane wave (one for which any acoustic variable has, at any instant of time, the same value anywhere in a plane perpendicular to the direction of propagation). For some acoustic considerations, such as reflection of a plane wave at a boundary, density times propagation speed has greater use as a descriptor of a medium than does either density or propagation speed alone. That is why the name "*characteristic* impedance" is applied.

Impedance in general is the ratio of force amplitude divided by its response amplitude. Impedance was first applied to electrical circuits, where it is the ratio of voltage amplitude to current amplitude. *Acoustic* impedance in general is pressure amplitude divided by particle velocity amplitude. Because pressure is force per unit area, acoustic impedance is impedance per unit area and thus is called specific acoustic impedance, with the term *specific* indicating "per unit amount" (area in this case).

Dividing the reflected (echo) intensity by the incident intensity yields the fraction of the incident intensity that is reflected. This fraction is called the **intensity**

reflection coefficient *(IRC)*. For example, if the incident intensity (I_i) is 10 mW/cm^2 and the echo, or reflected, intensity (I_r) is 1 mW/cm^2, the intensity reflection coefficient is one tenth, or 0.1. In this case, one tenth (10%) of the incident sound is reflected. Dividing the transmitted intensity (I_t) by the incident intensity yields the fraction of the incident intensity that is transmitted into the second medium. This fraction is called the **intensity transmission coefficient** *(ITC)*. For example, if the incident intensity is 10 mW/cm^2 and the transmitted intensity is 9 mW/cm^2, the intensity transmission coefficient is nine tenths, or 0.9. In this case, nine tenths (90%) of the incident sound is transmitted into the second medium. Reflection and transmission coefficients must add up to 1 (i.e., 100%) to account for all the incident sound intensity (what is not reflected at the boundary must be transmitted into the second medium). The two foregoing examples are really the same example, because if 10% of the sound is reflected back into the first medium, then 90% is transmitted into the second medium; that is, all (100%) of the incident sound arriving at the boundary is accounted for.

For perpendicular incidence, the reflection coefficient depends on the impedances as follows:

$$\text{IRC} = \frac{I_r \text{ (W/cm}^2)}{I_i \text{ (W/cm}^2)} = \left[\frac{(z_2 - z_1)}{(z_2 + z_1)}\right]^2$$

From this relationship between reflection coefficient and impedances, we see that the coefficient depends on the difference between the impedances. The more different the impedances are, the stronger the echo is. The more alike the impedances are, the weaker the echo is. If the media impedances are the same, there is no echo.

If the difference between the impedances increases, the intensity reflection coefficient (and echo intensity) increases.

The transmission coefficient depends on the reflection coefficient as follows:

$$\text{ITC} = \frac{I_t \text{ (W/cm}^2)}{I_i \text{ (W/cm}^2)} = 1 - \text{IRC}$$

Because the coefficients must add up to 1 (100%), larger reflection coefficients mean smaller transmission coefficients, and vice versa. As you would expect, if more of the incident sound is reflected (stronger echo), less remains to travel into the second medium.

If intensity reflection coefficient increases, intensity transmission coefficient decreases.

If the impedances are equal, there is no echo, and the transmitted intensity is equal to the incident intensity. This is what we expect: if no sound is reflected at a boundary, then all of it travels into the second medium as if there were no boundary. Conversely, we can conclude that *if there is no reflection, the media impedances must be equal.* If impedances are equal, then there is no echo, and the transmitted intensity equals the incident intensity.

For perpendicular incidence and equal impedances, there is no reflection, and the transmitted intensity equals the incident intensity. If there is a large difference between the impedances, there will be nearly total reflection (an intensity reflection coefficient close to 1, and an intensity transmission coefficient close to zero). An example of this is an air–soft tissue boundary. For this reason, a gel **coupling medium** is used to provide a good sound path from the transducer to the skin (eliminating the thin layer of air that would reflect the sound, preventing entrance of the sound into the body).

Example 2-7

For impedances of 40 and 60 rayls, determine the intensity reflection and transmission coefficients.

$$IRC = \left[\frac{(60-40)}{(60+40)}\right]^2 = \left(\frac{20}{100}\right)^2 = 0.2^2 = 0.2 \times 0.2 = 0.04$$

$$ITC = 1 - 0.04 = 0.96$$

In Example 2-7, the intensity reflection coefficient can be expressed as 4%, and the intensity transmission coefficient as 96%. The sum of the two coefficients is 100%, underscoring the fact that all of the incident intensity must be reflected or transmitted.

If the incident intensity is known, the reflected and transmitted intensities can be calculated by multiplying the incident intensity by the intensity reflection coefficient and the intensity transmission coefficient, respectively.

Example 2-8

For Example 2-7, if the incident intensity is 10 mW/cm², calculate the reflected and transmitted intensities.

From Example 2-7, the intensity reflection and transmission coefficients are 0.04 and 0.96, respectively, so that

$$I_r = 10 \times 0.04 = 0.4 \text{ mW/cm}^2$$

$$I_t = 10 \times 0.96 = 9.6 \text{ mW/cm}^2$$

The coefficients give the fractions of the incident intensity that are reflected and transmitted. By multiplying the coefficients by 100, these fractions are expressed in percentages. They must always add up to 1 (or 100%). In Example 2-8, all of the incident intensity is accounted for (0.4 mW/cm² reflected, 9.6 mW/cm² transmitted, for a total of 10 mW/cm², or 100% of the incident intensity).

ADVANCED CONCEPTS

Reflection and transmission of ultrasound at a boundary can be expressed in amplitude terms. For a plane wave, pressure amplitude and intensity are related as follows:

$$I = \frac{p^2}{z}$$

That is, intensity depends on pressure amplitude squared. Intensity reflection and transmission coefficients then depend on the square of the amplitude coefficients. Amplitude coefficients are slightly more involved because amplitudes can be positive or negative, whereas intensities are always positive. The amplitude reflection coefficient (*ARC*) is as follows:

$$ARC = \frac{p_r}{p_i} = \frac{(z_2 - z_1)}{(z_2 + z_1)}$$

where p_r is reflected pressure amplitude and p_i is incident pressure amplitude.
If z_2 equals z_1, there is no reflection (*ARC* = 0). If z_1 is greater than z_2, p_r is negative. The amplitude transmission coefficient is as follows:

$$ATC = \frac{p_t}{p_i} = \frac{2z_2}{(z_2 + z_1)}$$

where p_t is transmitted pressure amplitude.
If z_2 equals z_1, then *ATC* equals 1; that is, p_t equals p_i.
If z_1 is greater than z_2, then p_t is less than p_i.
The intensity transmission coefficient in terms of impedances is as follows:

$$ITC = \frac{4z_1z_2}{(z_2 + z_1)^2}$$

Oblique Incidence

Oblique incidence denotes a direction of travel of the incident ultrasound that is not perpendicular to the boundary between two media (Figure 2-24). This is a common situation in diagnostic ultrasound. The direction of travel with respect to the boundary is given by the **incidence angle** (θ_i) as shown in Figure 2-24. In geometry, angles are measured from a line perpendicular to the surface. For perpendicular incidence, the incidence angle is zero. The reflected and transmitted directions are given by the **reflection angle** (θ_r) and **transmission angle** (θ_t), respectively. The incidence angle equals the reflection angle.

$$\theta_i \text{ (degrees)} = \theta_r \text{ (degrees)}$$

This phenomenon is observed in optics also (e.g., a laser beam reflecting off a mirror). The transmission angle depends on the propagation speeds in the media. Note that for oblique incidence, the reflected sound does not return to the transducer but travels off in some other direction.

Refraction

If the direction of sound changes as it crosses a boundary, then the transmission angle is different from the incidence angle. A change in direction of sound when crossing a boundary is called **refraction** (from a Latin term meaning to turn aside). If the propagation speed through the second medium is greater than

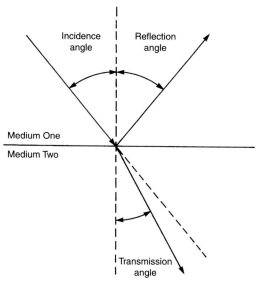

■ **FIGURE 2-24** Reflection and transmission at a boundary with oblique incidence. Incidence and reflection angles are equal. The transmission angle depends on the incidence angle and the media propagation speeds.

through the first medium, then the transmission angle is greater than the incidence angle (Figure 2-25). The changes are approximately proportional.

$$\text{If } c_1 < c_2, \text{ then } \theta_i < \theta_t. \text{ If } c_1 > c_2, \text{ then } \theta_i > \theta_t.$$

For example, if the speed increases by 1% as the sound enters the second medium, the transmission angle will be about 1% greater than the incidence angle. Similarly, if the speed in the second medium is less than in the first, the transmission angle is less than the incidence angle. No refraction occurs if the propagation speeds are equal. Also, if the incidence angle is zero (perpendicular incidence), there is no refraction, even though there may be different propagation speeds in the media. Thus the two requirements for refraction to occur are these:
1. Oblique incidence
2. Different propagation speeds on either side of the boundary

Refraction is important because when it occurs, lateral position errors (refraction artifacts) occur on an image.

Example 2-9

If the incidence angle is 20 degrees, the propagation speed in medium 1 is 1.7 mm/µs, and the propagation speed in medium 2 is 1.6 mm/µs, calculate the reflection and transmission angles.

The incidence and reflection angles are always equal, so the reflection angle is 20 degrees. The ratio of the media speeds is 1.6/1.7, which is equal to 0.94. This means that there is a 6% reduction in speed when crossing the boundary. Because the speed decreases by 6%, the transmission angle is 6% less than the incidence angle, that is, 94% of the incidence angle (0.94 × 20 = 19 degrees).

Refraction occurs with light and with sound. Refraction is the principle on which lenses operate.

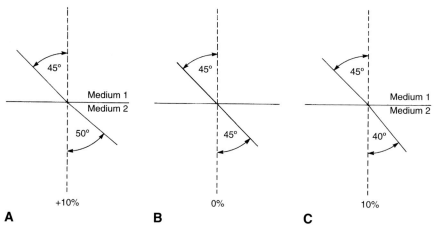

■ **FIGURE 2-25** Transmission angles for an incidence angle of 45 degrees and propagation speeds through medium 2 that are 10% greater than **(A)**, equal to **(B)**, and 10% less than **(C)** propagation speed through medium 1.

Refraction is also the cause of distortion when objects are seen in a fishbowl or swimming pool. As with sound, when light crosses a boundary obliquely and a change in the speed of the light occurs, the direction of the light changes.

ADVANCED CONCEPTS

The exact relationship between the incidence and transmission angles is known as Snell's law:

$$\left[\frac{sine\ (\theta_i)}{sine\ (\theta_t)}\right] = \frac{c_1}{c_2}$$

Where c_1 and c_2 are the propagation speeds in media 1 and 2, respectively, in Figure 2-25. This equation can be rearranged to yield the transmission angle:

$$\theta_t = sine^{-1}\left\{\frac{c_1}{c_2}\ [sine\ (\theta_i)]\right\}$$

The meaning of "$sine^{-1}(S)$" is the angle the sine of which is S.

Under the right conditions, there can be an angle at which there is *no* reflection (complete transmission into the second medium).

Because Snell's law involves ratios of sines and speeds, a good approximation allows the use of the ratio of the angles rather than the sines. This is why the angle ratio is approximately equal to the speed ratio as discussed previously. If Snell's law is used in the foregoing Example 2-9, the calculated incidence angle is 18.8 degrees, confirming validity of using the angles, rather than the sines, as an approximation.

For oblique incidence, the reflection equation involves angles in addition to impedances:

$$ARC = \frac{(z_2 \cos \theta_i) - (z_1 \cos \theta_t)}{(z_2 \cos \theta_i) + (z_1 \cos \theta_t)}$$

If c_2 is greater than c_1, there is a critical incidence angle (θ_c) beyond which there is *total* reflection (no transmission into the second medium):

$$\theta_c = sine^{-1}\left(\frac{c_1}{c_2}\right)$$

Scattering

The discussion thus far has assumed that a boundary is flat and smooth. The resulting reflections are called *specular* (from a Latin term meaning mirrorlike) reflections. If, however, the reflecting object is comparable in size to or smaller than the wavelength, or if a larger object does not have a smooth surface, the incident sound will be scattered. Scattering is the redirection of sound in many directions by rough surfaces or by heterogeneous media (Figure 2-26), such as (cellular) tissues, or particle suspensions, such as blood. These cases are analogous to light in which **specular reflections** occur at mirrors. But for rougher surfaces, such as a white wall, the light is scattered at the surface and mixed up as it travels back to the viewer's eyes. Therefore an observer does not see his or her reflected image when facing a wall. When light passes through fog, which is a suspension of water droplets in air, it is scattered as well. This limits the viewer's ability to see through fog. Although scattering inhibits vision (we cannot see ourselves reflected in a wall, and we cannot see well through fog), it is of great benefit in sonographic imaging. The reason is that with ultrasound, the goal is to see the "wall" (tissue interface), not a reflection of "oneself" (the transducer in this case). The sonographer also desires to see the "fog" (tissue parenchyma), not just the objects beyond it.

Backscatter (sound scattered back in the direction from which it originally came) intensities from rough surfaces and heterogeneous media vary with frequency and **scatterer** size. Normally, scatter intensities are less than boundary specular-reflection intensities, and they increase with increasing frequency. The intensity received by the sound source from specular reflections is highly angle dependent. Scattering from boundaries helps to make echo reception less dependent on incidence angle. Scattering permits ultrasound imaging of tissue boundaries that are not necessarily perpendicular to the direction of the incident sound (Figure 2-27, *A* and *B*). Scattering also allows imaging of tissue parenchyma (Figure 2-27, *C*) in addition to organ boundaries. Scattering is relatively independent of the direction of the incident sound and therefore is more characteristic of the scatterers. Most surfaces in the body are rough for our purposes. Reflections from smooth boundaries (e.g., vessel intima) depend not only on the acoustic properties at the boundaries but also on the angles involved.

Speckle

An ultrasound pulse, with its finite length and width, simultaneously encounters many scatterers at any location in its travel. Thus several echoes are generated simultaneously within the pulse as it interacts with these scatterers. They may arrive at the transducer in such a way that they reinforce (**constructive interference**) or partially or totally cancel (**destructive interference**) each other (Figure 2-28, *A* and *B*). As the ultrasound beam is scanned through the tissues with scatterers moving into and out of the beam, the **interference** alternates between constructive and destructive, resulting in a displayed dot pattern, a grainy appearance, that does not directly represent scatterers but rather represents the interference pattern of the scatterer distribution scanned. This phenomenon is called acoustic **speckle** and is similar to the speckle observed

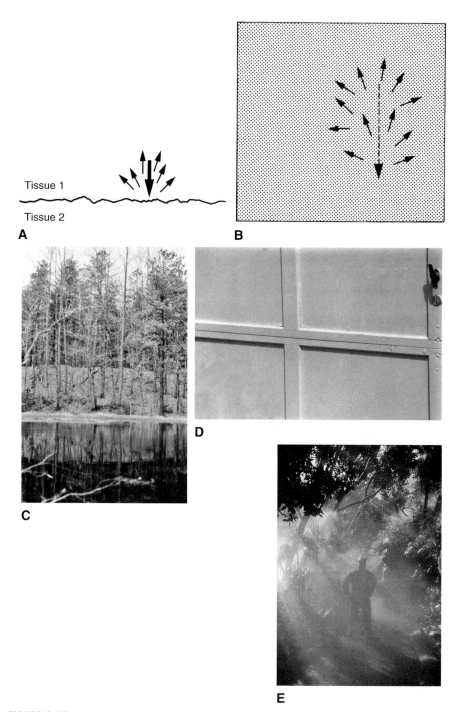

■ **FIGURE 2-26** A sound pulse may be scattered by a rough boundary between tissues **(A)** or within tissues due to their heterogeneous character **(B)**. The differences between a specular surface (smooth pond) **(C)**, a scattering surface (garage door) **(D)**, and a scattering medium (fog) **(E)** are illustrated.

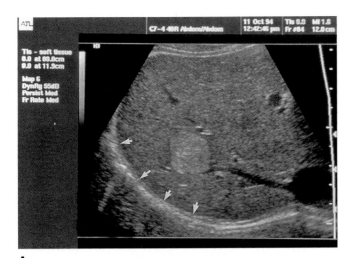

A

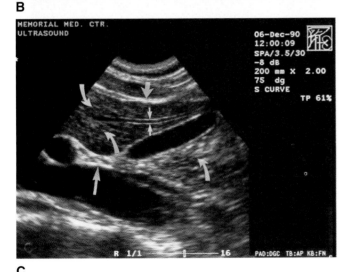

C

■ **FIGURE 2-27** **A,** Longitudinal abdominal scan in which the diaphragm is imaged even where it is not *(arrows)* perpendicular to the beam and scan lines. **B,** Strong echoes *(arrows)* from a tissue boundary. **C,** Abdominal scan showing echoes from tissue boundaries *(straight arrows)* and regions of scattering from within tissues *(curved arrows),* allowing parenchymal imaging.

with lasers. Speckle is a form of acoustic noise in sonographic imaging (Figure 2-28, *C*).

Contrast Agents

Liquid suspensions have been developed that can be injected into the circulation intravenously to increase echogenicity. These materials are called **contrast agents.**[7,8] Contrast agents must be capable of easy administration, be nontoxic and stable for a sufficient examination time, be small enough to pass through capillaries, and be large enough and echogenic enough to improve diagnostic ultrasound through an alteration in ultrasound-tissue interaction. Most agents contain microbubbles of gas that are stabilized by a protein, lipid, or polymer shell, although free gas microbubbles and solid particle suspensions also are used. These agents enhance echogenicity from vessels and perfused tissues in gray-scale sonography and Doppler ultrasound and "opacify" (fill normally anechoic regions with echoes) cardiac chambers (Figure 2-29). Contrast agents produce echoes because the impedance of the suspended particles differs from that of the suspending medium. Microbubbles in suspension are especially strong echo producers because the impedance of the gas is so much less than that of the suspending liquid. Bubbles also expand and contract unequally—that is, nonlinearly—under the influence of an ultrasound pulse. This means that echoes are produced that contain harmonics of the incident pulse frequency. Because bubbles generate stronger harmonics than tissue does, detecting harmonic frequency echoes increases the contrast between the contrast agent and surrounding tissue. This is called contrast harmonic imaging or harmonic contrast imaging. Encapsulation of the gas slows its diffusion back into solution, lengthening duration of the contrast effect. To further slow diffusion out of an encapsulated bubble, low-solubility gases such as perfluorocarbons are used. Three agents currently are approved for clinical cardiac use (left ventricular opacification and endocardial border detection) in the United States: Definity (nitrogen-containing lipisomes), Imagent (dimyristoyl lecithin), and Optison (perfluoropropane-filled albumin). In addition to these, others—such as Echovist, Levovist, and SonoVue—are in approved use in Canada, Europe, and Japan. Contrast agents (1) improve lesion detection when lesion echogenicity is similar to that of the surrounding tissue and (2) improve Doppler ultrasound detection when Doppler signals are weak (deep, slow, and small-vessel flows), often rescuing an otherwise failed examination. Ultrasound pulses of sufficiently high-pressure amplitude can fragment the bubbles, allowing the gas to dissolve and eliminating the contrast effect. Subsequent lower-amplitude imaging then can show the return of the contrast effect, giving an indication of tissue or organ perfusion rate.

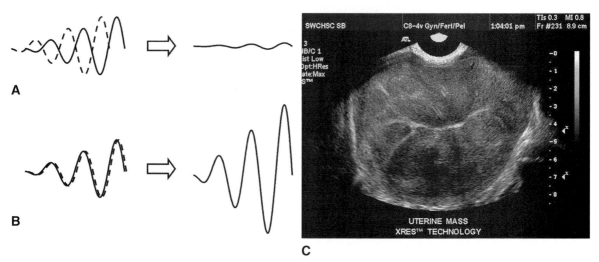

■ **FIGURE 2-28** **A,** Two similar echoes with slightly different arrival times sum to a nearly zero amplitude (destructive interference). **B,** Two similar echoes arriving nearly simultaneously sum to nearly double amplitude (constructive interference). **C,** Speckle, the grainy appearance of the tissues, is seen in this image.

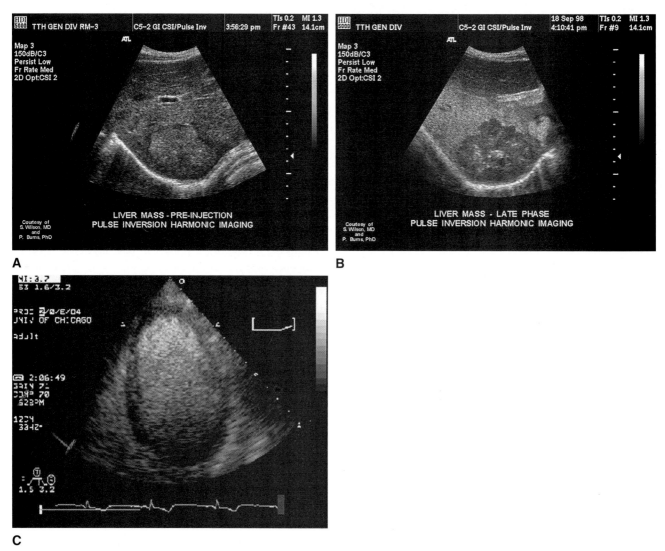

■ **FIGURE 2-29** Contrast agents enhance echogenicity from perfused tissues. Liver mass before **(A)** and after **(B)** injection of contrast agent. The agent has perfused the normal tissue better than the mass yielding and improved contrast difference between them. **C,** Left ventricular opacification with a contrast agent.

Range

Now that sound propagation, reflection, and scattering have been considered, we can discuss an important aspect of pulse-echo diagnostic ultrasound: the determination of the distance (range) from the transducer to an echo-generating structure and thus the appropriate location for the echo placement on the scan line. In sonography, pulses of ultrasound are sent into the body and echoes return from the body. To position the echoes properly on the display, two items of information are required:

1. The direction from which the echo came (which is assumed to be the direction in which the emitted pulse is launched)
2. The distance to the reflector or scatterer where the echo was produced

Regarding the second point, the instrument cannot measure distance directly; rather, it measures time and determines distance from it. Similarly, measuring the distance between two cities directly might be inconvenient (a long measuring tape might be required), but we could determine the distance by asking someone to drive from one city to the other and observe the time required. Of course, we would not know when the person arrived at the other city if we were not riding along, so we would instruct the driver to return immediately after arriving at the destination (Figure 2-30). Let us say that the round trip took exactly 4 hours. What was the distance traveled? We, of course, cannot determine the answer unless we know the speed traveled. If the driver was traveling at a speed of exactly 50 mph for the entire round trip (a difficult achievement), then we can determine that the distance traveled was 200 miles (50 mph × 4 hours). Therefore the distance to the city is 100 miles. Note that the total distance was halved because round-trip travel time was used to determine a one-way distance.

Thus the distance *(d)* to a reflector is calculated from the propagation speed and pulse round-trip travel time *(t)* according to the **range equation:**

$$d \text{ (mm)} = \tfrac{1}{2} \left[c \text{ (mm/}\mu\text{s)} \times t \text{ (}\mu\text{s)} \right]$$

 As round-trip time increases, calculated reflector distance increases.

To determine the distance from the source to the reflector, the propagation speed in the intervening medium must be known or assumed, and the pulse round-trip time must be measured. The reason that the

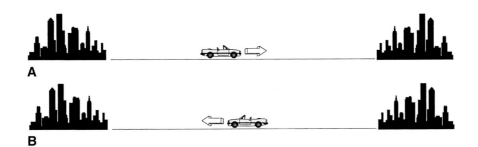

50 mph
4 hours

■ **FIGURE 2-30**   The distance between two cities can be determined by driving from one city to the other **(A)** and returning **(B)**. Multiplying the speed of travel by one half the round-trip travel time yields the distance between the cities. If the speed is 50 mph and the round-trip travel time is 4 hours, the distance between the cities is 100 miles. In this example, the *round-trip* distance traveled is 200 miles, obtained by multiplying the speed (50 mph) by the elapsed travel time (4 hours).

factor $\frac{1}{2}$ appears is that the round-trip time is the time for the pulse to travel to the reflector and return. However, only the distance *to* the reflector is desired. The average propagation speed in soft tissue (1.54 mm/μs) is assumed in using the range equation. For this case, the distance (millimeters) to the reflector can be calculated by multiplying 0.77 by the round-trip time (microseconds). Multiplying 1.54 by $\frac{1}{2}$ yields 0.77.

In the foregoing city separation distance problem, 50 mph is equivalent to 0.83 mile/min or 1.20 min/mile. Thus at this speed, 2.4 minutes of round-trip travel are required for each mile of distance separating the cities. Similarly, sound speed in tissue is 1.54 mm/μs, so 0.65 μs is required for each millimeter of travel; thus 6.5 μs are required for 1 cm of travel. Therefore 13 μs of round-trip travel time are required for each centimeter of distance from the transducer to the reflector. To confirm this, substitution of 13 μs for t in the foregoing range equation yields a reflector distance of 10 mm (1 cm):

$$d = \tfrac{1}{2}(c \times t) = \tfrac{1}{2}(1.54 \times 13) = \tfrac{1}{2}(20) = 10 \text{ mm} = 1 \text{ cm}$$

All this leads to the *important 13-μs/cm rule:* the pulse round-trip travel time is 13 μs for each centimeter of distance from source to reflector (Table 2-6; Figure 2-31). Figure 2-32 illustrates the correspondence between echo arrival time and reflector depth.

TABLE 2-6   Pulse Round-Trip Travel Time for Various Reflector Depths

Depth (cm)	Travel Time (μs)
0.5	6.5
1	13
2	26
3	39
4	52
5	65
10	130
15	195
20	260

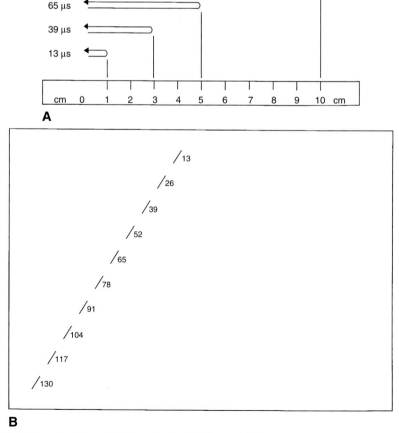

■ FIGURE 2-31   A, Echo arrival times for 1-, 3-, 5-, and 10-cm reflector distances. **B,** Echoes from 1-, 2-, 3-, 4-, 5-, 6-, 7-, 8-, 9-, and 10-cm depths arrive at the times (microseconds) indicated.

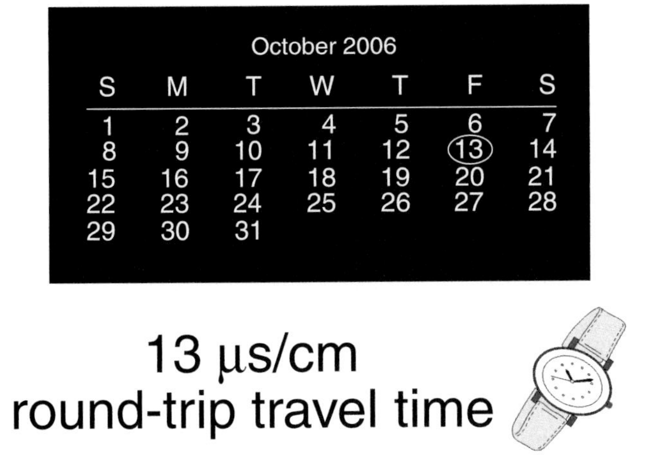

| October 2006 |
| S | M | T | W | T | F | S |

13 µs/cm
round-trip travel time

■ **FIGURE 2-32** Substituting the average speed of sound in soft tissues into the range equation yields the 13 µs/cm round-trip travel time rule.

TABLE 2-7   Sonographic Parameters in Tissue

Parameter	Symbol or Abbreviation	Range of Common Values
Frequency	f	2-15 MHz
Period	T	0.07-0.5 µs
Wavelength	λ	0.1-0.8 mm
Propagation speed	c	1.44-1.64 mm/µs
Impedance	z	1,300,000- 1,700,000 rayls
Pulse repetition frequency	PRF	4-15 kHz
Pulse repetition period	PRP	0.07-0.25 ms
Cycles per pulse	n	1-3
Pulse duration	PD	0.1-1.5 µs
Spatial pulse length	SPL	0.1-2.5 mm
Duty factor	DF	0.1% to 1%
Pressure amplitude	p	0.1-4 MPa
SPTA intensity	I_{SPTA}	0.01-100 mW/cm^2
SPPA intensity	I_{SPPA}	0.01-100 W/cm^2
Attenuation coefficient	a_c	1-8 dB/cm

TABLE 2-8   Dependence of Various Factors on Increasing (↑) Frequency

Parameter	Symbol or Abbreviation	Dependence (↑ Increase; ↓ Decrease)
Period	T	↓
Wavelength	λ	↓
Pulse duration	PD	↓
Spatial pulse length	SPL	↓
Attenuation	a	↑
Penetration	pen	↓

Example 2-10

If an echo returns 104 µs after a pulse was emitted by a transducer, at what depth is the structure located that produced the echo?

1. Using the range equation:

$$d \text{ (mm)} = 0.77 \text{ mm/µs} \times 104 \text{ µs} = 80 \text{ mm} = 8.0 \text{ cm}$$

2. Using the 13-µs/cm rule:

$$d \text{ (cm)} = \frac{104 \text{ µs}}{13 \text{ µs/cm}} = 8 \text{ cm}$$

Table 2-7 gives common values for several parameters of sonography. Table 2-8 summarizes how various parameters change with frequency.

REVIEW

The key points presented in this chapter are the following:

■ Sound is a wave of pressure and density variations and particle vibration.

■ Ultrasound is sound having a frequency greater than 20 kHz.

■ Frequency denotes the number of cycles occurring in a second.

■ Harmonic frequencies are generated as sound travels through tissue.

■ Wavelength is the length of a cycle of sound.

■ Propagation speed is the speed of sound through a medium.

■ The medium determines the propagation speed.

■ The average propagation speed of sound through soft tissue is 1.54 mm/µs.

■ Pulsed ultrasound is described by pulse repetition frequency, pulse repetition period, pulse duration, duty factor, and spatial pulse length.

■ Amplitude and intensity describe the strength of sound.

■ Six intensities (SATA, SPTA, SAPA, SPPA, SATP, and SPTP) are used to describe pulsed ultrasound.

■ Attenuation is the weakening of sound caused by absorption, reflection, and scattering.

■ Attenuation increases with frequency and path length.

■ The average attenuation coefficient for soft tissues is 0.5 dB/cm for each megahertz of frequency.

■ Imaging depth decreases with increasing frequency.

■ Impedance is the density of a medium times its propagation speed.

■ When sound encounters boundaries between media with different impedances, part of the sound is reflected and part is transmitted.

■ With perpendicular incidence, and if the two media have the same impedance, there is no reflection.

- The greater the difference in the impedances of the media at a boundary, the greater the intensity of the echo that is generated at the boundary.
- With oblique incidence, the sound is refracted at a boundary between media for which propagation speeds are different.
- Incidence and reflection angles at a boundary are always equal.
- Scattering occurs at rough media boundaries and within heterogeneous media.
- Contrast agents are used to enhance echogenicity in sonography and Doppler ultrasound.
- Pulse-echo round-trip travel time is 13 µs/cm. This time is used to determine the distance to a reflector.

EXERCISES

1. A wave is a traveling variation in quantities called _____ _____.
2. Sound is a traveling variation in quantities called _____ _____.
3. Ultrasound is sound with a frequency greater than _____ Hz.
4. Acoustic variables include _____, _____, and _____ _____.
5. Which of the following frequencies are in the ultrasound range? (There is more than one correct answer.)
   a. 15 Hz
   b. 15,000 Hz
   c. 15 MHz
   d. 30,000 Hz
   e. 0.04 MHz
6. Which of the following are acoustic variables? (There is more than one correct answer.)
   a. Pressure
   b. Frequency
   c. Propagation speed
   d. Period
   e. Particle motion
7. Frequency is a measure of how many _____ an acoustic variable goes through in a second.
8. The unit of frequency is _____, which is abbreviated _____.
9. Period is the _____ that it takes for one cycle to occur.
10. Period decreases as _____ increases.
11. Wavelength is the length of _____ over which one cycle occurs.
12. Propagation speed is the speed with which a _____ moves through a medium.
13. Wavelength is equal to _____ _____ divided by _____.
14. The _____ and _____ of a medium determine propagation speed.
15. Propagation speed increases if _____ is increased.
16. The average propagation speed in soft tissues is _____ m/s or _____ mm/µs.
17. Propagation speed is determined by
    a. frequency.
    b. amplitude.
    c. wavelength.
    d. period.
    e. medium.
18. Place the following in order of increasing sound propagation speed:
    a. Gas
    b. Solid
    c. Liquid
19. The wavelength of 7-MHz ultrasound in soft tissues is _____ mm.
20. Wavelength in soft tissues _____ as frequency increases.
21. It takes _____ µs for ultrasound to travel 1.54 cm in soft tissue.
22. Propagation speed in bone is _____ than in soft tissues.
23. Sound travels fastest in
    a. air.
    b. helium.
    c. water.
    d. steel.
    e. a vacuum.
24. Solids have higher propagation speeds than liquids because they have greater
    a. density.
    b. stiffness.
25. Sound travels slowest in _____.
26. Sound is a _____ _____ wave.
27. If propagation speed is doubled (a different medium) and frequency is held constant, the wavelength is _____.
28. If frequency in soft tissue is doubled, propagation speed is _____.
29. If wavelength is 2 mm and the frequency is doubled, the wavelength becomes _____ mm.
30. Waves can carry _____ from one place to another.
31. From given values for propagation speed and frequency, which of the following can be calculated?
    a. Amplitude
    b. Impedance
    c. Wavelength
    d. a and b
    e. b and c
32. If two media have different stiffnesses, the one with the higher stiffness will have the higher propagation speed. True or false?
33. The second harmonic of 3 MHz is _____ MHz.

34. Odd harmonics of 2 MHz are _____ MHz.
    a. 1, 3, 5
    b. 2, 4, 6
    c. 6, 9, 12
    d. 6, 10, 14
    e. 10, 12, 14
35. Even harmonics of 2 MHz are _____ MHz.
    a. 1, 3, 5
    b. 2, 4, 6
    c. 4, 8, 12
    d. 6, 10, 14
    e. 10, 12, 14
36. Nonlinear propagation means that
    a. the sound beam does not travel in a straight line.
    b. the propagation speed depends on frequency.
    c. the propagation speed depends on pressure.
    d. the waveform changes shape as it travels.
    e. more than one of the above.
37. As a wave changes from sinusoidal to sawtooth form, additional _____ appear that are _____ and _____ multiples of the _____. They are called _____.
38. If the density of a medium is 1000 kg/m^3 and the propagation speed is 1540 m/s, the impedance is _____ rayls.
39. If two media have the same propagation speed but different densities, the one with the higher density will have the higher impedance. True or false?
40. If two media have the same density but different propagation speeds, the one with the higher propagation speed will have the higher impedance. True or false?
41. Impedance is _____ multiplied by _____ _____.
42. What are the periods and frequencies shown in Figure 2-33?

43. If the wavelength in Figure 2-33, *A*, is 0.154 mm, the propagation speed is _____ mm/μs.
44. If the propagation speed is 1.54 mm/μs, the wavelength in Figure 2-33, *B*, is _____ mm.
45. The abbreviation CW stands for _____.
46. Pulsed ultrasound is ultrasound in the form of repeated short _____.
47. Pulse repetition frequency is the number of _____ occurring in 1 second.
48. The pulse repetition _____ is the time from the beginning of one pulse to the beginning of the next.
49. The pulse repetition period _____ as the pulse repetition frequency increases.
50. Pulse duration is the _____ it takes for a pulse to occur.
51. Spatial pulse length is the _____ of _____ that a pulse occupies as it travels.
52. _____ _____ is the fraction of time that pulsed ultrasound is actually on.
53. Pulse duration equals the number of cycles in the pulse multiplied by _____.
54. Spatial pulse length equals the number of cycles in the pulse multiplied by _____.
55. The duty factor of continuous wave sound is _____.
56. If the wavelength is 2 mm, the spatial pulse length for a three-cycle pulse is _____ mm.
57. The spatial pulse length in soft tissue for a two-cycle pulse of frequency 5 MHz is _____ mm.
58. The pulse duration in soft tissue for a two-cycle pulse of frequency 5 MHz is _____ μs.
59. For a 1-kHz pulse repetition frequency, the pulse repetition period is _____ ms.
60. For Exercises 58 and 59 together, the duty factor is _____.

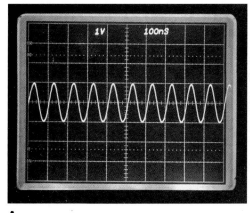
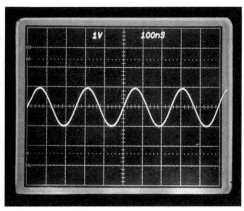

A   B

■ **FIGURE 2-33** Illustration to accompany Exercises 42 to 44. The total width of the screen represents 1 μs.

61. How many cycles are there in 1 second of continuous wave 5-MHz ultrasound?
    a. 5
    b. 500
    c. 5000
    d. 5,000,000
    e. None of the above
62. How many cycles are there in 1 second of pulsed 5-MHz ultrasound with a duty factor of 0.01 (1%)?
    a. 5
    b. 500
    c. 5000
    d. 5,000,000
    e. None of the above
63. In Exercise 62, how many cycles did pulsing eliminate?
    a. 100%
    b. 99.9%
    c. 99%
    d. 50%
    e. 1%
64. For pulsed ultrasound, the duty factor is always _____ _____ one.
65. Amplitude is the maximum _____ that occurs in an acoustic variable.
66. Intensity is the _____ in a wave divided by _____.
67. The unit for intensity is _____.
68. Intensity is proportional to _____ squared.
69. If power is doubled and area remains unchanged, intensity is _____.
70. If area is doubled and power remains unchanged, intensity is _____.
71. If both power and area are doubled, intensity is _____.
72. If amplitude is doubled, intensity is _____.
73. If a sound beam has a power of 10 mW and a beam area of 2 cm^2, the spatial average intensity is _____ mW/cm^2.
74. If the beam in Exercise 73 is focused to a beam area of 0.1 cm^2, the intensity becomes _____ mW/cm^2.
75. Multiplying pulse average intensity by duty factor yields _____ _____ intensity.
76. Which of the following intensities are equal for continuous wave sound?
    a. Spatial peak and spatial average
    b. Temporal peak and temporal average
    c. Spatial peak and temporal average
    d. Spatial average and temporal average
    e. None of the above
77. If the spatial peak–temporal average intensity is 1 mW/cm^2 and the duty factor is 0.01, calculate the spatial peak–pulse average intensity in mW/cm^2.

78. If pulsed ultrasound is on 50% of the time (duty factor = 0.5) and pulse average intensity is 4 mW/cm^2, the temporal average intensity is _____ mW/cm^2.
79. If the maximum value of an acoustic variable is 10 units and the normal (undisturbed) value is 7 units, the amplitude is _____ units. The minimum value of the acoustic variable is _____ units.
80. Attenuation is the reduction in _____ and _____ as a wave travels through a medium.
81. Attenuation consists of _____, _____, and _____.
82. The attenuation coefficient is attenuation per _____ of sound travel.
83. Attenuation and attenuation coefficient are given in units of _____ and _____, respectively.
84. For soft tissues, there is approximately _____ dB of attenuation per centimeter for each megahertz of frequency.
85. For soft tissues, the attenuation coefficient at 3 MHz is approximately _____.
86. The attenuation coefficient in soft tissue _____ as frequency increases.
87. For soft tissue, if frequency is doubled, attenuation is _____. If path length is doubled, attenuation is _____. If both frequency and path length are doubled, attenuation is _____.
88. If frequency is doubled and path length is halved, attenuation is _____.
89. Absorption is the conversion of _____ to _____.
90. Can absorption be greater than attenuation in a given medium at a given frequency?
91. Is attenuation in bone higher or lower than in soft tissue?
92. For average soft tissue, the attenuation is such that for each 1.5 cm traveled, a 4-MHz sound intensity is reduced by _____%. For 1 cm and 6 MHz, the reduction is _____%. For 4 cm and 3.5 MHz, the reduction is _____%. (Use Table 2-3.)
93. The attenuation coefficient for soft tissue at 10 MHz is _____ dB/cm.
94. The attenuation coefficient for soft tissue at 5 MHz is _____ dB/cm.
95. The attenuation coefficient (dB/cm) in soft tissue is approximately one half the _____ (MHz).
96. The imaging depth (penetration) _____ as frequency increases.
97. If the intensity of 4-MHz ultrasound entering soft tissue is 2 W/cm^2, the intensity at a depth of 4 cm is _____ W/cm^2.
98. If the intensity of 40-MHz ultrasound entering soft tissue is 2 W/cm^2, the intensity at a depth of 4 cm is _____ W/cm^2.

99. The depth at which half-intensity occurs in soft tissues at 7.5 MHz is
    a. 0.6 cm.
    b. 0.7 cm.
    c. 0.8 cm.
    d. 0.9 cm.
    e. 1.0 cm.
100. Give the logarithms of the following numbers:
    a. 10
    b. 0.1
    c. 100
    d. 0.001
101. If the intensity at point A is 40 mW/cm^2 and at point B it is 10 mW/cm^2, the attenuation from A to B is _____ dB.
102. If the intensities of traveling sound are 10 mW/cm^2 and 0.1 mW/cm^2 at two points 5 cm apart, the attenuation between the two points is _____ dB. The attenuation coefficient is _____ dB/cm.
103. If the intensity at the start of a path is 3 mW/cm^2 and the attenuation over the path is 2 dB, the intensity at the end of the path is _____ mW/cm^2. (Use Table 2-3.)
104. The intensities in order of decreasing values are
    a. SPTA, SATA, SPPA, and SPTP.
    b. SPTA, SPTP, and SPPA.
    c. SATA, SPTP, and SPPA.
    d. SPTP, SATA, and SPPA.
    e. SPTP, SPPA, SPTA, and SATA.
105. When ultrasound encounters a boundary with perpendicular incidence, the _____ of the tissues must be different to produce a reflection (echo).
106. With perpendicular incidence, two media _____ and the incident _____ must be known to calculate reflected intensity.
107. With perpendicular incidence, two media _____ must be known to calculate the intensity reflection coefficient.
108. For an incident intensity of 2 mW/cm^2 and impedances of 49 and 51 rayls, the reflected intensity is _____ mW/cm^2 and the transmitted intensity is _____ mW/cm^2.
109. For an incident intensity of 2 mW/cm^2 and impedances of 99 and 101 rayls, the reflected and transmitted intensities are _____ and _____ mW/cm^2, respectively.
110. For an incident intensity of 2 mW/cm^2 and impedances of 98 and 102 rayls, the reflected and the transmitted intensities are _____ and _____ mW/cm^2, respectively.
111. For an incident intensity of 5 mW/cm^2 and impedances of 45 and 55 rayls, the intensity reflection coefficient is _____, or _____%.
112. For impedances of 45 and 55 rayls, the intensity transmission coefficient is _____, or _____%.
113. For impedances of 45 and 55 rayls, the intensity reflection coefficient is _____ dB.
114. Given the following, calculate the reflected intensity (mW/cm^2):
    Incident intensity = 1 mW/cm^2
    Medium 1:
    Density = 1.0 kg/m^3
    Propagation speed = 1350 m/s
    Medium 2:
    Density = 1.0 kg/m^3
    Propagation speed = 1650 m/s
115. Given the following, calculate the reflected intensity (mW/cm^2):
    Incident intensity = 5 mW/cm^2
    Medium 1:
    Density = 1.00 kg/m^3
    Propagation speed = 1515 m/s
    Medium 2:
    Density = 1.01 kg/m^3
    Propagation speed = 1500 m/s
116. Given the following, calculate the reflected and transmitted intensities (milliwatts per square centimeter):
    Incident intensity = 5 mW/cm^2
    Medium 1 impedance = 2 rayls
    Medium 2 impedance = 0 rayls
117. If the impedances of the media are equal, there is no reflection. True or false?
118. If the densities of the media are equal, there is no reflection. True or false?
119. If propagation speeds of the media are equal, there is no reflection. True or false?
120. The intensity reflection and transmission coefficients depend on whether the sound is traveling from medium 1 into medium 2 or vice versa. True or false?
121. The intensity reflection coefficient at a boundary between soft tissue (impedance of 1,630,000 rayls) and air (impedance of 400 rayls) is _____.
122. A coupling medium is used to eliminate _____ between the transducer and the skin, thus eliminating a strong _____ at the transducer-air and air-skin boundaries.
123. The intensity reflection coefficient at a boundary between fat (impedance of 1,380,000 rayls) and muscle (impedance of 1,700,000 rayls) is _____.
124. The intensity reflection coefficient at a boundary between soft tissue (impedance of 1,630,000 rayls) and bone (impedance of 7,800,000 rayls) is _____.

125. With perpendicular incidence, the reflected intensity depends on
    a. density difference.
    b. impedance difference.
    c. impedance sum.
    d. b and c.
    e. a and b.

126. Refraction is a change in _____ of sound when it crosses a boundary. Refraction is caused by a change in _____ _____ at the boundary.

127. If the propagation speed through medium 2 is greater than the propagation speed through medium 1, the transmission angle will be _____ _____ the incidence angle, and the reflection angle will be _____ _____ the incidence angle.

128. If the propagation speed through medium 2 is less than the propagation speed through medium 1, the transmission angle will be _____ _____ the incidence angle, and the reflection angle will be _____ _____ the incidence angle.

129. If the propagation speed through medium 2 is equal to the propagation speed through medium 1, the transmission angle will be _____ _____ the incidence angle, and the reflection angle will be _____ _____ the incidence angle.

130. If the incidence angle is 30 degrees, the propagation speed through medium 1 is 1 mm/μs, and the propagation speed through medium 2 is 0.7 mm/μs, the reflection angle is _____ degrees and the transmission angle is _____ degrees.

131. If the incidence angle is 30 degrees, the propagation speed through medium 1 is 1 mm/μs, and the propagation speed through medium 2 is 1 mm/μs, the reflection angle is _____ degrees and the transmission angle is _____ degrees.

132. If the incidence angle is 30 degrees and the propagation speed through medium 2 is 30% higher than the propagation speed through medium 1, the reflection angle is _____ degrees and the transmission angle is _____ degrees.

133. Under what two conditions does refraction *not* occur?
    a. _____
    b. _____

134. The low speed of sound in fat is a source of image degradation because of refraction. If the incidence angle at a boundary between fat (1.45 mm/μs) and kidney (1.56 mm/μs) is 30 degrees, the transmission angle is _____ degrees.

135. Redirection of sound in many directions as it encounters rough media junctions or particle suspensions (heterogeneous media) is called _____.

136. With specular reflection, wavelength is small compared with boundary dimensions. True or false?

137. Scattering occurs when boundary dimensions are large compared with wavelength or when the boundary is smooth. True or false?

138. As frequency increases, backscatter strength
    a. increases.
    b. decreases.
    c. does not change.
    d. refracts.
    e. infarcts.

139. Backscatter helps make echo reception less dependent on incidence angle. True or false?

140. As frequency increases, specular reflections
    a. increase.
    b. decrease.
    c. do not change.
    d. refract.
    e. infarct.

141. The purpose of contrast agents is to
    a. strengthen the echogenicity of blood.
    b. strengthen the echogenicity of perfused organs.
    c. improve contrast between lesions and normal tissue.
    d. increase propagation speed.
    e. more than one of the above.

142. To calculate the distance to a reflector, the _____ _____ and the pulse round-trip travel _____ must be known.

143. If the propagation speed is 1.6 mm/μs and the pulse round-trip time is 5 μs, the distance to the reflector is _____ mm.

144. If the propagation speed is 1.4 mm/μs and the time for a pulse to travel to the reflector is 5 μs, the distance to the reflector is _____ mm.

145. When the pulse round-trip time is 10 μs, the distance to a reflector in soft tissue is _____ mm.

146. When the pulse round-trip time is 13 μs, the distance to a reflector in soft tissue is _____ cm.

146. If an echo arrives 39 μs after a pulse was emitted, at what depth should the echo be placed on its scan line?

147. When the pulse round-trip time is 130 μs, the distance to a reflector in soft tissue is _____ cm.

149. How long after a pulse is sent out by a transducer does an echo from an object at a depth of 5 cm return?

150. Which of the following is a characteristic of a medium through which sound is propagating?
    a. impedance
    b. intensity
    c. amplitude
    d. frequency
    e. period

151. Which of the following applies (apply) to continuous wave sound?
    a. Pulse duration
    b. Pulse repetition frequency
    c. Frequency
    d. Intensity
    e. c and d

152. Match the following:
    a. Frequency: _____   1. Time per cycle
    b. Period: _____   2. Maximum variation per cycle
    c. Wavelength: _____   3. Length per cycle
    d. Propagation speed: _____   4. Cycles per second
    e. Amplitude: _____   5. Speed of a wave through a medium

153. For Figure 2-34, give the pulse repetition period, pulse duration, duty factor, pulse repetition frequency, period, and frequency.

154. What must be known to calculate distance to a reflector?
    a. Attenuation, speed, and density
    b. Attenuation and impedance
    c. Attenuation and absorption
    d. Travel time and speed
    e. Density and speed

155. No reflection will occur with perpendicular incidence if the media _____ are equal.

156. Scattering occurs at smooth boundaries and within homogeneous media. True or false?

157. A 3-MHz instrument with an spatial peak–temporal average output intensity of 10 mW/cm^2 images to a maximum depth of 15 cm in soft tissue. To image to a depth of 18 cm, the output intensity of the instrument must be increased to _____ mW/cm^2.

158. Match the images in Figure 2-35 with the frequencies used.
    a. A _____   1. 2.0 MHz
    b. B _____   2. 3.5 MHz
    c. C _____   3. 5.0 MHz
    d. D _____   4. 7.5 MHz

159. Figure 2-36 shows the following:
    a. Attenuation
    b. Continous wave
    c. Pulsed wave
    d. a and b
    e. a and c

160. What fraction (percent) of the initial intensity returns to the surface from boundary 2 in Figure 2-37 if the intensity reflection coefficient at each boundary is 1% and 3 dB of attenuation occurs between each pair of boundaries?
    a. 3
    b. 0.3
    c. 0.06
    d. 0.003
    e. 0.0006

161. If bandwidth is 1 MHz and operating frequency is 3 MHz, determine the following:
    a. Fractional bandwidth _____
    b. Lowest frequency _____
    c. Highest frequency _____

162. Fractional bandwidth is expressed in
    a. megahertz.
    b. millimeters per millisecond.
    c. watts per square centimeter.
    d. all of the above.
    e. none of the above.

163. The range of _____ involved in an ultrasound pulse is called its bandwidth.

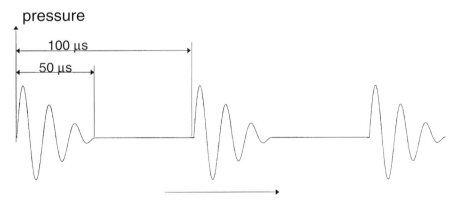

■ **FIGURE 2-34**   Illustration to accompany Exercise 153, showing pressure versus time for three pulses.

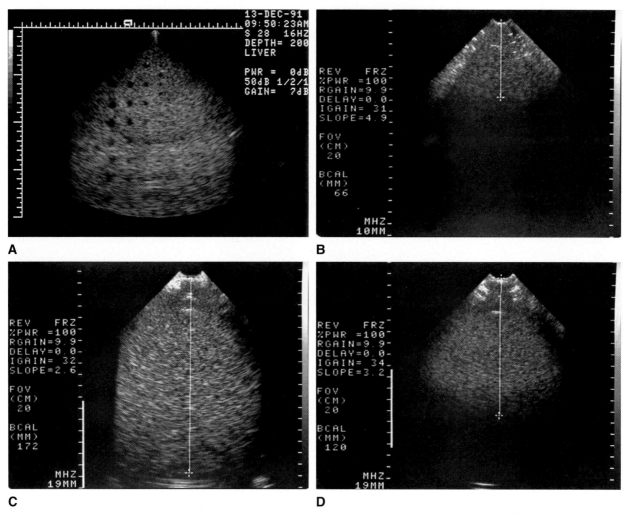

■ **FIGURE 2-35**   Illustration for Exercise 158, showing penetration at four frequencies: 20 cm **(A)**, 7 cm **(B)**, 17 cm **(C)**, and 12 cm **(D)**.

Distance

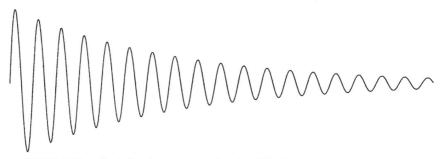

■ **FIGURE 2-36**   Illustration to accompany Exercise 159, showing pressure versus distance.

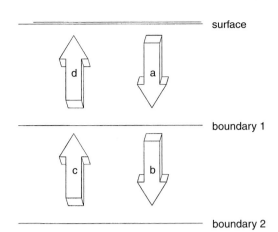

surface

boundary 1

boundary 2

■ **FIGURE 2-37** Illustration to accompany Exercise 160. Sound travels from the surface to boundaries 1 and 2, and then back through boundary 1 to the surface.

164. If the penetration of 3-MHz ultrasound in a specific tissue is 15 cm, the penetration at 5 MHz would be _____ cm.

165. The first even harmonic of 5 MHz is
   a. 2 MHz.
   b. 2.5 MHz.
   c. 5 MHz.
   d. 10 MHz.
   e. 50 MHz.

CHAPTER

3 Transducers

LEARNING OBJECTIVES

After reading this chapter, the student should be able to do the following:

- Describe the construction of a transducer and the function of each part.
- Explain how a transducer generates ultrasound pulses.
- Explain how a transducer receives echoes.
- Describe a sound beam and list the factors that affect it.
- Discuss how sound beams are focused automatically and scanned through tissue cross sections.
- Compare linear, convex, phased, and vector arrays.
- Define detail resolution.
- Differentiate between three aspects of detail resolution.
- List the factors that determine detail resolution.

KEY TERMS

The following terms are introduced in this chapter:

Aperture	Far zone	Near zone
Apodization	Focal length	Operating frequency
Array	Focal region	Phased array
Axial	Focal zone	Phased linear array
Axial resolution	Focus	Piezoelectricity
Beam	Fraunhofer zone	Probe
Composite	Fresnel zone	Resolution
Convex array	Grating lobes	Resonance frequency
Crystal	Lateral	Scanhead
Curie point	Lateral resolution	Sector
Damping	Lead zirconate titanate	Sensitivity
Detail resolution	Lens	Side lobes
Disk	Linear	Sound beam
Dynamic aperture	Linear array	Source
Dynamic focusing	Linear phased array	Transducer
Element	Linear sequenced array	Transducer assembly
Elevational resolution	Matching layer	Ultrasound transducer
f number	Natural focus	Vector array

This chapter describes transducers, the devices that generate and receive ultrasound. Transducers form the connecting link between the ultrasound-tissue interactions described in Chapter 2 and the instruments described in Chapters 4, 6, and 7. The sound produced by these transducers is confined in beams rather than traveling uniformly in all directions away from the **source.** These beams are focused and automatically are scanned through tissue by the transducers.

CONSTRUCTION AND OPERATION

A **transducer** converts one form of energy to another. **Ultrasound transducers** (Figure 3-1) convert electric energy into ultrasound energy and vice versa. The electric voltages applied to transducers are converted to ultrasound. Ultrasound echoes incident on the transducers produce electric voltages. Loudspeakers (Figure 3-2, *A*), microphones (Figure 3-2, *B*), and intercoms accomplish similar functions with audible sound.

Some transducers include parts of the electronics internally that are otherwise located in the instrument.

Piezoelectric Element

Ultrasound transducers operate according to the principle of **piezoelectricity.**[9] The word *piezoelectricity* is derived from the Greek *piezo*, to press, and *elektron*, meaning amber, which is the organic plant resin that was used in early electrical studies. This principle states that some materials (ceramics, quartz, and others) produce a voltage when deformed by an applied pressure. Conversely, piezoelectricity also results in production of a pressure when an applied voltage deforms these materials. Various formulations of **lead zirconate titanate** are used commonly as materials in the production of modern ultrasound transducer elements. Ceramics such as these are not *naturally* piezoelectric. They are made

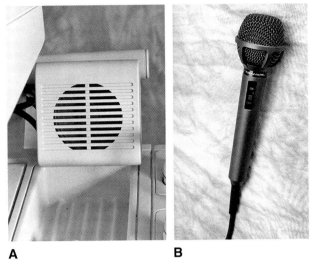

A   **B**

■ **FIGURE 3-2**   **A,** Loudspeaker. **B,** Microphone.

piezoelectric during their manufacture by being placed in a strong electric field while they are at a high temperature. If a critical temperature (the **Curie point**) subsequently is exceeded, the **element** will lose its piezoelectric properties. These ceramics often are combined with a nonpiezoelectric polymer to create materials that are called piezocomposites. These **composites** have lower impedance and improved bandwidth, **sensitivity,** and **resolution.**

> *Piezoelectric elements convert electric voltage into ultrasound pulses and convert returning echoes back into voltages.*

Single-element transducers take the form of **disks** (Figure 3-3, *A*). **Linear array** transducers contain numerous elements that have a rectangular shape (Figure 3-3, *B*). When an electric voltage is applied to the faces of either type, the thickness of the element increases or decreases, depending on the polarity of the voltage (Figure 3-3, *C*). The term *transducer element* (also called *piezoelectric element*, *active element*, or **crystal**) refers to the piece of piezoelectric material (Figure 3-3, *D*) that converts electricity to ultrasound and vice versa. Elements, with their associated case and **damping** and matching materials (Figure 3-3, *E*), are called the **transducer assembly, probe,** or **scanhead,** or are referred to simply as the transducer.

Transducers typically are driven by 1 cycle of alternating voltage for sonographic imaging. This single-cycle driving voltage produces a 2- or 3-cycle ultrasound pulse. Longer driving voltages, typically 5 to 30 cycles, are used for Doppler techniques. This operation produces an alternating pressure that propagates from the

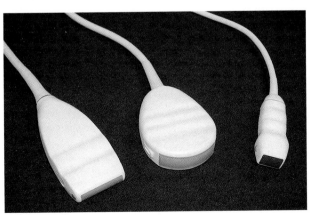

■ **FIGURE 3-1**   Transducers of various types.

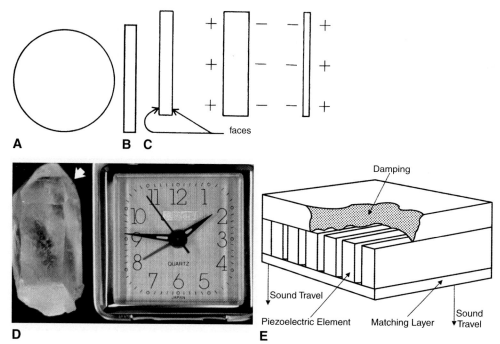

■ FIGURE 3-3   **A,** Front view of a disk transducer element. **B,** Front view of a rectangular element. **C,** Side view of either element with no voltage applied to faces (normal thickness), with voltage applied (increased thickness), and with opposite voltage applied (decreased thickness). **D,** Quartz crystals *(arrow)* are used in electric clocks, watches, and other devices. **E,** The internal parts of a transducer assembly (scanhead or probe). The damping (backing) material reduces pulse duration, thus improving axial resolution. The matching layer improves sound transmission into the tissues. Not included in this illustration are a lens and a protective/insulating layer that commonly are attached to the front of the assembly.

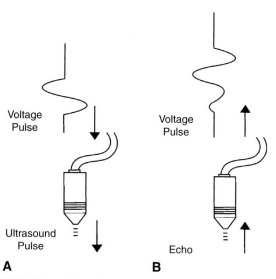

■ FIGURE 3-4   A transducer converts electric voltage pulses into ultrasound pulses **(A)** and converts received echoes into electric voltage pulses **(B).**

transducer as a sound pulse (Figure 3-4, *A*). The frequency of the sound produced is equal to the frequency of the driving voltage, which must be reasonably near the **operating frequency** *(f_o)* of the transducer for operation with acceptable efficiency. The operating frequency (sometimes called the **resonance frequency**) is the preferred, or natural, frequency of operation for the element. Operating frequency is determined by the following:

■ The propagation speed of the transducer material *(c_t)*
■ The element thickness *(th)* of the transducer element

The operating frequency is such that the thickness corresponds to half a wavelength in the element material. Typical diagnostic ultrasound elements are 0.2 to 1 mm thick (Table 3-1) and have propagation speeds of 4 to 6 mm/μs. Because wavelength decreases as frequency increases, thinner elements yield higher frequencies (Figure 3-5). This is analogous to smaller bells producing higher-pitched sounds (Figure 3-5, *C*). The transducer converts the returning echo into an alternating voltage pulse (Figure 3-4, *B*).

$$f_o \text{ (MHz)} = \left[\frac{c_t \text{ (mm/μs)}}{2 \times th \text{ (mm)}} \right]$$

Thinner elements operate at higher frequencies.

ADVANCED CONCEPTS

When a ceramic crystal is raised beyond the Curie point (about 350° C for lead zirconate titanate ceramics) the molecules in the crystal lattice can reorient with respect to each other. The molecules normally are oriented randomly, yielding no piezoelectric properties. If raised beyond the Curie point while in a strong electric field, the molecules (which are tiny electric dipoles) line up with the electric field. When the crystal is cooled below the Curie point while in the field, the crystal lattice is locked into the molecular structure that piezoelectric crystals naturally have, with the molecular dipoles lined up parallel to each other. Now if a voltage is applied to the front and rear faces of the element, it will get thicker or thinner as the dipoles together rotate toward or away (depending on the polarity of the voltage) from parallelism with the electric field produced by the voltage. If a polarized ceramic element is heated above the Curie point (not in an electric field), the molecules reorient randomly and the element loses its piezoelectric properties.

TABLE 3-1 Transducer Element Thickness* for Various Operating Frequencies

Frequency (MHz)	Thickness (mm)
2.0	1.0
3.5	0.6
5.0	0.4
7.5	0.3
10.0	0.2

*Assuming an element propagation speed of 4 mm/μs.

For wide-bandwidth transducers (e.g., those having a fractional bandwidth of at least 70%), voltage excitation can be used selectively to operate the same transducer at more than one frequency (Figure 3-6). The transducer is driven at one of two or three selectable frequencies by voltage pulses with the selected frequency. The two or three frequencies must fall within the transducer bandwidth. Choosing the higher frequency yields better **detail resolution.** If the resulting penetration is not sufficient for the study at hand, however, a lower frequency can be selected (resulting in some degradation in resolution). Push-button frequency switching is quicker and more convenient and cost-effective than changing of transducers. Wide bandwidth also allows harmonic imaging, where echoes of twice the frequency sent into the body are received to improve the image.

Damping Material

The pulse repetition frequency is equal to the voltage pulse repetition frequency. This is the number of voltage pulses sent to the transducer each second, which is determined by the instrument driving the transducer. The pulse duration is equal to the period multiplied by the number of cycles in the pulse. Damping (also called backing) material (a mixture of metal powder and a plastic or epoxy resin) is attached to the rear face of the transducer elements to reduce the number of cycles in each pulse (Figures 3-3, *E* and 3-7). Damping reduces pulse duration and spatial pulse length and improves resolution. This method of damping is analogous to packing foam rubber around a bell that is rung by a tap with a hammer. The rubber reduces the time that the bell rings following the tap. The rubber also reduces the loudness of the ringing. For ultrasound transducers, the damping material additionally reduces the ultra-

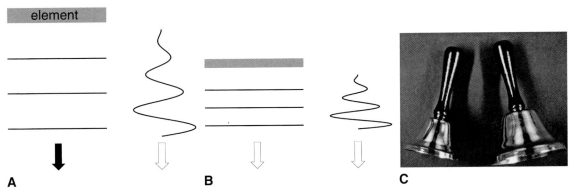

■ **FIGURE 3-5   A,** Thicker elements operate at lower frequencies. **B,** Thinner elements operate at higher frequencies. **C,** Smaller and larger bells ring with higher and lower pitches, respectively.

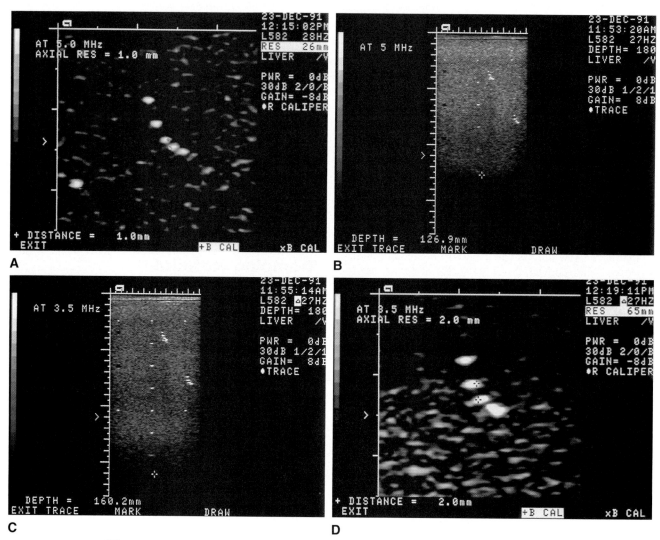

■ FIGURE 3-6 Multihertz operation allows the transducer to provide (at a higher frequency) selectively better detail resolution **(A)** with reduced penetration **(B)** or (at a lower frequency) deeper penetration **(C)** with some degradation of resolution **(D)**.

sound amplitude and thus decreases the efficiency and sensitivity (ability to detect weak echoes) of the system (an undesired effect). This is the price paid for reduced spatial pulse length (a desired effect resulting in improved resolution) with damping. Typically, pulses of two to three cycles are generated with (damped) diagnostic ultrasound transducers. Shortening the pulses broadens their bandwidth. Typical bandwidths for modern transducers range from 50% to 100%. An example of a 100% bandwidth is a 5-MHz operating frequency with a bandwidth of 5 MHz, that is, from 2.5 to 7.5 MHz.

Composites and damping material shorten pulses and improve resolution.

Transducers intended for continuous wave Doppler ultrasound use are not damped because pulses are not used in this application. These transducers have higher efficiencies because energy is not lost to damping material.

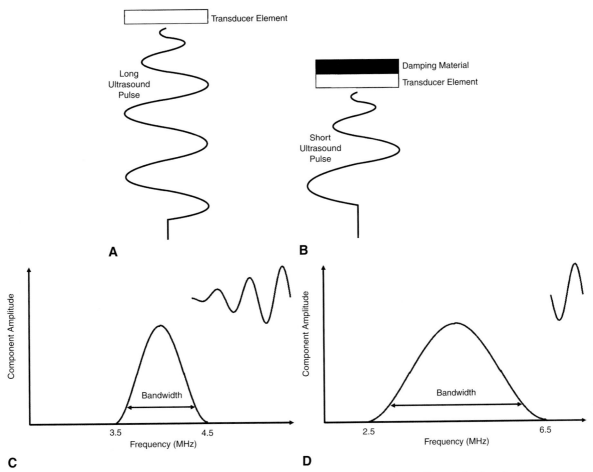

■ FIGURE 3-7 **A,** Without damping a transducer element produces a long ultrasound pulse of many cycles. **B,** With damping material on the rear face of the transducer element a short ultrasound pulse of a few cycles is produced. This figure shows each pulse traveling (down) away from the transducer in space so that the bottom end is the beginning or leading edge of the pulse as it travels down. **C** and **D,** Plots of the frequencies present in the ultrasound pulses (from **A** and **B,** respectively). Component amplitude is the amplitude of each frequency component present. Bandwidth is the frequency range within which the amplitudes exceed some reference value. Compare the frequency spectrum for a narrowband, undamped pulse **(C)** with the frequency spectrum for a broadband, damped pulse **(D).**

Matching Layers

Because the transducer element is a solid (having high density and sound speed), it has an impedance that is about 20 times that of tissues. Without compensation, this factor would cause about 80% of the emitted intensity to be reflected at the skin boundary. Thus most of the sound energy would not enter the body. A returning echo also would have about 80% of its intensity reflected, so that only a small portion would enter the transducer. Therefore because only about 20% of the intensity

enters and only about 20% of the echo intensity exits the body, the received echo intensity for a perfect (100%) reflector would be only 4% (0.2 × 1.00 × 0.2). To solve this problem, a **matching layer** commonly is placed on the transducer face (Figure 3-3, *E*). This material has impedance of some intermediate value between those of the transducer element and the tissue. The material reduces the reflection of ultrasound at the transducer element surface, thereby improving sound transmission across it. This is analogous to the coating on eyeglasses or camera lenses that reduces light reflection at the air-glass boundary. Many frequencies (the bandwidth) and wavelengths are present in short ultrasound pulses. Thus multiple matching layers improve sound transmission across the element-tissue boundary better than does a single layer. Typically, two layers are used, although in some cases, one or three layers are used. The lower impedance of piezocomposite elements assists in the impedance-matching process, allowing more of the ultrasound energy to exit the front of the element into the patient rather than being lost as heat in the damping material.

ADVANCED CONCEPTS

For continuous wave ultrasound, a single matching layer of quarter-wave thickness and impedance that is the geometric mean of the two impedances at the boundary provides the best match at the boundary. The geometric mean is the square root of the product of the two impedances. Because ultrasound pulses are characterized by a bandwidth rather than a single frequency, multiple layers (usually two for practical purposes) of varying impedance values and thicknesses match the impedances better than a single matching layer would. Even so, the matching layers still act as a bandpass filter, limiting the bandwidth of the pulses transmitted from the elements to the tissues.

Under development is a new class of transducer elements called capacitive microfabricated ultrasonic transducers or cMUTs. These elements are composed of thousands of microscopic silicon drums that include thin suspended membranes. Pulse generation is accomplished by applying a voltage to the drum. The voltage creates an electrostatic force on the membrane, causing it to vibrate and emit a pulse of ultrasound. Conversely, echoes arriving at the element cause the membrane to vibrate, producing the corresponding voltage that represents the echo in the electronics. One major advantage of cMUTs is that they have an impedance much lower than ceramic elements, easing the impedance-matching challenge and enabling broader bandwidth (exceeding 100%) pulses to be transmitted into tissues. Another advantage is that with semiconductor-based technology, the elements and electronics are combined in silicon. Thus more of the electronic components can be housed in the probe assembly, allowing more of the signal processing to be accomplished before sending of the electric signals through the probe cable to the instrument. A third advantage is that less energy is lost in the damping material because the pulse is coupled better to the tissues. This makes the transducer more efficient. Finally, the cMUT approach may allow flexible transducers to be fabricated that will conform to the surface of the patient more effectively and will allow a broader area of acoustic

coupling to the tissues. In summary, cMUTs will enable more efficient production and coupling of broader-band pulses to the patient.

Coupling Medium

Because of its very low impedance, even a very thin layer of air between the transducer and the skin surface reflects virtually all the sound, preventing any penetration into the tissue. For this reason, a coupling medium, usually an aqueous gel (Figure 3-8), is applied to the skin before transducer contact. This eliminates the air layer and facilitates sound passage into and out of the tissue. Thus the combination of matching layers with the coupling medium enables the efficient passage of ultrasound into the body and return of echoes from the body into the transducer.

Matching layers and coupling media facilitate the passage of the ultrasound across the transducer-skin boundary.

Invasive Transducers

Some transducers are designed to enter the body (Figure 3-9) via the vagina, rectum, esophagus, or a blood vessel (catheter-mounted type). These approaches allow the transducer to be placed closer to the anatomy of interest, thus avoiding intervening tissues (e.g., lung or

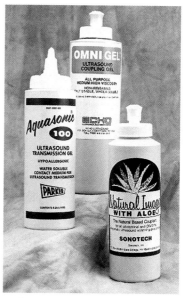

■ **FIGURE 3-8** Coupling gel improves sound transmission into and out of the patient by eliminating air reflection.

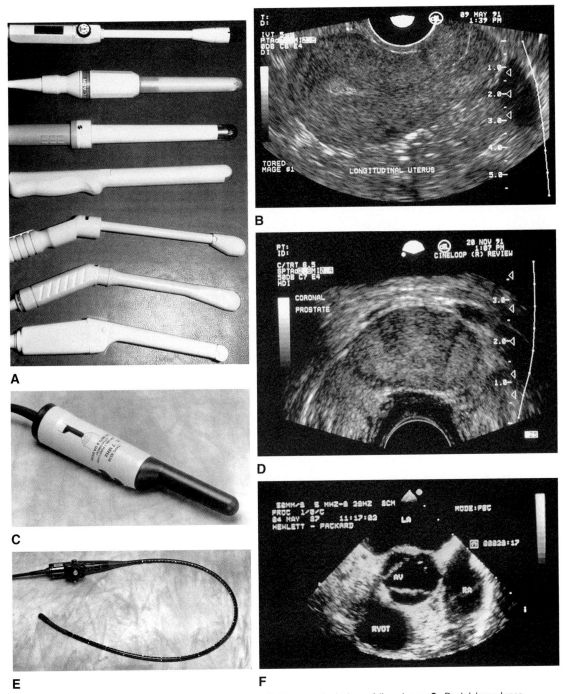

■ **FIGURE 3-9** **A,** Endovaginal transducers. **B,** Transvaginal view of the uterus. **C,** Rectal transducer. **D,** Transrectal view of the prostate. **E,** Transesophageal probe for echocardiography. **F,** Transesophageal view of the adult heart.

Continued.

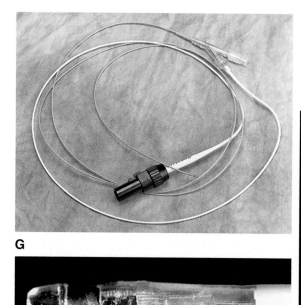

G

H

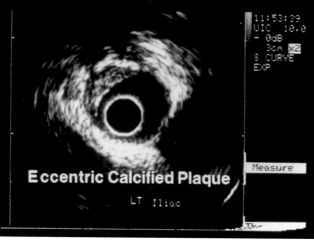

I

■ **FIGURE 3-9, cont'd** **G,** Catheter-mounted transducer for viewing the interior of a blood vessel. **H,** Close-up view of a catheter-mounted transducer. **I,** Interior view of a blood vessel with plaque.

gassy bowel) and reducing the sound transmission path length. This reduction in path length, yielding lower attenuation, allows higher frequencies to be used, with improved resolution.

BEAMS AND FOCUSING

A continuous wave ultrasound **beam** is filled with ultrasound similarly to a flashlight beam being filled with light. A pulsed beam is not. What is meant by "the beam," then, in the case of pulsed ultrasound? The beam is a description of the width of a pulse as it travels away from the transducer. Generally, the width in the scan plane is not the same as the width perpendicular to the scan plane. The width in the scan plane determines the **lateral resolution,** whereas the width perpendicular to the scan plane determines the extent of the section thickness artifact.

A single-element disk transducer operating in continuous wave mode provides a simple approximation to beams produced by sonographic transducers. The transducer produces a **sound beam** with a width that varies according to the distance from the transducer face, as shown in Figure 3-10.[10] The intensity is not uniform throughout the beam, but the beam shown includes nearly all the power in the beam. Sometimes, significant

intensity travels out in some directions not included in this beam. These additional beams are called **side lobes.** They are a source of artifacts.

Near and Far Zones

The region extending from the element out to a distance of one near-zone length is called the **near zone,** near field, or **Fresnel zone.** Near-zone length (*NZL;* also called near-field length) is determined by the size and operating frequency of the element. The near-zone length increases with increasing frequency or element size, which is also called **aperture** (a_p).

An ultrasound beam consists of near and far zones.

If aperture increases, near-zone length increases.

If frequency increases, near-zone length increases.

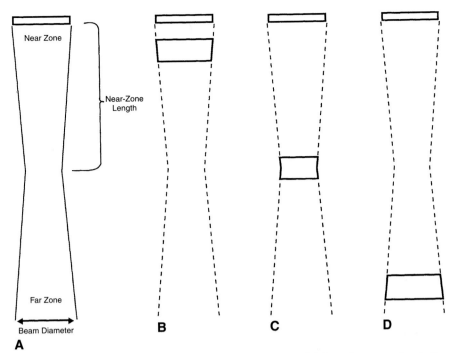

■ **FIGURE 3-10** **A,** Beam width for a single-element unfocused disk transducer operating in the continuous wave mode. The near zone is the region between the disk and the minimum beam width. The far zone is the region beyond the minimum beam width. Intensity varies within the beam, with intensity variations being greatest in the near zone. This beam approximates the changing pulse diameter as an ultrasound pulse travels away from a transducer. **B,** An ultrasound pulse shortly after leaving the transducer. **C,** Later, the ultrasound pulse is located at the end of the near-zone length, where its width is at a minimum. **D,** Still later, the pulse is in the far zone, where its width is increasing as it travels.

Table 3-2 lists near-zone lengths for various disk element frequencies and diameters. The region that lies beyond a distance of one near-zone length is called the **far zone,** far field, or **Fraunhofer zone.** The beam width increases with increasing distance from the transducer in the far zone.

TABLE 3-2 Near-Zone Length (NZL) for Unfocused Elements

Frequency (MHz)	Width (mm)	NZL (cm)
2.0	19	12
3.5	13	10
3.5	19	20
5.0	6	3
5.0	10	8
5.0	13	14
7.5	6	4
10.0	6	6

Aperture is the size of a source of ultrasound (single element or group of elements).

What is somewhat surprising but true is that even for this flat, unfocused transducer element, there is some beam narrowing. This narrowing sometimes is called **natural focus.** Modern diagnostic transducer **arrays** contain rectangular elements. Beams from rectangular elements are similar but not identical to those from disk elements.

Example 3-1

For a 10-mm, 5-MHz disk transducer, what are the beam widths at the near-zone length and at 2 times the near-zone length?

At the end of the near zone, the beam width is approximately equal to one half the width of the transducer element, or 5 mm. At double the near-zone length, the beam diameter is approximately equal to the diameter of the transducer element, or 10 mm.

ADVANCED CONCEPTS

The formation of a beam from an aperture of some size and shape is explained by the Huygens principle and the concept of diffraction. Diffraction is the deviation of the direction of a wave that is *not* attributable to reflection, scattering, or refraction. Diffraction occurs when a wave passes an obstacle or a small (similar to the wavelength) aperture. The Huygens principle states that all points on a wave front or at a source can be considered as point sources for the production of spherical secondary wavelets. As these wavelets propagate, the wave front location and orientation at later times can be constructed by the summation of these wavelets. This principle can be applied to the surface of a transducer to determine the beam profile of the wave that emanates from that surface.

The near-zone length is given by

$$NZL = \frac{(a_p)^2}{4\lambda} = \frac{(a_p)^2 f}{4c}$$

where a_p is the disk aperture, i.e., diameter, and c is the propagation speed.

The beam width (w_b) at any location depends on wavelength (λ), aperture (a_p), and distance from the transducer (d).

In the approximation of Figure 3-10, at the end of the near zone, the beam width is equal to one half the transducer width (Figure 3-11). At a distance of 2 times the near-zone length, the beam width is equal to the transducer diameter. Beyond this distance, the beam width increases in proportion to the distance. As a pulse travels through the near zone, its width decreases; as it travels through the far zone, its width increases. In the near zone,

$$w_b = a_p - \frac{2\lambda d}{a_p} = a_p - \frac{2cd}{f a_p}$$

where a_p is the diameter for a circular aperture. For a rectangular aperture the expression is more complicated. In the far zone,

$$w_b = \frac{2(\lambda \times d)}{a_p} = \frac{2cd}{f \times a_p}$$

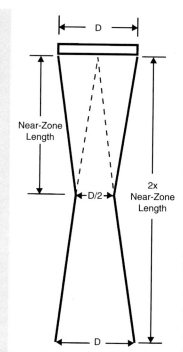

■ **FIGURE 3-11** Sound beam from a disk transducer. The beam width narrows to half the disk diameter (*D*) at the near-zone length and then widens to the disk diameter at twice the near-zone length.

The effects of frequency and aperture on near-zone length are shown in Figures 3-12 and 3-13, respectively. An increase in frequency or in aperture increases the near-zone length. At a sufficient distance from the transducer, increasing the frequency or the transducer size can *decrease* the beam diameter, as shown in the figures.

The beam in Figure 3-10, *A*, is for continuous wave mode, but it can be used to describe pulses in the rest of the figure. The beam for pulses is similar to, but not exactly the same as, that for continuous sound.

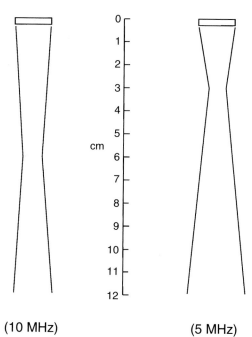

(10 MHz)   (5 MHz)

■ **FIGURE 3-12** Beams for disk transducers having a diameter of 6 mm at two frequencies. Higher frequencies produce smaller beam diameters (at a distance greater than 4 cm in this case) and longer near-zone lengths.

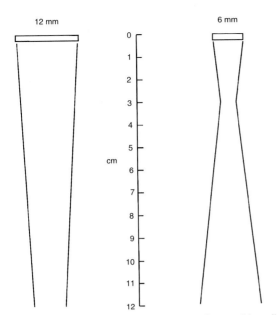

FIGURE 3-13 Beams for 5-MHz disk transducers of two diameters. The larger transducer *(left)* produces the longer near-zone length. A smaller transducer *(right)* can produce a larger-diameter beam in the far zone. In this example, the beam diameters are equal at a distance of 8 cm.

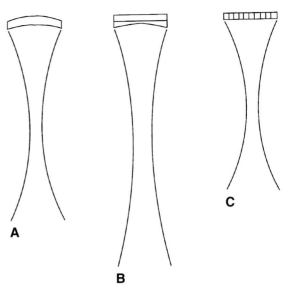

FIGURE 3-14 Sound focusing by a curved transducer element **(A)**, a lens **(B)**, or a phased array **(C)**. Lenses focus because the propagation speed through them is higher than that through tissues. Refraction at the surface of the lens forms the beam in such a way that a focal region occurs. The operation of phased arrays is described later in this chapter.

Focusing

To improve resolution, diagnostic transducers are focused. Focusing the sound in a manner similar to that used to focus light reduces beam width. Sound may be focused (Figure 3-14) by using curved (rather than flat) transducer elements, a **lens,** or by phasing. Focusing moves the end of the near zone toward the transducer and narrows the beam. Beam width is decreased in the **focal region** and in the area between it and the transducer, but it is *widened* in the region beyond (Figure 3-15). **Focal length** *(fl)* is the distance from the transducer to the center of the focal region. Focusing can be accomplished only in the near-zone of a transducer. **Focal zone** length (called depth of field in photography) is the distance between equal beam widths that are some multiple (e.g., ×2) of the minimum value (at the **focus**).

Focusing can be achieved only in the near zone of a beam.

As the element or lens is increasingly curved (or phase-delay curvature in a **phased array** is increased), the focus moves closer to the transducer and becomes "tighter" (i.e., the beam width at the focus decreases). The limit to which a beam can be narrowed depends on the wavelength, aperture, and focal length.

For a rectangular aperture, the minimum beam width (at the focus)—that is, the focal beam diameter (*d*ₜ)—can be obtained by multiplying twice the wavelength by the **f number** *(F),* which is the focal length divided by the aperture.

$$d_f = 2 \times \lambda \times F = \frac{2(\lambda \times fl)}{a_p}$$

As the aperture is increased, the focus narrows, improving the resolution. Also, as frequency is increased, wavelength decreases, again narrowing the focus and improving resolution. Table 3-3 shows f number ranges in use. The best practical focus is with an f number of 2, yielding $d_f = 4\lambda$. Thus the best lateral resolution is about 4 times the best **axial resolution** (which is wavelength for a two-cycle pulse).

TABLE 3-3	f-Number Ranges
Focus	**f Number**
Weak	>6
Moderate	2-6
Strong	<2

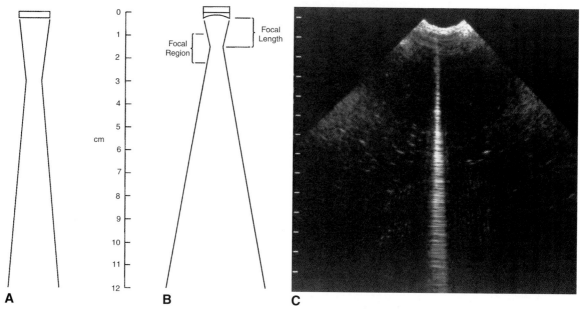

■ FIGURE 3-15   Beam diameter for a 6-mm, 5-MHz transducer without **(A)** and with **(B)** focusing. Focusing reduces the minimum beam width compared with that produced without focusing. However, well beyond the focal region, the width of the focused beam is *greater* than that of the unfocused beam. **C,** A focused beam. This is an ultrasound image of a beam profile test object containing a thin vertical scattering layer down the center. Scanning this object generates a picture of the beam (the pulse width at all depths). In this case the focus occurs at a depth of about 4 cm (this image has a total depth of 15 cm). Depth markers (in 1-cm increments) are indicated on the left edge of the figure.

AUTOMATIC SCANNING

Not only must the transducer emit ultrasound pulses and receive echoes, but also it is responsible for sending the pulses through the many paths required to generate a cross-sectional image. This sometimes is called scanning, sweeping, or steering the beam through the tissue cross section to be imaged. Scanning is done rapidly and automatically so that many images, called frames, can be acquired and presented in rapid sequence within a second of time. Presenting images in a rapid sequential format, like a movie, is called real-time sonography.

Automatic scanning of a sound beam is performed electronically, providing a means for sweeping the sound beam through the tissues rapidly and repeatedly.

Electronic scanning is performed with arrays. Transducer arrays are transducer assemblies with several transducer elements. The elements are rectangular and are arranged in a straight line (**linear array;** Figure 3-3, *E*) or curved line (**convex array;** Figure 3-16). **Linear** is the adjectival form of line. *Convex* means bowed out.

Linear Array

Arrays are operated in two ways, called sequencing and phasing. A more complete name for what commonly is called a linear array is **linear sequenced array.** This array contains a straight line of rectangular elements, each about a wavelength wide, and is operated by

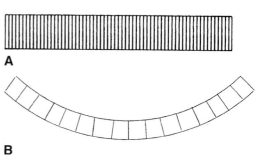

■ FIGURE 3-16   **A,** Front view of a linear array with 64 rectangular elements. **B,** Side view of a convex array with 16 elements.

applying voltage pulses to groups of elements in succession (Figure 3-17). Each group of elements acts like a larger transducer element, providing a large enough aperture to confine the ultrasound to a fine enough beam for satisfactory resolution. As different groups are energized, the origin of the sound beam moves across the face of the transducer assembly from one end to the other, thus producing the same effect as would manual linear scanning with a single element the size (aperture) of the energized groups. Such electronic scanning, however, can be done rapidly and consistently without involving moving parts or a coupling liquid. If this electronic scanning is repeated rapidly enough, real-time presentation (many images per second) of visual information can result. Real-time presentation requires scanning the beam across the transducer assembly several

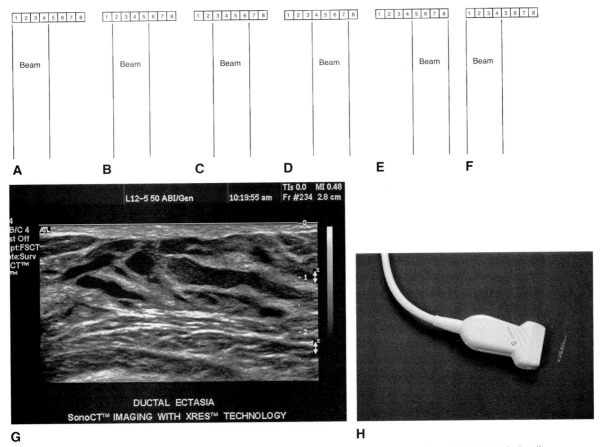

■ **FIGURE 3-17** A linear sequenced array (side view). A voltage pulse is applied simultaneously to all elements in a small group: first to elements 1 to 4 (for example) as a group **(A)**, then to elements 2 to 5 **(B)**, and so on across the transducer assembly **(C** to **E)**. The process then is repeated **(F). G,** An image generated from a linear array. **H,** A linear array transducer.

times per second. The aperture is the size of the group of elements energized to produce one pulse. The width of the entire image is approximately equal to the length of the array (Figure 3-18). The linear image consists of parallel scan lines produced by pulses originating at different points across the surface of the array but all traveling in the same direction (parallel). This produces a rectangular image, as shown in Figures 3-17, G, and 3-18.

A linear array produces rectangular images composed of many vertical, parallel scan lines.

The pulsing sequence described in Figure 3-17 (eight elements, pulsed in groups of four) yields only five scan lines to make up the image. This would certainly be a poor-quality image. A 128-element array pulsed in groups of four would yield a 125-line display. Pulsing these elements individually (rather than in groups of four) would yield a 128-line display, but the small aperture (a single element less than 1 mm in size) would cause excessive beam spreading and poor resolution. If

the pulsing sequence alternated groups of three and four elements (e.g., elements 1 to 3, then 1 to 4, then 2 to 4, 2 to 5, 3 to 5, 3 to 6, 4 to 6, 4 to 7, and on through the array), the number of scan lines would be doubled, to 250, thereby improving the quality of the image.

Convex Array

A convex array, also called a curved array, is constructed as a curved line of elements rather than a straight one. The operation of a convex array is identical to that of the linear sequenced array (sequencing groups of elements from one end of the array to the other), but because of the curved construction, the pulses travel out in different directions, producing a sector-type image (Figure 3-19). A complete name for this transducer is convex sequenced array.

The convex array operates similarly to the linear array but produces a sector image.

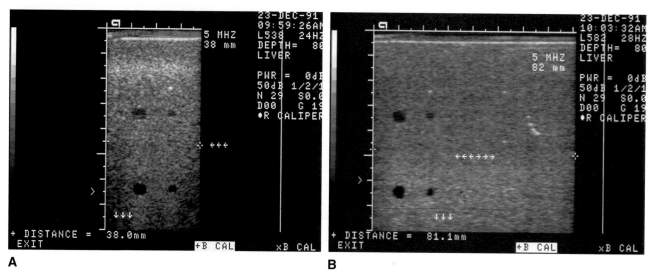

■ **FIGURE 3-18**   The linear image width is determined by the length of the linear array used. **A,** In this example, a 5-MHz, 38-mm linear array (L538) produces an image that is 38 mm wide. **B,** A 5-MHz, 82-mm linear array (L582) produces an image that is 81 mm wide.

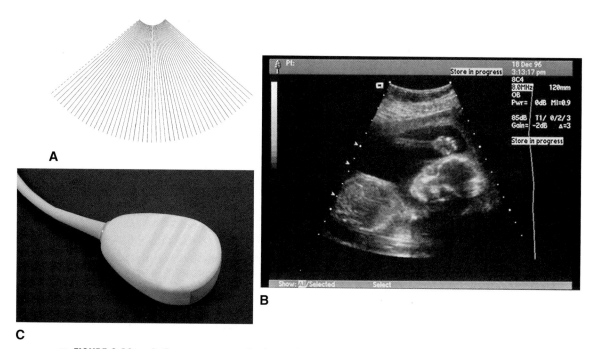

■ **FIGURE 3-19**   **A,** Convex arrays send pulses out in different directions from different points across the curved array surface. **B,** A sector-type image with a curved top is produced by a convex array. **C,** A convex array transducer.

Phased Array

A **linear phased array** (commonly called a phased array) contains a compact line of elements, each about one quarter of a wavelength wide. The linear phased array is operated by applying voltage pulses to most or all elements (not a small group) in the assembly, but with small (less than 1 μs) time differences (called phasing) between them, so that the resulting sound pulse is sent out in a specific path direction, as shown in Figure 3-20. If the same time delays were used each time the process was repeated, the subsequent pulses would travel out in the same direction repeatedly. However, the time delays automatically are changed slightly with each successive repetition so that subsequent pulses travel out in slightly different directions, and the beam direction continually changes (Figure 3-21). This process results in sweeping of the beam, with beam

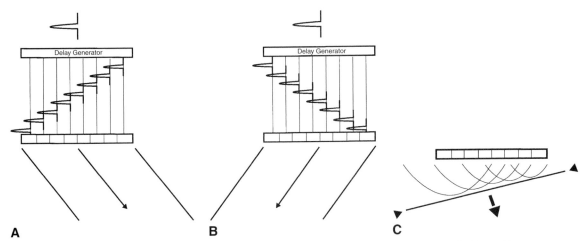

■ **FIGURE 3-20** A linear phased array *(side view)*. **A,** When voltage pulses are applied in rapid progression from left to right, one ultrasound pulse is produced that is directed to the right. **B,** Similarly, when voltage pulses are applied in rapid progression from right to left, one ultrasound pulse is produced that is directed to the left. **C,** The delays in **A** produce a pulse the combined pressure wavefront of which *(arrowheads)* is angled from lower left to upper right. A wave always travels perpendicular to its wavefront, as indicated by the arrow.

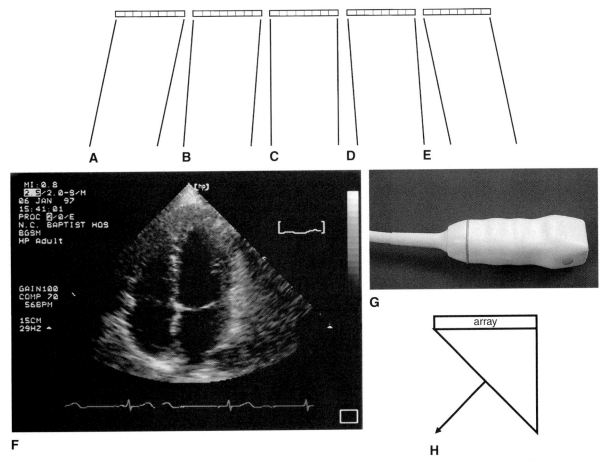

■ **FIGURE 3-21** A five-pulse sequence in which each pulse travels out in a different direction. **A,** The rapid voltage-application progression is from right to left across the array. **B,** A right-to-left progression with slightly shorter time delays. **C,** No delays (all elements energize simultaneously). **D,** A left-to-right progression. **E,** A left-to-right progression with slightly longer delays. **F,** A cardiac sector image produced by a phased array. The image comes to a point at the top. **G,** A phased array transducer. **H,** Diagram for calculation of phase delay.

direction changing with each pulse, to produce a sector image (Figure 3-21, *F*). The phased array sometimes is called an electronic sector transducer.

A phased array scans the beam in sector format with short time delays.

Phasing is applied to some linear and convex arrays to steer the beam from each element group in several directions by sending out several pulses from each group with different phasing. Thus echoes can be generated from a specific anatomic location with several viewing angles. The echo information from these multiple views is processed to present an improved-quality image. This is a form of electronic "compounding" of the image.

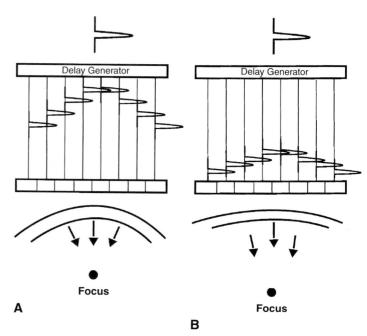

■ **FIGURE 3-22** By putting curvature in the phase delay pattern, a pulse is focused. **A,** Greater curvature places the focus closer to the transducer. **B,** Less curvature moves the focus deeper.

ADVANCED CONCEPTS

As an example of the required delay to steer a beam (and scan line) in a specific direction, let us consider a 40-mm aperture containing 128 elements. We will calculate the case for a beam directed out at a 45-degree angle to the left of the transducer axis. The tangent of 45 degrees is 1; that is, the opposite and adjacent are equal (Figure 3-21, *H*). The hypotenuse is the wave front. The arrow shows the direction of travel that is always perpendicular to the orientation of the wave front.

The length of the adjacent side of the triangle (also the length of the array aperture) is 40 mm. Thus the length of the opposite side is also 40 mm. Thus the time required for that portion of the pulse to travel from the right-most element to a depth of 40 mm is $t = 40 \div 1.54 = 26$ μs. At this instant in time the left-most element has emitted its contribution to the pulse. Thus the total delay from right to left in energizing the elements is 26 μs. Because the transducer has 128 elements in the 40-mm array, it has a 0.2-μs element-to-element delay ($26 \div 128$) to achieve a pulse directed at 45 degrees off the array axis.

Electronic Focus

In addition to steering the beam by phasing, the phased array can focus the beam by phasing (Figure 3-22). An increase in the curved delay pattern (greater time delays between elements) moves the focus closer to the transducer, whereas a decrease (shorter delays) in curvature moves it deeper. Thus phasing provides electronic control of the location of the focus (Figure 3-23). Multiple foci can be used to achieve, in effect, a long focus (Figure 3-24). One pulse can be focused at only one depth. Therefore multiple foci require multiple

pulses (per scan line), each focused at a different depth. Echoes from the focal region of each pulse are displayed and the rest are discarded. The resulting image is a montage of the focal regions of the different pulses. However, using multiple pulses per scan line takes more time, and the frame rate is reduced, thereby degrading temporal resolution. Thus temporal resolution is sacrificed for an improvement in detail resolution.

Electronic focusing is accomplished with a curved pattern of phased delays. An increase or decrease in the curvature of the delay pattern moves the focus shallower or deeper, respectively.

Phasing also is applied to linear arrays to provide electronic focal control (Figure 3-25). The term **phased linear array** indicates that phased focus control is applied to a linear sequenced array. Rather than each group of elements being pulsed simultaneously, as in Figure 3-17, the outer elements are pulsed slightly ahead of the inner ones (Figure 3-25, *C*). This produces a curved pulse that is focused at a depth determined by the delay between the firing of the outer and inner elements. These pulses are focused, but not steered, by phasing. They still travel straight down to produce parallel vertical scan lines and a rectangular display. In a similar way, phased focusing is applied to convex arrays.

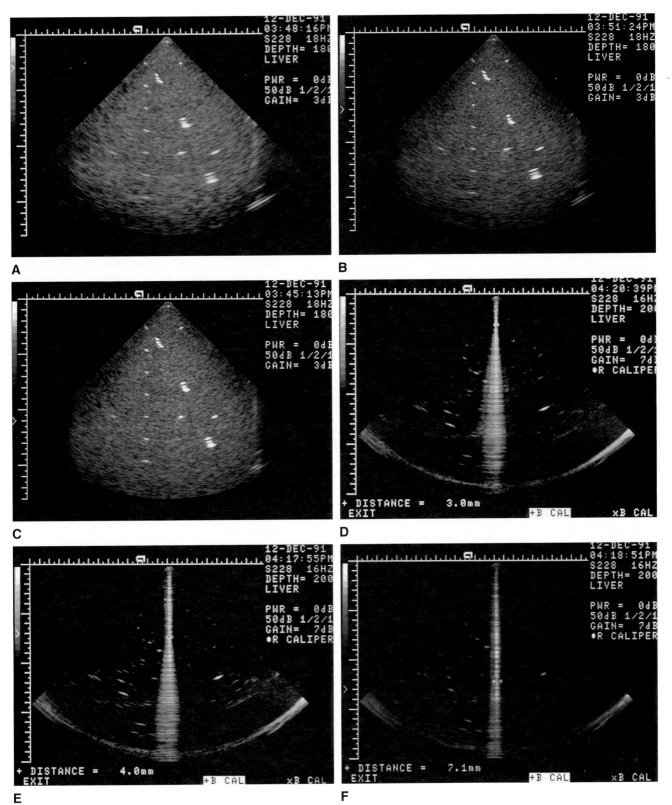

■ **FIGURE 3-23** Phase control of focal length. Focus located at 3 cm **(A)**, 7 cm **(B)**, and 11 cm **(C)**. The arrowhead on the left shows the location of the focus. Beam profiles show foci located at 3 cm **(D)**, 7 cm **(E)**, and 13 cm **(F)**.

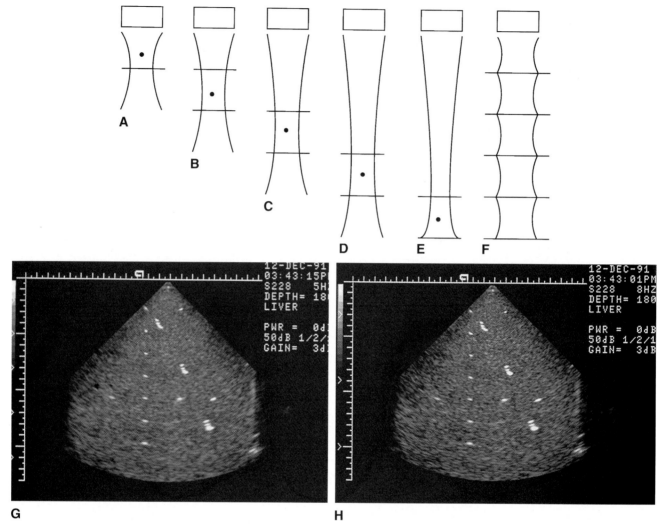

■ **FIGURE 3-24**   Multiple-transmit focus uses a pulse for each focus. In this example, five pulses focused at different depths (**A** to **E**) are needed to produce a montage image (**F**) with an effectively long focus (narrow beam). Only the echoes from the focal region of each pulse are used to produce the image. The rest are discarded. **G,** Five foci at 2, 5, 8, 12, and 16 cm. **H,** Triple foci at 3, 9, and 15 cm. Note the reduced frame rates (5 and 8 Hz, compared with 18 and 16 Hz in Figure 3-23).

Variable Aperture

Recall that the aperture, focal length, and wavelength determine the beam width at the focus. To maintain the same beam width at the focus for increasing focal lengths, the aperture must be increased also. This means that in fact not all elements of a phased array are used to generate all pulses. Smaller groups are used for short focal lengths, whereas larger groups are used for foci of increasing depth (Figure 3-26).

Section Thickness Focus

A single line of elements can focus or steer electronically only *in* the scan plane. Focus (fixed at one depth) can be achieved in the third dimension with a lens or with curved elements. With at least three rows of elements—

that is, a two-dimensional array—phasing can be applied to focus the third dimension electronically. Electronic focusing in the third dimension eliminates the need for a lens or curved elements. Two-dimensional arrays as large as 3000 elements are commercially available. This dimension, perpendicular to the scan plane, is called the slice thickness or section thickness dimension. Beam width in this dimension is important regarding section thickness artifacts, also called partial-volume artifacts. This third dimension and its associated section thickness are shown in Figures 1-7, *A*, and 1-9, *A*.

Grating Lobes

In addition to side lobes, which single-element transducers have, arrays have **grating lobes,** which are additional beams resulting from their multielement structure.

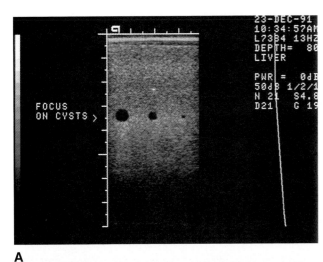

A

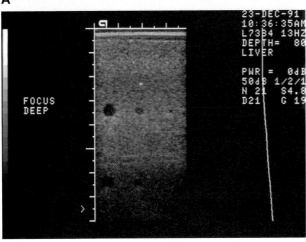

B

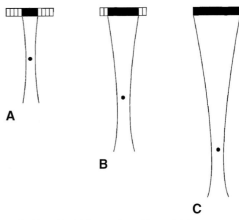

■ FIGURE 3-26   *Variable aperture. To maintain comparable focal beam width at different depths, more array elements are used (increasing the aperture) as the focus is moved deeper.* **A,** *Four elements.* **B,** *Eight elements.* **C,** *Twelve elements.*

Grating lobes can be reduced by driving the elements in a group nonuniformly (i.e., with different voltage amplitudes). Outer elements are driven at lower amplitudes than the inner elements. The echo-reception sensitivity also is less for the outer elements. This is called **apodization.** Because optimum apodization changes continually with focusing and steering, it is called dynamic apodization. The downside of apodization is that there is some broadening of the main beam with degradation of resolution. Subdicing of each element into a group of smaller crystals is also done to weaken grating lobes and to reduce interelement interaction for improved electronic focusing. The subelements are tied together electrically so that they function as one element.

Vector Array

Phasing can be applied to each element group in a linear sequenced array to steer pulses in various directions, in addition to initiating them at various starting points across the array. **Vector array** is the name applied to this type of transducer (Figure 3-27). This transducer converts the image format for a linear array from rectangular to **sector.** Scan lines originate from different points across the top of the display *and* travel out in different directions. The image format is similar to that for the convex array except that the contact surface (footprint) is smaller and the top of the display is flat. More elements can be used at a time, allowing for larger apertures than can be achieved with convex arrays. Phasing also can be applied to linear sequenced arrays in such a way that each pulse travels in the *same* direction (but not straight down). This converts a rectangular display to a parallelogram-shaped display useful in color Doppler imaging (Figure 3-27, *D,* and Color Plate 2).

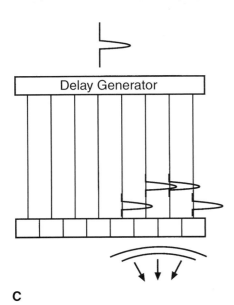

C

■ FIGURE 3-25   **A,** *A phased linear array with the focus located at 3.5 cm produces a clear image of the small cystic object.* **B,** *When the focus is located at 7.5 cm (less phase delay curvature), a loss of image quality results for cystic objects.* **C,** *Phased delays are applied to each element group to focus the pulse.*

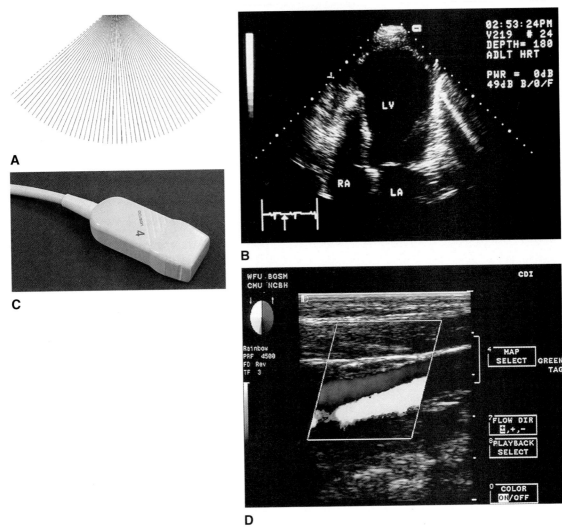

■ **FIGURE 3-27** **A,** A vector array sends pulses out in different directions from different starting points across the flat surface of the array. **B,** A cardiac scan produced by a vector array. **C,** A vector array transducer. **D,** A phased linear array producing a parallelogram-shaped color Doppler display (see Color Plate 2).

The vector array is a combination of linear and phased array operations. It presents a sector display with a nonzero width at the top.

Reception Steering, Focus, and Aperture

When an array is receiving echoes, the electric outputs of the elements can be timed so that the array is sensitive in a particular direction, with a listening focus at a particular depth (Figure 3-28). This reception focus depth may be increased continually as the transmitted pulse travels through the tissues and the echoes arrive from deeper and deeper locations. This continually changing reception focus is called **dynamic focusing.**

Dynamic focusing is similar to the continual change in focusing that occurs with a camcorder when filming a child riding away on a bicycle. The combination of transmission focus (particularly multizone focusing) and dynamic reception focus improves detail resolution over large depth ranges in images. As the focus continually changes during echo reception, the aperture increases to maintain a constant focal width. This is called **dynamic aperture.** The terms used to describe arrays describe their construction and function as shown in Table 3-4. Boxes 3-1 and 3-2 and Tables 3-5 and 3-6 summarize transducer types, terminology, characteristics, and display formats.

With phasing, the reception beam is steered and dynamically focused.

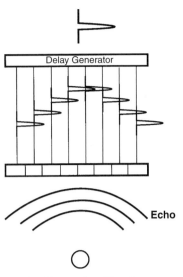

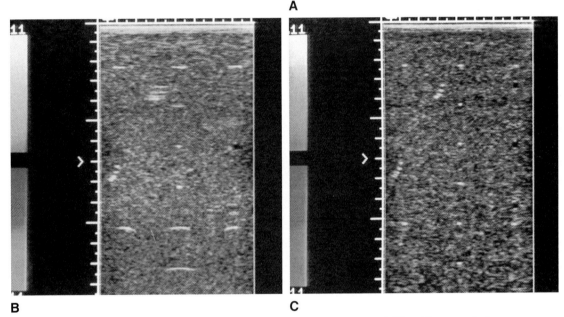

B   **C**

■ **FIGURE 3-28** **A,** A spherically shaped echo arrives at array elements at different times, producing non-coincident voltages in the various channels. If simply combined, a weak, long voltage (with poor resolution and sensitivity) would result. However, with proper delays, the voltages are made to coincide, producing a strong, short (good resolution and sensitivity) voltage. As echoes return from deeper and deeper locations, their curvature is reduced. Thus the delay correction must be reduced as echoes return. This is called dynamic focusing. **B,** Dynamic focus is off. **C,** When the dynamic focus is on, resolution improves.

TABLE 3-4   Terms Used to Describe Arrays

Term	Construction	Scanning	Focusing
Array	√		
Linear	√		
Sequenced		√	
Convex	√		
Phased		√	√

TABLE 3-5   Transducer Characteristics

Type	Beam Scanned by Sequencing	Beam Scanned by Phasing	Beam Focused by Phasing
Linear array	√		√
Convex array	√		√
Phased array		√	√
Vector array	√	√	√

TABLE 3-6   Display Formats

Type	Rectangle or Parallelogram	Sector	Flat Top	Curved Top	Pointed Top
Linear array	√		√		
Convex array		√		√	
Phased array		√			√
Vector array		√	√		

BOX 3-1   Common Transducer Types

Linear array
Convex array
Phased array
Vector array

BOX 3-2   Array Terminology

(Phased) linear (sequenced) array
(Phased) convex (sequenced) array
(Linear) phased array
(Phased and sequenced) (linear) vector array
The words in parentheses are implied in the abbreviated common terminology.

DETAIL RESOLUTION

Imaging resolution has three aspects:

■ Detail
■ Contrast
■ Temporal

Contrast and temporal resolutions relate more directly to instruments. *Detail resolution* (Figure 3-29) relates more directly to transducers and is thus discussed in this section. If two reflectors are not separated sufficiently, they produce overlapping (not distinct) echoes that are not separated on the instrument display. Rather, the echoes merge together and appear as one. Thus the echoes are not resolved. If distinct (separated by a gap) echoes are not generated initially in the anatomy, the reflectors will not be separated on the display. In ultrasound imaging, the two aspects to detail resolution are **axial** and **lateral**. These aspects depend on different characteristics of the ultrasound pulses as they travel through the tissues.

Axial Resolution

Axial resolution is the minimum reflector separation required along the direction of sound travel (along the scan line) to produce separate echoes (Figure 3-30). The important factor in determining axial resolution is the spatial pulse length. Axial resolution is equal to half the spatial pulse length.

$$\text{Axial resolution (mm)} = \frac{\text{spatial pulse length}}{2}$$

Axial resolution is the minimum reflector separation necessary to resolve reflectors along scan lines. Axial resolution (millimeters) equals spatial pulse length (millimeters) divided by 2.

Note that the numeric value for detail resolution *decreases* as frequency increases. Axial resolution is like product pricing or a golf score: smaller is better. The smaller the axial resolution, the finer the detail that can be displayed and the closer two reflectors can be along the sound path and still be seen distinctly, thereby allowing tinier objects to be displayed. To improve axial resolution, spatial pulse length must be reduced. Because spatial pulse length is wavelength multiplied by the number of cycles in the pulse, one or both of these factors must be reduced. Wavelength is reduced by increasing frequency. The number of cycles in each pulse is reduced by transducer damping. Because the number of cycles per pulse has been reduced to a minimum (one to three) by transducer design, the only way the instrument operator can improve axial resolution further is to increase frequency. With an increase in frequency, however, comes a reduction in penetration (imaging depth) because attenuation increases as frequency increases.

Lateral Resolution

Lateral resolution is the minimum reflector separation in the direction perpendicular to the beam direction (that is, across scan lines) that can produce two separate echoes when the beam is scanned across the reflectors (Figure 3-31). Lateral resolution is equal to the beam width in the scan plane.

$$\text{Lateral resolution} = \text{beam width (mm)}$$

Lateral resolution is the minimum reflector separation necessary to resolve reflectors across scan lines. Lateral resolution (millimeters) equals beam width (millimeters).

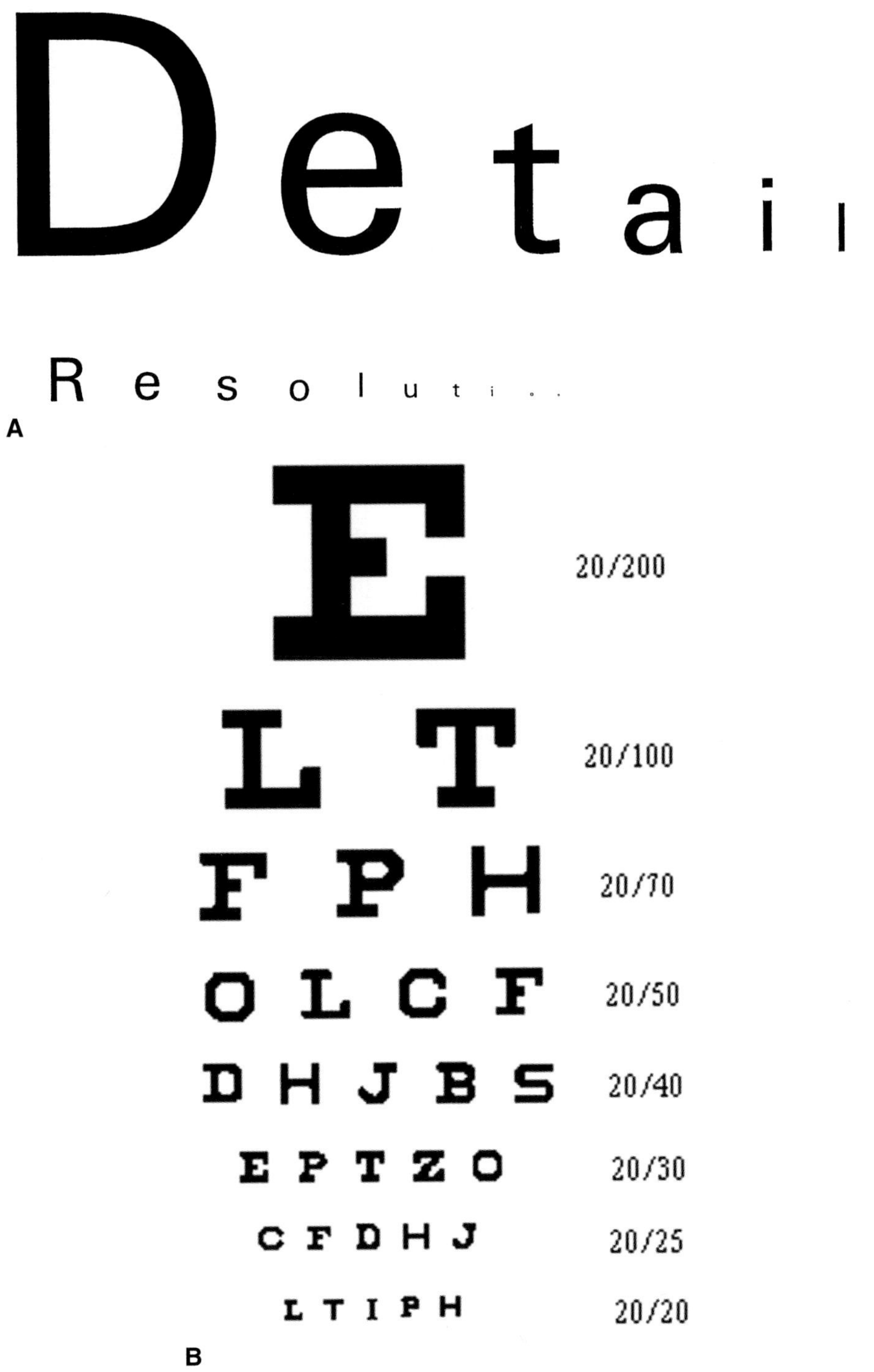

Detail

Resoluti..

A

E 20/200

L T 20/100

F P H 20/70

O L C F 20/50

D H J B S 20/40

E P T Z O 20/30

C F D H J 20/25

L T I P H 20/20

B

■ **FIGURE 3-29**   **A,** Excellent detail resolution is the ability to image fine detail. Smaller is better, meaning that tinier details can be discerned. **B,** Snellen vision testing chart.

As with axial resolution, smaller lateral resolution is better. A smaller value indicates an improvement (finer detail and the ability to image tinier objects). Just as beam width varies with distance from the transducer, so too does lateral resolution. If the lateral separation between two reflectors is greater than the beam diameter, two separate echoes are produced when the beam is scanned across them. Thus the echoes are resolved, or detected, as separate reflectors.

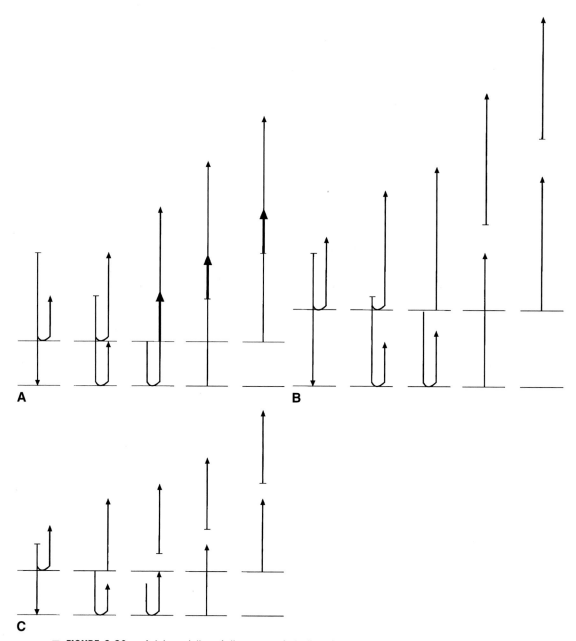

■ **FIGURE 3-30** Axial resolution. Action proceeds in time from left to right in each part of the figure. **A,** The separation of the reflectors is less than half the spatial pulse length, so echo overlap occurs. Separate echoes are not produced. The reflectors are not resolved on the display. **B,** The reflector separation is increased so that it is greater than half the spatial pulse length. Echo overlap does not occur. Separate echoes are produced, and the reflectors are resolved on the display. **C,** The reflector separation is the same as in **A,** but resolution is achieved by shortening the pulse so that separate echoes are produced.

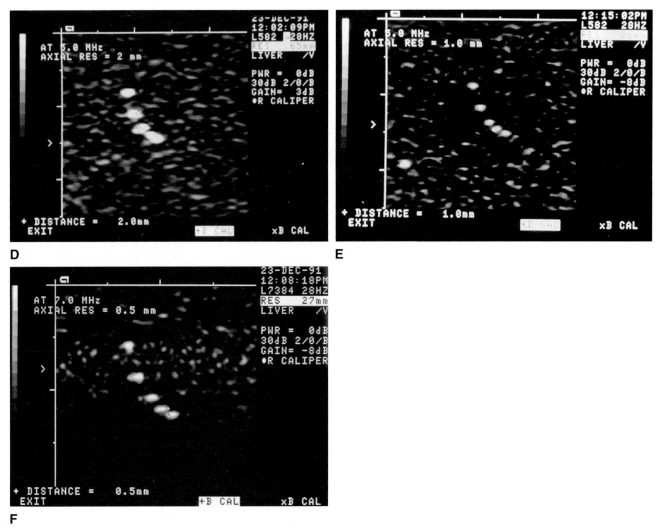

■ **FIGURE 3-30, cont'd** **D** to **F,** Axial resolution improves as frequency increases. **D,** 3.5 MHz, with a resolution of 2.0 mm. **E,** 5.0 MHz, with a resolution of 1.0 mm. **F,** 7.0 MHz, with a resolution of 0.5 mm.

With detail resolution, smaller is better.

If frequency increases, detail resolution improves but penetration decreases.

Lateral resolution is improved by reducing the beam diameter, that is, focusing (Figure 3-32). Figure 3-33 shows a focused beam. The lateral smearing of a thin layer of scatterers indicates the beam width and lateral resolution at various depths. The best resolution is obtained at the focus (Figure 3-34; see also Figure 3-25). Diagnostic ultrasound transducers often have better axial resolution than lateral resolution, although the two may be comparable in the focal region of strongly focused beams. Figure 3-35 shows examples of typical detail resolution.

Section thickness can be considered a third aspect of detail resolution and thus sometimes is called **elevational resolution.** Elevational resolution contributes to section thickness artifact, also called partial-volume artifact. This artifact is a filling in of what should be anechoic structures, such as cysts. This filling in occurs when the section thickness is larger than the size of the structure. Thus echoes from outside the structure are included in the image and the structure appears to be echoic. The thinner the section thickness, the less its negative impact on sonographic images. Focusing in the section-thickness plane reduces section thickness artifacts.

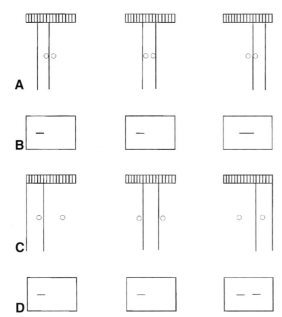

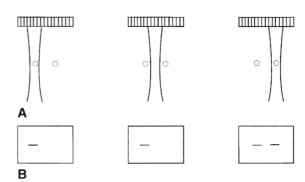

■ **FIGURE 3-32**   **A,** Two separate echoes are generated because the beam is focused and is narrower than the reflector separation. **B,** The two reflectors are resolved on the display. Without focusing in this case, they would not have been resolved.

■ **FIGURE 3-31**   Lateral resolution. Reflector separation (perpendicular to beam direction) is less than beam diameter in **A** and **B,** whereas in **C** and **D,** reflector separation is greater than beam diameter. Action proceeds in time from left to right in each part of the figure. **A,** The beam first encounters the left reflector, then is reflected by both reflectors, and finally is reflected by the right reflector. **B,** This scanning sequence results in continual reflection from one or both reflectors. Separate echoes are not produced, and the reflectors are not resolved. **C,** The beam encounters the left reflector, then fits between both reflectors (yielding no echo), and finally is reflected by the right reflector. **D,** Separate echoes are produced, and the reflectors are resolved on the display.

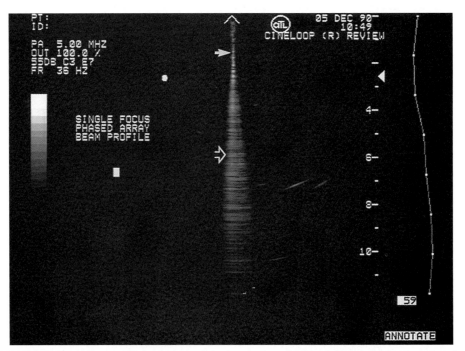

■ **FIGURE 3-33**   Beam width is shown as lateral smearing of a thin vertical scattering layer in a test object. The beam indicates the lateral resolution at each depth. In this example, beam width is about 2 mm at the focus *(closed arrow)* and about 10 mm at a depth of 6 cm *(open arrow),* well beyond the focus.

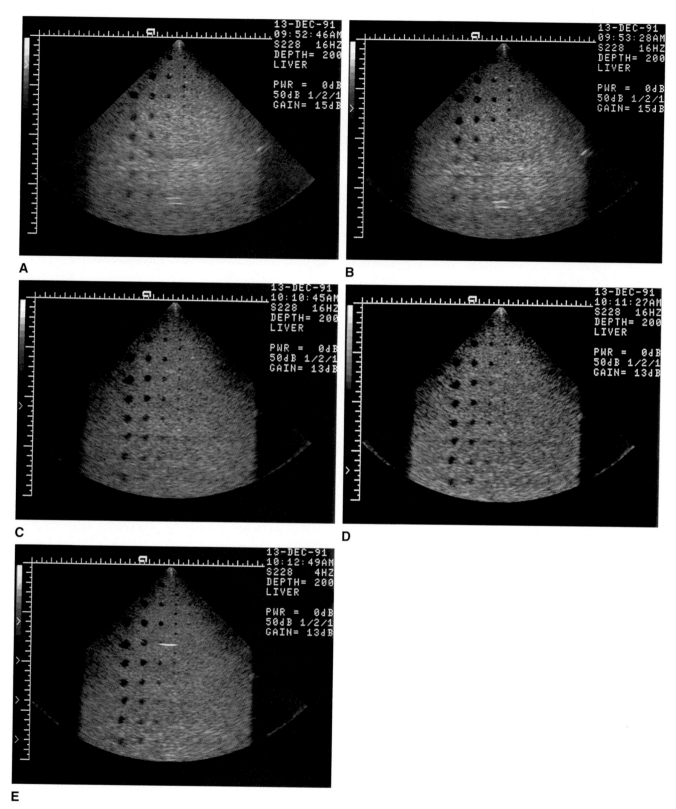

■ **FIGURE 3-34** Imaging of small cysts involves both aspects of detail resolution: axial and lateral. Resolution improves at various depths as the focus is located there. Focus at 3 cm **(A)**, 7 cm **(B)**, 11 cm **(C)**, and 17 cm **(D)**. With multiple foci **(E)**, resolution is improved throughout depth.

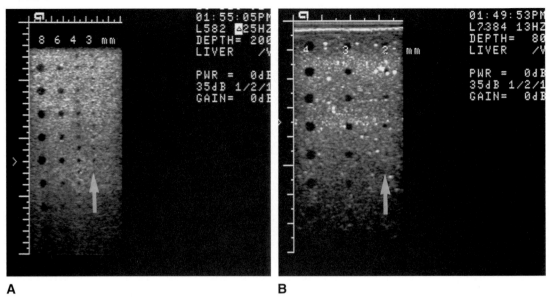

A **B**

■ **FIGURE 3-35** **A,** An image of a resolution penetration phantom that contains circular anechoic regions ("cysts") in tissue-equivalent material. From left to right, the cysts are 8, 6, 4, 3, and 2 mm in diameter and occur every 1 or 2 cm in depth of the image. Close examination reveals that the 3-mm cysts are the smallest that can be resolved. This image was produced using a 3.5-MHz transducer. **B,** The same phantom is imaged with a 7.0-MHz transducer. In this instance the 2-mm cysts can be seen. Note the loss of penetration compared with that in **A** (8 cm versus 20 cm). Detail resolution can be improved by increasing the frequency of the ultrasound beam, but at the expense of decreasing the imaging depth.

TABLE 3-7 Typical Imaging Depth and Axial Resolution (Two-Cycle Pulse) in Tissue

Frequency (MHz)	Imaging Depth (cm)	Axial Resolution (mm)
2.0	30	0.77
3.5	17	0.44
5.0	12	0.31
7.5	8	0.20
10.0	6	0.15
15.0	4	0.10

Useful Frequency Range

To meet resolution and penetration requirements reasonably, the useful frequency range for most diagnostic applications is 2 to 15 MHz. The lower portion of the range is useful when increased depth (e.g., in an obese subject) or high attenuation (e.g., in transcranial studies) is encountered. The higher portion of the frequency range is useful when little penetration is required (e.g., in imaging breast, thyroid, or superficial vessels or in pediatric imaging). In most large patients, 3-5 MHz is a satisfactory frequency, whereas in thin patients and in children, 5 and 7.5 MHz often can be used. If frequencies less than 2 MHz are used, axial resolution is insufficient. If frequencies higher than

15 MHz (less than 15 MHz in deeper applications) are used, the depth is not sufficient. In the case of ophthalmologic, dermatologic, and intravascular imaging (the latter involving use of catheter-mounted transducers), frequencies up to 50 MHz are used because penetration of only a few millimeters is needed. Table 3-7 lists values for typical imaging depths and axial resolution for various frequencies.

REVIEW

The key points presented in this chapter are the following:
- Transducers convert energy from one form to another.
- Ultrasound transducers convert electric energy to ultrasound energy and vice versa.
- Transducers operate on the piezoelectric principle.
- Transducers are operated in pulse-echo mode.
- The operating frequency depends on the element thickness.
- Axial resolution is equal to one half the spatial pulse length.
- Pulsed transducers have damping material to shorten the spatial pulse length for acceptable resolution.
- Transducers produce sound in the form of beams with near and far zones.
- Lateral resolution is equal to beam width.
- Beam width can be reduced by focusing to improve resolution.

- Detail resolution improves with increasing frequency.
- Linear and convex are types of array construction.
- Sequenced, phased, and vector are types of array scanning operations.
- Phasing also enables electronic control of focus.

EXERCISES

1. A transducer converts one form of _____ to another.
2. Ultrasound transducers convert _____ energy into _____ energy and vice versa.
3. Ultrasound transducers operate on the _____ principle.
4. Single-element transducers are in the form of _____
5. The _____ of a transducer element changes when a voltage is applied to its faces.
6. The term *transducer* is used to refer to a transducer _____ or to a transducer _____.
7. A transducer _____ is part of a transducer _____.
8. An electric voltage pulse, when applied to a transducer, produces an ultrasound _____ of a _____ that is equal to that of the voltage pulse.
9. The resonance frequency of an element is determined by its _____
10. Operating frequency _____ as transducer element thickness is increased.
11. Addition of damping material to a transducer reduces the number of _____ in the pulse, thus improving _____ _____. It increases the _____.
12. Damping material reduces the _____ of the transducer and _____ of the diagnostic system.
13. Ultrasound transducers typically generate pulses of _____ or _____ cycles.
14. For a particular transducer element material, if a thickness of 0.4 mm yields an operating frequency of 5 MHz, the thickness required for an operating frequency of 10 MHz is _____ mm.
15. A transducer with which frequency would have the thinnest elements?
    a. 2 MHz
    b. 3 MHz
    c. 5 MHz
    d. 7 MHz
    e. 10 MHz
16. The matching layer on the transducer surface reduces _____ caused by impedance differences.
17. A coupling medium on the skin surface eliminates reflection caused by _____.
18. Damping lengthens the pulse. True or false?

19. Damping increases the efficiency. True or false?
20. The damping layer is in front/back of the element.
21. The matching layer is in front/back of the element.
22. The matching layer has _____ impedance.
23. Elements in linear arrays are in the form of _____.
24. Transducer assemblies are also called
    a. transducers.
    b. probes.
    c. scanheads.
    d. scan converters.
    e. skinheads.
    f. more than one of the above.
25. Operating frequency is also called _____ _____.
26. Mixtures of a piezoelectric ceramic and a non-piezoelectric polymer are called _____.
27. To operate a transducer at more than one frequency requires _____ _____.
28. Is it practical to attempt to operate a 5-MHz transducer with a bandwidth of 1 MHz at 6 MHz?
29. Is it practical to attempt to operate a 5-MHz transducer with a bandwidth of 2.5 at 3 and 7 MHz?
30. A beam is divided into two regions, called the _____ zone and the _____ zone.
31. The dividing point between the two regions referred to in Exercise 30 is at a distance from the transducer equal to the _____ _____ length.
32. Transducer size is also called _____.
33. Beam width depends on _____, element _____, and _____ from the source.
34. Near-zone length increases with increasing source _____ and _____.
35. At a distance of one near-zone length from the transducer, beam width is equal to _____ the transducer width.
36. At a distance of _____ times the near-zone length, beam width is equal to transducer width.
37. In the near zone, beam width _____ as distance from the transducer increases.
38. In the far zone, beam width _____ as distance from the transducer increases.
39. If a 5-MHz transducer with a near-zone length of 10 cm is increased in size, the near-zone length _____.
40. Which transducer element has the longest near zone?
    a. 6 mm, 5 MHz
    b. 6 mm, 7 MHz
    c. 8 mm, 7 MHz
41. A 6-mm, 10-MHz transducer has a near-zone length of 60 mm. If frequency is reduced to 5 MHz, near-zone length is _____ mm.

42. For Exercise 41 (10 MHz), the beam diameters at 60, 120, and 180 mm from the transducer are _____, _____, and _____ mm, respectively.
43. A higher-frequency transducer produces a _____ near-zone length.
44. A smaller transducer produces a _____ near-zone length.
45. A transducer with a near-zone length of 10 cm can be focused at 12 cm. True or false?
46. Which of the following transducer(s) can focus at 6 cm?
    a. 5 MHz, near-zone length of 5 cm
    b. 4 MHz, near-zone length of 6 cm
    c. 4 MHz, near-zone length of 10 cm
    d. b and c
    e. None of the above
47. Doubling the aperture _____ the near-zone length.
48. Doubling the frequency _____ the near-zone length.
49. If transducer diameter is doubled, the near-zone length is _____.
50. Sound may be focused by using a
    a. curved element.
    b. lens.
    c. phased array.
    d. more than one of the above.
51. Focusing reduces the beam diameter at all distances from the transducer. True or false?
52. The distance from a transducer to the location of the narrowest beam width produced by a focused transducer is called the _____.
53. For a wavelength of 0.5 mm and an f number of 4, the focal beam width is _____ mm.
    a. 0.5
    b. 1
    c. 2
    d. 4
    e. 8
54. For a 5-MHz transducer with an aperture of 25 mm and a focal length of 5 cm, the f number is _____ and the focal beam width is _____ mm.
    a. 0.5, 0.3
    b. 2, 1.2
    c. 3, 1.0
    d. 3, 2.0
    e. 5, 3.0
55. Match the following f numbers with the appropriate description of the resulting focus:
    a. f = 1 _____   1. Weak
    b. f = 3 _____   2. Moderate
    c. f = 5 _____   3. Strong
    d. f = 7 _____
    e. f = 9 _____

56. Transducer arrays are transducer assemblies with several transducer _____.
57. Linear arrays scan beams by _____ element groups.
58. Match the following (answers may be used more than once):
    a. A linear sequenced array can _____ the beam.
    b. Without phasing, a linear sequenced array cannot _____ or _____ the beam.
    c. A linear phased array can _____ and _____ the beam.
    d. A phased linear sequenced array can _____, _____, and _____ the beam.
    e. A convex array can _____ the beam.
    f. A phased convex array also can _____ the beam.
    g. A vector array can _____, _____, and _____ the beam.
    1. Scan (slide beam across array surface)
    2. Electronically steer
    3. Electronically focus
59. A phased linear array with a single line of elements can focus in _____ dimension(s).
60. Focusing in section thickness can be accomplished with _____ elements or a _____.
61. Electronic focusing in section thickness requires multiple rows of _____.
62. Match the following (answers may be used more than once):
    a. Linear array _____   1. Voltage pulses are applied in succession to groups of elements across the face of a transducer.
    b. Phased array _____   2. Voltage pulses are applied to most or all elements as a group, but with small time differences.
    c. Convex array _____
63. If the elements of a phased array are pulsed in rapid succession from right to left, the resulting beam is
    a. steered right.
    b. steered left.
    c. focused.
64. If the elements of a phased array are pulsed in rapid succession from outside in, the resulting beam is
    a. steered right.
    b. steered left.
    c. focused.

65. _____ and _____ describe how arrays are constructed.
    a. Linear
    b. Phased
    c. Sequenced
    d. Vector
    e. Convex

66. _____, _____, and _____ describe how arrays are operated.
    a. Linear
    b. Phased
    c. Sequenced
    d. Vector
    e. Convex

67. Shorter time delays between elements fired from outside in results in _____ curvature in the emitted pulse and a _____ focus.
    a. No, weak
    b. Less, shallower
    c. Less, deeper
    d. Greater, shallower
    e. Greater, deeper

68. A rectangular image is a result of linear scanning of the beam. This means that pulses travel in _____ _____ direction from _____ starting points across the transducer face.

69. A sector image is a result of sector steering of the beam. This means that pulses travel in _____ directions from a common _____ at the transducer face.

70. In _____ and _____ arrays, pulses travel out in different directions from different starting points on the transducer face.

71. Axial resolution is the minimum reflector separation required along the direction of the _____ _____ to produce separate _____.

72. Axial resolution depends directly on _____ _____ _____.

73. Smaller axial resolution is better. True or false?

74. If there are three cycles of a 1-mm wavelength in a pulse, the axial resolution is _____ mm.

75. For pulses traveling through soft tissue in which the frequency is 3 MHz and there are four cycles per pulse, the axial resolution is _____ mm.

76. If there are two cycles per pulse, the axial resolution is equal to the _____. At 5 MHz in soft tissue, this is _____ mm.

77. Doubling the frequency causes axial resolution to be _____.

78. Doubling the number of cycles per pulse causes axial resolution to be _____.

79. When studying an obese subject, a higher frequency likely will be required. True or false?

80. If better resolution is desired, a lower frequency will help. True or false?

81. If frequencies less than _____ MHz are used, axial resolution is not sufficient.

82. If frequencies higher than _____ MHz are used, penetration is not sufficient.

83. Increasing the frequency improves resolution because _____ is reduced, thus reducing _____ _____ _____.

84. Increasing the frequency decreases the penetration because _____ is increased.

85. Lateral resolution is the minimum _____ between two reflectors at the same depth such that when a beam is scanned across them, two separate _____ are produced.

86. Lateral resolution is equal to _____ _____ in the scan plane.

87. Lateral resolution does *not* depend on
    a. frequency.
    b. aperture.
    c. phasing.
    d. depth.
    e. f number.
    f. damping.

88. For an aperture of given size, increasing the frequency improves lateral resolution. True or false?

89. Lateral resolution varies with distance from the transducer. True or false?

90. For a given frequency, a smaller aperture always yields improved lateral resolution. True or false?

91. Lateral resolution is determined by (more than one correct answer)
    a. damping.
    b. frequency.
    c. aperture.
    d. number of cycles in the pulse.
    e. distance from the transducer.
    f. focusing.

92. Match the following transducer assembly parts with their functions:
    a. Cable _____   1. Reduces reflection at transducer surface
    b. Damping material _____   2. Converts voltage pulses to sound pulses
    c. Piezoelectric element _____   3. Reduces pulse duration
    d. Matching layer _____   4. Conducts voltage pulses

93. Which of the following improve sound transmission from the transducer element into the tissue (more than one correct answer)?
    a. Matching layer
    b. Doppler effect
    c. Damping material
    d. Coupling medium
    e. Refraction

94. A 5-MHz unfocused transducer with an element thickness of 0.4 mm, an element width of 13 mm, and a near-zone length of 14 cm produces two-cycle pulses. Determine the following:
    a. Operating frequency if thickness is reduced to 0.2 mm: _____ MHz
    b. Axial resolution in the case of (a): _____ mm
    At 5 MHz:
    c. Depth at which lateral resolution is best: _____ cm
    d. Lateral resolution at 14 cm: _____ mm
    e. Lateral resolution at 28 cm: _____ mm
    f. This transducer can be focused at depths less than _____ cm.
95. Lateral resolution is improved by
    a. damping.
    b. pulsing.
    c. focusing.
    d. matching.
    e. absorbing.
96. For an unfocused transducer, the best lateral resolution (minimum beam width) is _____ the transducer width. This value of lateral resolution is found at a distance from the transducer face that is equal to the _____ _____ length.
97. For a focused transducer, the best lateral resolution (minimum beam width) is found in the _____ region.
98. An unfocused 3.5-MHz, 13-mm transducer will yield a minimum beam width (best lateral resolution) of _____ mm.
99. An unfocused 3.5-MHz, 13-mm transducer produces three-cycle pulses. The axial resolution in soft tissue is _____ mm.
100. In Exercises 98 and 99, axial resolution is better than lateral resolution. True or false?
101. Axial resolution is often not as good as lateral resolution in diagnostic ultrasound. True or false?
102. The two resolutions may be comparable in the _____ region of a strongly focused beam.
103. Beam diameter may be reduced in the near zone by focusing. True or false?
104. Beam diameter may be reduced in the far zone by focusing. True or false?
105. Match each transducer characteristic with the sound beam characteristic it determines (answers may be used more than once):
    a. Element thickness: 1. Axial resolution
       _____, _____,   2. Lateral resolution
       and _____   3. Operating
    b. Element width: frequency
       _____

    c. Element shape (flat or curved): _____
    d. Damping: _____
106. The principle on which ultrasound transducers operate is the
    a. Doppler effect.
    b. Acoustooptic effect.
    c. Acoustoelectric effect.
    d. Cause and effect.
    e. Piezoelectric effect.
107. Which of the following is *not* decreased by damping?
    a. Refraction
    b. Pulse duration
    c. Spatial pulse length
    d. Efficiency
    e. Sensitivity
108. Which three things determine beam diameter for a disk transducer?
    a. Pulse duration
    b. Frequency
    c. Aperture
    d. Distance from disk face
    e. Efficiency
109. A two-cycle pulse of 5-MHz ultrasound produces separate echoes from reflectors in soft tissue separated by 1 mm. True or false?
110. The lower and upper limits of the frequency range useful in diagnostic ultrasound are determined by _____ and _____ requirements, respectively.
111. The range of frequencies useful for most applications of diagnostic ultrasound is _____ to _____ MHz.
112. Because diagnostic ultrasound pulses are usually two or three cycles long, axial resolution is usually equal to _____ to _____ wavelengths.
113. What is the axial resolution in Figure 3-36, *A* and *B*?
114. The best lateral resolution in Figure 3-15, *C,* is at what depth?
115. Match the transducer type with the display formats in Figure 3-37.
    a. Linear array _____
    b. Convex array _____
    c. Phased array _____
    d. Vector array _____
    e. Phased linear array _____

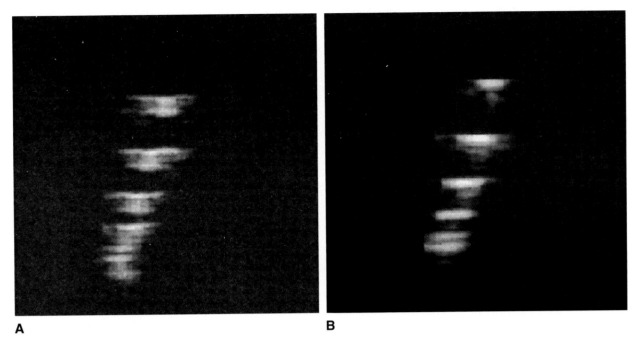

A   B

■ **FIGURE 3-36** Illustration to accompany Exercise 113. **A,** An image of a set of six rods in a test object. They are separated by 5, 4, 3, 2, and 1 mm from top to bottom. This scan was made using a transducer that produces 3.5-MHz ultrasound. The first three rods have been separated, whereas the images of the last three rods have merged. This image also shows small reverberation echoes behind each rod. **B,** The same rods imaged with a 5-MHz transducer. Higher-frequency transducers produce shorter pulse lengths and therefore provide improved axial resolution.

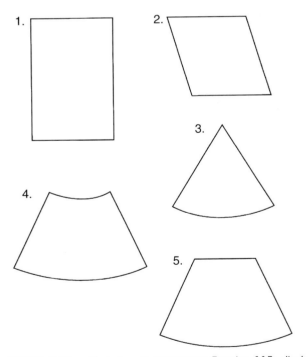

■ **FIGURE 3-37** Illustration to accompany Exercise 115; display formats.

4 Imaging Instruments

LEARNING OBJECTIVES

After reading this chapter, the student should be able to do the following:

- Explain how sonographic instruments work.
- List the primary components of sonographic instruments.
- List the functions of each component.
- Discuss the purposes of coded excitation, gain, compensation, detection, and compression.
- Describe how images are stored electronically.
- Compare preprocessing and postprocessing.
- Compare signal processing and image processing.
- Define contrast resolution and list the factors that influence it.
- Explain how displays work.
- List the common display modes.
- Define temporal resolution and list the factors that influence it.

KEY TERMS

The following terms are introduced in this chapter:

A mode
Amplification
Amplifier
Analog
Analog-to-digital converter
B mode
B scan
Beam former
Bistable
Bit
Cathode-ray tube
Channel
Cine loop
Coded excitation
Compensation
Compression
Contrast resolution
Demodulation
Depth gain compensation

Detection
Digital
Digital-to-analog converter
Display
Dynamic range
Filter
Flat-panel display
Frame
Frame rate
Freeze-frame
Gain
Gray scale
Image memory
Image processor
Lateral gain control
M mode
Panoramic imaging
Persistence

Picture archiving and
communications systems
Pixel
Postprocessing
Preprocessing
Radio frequency
Real-time
Real-time display
Refresh rate
Scan converter
Scan line
Scanning
Signal
Signal processor
Spatial compounding
Temporal resolution
Time gain compensation
Video

n the preceding chapters, the means by which ultrasound is generated and how it interacts with tissues were described. We now consider the instruments that receive echo voltages from the transducer and display them in the form of anatomic images. Diagnostic ultrasound systems are pulse-echo instruments. They determine echo strengths and locations of echo-generation sites. The directions and arrival times of echoes returning from the tissues determine the locations of echo generation sites. This chapter describes how the instrument drives the transducer and what it does with the returning echoes.

Sonographic systems (Figure 4-1) produce visual displays from the echo voltages received from the transducer. Figure 4-1, *A*, presents a diagram of the organization of a pulse-echo sonographic imaging system and examples of operational controls. The instrument is composed of a **beam former**, a **signal processor**, an **image processor**, and a **display**.

BEAM FORMER

The beam former is where the action originates. The beam former is diagrammed in Figure 4-2. It consists of a pulser, pulse delays, transmit/receive (T/R) switch, amplifiers, analog-to-digital converters, echo delays, and a summer. Box 4-1 lists the functions of a beam former.

Pulser

The pulser produces electric voltages (Figure 4-3) that drive the transducer, forming the beam that sweeps through the tissue to be imaged. The driving voltages are in the form of electric pulses of a cycle or two of voltage. In response, the transducer produces ultrasound pulses that travel into the patient. The frequency of the voltage pulse determines the frequency of the resulting ultrasound pulse (Figure 4-3, *C* and *D*). The frequency ranges from 2 to 15 MHz for most applications.

The pulser generates the voltages that drive the transducer.

BOX 4-1 **Functions of the Beam Former**
Generate voltages that drive the transducer.
Determine pulse repetition frequency, coding, frequency, and intensity.
Scan, focus, and apodize the transmitted beam.
Amplify the returning echo voltages.
Compensate for attenuation.
Digitize the echo voltage stream.
Direct, focus, and apodize the reception beam.

The pulse repetition frequency (PRF) is the number of voltage pulses sent to the transducer each second and thus the number of ultrasound pulses produced per second. The PRF ranges from 4 to 15 kHz. The ultrasound PRF is equal to the voltage PRF because one ultrasound pulse is produced for each voltage pulse. Similarly, the ultrasound pulse repetition period is equal to the voltage pulse repetition period. This is the time from the beginning of one pulse to the beginning of the next. The operator does not normally have direct control of the PRF. Rather, the pulser adjusts the PRF appropriately for the current imaging depth. To receive information for display at a rapid rate, a high PRF is desirable. Pulse repetition frequency, however, must be limited to provide proper display of returning echoes. The timing sequence that is initiated by the pulse is shown in Figure 4-4. To avoid echo misplacement, all echoes from one pulse must be received before the next pulse is emitted. For deeper imaging, echoes take longer to return, thus forcing a reduction in the PRF and the number of images that are generated each second, called the **frame rate**. Imaging depth—that is, penetration *(pen)* in centimeters—multiplied by *PRF* (in kilohertz) must not exceed 77 if echo misplacement is to be avoided.

$$\text{pen (cm)} \times \text{PRF (kHz)} \leq 77 \text{ (cm/ms)}$$

The symbol $\leq$ means "less than or equal to."

ADVANCED CONCEPTS
The 77 is derived as follows. The time required for the ultrasound pulse to travel to the maximum imaging depth (penetration) and return is
$$t \, (\mu s) = \frac{[2 \times \text{pen (mm)}]}{c \, (\text{mm}/\mu s)} = \frac{2 \times \text{pen}}{1.54} = \frac{\text{pen}}{0.77}$$
where *t* is time (in microseconds) and *c* is propagation speed (in millimeters per microsecond). This is the minimum allowable time in microseconds between pulses (the pulse repetition period, or *PRP*). In milliseconds, *t* = pen/770. The reciprocal is the maximum allowable PRF (kilohertz) to avoid echo misplacement; that is, $PRF_{max} = 1/PRP_{min} = 770/pen$. Thus $pen \times PRF_{max} = 770$. Converting pen from millimeters to centimeters, $pen \times PRF_{max} = 77$. Thus *pen* (cm) $\times$ *PRF* (kHz) ≤ 77.

The instrument automatically achieves the highest PRF while avoiding echo misplacement. As operating frequency is reduced and penetration increases, the PRF must be reduced to avoid echo misplacement.

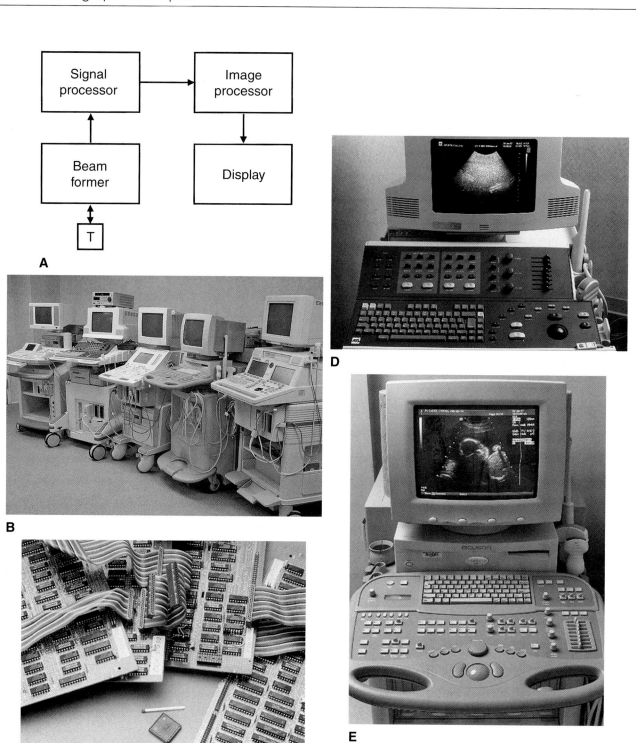

■ FIGURE 4-1 **A,** The organization of a pulse-echo imaging system. The beam former produces electric pulses that drive the transducer *(T)* and performs initial functions on returning echo voltages from the transducer. The transducer produces an ultrasound pulse for each electric pulse applied to it. For each echo received from the tissues, an electric voltage is produced by the transducer. These voltages go through the beam former to the signal processor, where they are processed to a form suitable for input to the image processor. Electric information from image processor drives the display, which produces a visual image of the cross-sectional anatomy interrogated by the system. **B,** Sonographic instruments from various manufacturers. **C,** Sonographic instruments contain hundreds of electronic components. **D** and **E,** Instrument control panels. Point-and-click software controls are available for gray-scale signal processing

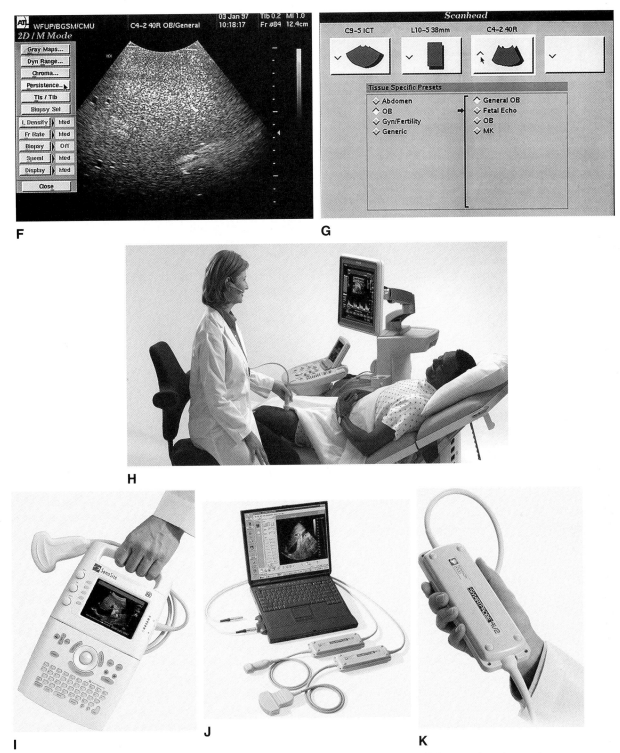

■ **FIGURE 4-1, cont'd** **(F)**, transducer selection **(G)**, and other functions. **H,** Some systems have voice-activated controls to allow hands-free operation. **I,** Portable systems are commercially available. **J** and **K,** Microsystems attach to a laptop computer.

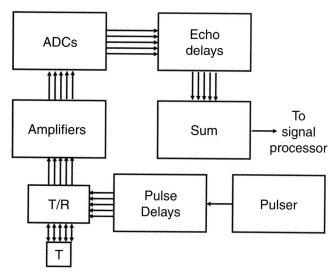

■ **FIGURE 4-2** The beam former consists of a pulser, delays, a transmit/receive (T/R) switch, amplifiers, analog-to-digital converters (ADCs), and a summer. The beam former sends digitized echo voltages to the signal processor. T is the transducer.

The greater the voltage amplitude produced by the pulser, the greater the intensity of the ultrasound pulse produced by the transducer. Transducer driving-voltage amplitudes range up to about 100 V. Output level sometimes is shown on the display in terms of a percentage or decibels relative to maximum (100% or 0 dB) output (Figure 4-5). Other output indicators account for relevant risk mechanisms.

Reduction of acoustic output reduces received echo amplitude (Figure 4-5, G). Increasing amplifier gain can compensate for this. A reduction in imaging depth also occurs, but this is surprisingly small.[11] For example, a reduction of 50% in output from a 5-MHz transducer corresponds to only a 5% penetration reduction (from about 12.0 to 11.4 cm).

Pulse Delays

Thus far the job of the beam former appears simple, but we must remember that for arrays, complicated sequencing and phasing operations are involved. The sequencing, phase delays, and variations in pulse amplitudes that are necessary for the electronic control of beam **scanning,** steering, transmission focusing, aperture, and apodization must be accomplished. The pulser and pulse delays carry out all these tasks.

Coded Excitation

More sophisticated instruments use, in some cases, more complicated driving voltage–pulse forms called **coded excitation.**[12] This approach accomplishes functions such as multiple transmission foci, separation of

harmonic echo bandwidth from the transmitted pulse bandwidth, increased penetration, reduction of speckle with improved **contrast resolution,** and gray-scale imaging of blood flow (called B-flow). In straightforward pulsing, the pulser drives the transducer through the pulse delays with one voltage pulse per **scan line.** In coded excitation, ensembles of pulses drive the transducer to generate a single scan line. For example, instead of a single pulse, a series (such as three pulses, followed by a missing pulse [a gap], followed by two pulses, followed by another gap, followed by two pulses) could be used (Figure 4-6). A decoder in the receiving portion of the beam former recognizes and disassembles the coded sequence in the returning echoes and stacks up the individual pulses in the sequence to make a short, high-intensity echo out of them. The result is equivalent to having a much higher-intensity driving pulse or a much more sensitive receiving system. Thus for example in the case of blood flow, weak echoes from blood are imaged and flow can be seen in **gray scale** along with the much stronger tissue echoes (Figure 4-6, C).

Coded excitation uses a series of pulses and gaps rather than a single driving pulse.

ADVANCED CONCEPTS

Coded excitation has been applied in radar for decades. A coded pulse is one that has internal amplitude, frequency, or phase modulation used for pulse compression. Pulse compression is the conversion, using a matched **filter,** of a relatively long coded pulse to one of short time duration, excellent resolution, and equivalent high intensity and sensitivity. A matched filter maximizes the signal-to-noise ratio of the returning **signal.** The longer the coded pulse, the higher the signal-to-noise ratio in matched-filter implementations will be. The intrapulse coding is chosen to attain adequate axial resolution, and the pulse duration is chosen to achieve the desired sensitivity. The matched-filter decoding process can be thought of as a sliding correlation of the parts of the coded pulse with the matched filter. The result of this process is, in effect, a shorter and stronger pulse (Figure 4-7) yielding good resolution and sensitivity while conforming to transmitted pulse amplitude and intensity limitations imposed by technologic and safety considerations. Such coding schemes are called Barker codes. An even better match can be achieved by Golay codes that use pairs of transmitted pulses with the second being a bipolar sequence in which the latter portion of the pulse is the inverse of the first.

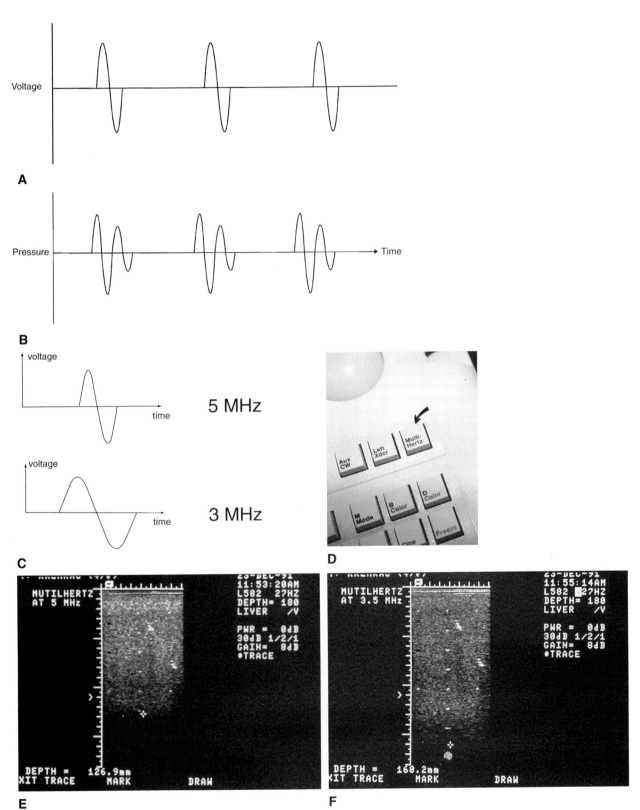

■ **FIGURE 4-3** With every voltage pulse applied **(A)**, an ultrasound pulse **(B)** is produced by the transducer. Voltage pulses of different frequencies **(C)** produce ultrasound pulses of different frequencies. By pressing the control-panel button **(D,** *arrow*), the operator can change the operating frequency without changing transducers. **E** and **F,** Images using 5- and 3-MHz frequencies, respectively.

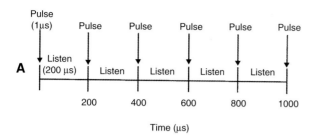

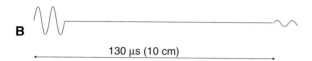

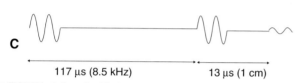

■ **FIGURE 4-4** **A,** Timing sequence for pulse-echo ultrasound imaging. The sequence is initiated by the production of a 1-μs pulse of ultrasound when the pulser sends a voltage pulse to the transducer. This is followed by a period of up to 250 μs, during which echoes are received from the tissue by the transducer. The length of this time is determined by the maximum depth from which the echoes return. For example, at a frequency of 5 MHz, echoes can return from as deep as 15 cm. The round-trip travel time (13 μs/cm × 15 cm) to this depth is 195 μs. This listening period is followed (5 μs later) by the next pulse. In this illustration the listening period is 200 μs; that is, the pulse repetition period is 200 μs (the pulse repetition frequency [PRF] is 5 kHz). If the PRF were greater, the pulse repetition period would be decreased, resulting in emission of the next pulse before the reception of all the (deeper) echoes from the previous pulse. This would produce range-ambiguity artifact (see Chapter 8) and thus should be avoided. The PRF automatically is adjusted to avoid this problem: higher PRFs are used for superficial imaging, whereas lower PRFs are used for deep imaging (to allow for the longer time required for the arrival of deeper echoes). The latter causes a reduction in frame rate. **B,** An echo (from a 10-cm depth) arrives 130 μs after pulse emission. **C,** If the pulse repetition period were 117 μs (corresponding to a PRF of 8.5 kHz), the echo in **B** would arrive 13 μs after the next pulse was emitted. The instrument would place this echo at a 1-cm depth rather than the correct value. This is known as the range-ambiguity artifact.

Channels

The pulse delays have a single input from the pulser but multiple outputs to the transducer elements; that is, there are actually many delay paths in the pulse delay circuitry. The reason for this is that the many elements in the array each need a different delay to form the ultrasound beam properly. Each independent delay and element combination constitutes a transmission **channel** (Figure 4-8). An increased number of channels allows more precise control of beam characteristics. On reception, each independent element, **amplifier, analog-to-digital converter,** and delay path constitutes a reception

channel. Typical numbers of channels in modern sonographic instruments are 64, 128, and 192. Larger numbers sometimes are advertised, but a looser definition (than the one presented here) of channel is used in such cases. Normally, the number of channels does not exceed the number of elements in the transducer.

> *A channel is an independent signal path consisting of a transducer element, delay, and possibly other electronic components.*

Transmit/Receive Switch

The T/R switch directs the driving voltages from the pulser and pulse delays to the transducer during transmission and then directs the returning echo voltages from the transducer to the amplifiers during reception (Figure 4-9). The T/R switch protects the sensitive input components of the amplifiers from the large driving voltages from the pulser.

Amplifiers

Amplifiers increase voltage amplitude. The beam former has one amplifier for each channel. **Amplification** is the conversion of the small voltages received from the transducer elements to larger ones suitable for further processing and storage (Figure 4-10). **Gain** is the ratio of amplifier output to input electric power. The power ratio, which is expressed in decibels, is equal to the voltage ratio squared, because electric power depends on voltage squared. For example, if the input voltage amplitude to an amplifier is 2 mV and the output voltage amplitude is 200 mV, the voltage ratio is 200/2, or 100. The power ratio is 100^2, or 10,000. From Table 4-1, the gain is seen to be 40 dB. Beam former amplifiers typically have 60 to 100 dB of gain. Voltages from transducers to these amplifiers range from a few microvolts (μV; e.g., from blood) to a few hundred millivolts (mV; e.g., from bone or gas). For a 60-dB gain amplifier, the output power is 1,000,000 times the input power, and the output voltage is 1000 times the input. For a 10-μV voltage input, the output voltage is 10 mV. If the gain of this amplifier is increased to 100 dB, the output voltage increases to 1 V.

> *Amplifiers increase voltage amplitudes. This is called gain.*

Text continued on p. 99.

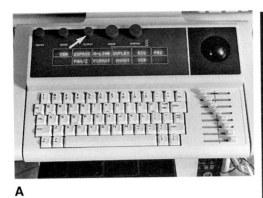

A

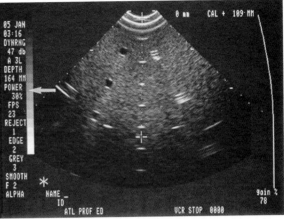

B

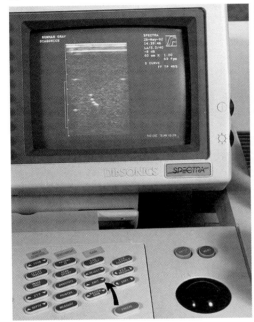

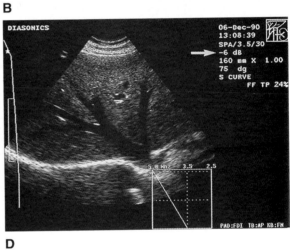

D

C

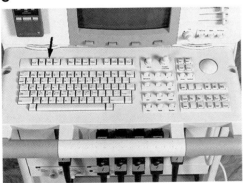

E

■ **FIGURE 4-5** The output controls of three instruments are shown (**A** and **E**, *straight arrows*; **C**, *curved arrow*). **B,** The output indicator *(arrow)* shows a percentage relative to the maximum (30% in this example). **D,** The output indicator *(arrow)* shows decibels relative to the maximum. In this example, the value is –6 dB, which corresponds to 25% of maximum.

Continued.

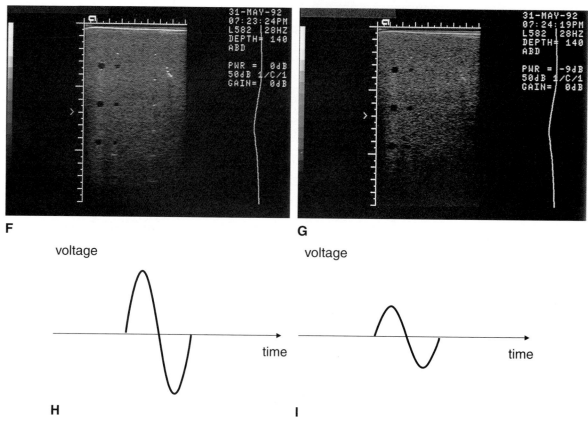

F   **G**

voltage   voltage

                time   time

H   **I**

■ **FIGURE 4-5, cont'd**   An output of 0 dB **(F)** is compared with one of –9 dB **(G),** in which the weaker echoes produce a darker image. **H** and **I,** Driving voltages from pulser to transducer for 0 and –6 dB, respectively. The voltage amplitude in **I** is half that in **H,** yielding one fourth the power and intensity, thus –6 dB output compared with **H.**

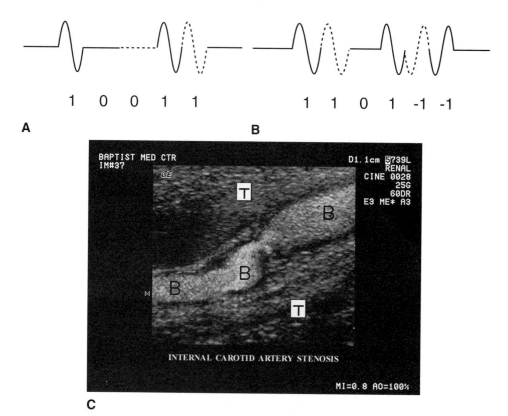

A   **B**

C

■ **FIGURE 4-6**   Examples of coded pulse sequences. Each pulse consists of a cycle of pressure variation. **A,** This sequence includes a pulse, two gaps, and two final pulses. **B,** This sequence includes two pulses, a gap, and one pulse followed by two inverted pulses. **C,** Blood flow imaging, in which weak echoes from flowing blood *(B)* are imaged along with much stronger tissue echoes *(T).*

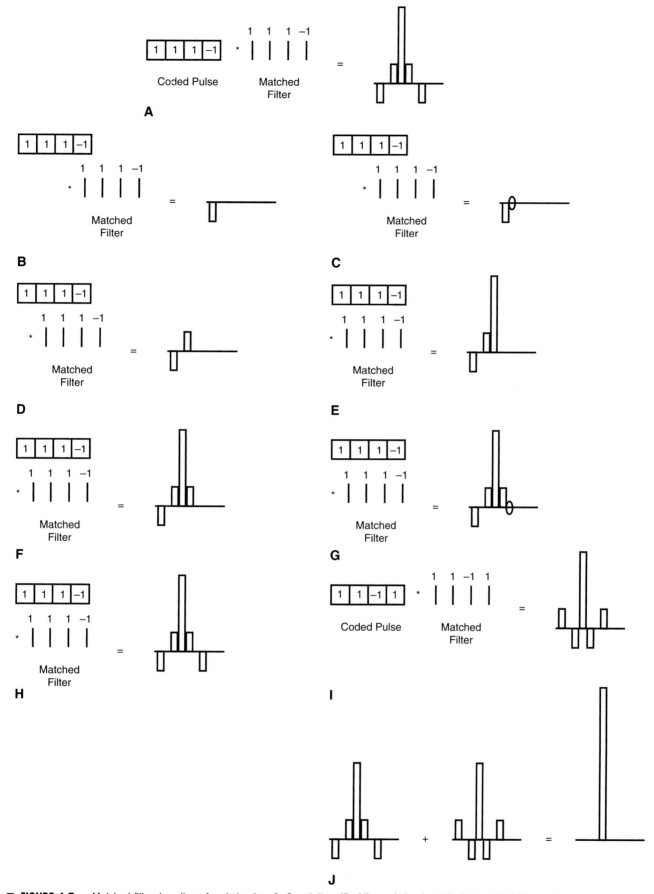

■ FIGURE 4-7 Matched filter decoding of coded pulse. **A,** Correlation (*) of the coded pulse with the matched filter yields a result that has a peak amplitude 4 times (16 times for intensity) that for a comparable uncoded pulse. This is accomplished by sliding the coded pulse in time over the matched filter characteristic and multiplying the two. **B,** Multiplying the first part of the coded pulse (−1) with the first part of the matched filter (+1) yields the result of −1, seen to the right of the equals sign. **C,** With the coded pulse slid more to the right (two portions overlap) there are two multiplications (−1 × +1 and +1 × +1). Summing the results yields 0. **D,** Sliding further to the right yields three multiplications the sum of which is +1. **E,** The sum of four multiplications [(−1) × (−1), 1 × 1, 1 × 1, 1 × 1] is 4. **F to H,** The next results are +1, 0, and −1. To make the result even stronger and sharper, a pair of codes (called a Golay code pair) can be used. The appropriate coded sequence to use with **A** is shown in **I. J,** When the two results (**A** and **I**) are summed, there is a sharp, strong result (amplitude 8 compared with the individual amplitudes of 1 in the coded sequence and the amplitude of 4 in the result in **A**).

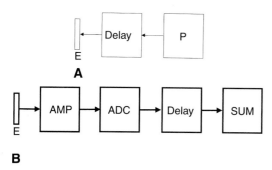

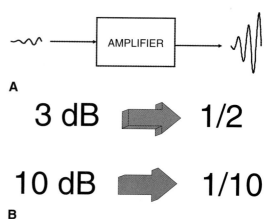

■ **FIGURE 4-8** **A,** A transmission channel consists of an independent delay and transducer element *(E)* combination. Several channels emanate from the pulser *(P)*. **B,** A reception channel consists of an independent element *(E)*, amplifier *(AMP)*, analog-to-digital converter *(ADC)*, and delay. The signals from many channels are combined in the summer *(SUM)*.

■ **FIGURE 4-10** Gain. **A,** Amplification (gain) increases voltage amplitude and electric power. **B,** A gain of 3 dB corresponds to an output power equivalent to input power ×2; 10 dB corresponds to an input power ×10.

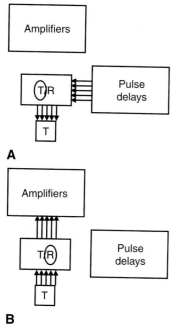

■ **FIGURE 4-9** Transmit/receive *(T/R)* switch. **A,** During transmission (energizing the transducer to send a pulse into the body), the T/R switch opens the path from the pulser to the transducer elements. **B,** During echo reception, the T/R switch opens the path from the elements to the reception amplifiers.

TABLE 4-1 Gain (Expressed in Decibels) and Corresponding Power and Amplitude Ratios*		
Gain (dB)	**Power Ratio**	**Amplitude Ratio**
0	1.0	1.0
1	1.3	1.1
2	1.6	1.3
3	2.0	1.4
4	2.5	1.6
5	3.2	1.8
6	4.0	2.0
7	5.0	2.2
8	6.3	2.5
9	7.9	2.8
10	10	3.2
15	32	5.6
20	100	10
25	320	18
30	1,000	32
35	3,200	56
40	10,000	100
45	32,000	180
50	100,000	320
60	1,000,000	1,000
70	10,000,000	3,200
80	100,000,000	10,000
90	1,000,000,000	32,000
100	10,000,000,000	100,000

*The power (amplitude) ratio is output power (amplitude) divided by input power (amplitude).

Two useful decibel values to remember are 3 and 10 (Figure 4-10, *B*). Whereas 3 dB corresponds to a power gain of ×2, 10 dB corresponds to ×10. Values also can be combined; for example, 6 dB corresponds to two doublings (×4); 20 dB corresponds to ×10×10, or ×100; and 13 dB corresponds to ×10×2, or ×20.

The gain control (Figure 4-11) determines how much amplification is accomplished in the amplifier. Gain control is similar in function to the level control on your sound system at home. With too little gain, weak echoes are not imaged. With too much gain, saturation occurs; that is, most echoes appear bright and differences in echo strength are lost.

Gain is set subjectively so that echoes appear with appropriate brightnesses.

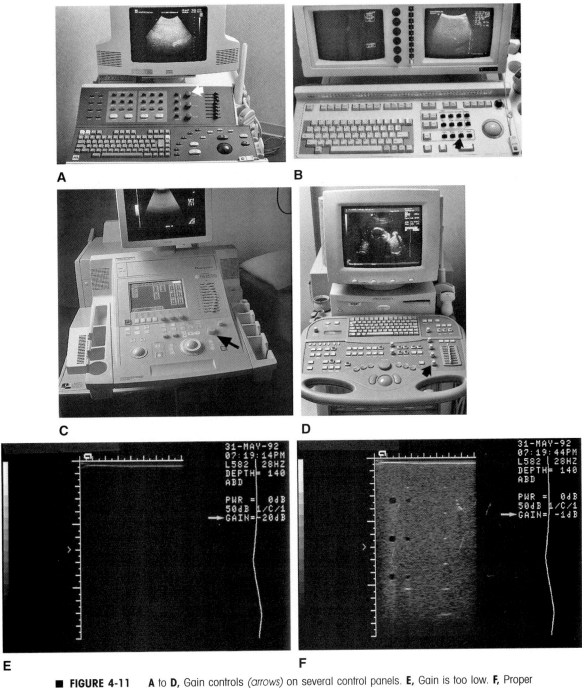

■ **FIGURE 4-11** **A** to **D,** Gain controls *(arrows)* on several control panels. **E,** Gain is too low. **F,** Proper gain.

Continued.

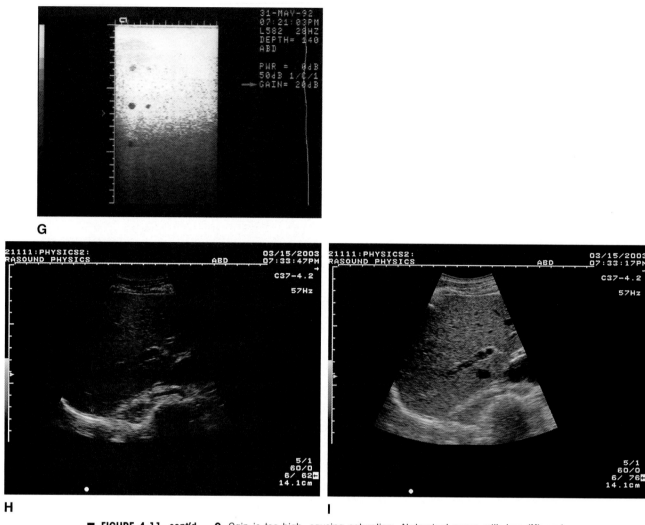

■ **FIGURE 4-11, cont'd**   **G,** Gain is too high, causing saturation. Abdominal scans with low **(H)** and proper **(I)** gain.

The amplifiers also must compensate for the effect of attenuation on the **image. Compensation** (also called **time gain compensation** [TGC] and **depth gain compensation**) equalizes differences in received echo amplitudes caused by different reflector depths. Reflectors with equal reflection coefficients will not result in echoes of equal amplitude arriving at the transducer (Figure 4-12) if their travel distances are different (i.e., if the distance between the transducer and the reflectors is different) because sound weakens as it travels (attenuation). Display of echoes from similar reflectors in a similar way is desirable. Because these echoes may not arrive with the same amplitude because of different path lengths, their amplitudes must be adjusted to compensate for differences in attenuation. Longer path lengths result in greater attenuation *and* later arrival times. Therefore if voltages from echoes arriving later are amplified correctly to a

greater degree than are earlier ones, attenuation compensation is accomplished. This is the goal of compensation (Figure 4-13). In other words, the later an echo arrives, the farther it has traveled and the weaker it will be. However, the later it arrives, the more it will be amplified. If this compensation is done properly, the resulting amplitude will be the same as if there had been no attenuation.

The increase of gain with depth commonly is called the TGC slope because it sometimes is displayed graphically as a line with increasing deflection to the right (Figure 4-13, *B*). This slope can be expressed in decibels of gain per centimeter of depth. When properly adjusted, the slope should correspond to the average attenuation coefficient in the tissue, expressed in decibels per centimeter of depth. Remember that each centimeter of depth corresponds to 2 cm of round-trip

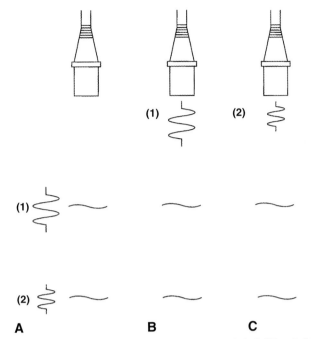

■ FIGURE 4-12 Two identical reflectors are located at different distances from the transducer. **A,** The echo at the second reflector is weaker because the incident pulse had to travel farther to get there, thereby increasing attenuation. **B,** The echo from the first reflector arrives at the transducer. The echo is weaker than it was in **A** because of attenuation on the return trip. **C,** The echo from the second reflector arrives at the transducer later and in a weaker form than the first one did because of the longer path to the second reflector.

sound travel, so that the resulting slope should be about 1 dB/cm-MHz because average attenuation in soft tissue is 0.5 dB/cm-MHz. The former refers to centimeters of depth, whereas the latter refers to centimeters of travel. Because the attenuation depends on the frequency of the ultrasound beam, the operator subjectively adjusts the TGC to compensate for the frequency used and the attenuation of the tissues being imaged. Time gain compensation is set by the operator to achieve, on average, uniform brightness throughout the image. The average attenuation in the tissue cross section at the operating frequency has been compensated when this is accomplished.

Time gain compensation compensates for the effect of attenuation on an image.

Typical TGC amplifiers compensate for about 60 dB of attenuation. At the depth at which maximum gain has been achieved, the echo brightness begins to decrease because the TGC can no longer compensate (the amplifier gain cannot be increased further). Thus the attenuation and maximum amplifier gain determine the maximum imaging depth. The maximum amplifier gain is determined by noise. Electronic noise (Figure 4-14, *A* and *B*) exists in all electronic circuits. High-quality input amplifier circuit noise levels are a few microvolts in amplitude. At maximum gain, the amplifier noise and the weak echoes being amplified have comparable amplitude. Any further increase in gain would only increase the noise, with weaker echoes being lost in the noise and thus being unobservable.

Some instruments have **lateral gain control,** which allows adjustment of gain laterally across the image (Figure 4-14, *C* and *D*). Regions with different attenuation values located laterally to each other can be compensated to yield similar image brightnesses.

The overall gain control is adjusted first to yield a perceptible image on the display. Then the TGC (and possibly the lateral gain control) controls are adjusted to yield on-average uniform brightness over the image. Attenuation variations throughout the image thus are compensated out, yielding a good representation of the tissue cross section imaged.

Analog-to-Digital Converters (Digitizers)

After amplification the echo voltages are digitized; that is, they pass through analog-to-digital converters (ADC). An ADC (also called a digitizer) converts the voltage from **analog** to **digital** form (Figure 4-15). Analog means proportional, and digital means in the form of discrete numbers. Thus far in the instrument, the echo voltage has been proportional to the echo pressure. After the ADC, numbers represent echo voltages, and further manipulation of the echoes is accomplished as digital signal processing (mathematical manipulation of numbers representing echoes). This is similar to what is done in all digital electronics such as CD and DVD players and digital cellular telephones that handle, store, and process sound and pictures in digital form. The ADC interrogates the incoming voltage at regular intervals and determines its value at each interrogation instant. The interrogation rate must be twice the highest frequency involved in the interrogated voltage to preserve (in the subsequent digital number stream) all the harmonics contained in the interrogated voltage. For example, to digitize a 5-MHz continuous wave voltage properly, the digitizing rate must be at least 10 MHz; that is, the voltage is interrogated 10 million times per second, yielding a stream of 10 million digitized values per second describing the original analog voltage.

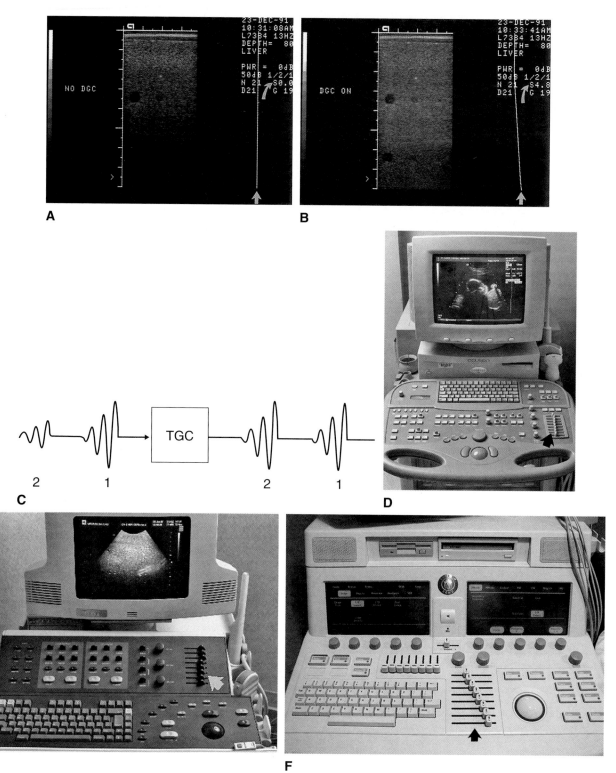

■ **FIGURE 4-13** Time gain compensation (TGC). Two scans of a tissue-equivalent phantom imaged at 7 MHz without **(A)** and with **(B)** depth gain compensation *(DGC)*. Without DGC, the echo brightness (amplitude, intensity, strength) declines with depth *(top to bottom)*. On the display, DGC settings are shown graphically *(straight arrows)*. The slopes *(curved arrows)* are 0 dB/cm **(A)** and 4.8 dB/cm **(B)**. Average tissue attenuation is 0.5 dB/cm-MHz. This is calculated per centimeter of sound propagation. Average attenuation then is 1 dB/cm-MHz when the centimeter value is the distance from the transducer to the reflector. The sound must travel twice this distance (round-trip), so the attenuation number doubles. Typical DGC slopes then will be about 1 dB/cm-MHz. **C,** Uncompensated echoes from identical structures at differing depths enter the TGC amplifier. The second (2) is weaker than the first (1) because it has come from a deeper site and has experienced more attenuation. After TGC the amplitudes are identical. **D** to **F,** Time gain compensation controls *(arrows)* on several instruments.

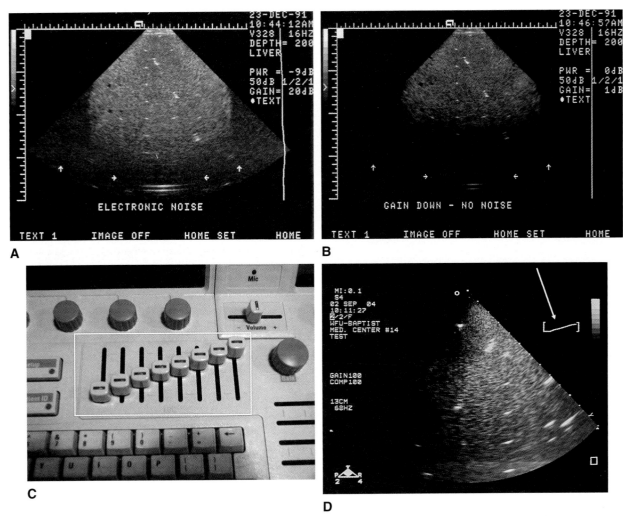

■ FIGURE 4-14 **A,** Under conditions of high gain, electronic noise (with its fuzzy appearance) can be seen on the display *(arrows)*. **B,** With reduced gain, these weak voltages are not amplified enough to be visualized. **C,** Lateral gain controls. **D,** Lateral gain adjusted to increase gain from left to right.

ADVANCED CONCEPTS

The voltage precision of the digitizer depends on the number of bits of the digitized binary number. For example, an 8-bit digitizer can yield any decimal number from 0 to 255. If the maximum voltage amplitude to be digitized is 10 volts, the digitizer can determine its value at any interrogation to a precision of 10/255 or 0.039 volt (0.4%). The temporal precision of the digitizer is determined by the digitizing frequency. Each cycle of the voltage must be interrogated at least twice to determine its frequency. Thus changes in the interrogated voltage that occur at a faster rate than half the digitizing frequency cannot be followed by the digitizer and will be lost in the digitizing process. A 10-MHz digitizer interrogates 10 million times per second. Voltage frequencies of 5 MHz or less can be digitized properly in this case.

Analog-to-digital converters convert the analog voltages representing echoes to numbers for digital signal processing and storage.

Echo Delays

After amplification and digitizing, the echo voltages pass through digital delay lines to accomplish reception dynamic focus and steering functions.

Summer

After all the channel signal components are delayed properly to accomplish the focus and steering functions, they are added together in the summer to produce the

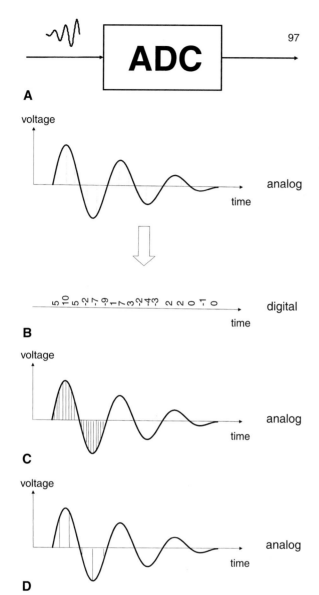

■ FIGURE 4-15 **A,** The analog-to-digital converter *(ADC)* converts **(B)** the analog (proportional) echo voltage into a series of numbers representing the sampled voltage. The higher the sampling rate of the analog-to-digital converter, the better the temporal detail of the voltage is preserved. **C,** High sampling rate. **D,** Low sampling rate.

resulting scan line that, along with all the others, will be displayed after signal processing and image processing. Reception apodization and dynamic aperture functions also are accomplished as part of this summing process.

The beam former is responsible for electronic beam scanning, steering, focusing, apodization, and aperture functions with arrays.

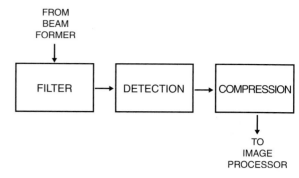

■ FIGURE 4-16 The signal processor performs filtering, detection, and compression functions. The processor receives digital signals from the beam former and, after processing, sends them on to the image processor.

BOX 4-2   Functions of the Signal Processor
Bandpass filtering
Amplitude detection (radio frequency to video)
Compression (dynamic range reduction)

SIGNAL PROCESSOR

The reception portion of the beam former has amplified and combined the contributions from the individual elements and channels to form the stream of echoes returning from each transmitted pulse and sends them on to the signal processor. Here operations are carried out that include filtering, **detection,** and **compression.** The signal processor is diagrammed in Figure 4-16. Box 4-2 lists the functions of the signal processor.

Filtering

Tuned amplifiers often are used to reduce noise in the electronics. They operate at a specific frequency with a bandwidth that includes the frequencies in the returning echoes and eliminates the electronic noise outside that bandwidth. A tuned amplifier is simply an amplifier with an electronic filter called a bandpass filter. A bandpass filter is one that passes a range of frequencies (its bandwidth) and rejects those above and below the acceptance bandwidth (Figure 4-17). Some tuned amplifiers dynamically move the frequency range of the filter to track the bandwidth of the returning series of echoes from a pulse. The echo bandwidth decreases as the echoes return because the higher frequencies in the bandwidth are attenuated more than are the lower ones. The box in the lower right corner of Figure 4-18 describes such a tracking-filter-tuned-amplifier operation.

Filtering eliminates frequencies outside the echo bandwidth while retaining those that are most useful in a given type of operation.

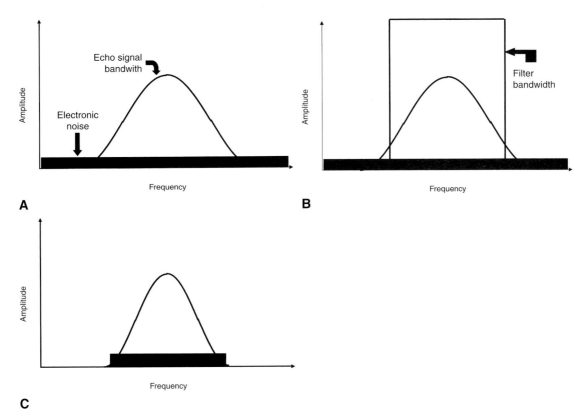

A

B

C

■ **FIGURE 4-17** **A,** Input to filter includes the echo signal bandwidth and the electronic noise with unlimited bandwidth. **B,** The filter bandwidth is designed to accommodate the signal bandwidth. **C,** The output from the filter has the frequencies above and below its bandwidth removed. Only the noise frequencies within the filter bandwidth remain.

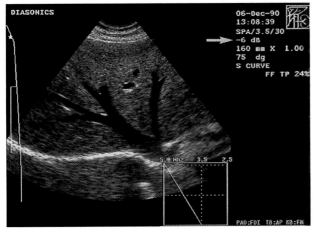

■ **FIGURE 4-18** The box in the lower right corner shows the decreasing frequency bandwidth of a tracking filter with increasing depth of the returning echoes.

Harmonic Imaging

A second type of filtering occurs with harmonic imaging, in which the fundamental (transmitted) frequency is filtered out and the second harmonic frequency echoes are passed. (The generation of har-

monic frequencies in tissue is discussed in Chapter 2.) At this point the bandpass filter is centered at the second harmonic frequency with an appropriate bandwidth to include the bandwidth of the second harmonic echo signal (Figure 4-19, *A* to *D*). Harmonic imaging improves the image quality in three primary ways (Figure 4-19, *E* to *G*):

■ The primary beam is much narrower, improving lateral resolution, because harmonics are generated only in the highest-intensity portion of the beam.

■ Grating lobe artifacts are eliminated because these extra beams are not sufficiently strong to generate the harmonics.

■ Because the harmonic beam is generated at a depth beyond where some of the artifactual problems occur (e.g., superficial reverberation), the image degradation that they cause is reduced or eliminated.

Because the fundamental and second harmonic bandwidths must fit within the overall transducer bandwidth (Figure 4-19, *G*), they must be reasonably narrow. This means that the corresponding ultrasound pulses must be somewhat longer than otherwise, causing some degradation in axial resolution. A solution to this degradation in image quality is to use pulse inversion, a technique that uses two pulses per scan line

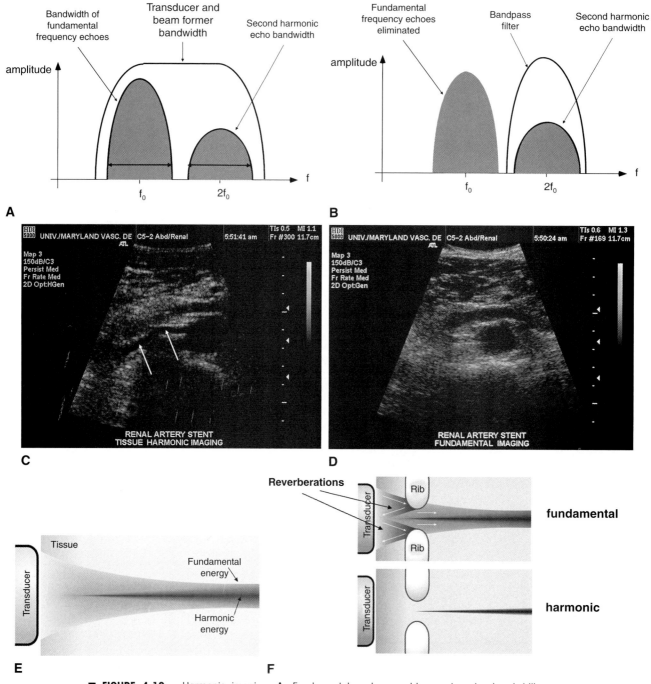

■ **FIGURE 4-19** Harmonic imaging. **A,** Fundamental and second-harmonic echo bandwidths are shown. The beam former and transducer must pass both to generate the ultrasound beam and to accomplish harmonic imaging. **B,** For harmonic imaging the bandpass filter eliminates the fundamental frequency echoes and passes the second harmonic echoes. The harmonic image **(C)** has improved quality compared with the fundamental image **(D)**. **E,** The harmonic beam is much narrower than the fundamental. **F,** Reverberations are reduced with the harmonic beam.

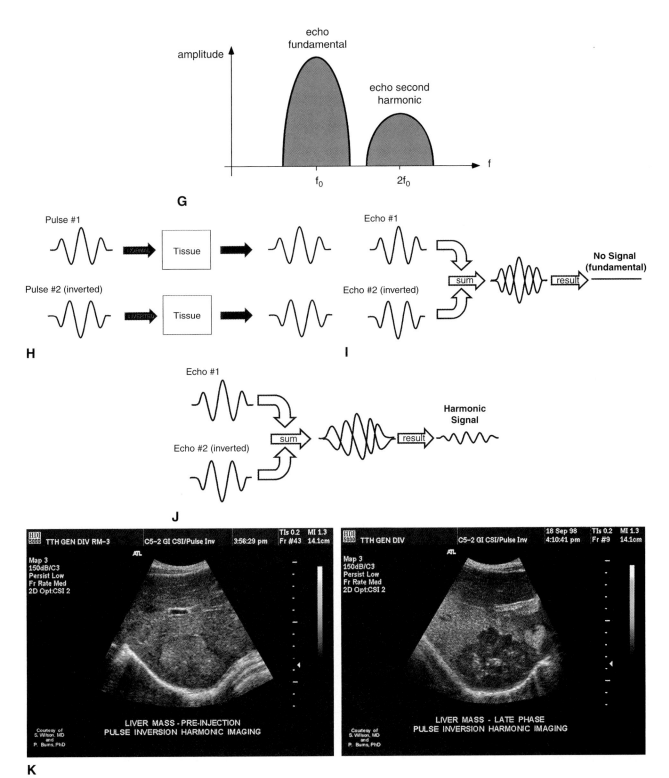

■ **FIGURE 4-19, cont'd** **G,** In harmonic imaging two bandwidths (fundamental and second harmonic) must fit within the transducer bandwidth and not overlap so that the fundamental frequency echoes can be eliminated from the second harmonic image. **H,** In pulse inversion harmonic imaging, a normal pulse of ultrasound is followed by an inverted pulse. Two series of echoes return from these two pulses (only one echo is shown for each pulse in this drawing). When the echoes from the two pulses are summed, the fundamental frequency echoes cancel **(I),** whereas the second harmonic echoes are not canceled **(J).** **K,** Pre- and post-injection abdominal images using a contrast agent and pulse inversion harmonic imaging.

rather than one. The second pulse is the inverse of the first. The echo sequences from the two pulses (Figure 4-19, *H*) are added together to yield the resulting scan line. Fundamental frequency echoes cancel (Figure 4-19, *I*), and the second harmonic echoes remain (Figure 4-19, *J*). This technique allows broad-bandwidth, short pulses to be used so that detail resolution is not degraded (Figure 4-19, *K*). Instead, frame rate is reduced, with some degradation of **temporal resolution.**

Detection

Detection (also called **demodulation**) is the conversion of echo voltages from **radio frequency** form to **video** form (Figure 4-20). This is done by detecting and connecting together the maxima of the cyclic variations. The cyclic voltage form is called radio frequency because it is similar to voltages found in a radio receiver, and the frequencies are similar to those in the low end of the shortwave radio band. The detected form retains the amplitudes and is called video because such a process is accomplished in television sets. Because diagnostic ultrasound pulses do not have constant amplitude, when demodulated, they do not have the simplified blocked appearance shown in Figure 4-20. Detection is not an operator-controllable function.

Detection is the conversion of echo voltages from radio frequency to video form. Video form retains amplitudes of the echo voltages.

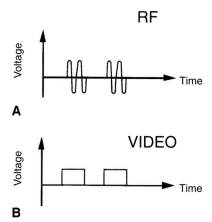

A

B

■ **FIGURE 4-20** Echo voltages are produced in a complicated cyclic form **(A)** called radio frequency *(RF)*, which would be difficult to store and display. Furthermore, only the amplitude of each echo is needed for a gray-scale display of anatomy. Thus the radio frequency form is converted to video form **(B)**, which retains the amplitude of each echo voltage.

Compression

The ratio of the largest to the smallest amplitude or power that a system can handle is called the **dynamic range** (Figure 4-21). Dynamic range is expressed in decibels. For example, if an amplifier is insensitive to voltage amplitudes of less than 0.01 mV (because they are buried in the electronic noise) and cannot properly handle voltage amplitudes of greater than 1000 mV, the ratio of usable voltage extremes is 1000/0.01, or 100,000. The power ratio is equal to the square of the voltage ratio: $100,000^2$, or 10,000,000,000. According to Table 4-1, the dynamic range of the amplifier is 100 dB. Amplifiers have dynamic ranges typically of 100 to 120 dB. System dynamic ranges are claimed as high as 170 dB. Greater values indicate the ability to detect weaker echoes, that is, greater sensitivity. The higher dynamic ranges assume some bandwidth reduction (to reduce electronic noise) and improvement yielded from the reception beam-forming process with several reception channels. Other portions of the electronics (especially the display) have much smaller dynamic range capability. Displays have dynamic ranges of up to 30 dB. Furthermore, human vision is limited to a dynamic range of about 20 dB. The largest power (brightness) can be only about 100 times the smallest for our viewing of the display. Thus the largest voltage amplitude can be only about 10 times the smallest. The echo dynamic range remaining after compensation is typically 50 to 100 dB. Compression is the process of decreasing the differences between the smallest and largest echo amplitudes to a usable range (Figure 4-22). Amplifiers that amplify weak inputs more than strong ones accomplish this. A compressor would have to compress the intensity ratio (100,000) corresponding to 50 dB to an intensity ratio of 100 (acceptable for the display).

Compression reduces dynamic range with logarithmic amplification.

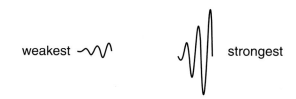

weakest   strongest

■ **FIGURE 4-21** Dynamic range is the relationship between the weakest and strongest echoes and is expressed in decibels.

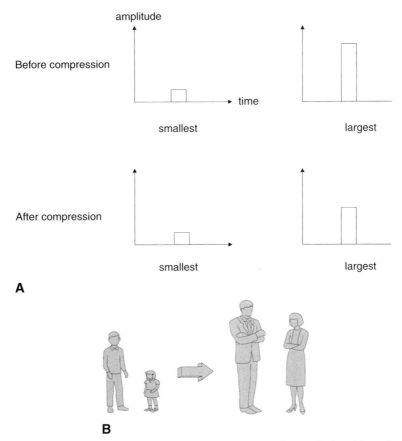

Before compression

amplitude

smallest

largest

time

After compression

smallest

largest

A

B

■ **FIGURE 4-22** Compression decreases the difference between the smallest and largest amplitudes passing through the system. **A,** In this example, the ratio of largest to smallest amplitudes before compression is 5. After compression, the ratio is 3. **B,** A family illustration of compression amplification. Big brother (age 15 years) is twice as tall (large dynamic range) as little sister (age 5 years). Fifteen years later, brother (age 30 years) is just slightly taller than sister (age 20 years). Both have grown (amplification), but the shorter child grew more than the taller one, reducing the difference between them (compression).

Compression is operator adjustable as a dynamic range control (Figure 4-23). This control reduces dynamic range by assigning some weak echo amplitude values to zero or by assigning some of the strongest to maximum. Reassigned echoes may be at either end of the dynamic range or at both ends (Figure 4-23, *I* to *K*). A smaller dynamic range setting presents a higher-contrast image. The gain control moves the dynamic range curve to the left or right (down or up the dynamic range) as gain is increased or decreased (Figure 4-23, *L* and *M*).

Signal processing includes digital filtering, detection, and compression of echo data.

IMAGE PROCESSOR

Up to this point (through the beam former and signal processor), the echo data are travelling in scan-line form serially through the system, that is, one scan line at a time. No image has yet been formed. The image processor converts the digitized, filtered, detected, and compressed serial scan line data into images that are processed before and following storage in **image memory,** all in preparation for presentation on the instrument display. Following detection of the echo voltage amplitude in the signal processor, the scan line data enter the image processor, where they are converted into image form by scan conversion and then are processed in image form (Figure 4-24). Box 4-3 lists the functions of the image processor.

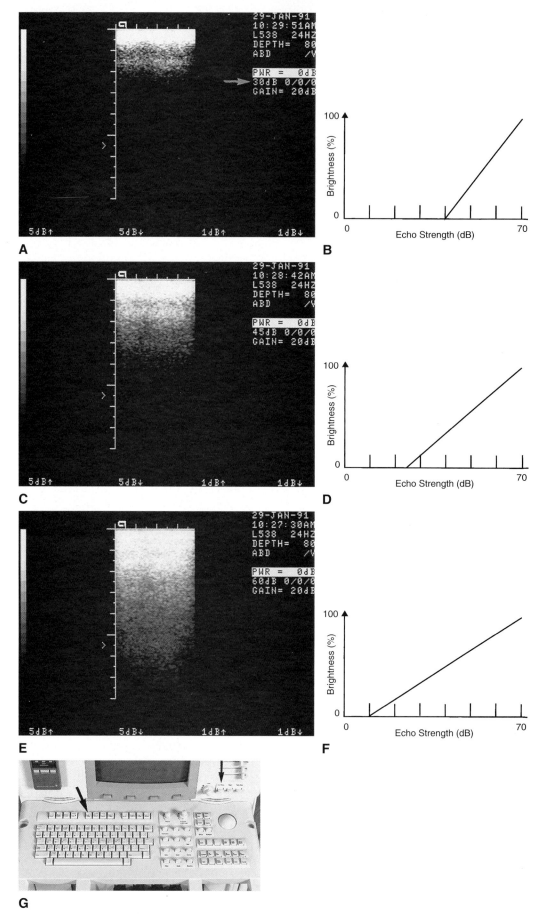

■ **FIGURE 4-23** **A,** The dynamic range setting *(arrow)* is 30 dB. The lower 40 dB of echoes returning from a tissue-equivalent phantom are set to 0 *(black portion)*. The remainder show high contrast, with brightness progressing from black for 40-dB echoes to white for 70-dB echoes. **B,** A 30-dB dynamic range setting assigns the weakest 40 dB of echo dynamic range to zero *(black)* and the remaining 30 dB of dynamic range to linearly higher brightnesses. **C,** A display with a dynamic range of 45 dB. **D,** Brightness assignment for a 45-dB dynamic range. **E,** A display with a dynamic range of 60 dB. **F,** Brightness assignment for a 60-dB dynamic range. **G,** Compression control *(arrows)*.

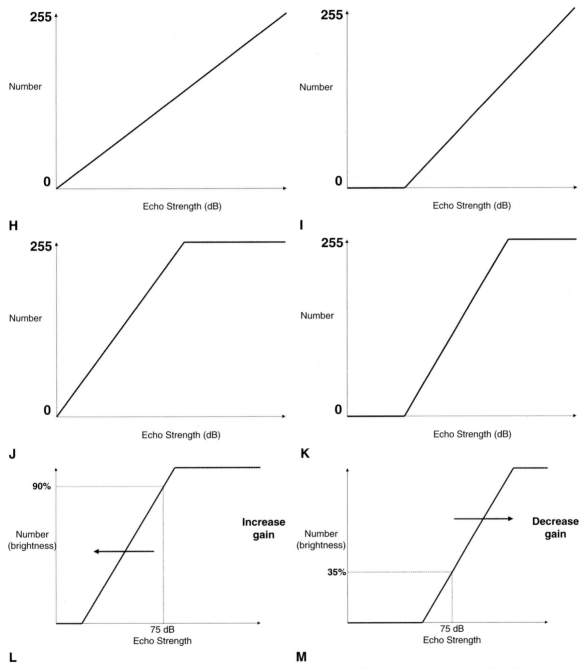

■ **FIGURE 4-23, cont'd** **H,** Full system dynamic range displayed. **I,** Dynamic range reduced by setting a weaker portion to 0 *(black).* **J,** Dynamic range reduced by setting a stronger portion to maximum *(white).* **K,** Dynamic range reduced by setting weaker and stronger portions to black and white, respectively. **L,** This curve of brightness versus echo strength moves to the left as gain is increased. A midrange echo appears bright. **M,** The curve moves to the right for decreasing gain. The midrange echo appears dark.

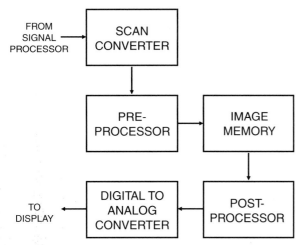

■ **FIGURE 4-24** The image processor converts scan line data into images, processes the images before storing them in image memory, processes them as they come out of memory, converts them from digital to analog form, and sends them on to the display.

BOX 4-3   Functions of the Image Processor

Scan conversion
Preprocessing
    Persistence
    Panoramic imaging
    Spatial compounding
    Three-dimensional acquisition
Storing image frames
    Cine loop
Postprocessing
    Gray scale
    Color scale
    Three-dimensional presentation
Digital-to-analog conversion

Scan Conversion

Using a computer monitor scan format, digital scan converters provide means for displaying information acquired in a linear or sector ultrasound scan line format. Information regarding the direction of each scan line and the location of echoes in depth down each scan line is used to determine the proper location in memory (and thus on the display) for each echo. For example, a pulse emitted from the transducer straight down into the body will result in a series of echoes that are located in appropriate memory locations straight down a column in memory at various depths, that is, various row locations (Figure 4-25, *A*). A pulse emitted in a direction off vertical will result in a series of echoes

that must be located in various rows and columns (Figure 4-25, *B*). The **scan converter** properly locates each series of echoes corresponding to each scan line for each pulse emitted from the transducer, filling up the memory with echo information. This is accomplished in a fraction of a second, yielding one scan or **frame** of image information. This process is repeated several times per second to produce a rapid sequence of frames stored in memory and presented on the display. This rapid-sequence presentation is called a **real-time display**, and the entire process is called **real-time** sonography. The image depth control determines the depth to be displayed and thus the depth range covered by the image memory in the scan conversion process.

The scan converter reformats echo data into image form for image processing, storage, and display.

Preprocessing

As part of the scan conversion process, various processing may be performed on the image. This is called **preprocessing** because it occurs before the echo data are stored in image memory. Examples of preprocessing include edge enhancement (a function that sharpens boundaries to make them more detectable and measurements more precise), pixel interpolation, **persistence, panoramic imaging, spatial compounding,** and three-dimensional (3D) acquisition. Preprocessing includes functions that are performed as part of scan conversion.

Preprocessing is signal and image processing done as echo data are stored in memory.

Pixel Interpolation

Image improvement can be accomplished by filling in missing pixels. A common situation where this occurs is in sector scans in which scan lines have increasing separation with distance from the transducer and intervening pixels are left out. Interpolation assigns a brightness value to a missed **pixel** based on an average of brightnesses of adjacent pixels (Figure 4-25, *C*).

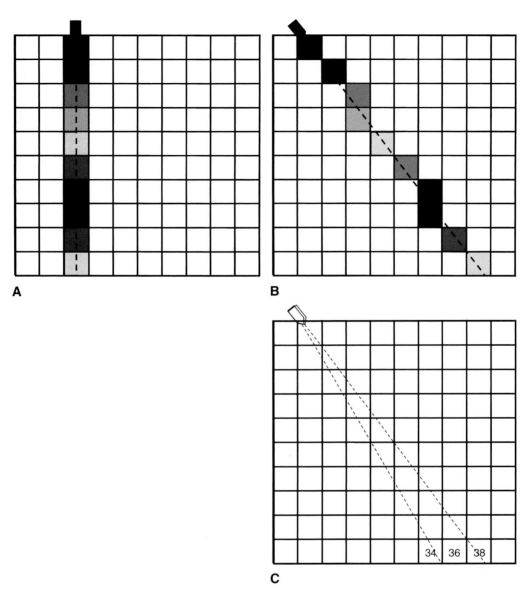

■ **FIGURE 4-25** **A,** A pulse emitted straight down into the body *(arrowhead and dashed line)* results in echoes located in a column of memory locations. **B,** A pulse emitted in another direction results in echoes located in various rows and columns. **C,** Pixel interpolation. Part of the image memory pixel grid is shown along with the paths of two pulses. At the bottom of the grid the paths have separated sufficiently so that the pixel between them is missed. The interpolation calculation determines the mean value of the two adjacent pixels (34 and 38) which is 36. That value then is entered in the intervening pixel.

Persistence

Persistence is the averaging of sequential frames for the purpose of providing a smoother image appearance and reduction of noise (Figure 4-26). Noise, primarily speckle, is reduced because it is a random process. When several frames containing random content are averaged, the random content is reduced. Speckle reduction improves dynamic range and contrast resolution. But frame averaging in effect reduces the frame rate because averaged frames are no longer independent. Operator control permits averaging of a selectable number of sequential frames from zero up to some maximum. Lower levels of persistence, or none at all, are appropriate for following rapidly moving structures. Higher levels are appropriate for slower-moving structures.

Persistence reduces noise and smoothes the image by frame averaging.

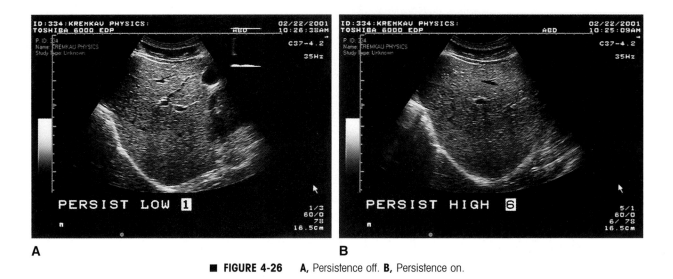

■ **FIGURE 4-26** **A,** Persistence off. **B,** Persistence on.

Panoramic Imaging

Panoramic imaging provides a way to produce an image that has a wider field of view than what is available on an individual frame from a transducer. Panoramic imaging is achieved by sliding the transducer and the scan plane in a direction parallel to the scan plane. At the same time, the old echo information from previous frames is retained while the new echoes are added to the image in the direction in which the scan plane is moving. The result is a larger field of view allowing presentation of large organs and regions of anatomy on one image (Figure 4-27). The addition of the new echoes to the existing image as the transducer is moved requires their proper location relative to the existing image. This is accomplished by correlating locations of echoes common to adjacent frames (i.e., the overlap) so that the new information on the new frame is located properly (Figure 4-28).

> *Panoramic imaging expands the image beyond the normal limits of the field of view of the transducer.*

Spatial Compounding

Spatial compounding is a technique in which scan lines are directed in multiple directions by phasing so that structures are interrogated more than once by the ultrasound beam (Figure 4-29). Averaging sequential frames, up to nine typically, improves the quality of the image in several ways:

■ As in persistence, speckle is reduced.
■ Clutter caused by artifacts is reduced.

■ Smooth (specular) surfaces are presented more completely because they are interrogated at more than one angle, increasing the probability that close to 90-degree incidence is achieved (which is necessary to receive echoes from them).
■ Structures previously hidden beneath highly attenuating objects can be visualized.

> *Spatial compounding is the averaging of frames that view anatomy from different angles.*

Three-Dimensional Imaging

Three-dimensional imaging is accomplished by acquiring many parallel two-dimensional (2D) scans (Figure 4-30) and then processing this 3D volume of echo information in appropriate ways for presentation on 2D displays. The multiple 2D frames are obtained by (1) manual scanning of the transducer, with position-sensing devices keeping track of scan-plane location and orientation, (2) automated mechanically scanned transducers, or (3) electronic scanning with 2D element-array transducers. Common ways of presenting the 3D echo data include surface renderings, 2D slices through the 3D volume, and transparent views. The advantage of the 2D slice presentation is that image plane orientations can be presented that are impossible to obtain with conventional 2D scanning. Surface renderings are popular in obstetric imaging. Transparent views allow "see-through" imaging of anatomy similar to plain film radiographs.

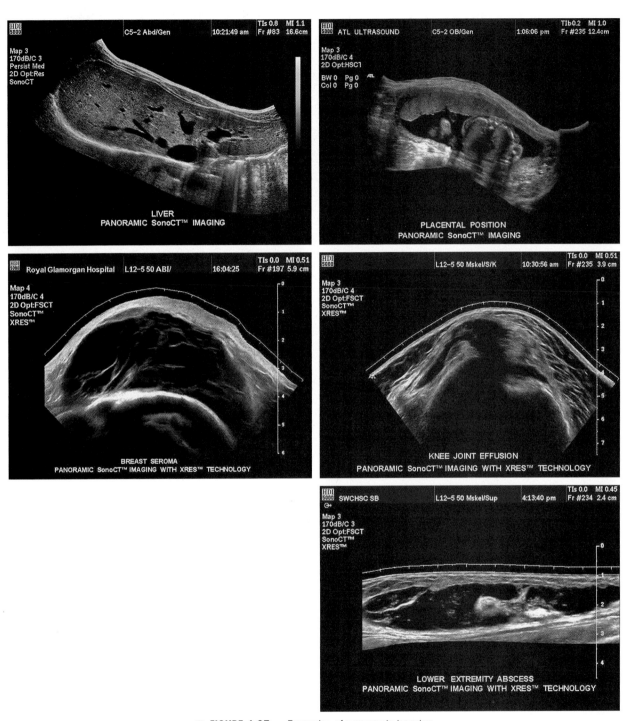

■ FIGURE 4-27 Examples of panoramic imaging.

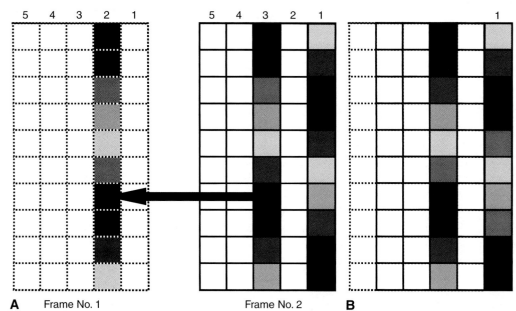

■ **FIGURE 4-28**   *Panoramic imaging is accomplished by adding new information to one end of an image, spatially correlating the overlapping old echoes to properly locate the new ones.* **A,** *Two sequential frames are shown; frame No. 2 temporally follows frame No. 1. Frame No. 2 is located slightly to the right of frame No. 1 in the anatomy by manual movement of the transducer by the sonographer. Thus a new scan line is added to frame No. 2. Scan line No. 3 in the new frame corresponds to scan line No. 2 in the previous frame. A spatial correlation process in the image processor identifies the equality of these two scan lines. Frame No. 2 then is slid to the left over the top of frame No. 1 so that the identical scan lines in the two frames overlap.* **B,** *The new scan line thus is added properly to the old frame. This process is repeated many times as the transducer is moved in a direction parallel to the scan plane. The old scan lines are retained as the new ones are added to the image.*

Three-dimensional images are acquired by assembling several 2D scans into a 3D volume of echo information in image memory.

Three-dimensional images can be acquired at rates of up to 30 volumes per second and thus are considered "live" or real-time presentations. The current tendency is to call this "4D imaging" where the fourth dimension is time. Although this term sounds fashionable for marketing purposes, it is inconsistent with previous terminology; that is, real-time 2D imaging is not called 3D. Nevertheless, the moniker appears to be catching on.

Image Memory

After echo data are scan-converted into image form and preprocessed, the image frames are stored in image memory. Storing each image in memory as the sound beam is scanned through the anatomy permits display of a single image (frame) out of the rapid sequence of several frames acquired each second in real-time sonographic instruments. Holding and displaying one frame out of the sequence is known as the **freeze-frame** (Figure 4-30, *D*). Most instruments store the last several frames acquired before freezing. This is called the **cine loop,** cine review, or image review feature.

Pixels and Bits

Image memories used in diagnostic ultrasound instruments are digital; that is, they are computer memories that store numbers (digits) as digital cameras do (Figure 4-31, *A*). The 2D image plane is divided like a checkerboard (Figure 4-31, *B*) into squares called pixels (picture elements), in a rectangular matrix such as 1024 × 768 or 512 × 384. The pixels number several thousand (786,432 and 196,608 in the previous examples), so they are tiny and not normally noticed unless magnified sufficiently. In each of the pixel locations in memory, a number is stored that corresponds to the echo strength received from the location within the anatomy corresponding to that memory position (Figure 4-31, *C*). The more pixels there are, the finer the spatial detail in the stored image (Figure 4-31, *D* to *F*). If the digital memory were composed of a single-layer matrix checkerboard, each pixel location could store only one of two numbers: a zero or a one. The reason is that the memory element

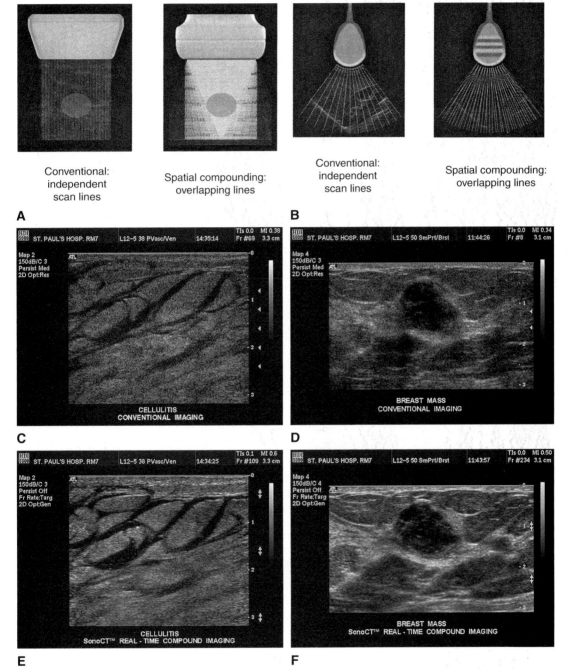

■ **FIGURE 4-29** Conventional scan lines and spatial compounding with **(A)** linear array and **(B)** convex array. A comparison of conventional imaging **(C** and **D)** with compound imaging **(E** and **F)** shows improvement in image quality.

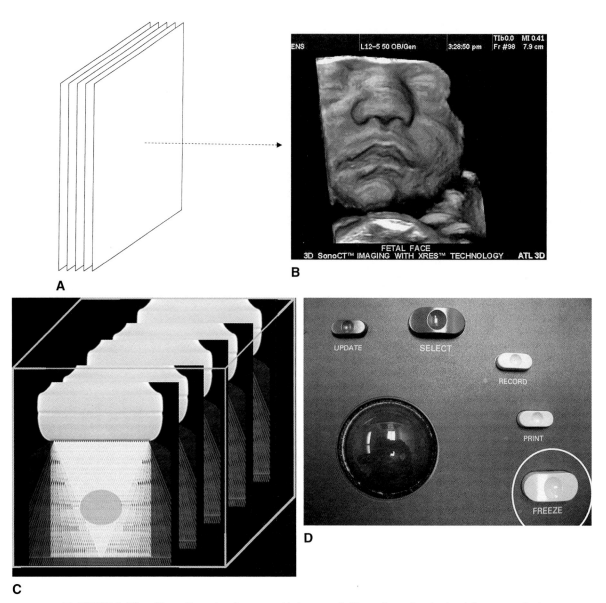

A

B

C

D

■ **FIGURE 4-30** Three-dimensional sonographic images. **A,** Three-dimensional echo data are acquired by obtaining many parallel two-dimensional sections of echo information from the imaged anatomy yielding **(B)** a three-dimensional image. **C,** Another representation of the building up of a three-dimensional volume of echo information from successive parallel two-dimensional scans. **D,** The freeze button stops scanning and saves the last several image frames in image memory.

assigned to each pixel is an electronic device that is binary (*bi* meaning two), like an on-off switch (Figure 4-32, *A*) and so can operate only in two conditions corresponding to one or zero. This would allow only **bistable** (black-and-white) imaging (Figure 4-32, *B* and *C*). To image gray scale (several shades of gray or brightness, in addition to black and white), storage of one of *several* possible numbers in each memory location is necessary. This requires the memory to have more than one matrix. These "checkerboards" can be thought of as being layered back to back. In a four-binary-digit memory, there are four checkerboards back to back

(Figure 4-32, *D*) so that each pixel has 4 **bits** (binary digits) associated with it. In the binary numbering system, this allows numbers from 0 to 15 to be stored (a 16-shade system). Thus a 4-bit memory is a 16-shade memory. A 4-bit memory has four binary digits assigned to each pixel, that is, four layers of memory.

The memory divides the image into pixels, such as a matrix of 512 × 384.

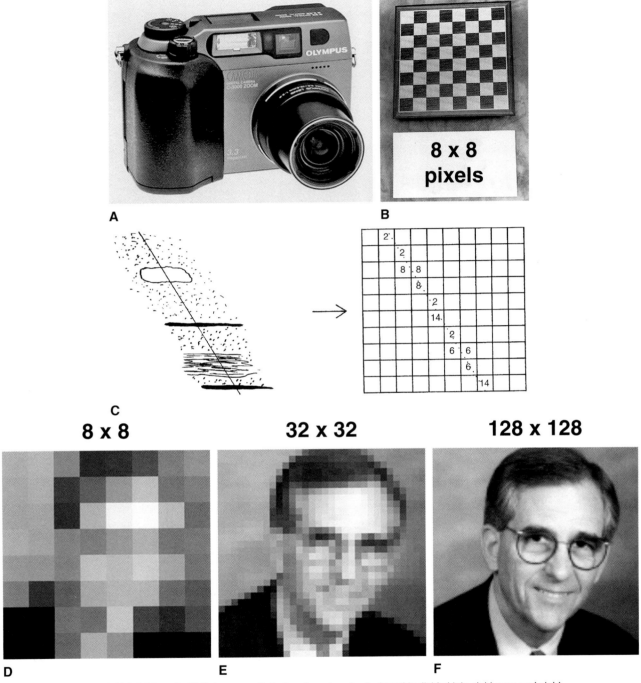

■ **FIGURE 4-31** **A,** Digital camera. **B,** A chessboard or checkerboard is divided into eight rows and eight columns of squares, for a total of 64 "pixels." **C,** Anatomic cross section to be scanned, and the front view of a portion of the image memory. Numbers are stored in the memory elements according to the intensity of the echoes received from corresponding anatomic locations as an ultrasound pulse passes through them. **D** to **F,** Digital photos at pixel resolutions of 8×8, 32×32, and 128×128, respectively.

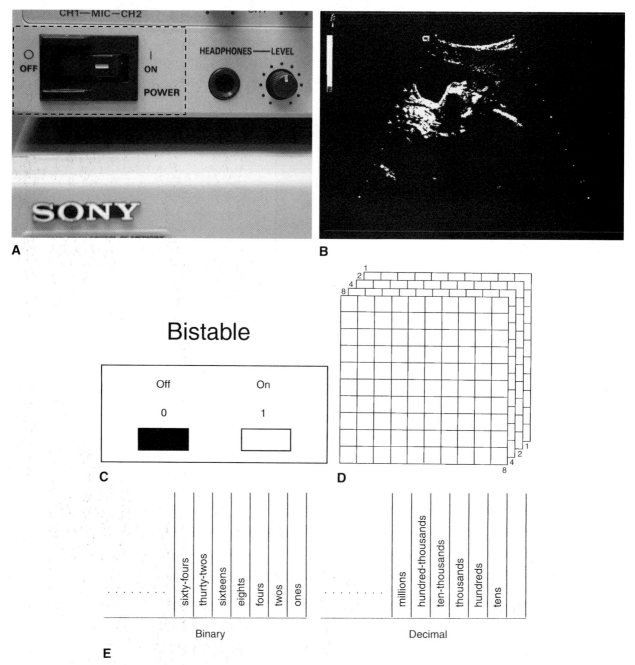

■ **FIGURE 4-32** **A,** Each digital memory element is like a switch, with 1 as on and 0 as off. **B,** Bistable image of fetal head and neck. **C,** In bistable imaging, only two values are used: memory element off represents 0 and is presented as black; memory element on represents 1 and is presented as white. **D,** A 10 × 10-pixel, 4-bit-deep (4 bits per pixel) digital memory. **E,** Columns in decimal numbers represent multiples of 10, whereas those in binary numbers represent multiples of 2.

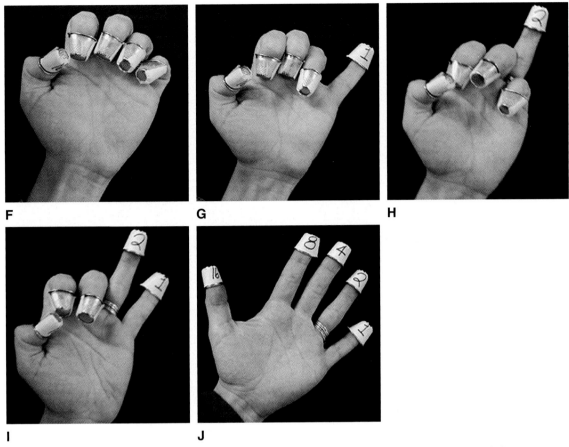

■ FIGURE 4-32, cont'd **F** to **J**, Conventional counting with fingers assigns the value 1 to each finger. Counting is much more efficient if different values are assigned to different fingers. Using the binary assignment procedure, each finger represents double the value of the previous finger. Normally we count only to 5 on one hand, but in this manner we can count to 31 (1 + 2 + 4 + 8 + 16) and to 1023 on two hands.

Binary Numbers

Because the memory elements are binary, digital memories use the binary numbering system to store echo information in image memory. Computer memories and processors use binary numbers in carrying out their functions because they contain electronic components that operate in only two states, representing the numbers 0 and 1.

Binary digits (bits) consist of only zeros and ones, represented by their respective numeric symbols, 0 and 1. Other values must be represented by moving these symbols to different positions (columns). In the decimal system, in which there are 10 different symbols, 0 through 9, there is no single symbol for the number 10 (9 is the largest number for which there is a single symbol). To represent 10 in symbolic form then, the symbol for one is used, but it is moved to the left, to the second column. A 0 is placed in the right column to clarify this, resulting in the symbol 10. The same symbol used to represent one is used, but in such a way—that is, in the second column—that it no longer represents one but rather ten.

A similar procedure is used in the binary numbering system. The symbol 1 represents the largest number (one) for which there is a symbol in this system. To represent the next number (two), the same thing is done as in the decimal system; that is, the symbol 1 is placed in the next column to represent the number 2. In this case, a 1 in the second column represents a value of 2 rather than 10, as in the decimal system. Columns in the two systems represent values as shown in Figure 4-32, *D* to *J*. In the decimal system, each column represents 10 times the column to its right. In the binary system, each column represents 2 times the column to its right.

Table 4-2 lists the binary forms of the decimal numbers 0 to 63. Numbers 64 to 127 would have one additional digit (representing the sixty-fourth column), and so forth with higher multiples of 2.

TABLE 4-2 Binary and Decimal Number Equivalents

Decimal	Binary	Decimal	Binary
0	000000	32	100000
1	000001	33	100001
2	000010	34	100010
3	000011	35	100011
4	000100	36	100100
5	000101	37	100101
6	000110	38	100110
7	000111	39	100111
8	001000	40	101000
9	001001	41	101001
10	001010	42	101010
11	001011	43	101011
12	001100	44	101100
13	001101	45	101101
14	001110	46	101110
15	001111	47	101111
16	010000	48	110000
17	010001	49	110001
18	010010	50	110010
19	010011	51	110011
20	010100	52	110100
21	010101	53	110101
22	010110	54	110110
23	010111	55	110111
24	011000	56	111000
25	011001	57	111001
26	011010	58	111010
27	011011	59	111011
28	011100	60	111100
29	011101	61	111101
30	011110	62	111110
31	011111	63	111111

Binary numbers use only the digits 0 and 1. Each column of a binary number represents double the column to its right.

Table 4-3 gives several examples of digital memories. Figure 4-32, *D*, shows a 10 × 10, 4-bit (per pixel) memory. Table 4-4 gives the total number of memory elements in various digital memories. A group of 8 bits is called a byte, and 1024 bytes (8192 bits) are called a kilobyte. Common in ultrasound instruments today are 6-, 7-, and 8-bit memories. Human vision can differentiate about 100 gray levels. More than the 256 shades of an 8-bit system are not appreciated directly in human vision.

In summary then, the procedure for entering the echo information required for display of the 2D cross-sectional image into a digital memory is as follows:

■ The beam is scanned through the patient in such a way that it "cuts," like a knife, through the tissue cross section.

■ Echoes received from all points on this cross section are converted to numbers that are stored at corresponding pixel locations in the digital memory.

■ All the information necessary for displaying this cross-sectional image now is stored in memory.

■ The information then can be taken out of memory and presented on a 2D display and in such a way that the numbers coming out of memory are displayed with corresponding pixel brightnesses on the face of the display (Figure 4-33).

Figure 4-34 shows examples of such presentations. To enlarge the pixels, read magnification (sometimes called zoom) is used. In this presentation, rather than viewing all the pixels in memory, the monitor shows a smaller group of pixels in expanded (magnified) fashion. This increases pixel size, making the pixel composition of the image more obvious. Write magnification is also available on some instruments. This allows a smaller anatomic field of view to be written into the entire memory, thereby enlarging the image without enlarging pixel size (Figure 4-35). Write zoom is a preprocessing function.

Digital (derived from the Latin term *digitus*, meaning finger or toe) memories are discrete rather than continuous, which means that they can store only whole numbers in each pixel location. These numbers range

TABLE 4-3 Characteristics of Digital Memories

Bits per Pixel	Lowest Number Stored		Highest Number Stored		No. of Shades
	Decimal	Binary	Decimal	Binary	
4	0	0000	15	1111	16
5	0	00000	31	11111	32
6	0	000000	63	111111	64
7	0	0000000	127	1111111	128
8	0	00000000	255	11111111	256

TABLE 4-4 Bits (Binary Digits or Memory Elements) in Digital Memories with 512 × 512 (262,144) Pixels

Bits per Pixel	Total Bits	Total Kilobytes*
4	1,048,576	128
5	1,310,720	160
6	1,572,864	192
7	1,835,008	224
8	2,097,152	256

*1 byte = 8 bits; 1 kilobyte = 1024 bytes, or 8192 bits.

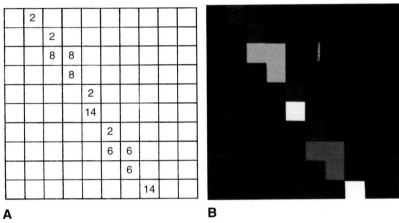

A **B**

■ **FIGURE 4-33** For display of scanned anatomic structures, numbers are read out of pixel locations in digital memory **(A)** and applied to the display in such a way that pixel brightness corresponds to those stored numbers **(B).** The display for the scan line acquired in Figure 4-31, C, is shown.

TABLE 4-5 Contrast Resolution of Digital Memories

	40-dB Dynamic Range		60-dB Dynamic Range	
Bits per Pixel	Decibels per Shade	Intensity Difference (%)*	Decibels per Shade	Intensity Difference (%)*
4	2.5	78	3.8	140
5	1.2	32	1.9	55
6	0.6	15	0.9	23
7	0.3	7	0.5	12
8	0.2	5	0.2	5

*The average difference required between two echoes for the echoes to be assigned different shades.

from zero to a maximum that is determined by the number of bits per pixel (Table 4-3).

For a 256 × 512 matrix in which the represented anatomic width and depth are 10 and 20 cm, respectively, each pixel represents an anatomic dimension of 0.4 mm. This represents the spatial (detail) resolution of the memory matrix. If the width and depth are 5 and 10 cm, then the memory spatial resolution is 0.2 mm. Detail resolution usually is limited by spatial pulse length and beam width rather than by pixel density in the memory.

Contrast Resolution

For linear assignment of echo intensities to numbers in memory, the echo dynamic range is equally divided throughout the gray levels of the system. Table 4-5 gives, for 4- to 8-bit systems, the number of decibels of dynamic range covered by each shade (for two different echo dynamic range values, 40 dB and 60 dB, after attenuation compensation) and the average intensity difference between two echoes for them to be assigned to different shades (different numbers) in memory. This relates to

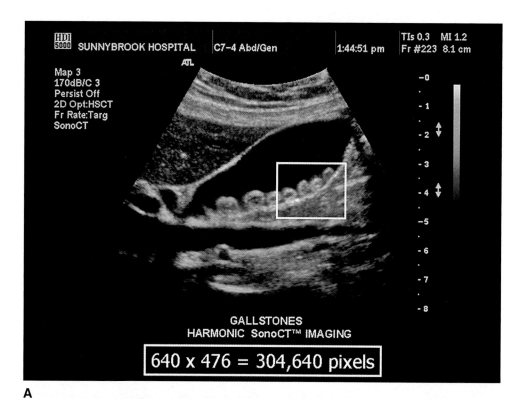

A

B

■ **FIGURE 4-34** Displays of pixels of various brightnesses representing various numbers in the corresponding memory locations. The display is magnified (zoom) here to make the square pixels more easily discernible. Normally the pixels are too small and numerous to be noticed individually. **A,** Unmagnified abdominal image containing 304,640 unresolved pixels. The box encloses the region magnified in **B.** Magnification reveals the 7722 pixels included within the box in **A.** The circle and the box enclose regions of small and large numbers in image memory, respectively.

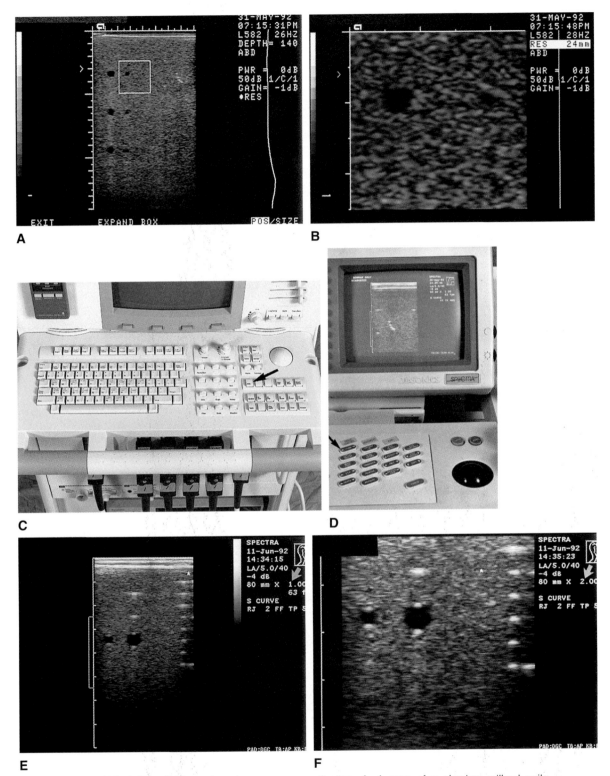

■ **FIGURE 4-35** Write and read zoom or magnification. **A,** A scan of a phantom without write magnification. **B,** A scan using write magnification. Included are 4- and 2-mm simulated cysts. **C,** On this control panel, write magnification is indicated by RES *(arrow)*, meaning regional expansion selection. **D,** Read magnification, or zoom *(arrow)*, when applied to an "unzoomed" image **(E)**, magnifies the stored pixels **(F).**

contrast resolution, the ability visually to observe subtle echo strength differences between adjacent tissues. Increasing the number of bits per pixel (more gray shades) improves contrast resolution. For a 4-bit, 40-dB dynamic range system, an echo must have nearly twice the intensity of another one for it to be assigned a different shade. With a 60-dB dynamic range, more than twice the intensity would be required. For a 6-bit, 40-dB system, only a 15% difference is required. For an 8-bit, 60-dB system, a 5% difference is sufficient. Table 4-5 and Figure 4-36 show how a greater number of shades or a reduced dynamic range improves contrast resolution.

Contrast resolution is the ability of a gray-scale display to distinguish between echoes of slightly different intensities. Contrast resolution depends on the number of bits per pixel in the image memory.

Postprocessing

Signal processing and image processing done before storing of the echo information in image memory are called preprocessing. In general, preprocessing includes all that is done to echoes before they are stored in memory (Figure 4-37). Image processing accomplished after memory is called **postprocessing**. In general, postprocessing includes everything done with echoes as they are brought out of memory to be displayed. Read magnification is an example. Sometimes these terms are used in a more restricted sense to include only *digital* processing, that is, those processes that occur between the ADC and the **digital-to-analog converter**. An even more restrictive definition includes only those processes executed after the formation of the image (after scan conversion). Embedded in all this is another definition of preprocessing, that is, the determination of specific numbers to be assigned to echo intensities as they are stored in memory (Figure 4-36). Postprocessing is the assignment of specific display brightnesses to numbers retrieved from memory (Figure 4-38). Some aspects of preprocessing such as persistence and image depth are operator controllable. Postprocessing is also an operator-controllable operation.

Postprocessing is image processing performed on image data retrieved from memory. Postprocessing determines how echo data stored in memory will appear on the display.

One can easily determine whether a function is preprocessing or postprocessing. If the function cannot be performed on a frozen image, it is probably a preprocessing function (e.g., image depth and write magnification). If the function can be performed on a frozen image, it is a postprocessing function. In rare cases a postprocessing function cannot be performed on a frozen image because of operational or regulatory reasons.

Preprocessing functions cannot be performed on frozen images. Postprocessing functions can be performed on frozen images.

ADVANCED CONCEPTS

A complication to the previous statement is that when the freeze button is activated, some instruments store the serial scan line data before scan conversion. In that case, gain and other preprocessing functions *can* be performed on the frozen image because these control functions *follow* the stored echo data in the processing chain.

On most instruments, preprogrammed postprocessing brightness assignment schemes are selectable by the operator. On some, the postprocessing curve may be designed as desired by the operator using panel controls. A linear assignment (Figure 4-38) equally divides the display brightness range among the stored gray levels of the system. This can be in white-echo (Figure 4-38, *D*) or black-echo (Figure 4-38, *E*) form although the latter is seldom used. The assignment rules for these two schemes are the inverse of each other (Figure 4-38, *A* and *B*). Other schemes (Figure 4-39) may be used that allow assignment of more of the brightness range to certain portions of the stored number range capability of the system. This can improve the presentation and perception of small echo strength differences stored in memory (improved contrast resolution). Liver metastases (Figure 4-40) illustrate the importance of contrast resolution, because they can be just slightly more or less echogenic than the surrounding normal liver tissue. The less difference in echogenicity, the more difficult it is to detect the masses. First, more gray shades (more bits per pixel) will be required to store the echoes emanating from metastases with different numbers in memory than those for the surrounding liver. Even then, if a linear postprocessing assignment is used, these small number differences in memory may not be observed in the display. For example, in Figure 4-40, *E*, in which more gray-scale range is assigned to the weaker echoes, if normal and abnormal tissue echoes differed by one digit in memory (e.g., normal = 40; abnormal = 41), there would be a 1.2% difference in brightness (gray

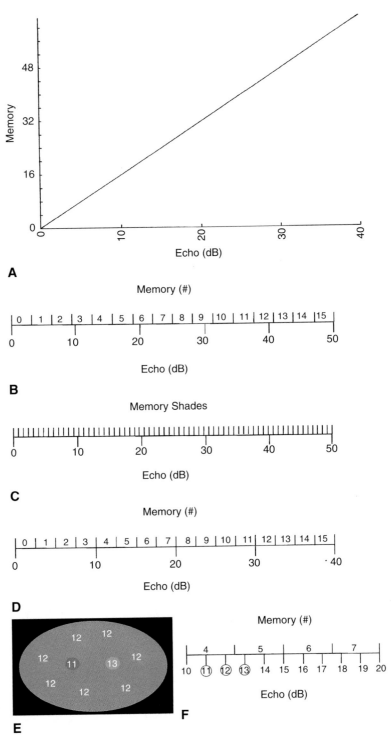

■ **FIGURE 4-36** **A,** Assignment of numbers (to be stored in memory) to echo intensities. Echo intensity is expressed in decibels in the form of a straight-line assignment (relative to the weakest echo, which is represented as 0 dB). The strongest echo is 40 dB, which is 10,000 times the intensity of the weakest). An instrument dynamic range of 40 dB and a 6-bit (64-shade) memory are assumed. **B,** With a 4-bit memory, a 50-dB dynamic range is divided into 16 regions (shades). **C,** With a 6-bit memory, a 50-dB dynamic range is divided into 64 regions, which are numbered 0 to 63. **D,** With a 4-bit memory, a 40-dB dynamic range is divided into 16 regions. **E,** Liver echoes are 12 dB in strength on the dynamic range scale, whereas two metastasic regions have strength 11 and 13 dB. These regions should be displayed slightly darker and lighter as shown. **F,** The 10- to 20-dB dynamic range portion of **D** is expanded. If normal liver echoes were 12 dB (assigned 4 in memory) and metastases were 13 dB (slightly hyperechoic; assigned 5), the normal and abnormal would be different in memory and would appear with different brightness on the display. If the metastases were 11 dB (slightly hypoechoic), they would be assigned 4 in memory, just as would the normal echoes, and the difference would be lost (identical displayed brightnesses).

Continued.

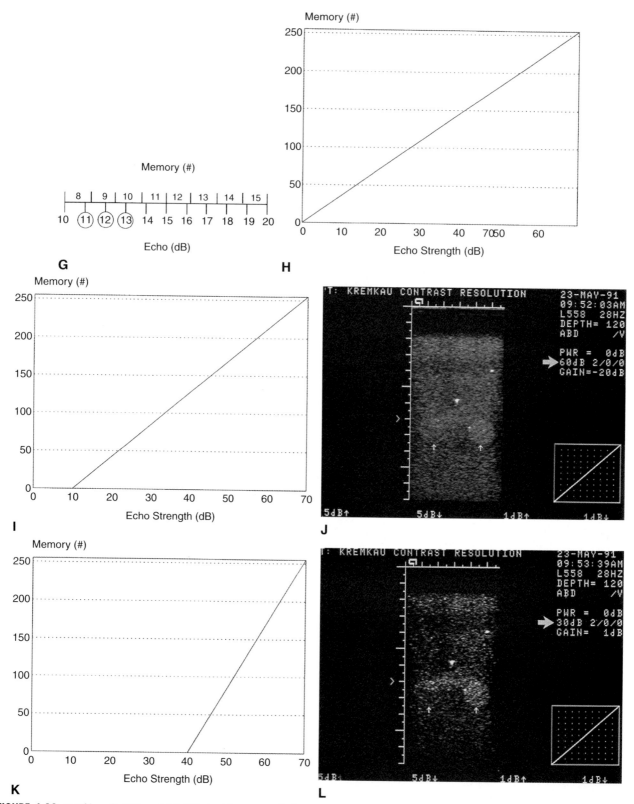

■ **FIGURE 4-36, cont'd** **G,** With a 5-bit (32-shade) memory, both metastatic regions in **E** would be assigned numbers different from those for normal liver and different from each other; that is, contrast resolution would be maintained for both. A dynamic range or compression (preprocessing) control reassigns echo intensities in memory, with the weaker portion as zeros and the remainder in linear fashion. The compression control is set at maximum (70 dB; **H**), 60 dB (**I** and **J**), and 30 dB (**K** and **L**). With decreasing dynamic range, more of the weaker portion is assigned to zero in memory *(black on the display)*, and the contrast of the remainder *(displayed)* is enhanced with improved contrast resolution.

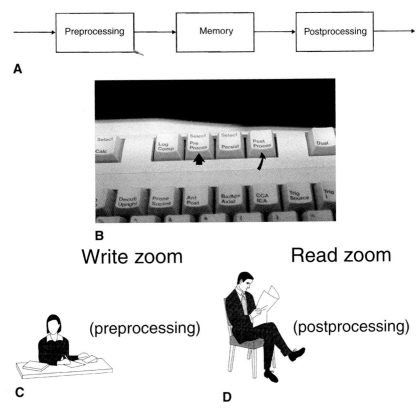

■ **FIGURE 4-37**   **A,** Preprocessing (*straight arrow* in **B**) includes operations performed on echoes before storage in memory. Postprocessing (*curved arrow* in **B**) includes operations performed after information is stored in memory. Write (**C;** see Figure 4-35, *B*) and read (**D;** see Figure 4-35, *F*) magnification are examples of preprocessing and postprocessing, respectively.

level) between the two on the display. This difference could be observed. However, with linear postprocessing (see Figure 4-40, *D*), there would be only a 0.4% brightness difference, which would go unnoticed. In Figure 4-40, *E*, the improvement in contrast resolution for weaker echoes (because of the steeper slope for echoes assigned values 0 to 64 in memory) is accomplished at the cost of degraded contrast resolution for the remainder of the dynamic range (shallow slope for echoes assigned values 65 to 255 in memory). Figure 4-41, *A* and *B*, shows a hemangioma the presentation of which is enhanced by using a specially crafted, steep postprocessing assignment at the echo level corresponding to the hemangioma echogenicity. The contrast between the abnormal and normal tissues is greatly increased. If the mass were not obvious with linear postprocessing, the steep slope assignment likely would have made it visible.

B Color

Some instruments have the postprocessing ability to present different echo intensities in various colors rather than in gray shades, that is, the ability to colorize echoes. In this case, various colors, rather than gray levels, are assigned to various echo intensities. Because the eye can differentiate more color tints than gray shades, color displays offer improved contrast resolution capability. This process is called B color or color scale (compared with gray scale). A color bar is included in such displays to show how colors are assigned to various echo strengths. Figure 4-41, *C* to *E*, shows examples. See Color Plate 3.

B color is a form of postprocessing that improves contrast resolution by assigning colors, rather than gray shades, to different echo strengths.

Three-Dimensional Presentation

Common ways of presenting 3D echo data (Figure 4-42) include surface renderings, 2D slices through the 3D volume, and transparent views. The advantage of the 2D slice presentation is that image plane orientations can be presented that are impossible to obtain with conventional 2D scanning. Surface renderings are popular in obstetric imaging. Transparent views allow

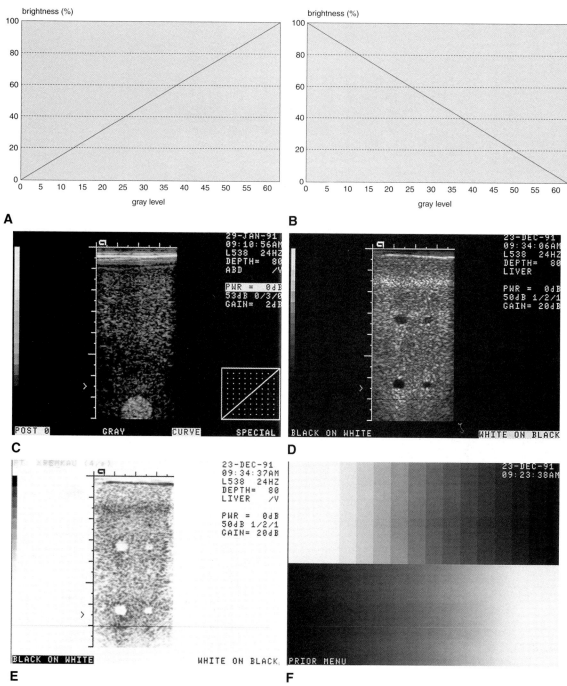

■ **FIGURE 4-38**   Postprocessing is the assignment of specific display brightnesses to numbers derived from specific pixel locations in memory. **A,** Brightness increases with increasing echo intensity (i.e., gray level stored in memory). This is called a white-echo display. **B,** Brightness increases with decreasing echo intensity (black-echo display). Both forms of display were common in the early days of gray-scale imaging. The latter is now seldom used because the white-echo display has been shown to be superior. **C** and **D,** Examples of the numerical assignment shown in **A. E,** Example of the numerical assignment shown in **B. F,** The upper portion shows 16 shades using a numerical assignment similar to that of **B.** The lower portion shows 256 shades and uses a numerical assignment similar to that of **A.** In both cases, echo strength increases to the right.

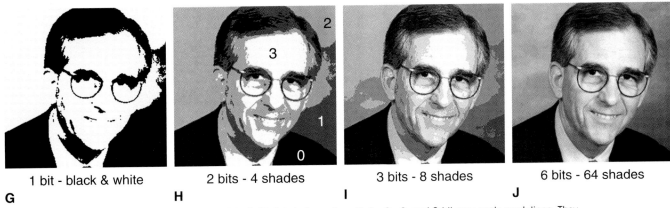

1 bit - black & white   2 bits - 4 shades   3 bits - 8 shades   6 bits - 64 shades

G   **H**   **I**   **J**

■ **FIGURE 4-38, cont'd**   **G** to **J,** Digital photographs with 1-, 2-, 3- and 6-bit gray-scale resolutions. They yield 2 (black and white), 4, 8, and 64 shades, respectively.

"see-through" imaging of anatomy similar to plain film radiographs. These presentation choices are postprocessing choices that present the stored 3D volume of echo information in different ways on the display.

> *A 3D volume of echo data can be displayed in several ways, including 2D slices, surface renderings, and transparent views.*

Digital-to-Analog Converter

After numbers are retrieved from memory and postprocessed, they are converted into voltages that determine the brightnesses of echoes on the display. This task is accomplished by the digital-to-analog converter. The digital-to-analog converter converts the digital data received from the image processor to analog voltages that are fed to the display to determine the echo brightnesses displayed (Figure 4-42, *H*)

DISPLAY

The information delivered to the display can be presented in several ways. Common to all clinical applications is brightness mode, also called **B mode, B scan,** or gray-scale sonography. In echocardiography, motion mode **(M mode)** also is used. In ophthalmology, amplitude mode **(A mode)** also is used.

Cathode-Ray Tube

The display device commonly used is a **cathode-ray tube** (CRT). This tube generates a sharply focused beam of electrons that produces a spot of light on the phosphor-coated, fluorescent, inner front face of the tube (Figure 4-43). The beam can be moved across or up and down the face by applying electric currents to electromagnetic deflection coils surrounding the neck of the tube. If the currents are varied properly, the spot can be made to move across the face in a specific pattern. At the completion of this pattern (i.e., when a display image is completed), the spot jumps rapidly back to the starting point and the next image is begun. The number of images presented per second is called the **refresh rate** of the display.

The brightness of the spot at any location is determined by the strength of the electron beam. Because we do not want to display the *numbers* that represent the echo intensities in the image memory but rather pixels with proportional brightnesses, these numbers must be converted by the digital-to-analog converter to proportional voltages that control the electron beam strength in the CRT.

> *The common display is a CRT that presents an image by scanning a spot of light in horizontal lines from upper left to lower right, left to right, top to bottom.*

The entire chain of events covered thus far is illustrated in Figure 4-44. B mode operation causes a brightening of the spot for each echo in memory. The brightness (gray scale) is proportional to the echo strength. The memory is filled with echoes from many pulses as the beam is scanned through the tissue cross section to be imaged. The B scan is a brightness image that represents an anatomic cross section in the scanning plane, as if the sound beam cuts a section through the tissue like a knife. Each individual image is called a frame. Because several frames can be acquired and

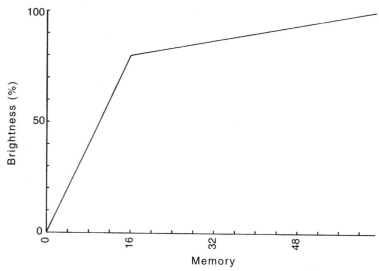

A

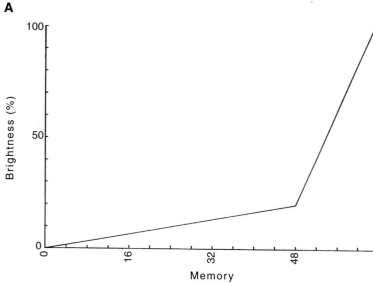

B

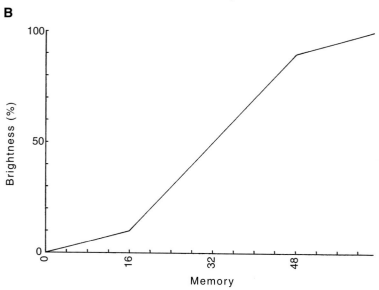

C

■ **FIGURE 4-39** Nonlinear postprocessing assignment schemes. A large brightness range is reserved for weak **(A)**, strong **(B)**, and intermediate-strength **(C)** echoes. Each area has improved contrast resolution at the expense of poorer contrast resolution in the remainder of the dynamic range.

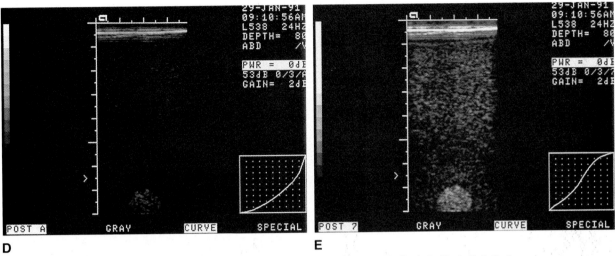

■ FIGURE 4-39, cont'd **D,** A display using a postprocessing curve similar to that in **B. E,** A display using a postprocessing curve similar to that in **C.** Compare **D** and **E** with the linear case in Figure 4-38, C.

presented in each second of time, this is called a real-time display.

In summary, the frame rate is the number of sonographic images entered into image memory per second, while the refresh rate is the number of times per second that images are retrieved from memory and presented on the display. They can be, but are not necessarily, equal.

Computer Monitor

Sonographic images are presented on computer monitors because they represent digital information that is stored in image memory. Computer monitors present image information in the form of horizontal lines on the display (Figure 4-45, A). The electron beam in the CRT scans in a left-to-right, top-to-bottom format, starting at the top left and ending at the bottom right. Each horizontal display scan line corresponds to a row of digital data in image memory. The information is read out of memory, row by row (much as we read a page of text), and is written on the display, line by line, like writing on a lined sheet of paper. Because the display includes more than the sonographic image (such as alphanumeric data, icons, and Doppler spectral display), the data in memory are of various types. But whatever is stored in a given pixel in memory (whether it be part of a gray-scale anatomic image, part of an alphabetic letter, or anything else) will appear at the corresponding pixel location on the display with the appropriate brightness and color.

Because color is used in some cases, such as B color and color Doppler, color displays are common in sonographic instruments. Color CRTs include three cathodes and thousands of triple-groups of tiny, colored (red, green, blue) phosphor dots on the inside face of the tube. As the instrument scans the echo data in image memory, each of the three electron beams is aimed at corresponding colored dots; that is, the "red" beam is aimed at the red dots, the "green" beam at the green dots, and the "blue" at the blue. The dots in each group are so tiny and close together that we see them merged together as one. Red, green, and blue are known as primary additive colors because various combinations of them can produce nearly any color desired. For example, red and green, mixed equally, produce yellow. Green and blue produce cyan, the technical term for aqua. Red and blue produce magenta. Red, green, and blue, equally mixed, produce white (or gray, depending on brightness).

Various standards are used in computer displays. An example is the SVGA (super video graphics array) standard in which the pixel matrix can be, among other values, 1024 by 768 and the display refresh rate is 60 Hz.

> *A computer monitor is a CRT that presents data retrieved from memory in a 2D pixel matrix, refreshing the display often (e.g., 60 times per second).*

Flat-Panel Display

Flat-panel displays have been on notebook (laptop) computers from the start and recently have begun to appear with desktop computers and television sets. They now are beginning to be used on sonographic

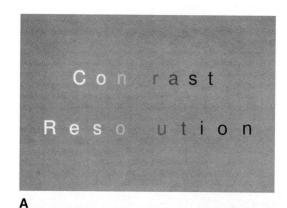

A

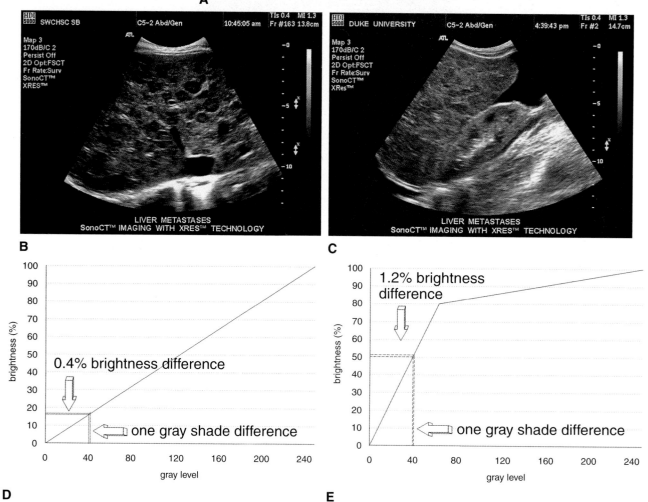

■ **FIGURE 4-40** **A,** Contrast resolution is the ability of a gray-scale display to distinguish between echoes of slightly different amplitudes or intensities. **B,** Normal liver and kidney. **C,** Liver metastases that are less echogenic (and therefore darker) than the surrounding liver tissue. Two tissue regions with slightly different echogenicities require good contrast resolution to be observed with different brightnesses. This requires enough gray levels so that echoes from the two regions are stored in memory with different numbers to indicate their different strengths (echogenicities). However, even then the differences may not be observed on the display if they are minimal. **D,** In this example, one tissue region has echoes stored as gray level 40, whereas an adjacent region has echoes stored at gray level 41. These two regions would differ in brightness by 0.4% using a linear postprocessing assignment. This difference would not be noticed by a human observer. **E,** Using a different postprocessing choice, the brightness difference is 1.2%, which could be observed.

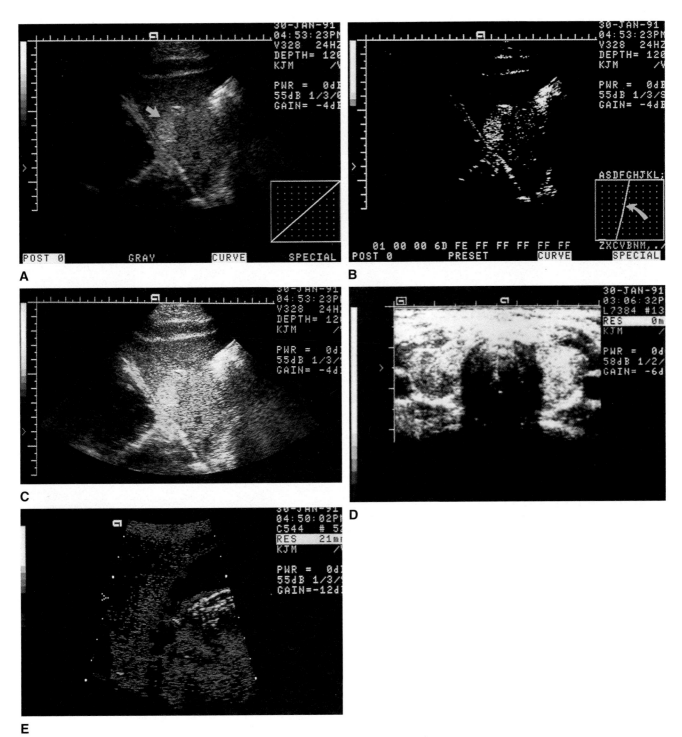

■ **FIGURE 4-41** **A,** An image of a hemangioma *(arrow)* obtained using linear postprocessing. **B,** An image of a hemangioma with a steep postprocessing assignment *(curved arrow)* designed to produce a great contrast between these normal and abnormal tissue echoes. **C** to **E,** Color displays of a hemangioma (**C;** compare with **A** and **B**), thyroid **(D)**, and gallbladder **(E)**. Color assignments, shown in the color bars on the left, are designated as follows: **(C)** temperature (increasing intensity assigned dark orange through yellow to white), **(D)** magenta (dark magenta through light magenta to white), and **(E)** rainbow (dark violet through various colors to white). (See Color Plate 3.)

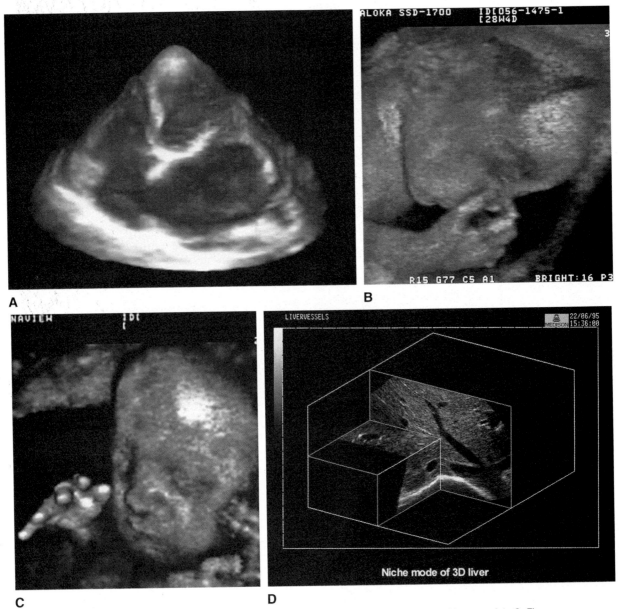

■ FIGURE 4-42 Various postprocessing choices for presented three-dimensional images. **A** to **C**, Three-dimensional surface renderings. **A**, Cardiac image. **B**, Fetus holding nose. **C**, Fetal head and hands. **D**, Three orthogonal two-dimensional slices through the three-dimensional liver echo volume.

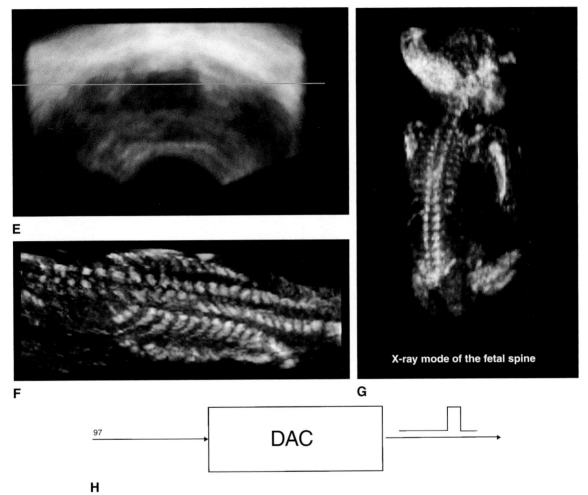

X-ray mode of the fetal spine

97 → DAC → ⊓

■ FIGURE 4-42, cont'd **E** to **G,** Transparent (x-ray) mode. **E,** All echoes in the volume can be included, as in this image of the prostate, or (**F** and **G**) only the strongest ones. **H,** The digital-to-analog converter (*DAC*) converts the numbers (digital) stored in memory to proportional (analog) voltages that control the brightness of the echo on the display.

instruments (Figure 4-45, *B* and *C*). Advantages include lighter weight, slim profile (i.e., less bulky), and less power consumption and heat generation. A **flat-panel display** is a backlighted liquid crystal display, or LCD. Such a display is composed of a rectangular matrix of thousands (e.g., a 1024 × 768 matrix contains 786,432) of LCD elements. These elements can be electrically turned on or off individually, acting as tiny light valves for blocking or passing the light from the light source underneath the matrix. More specifically, the elements can be turned on *partially* to allow a measured amount of light through, usually in 256 steps of luminance; that is, 256 displayed gray levels from black to white. Groups of red, green, and blue elements allow what is called 24-bit color (8 bits or 256 luminance values for each primary color element) yielding 16,777,216 possible colors presented at each pixel location.

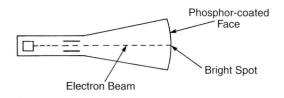

A

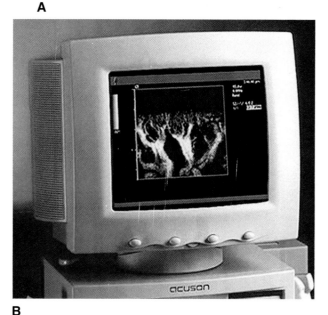

B

■ **FIGURE 4-43** **A**, A cathode-ray tube *(side view)*. The electron beam, generated by a cathode *(the square at left)*, produces a spot of light where it strikes the phosphor-coated (fluorescent) inner front face of the tube. **B**, Sonographic instrument cathode-ray tube display.

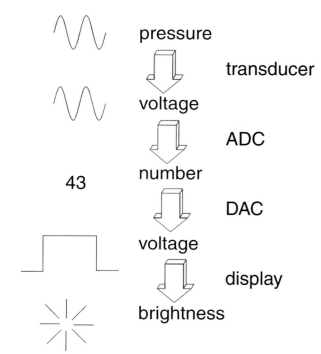

■ **FIGURE 4-44** Information chain from the echo (pressure), through the transducer and electronics, to the display. The analog-to-digital converter *(ADC)* is part of the beam former. An echo is stored as a number in image memory (part of the image processor). The digital-to-analog converter *(DAC)* is part of the image processor.

ADVANCED CONCEPTS

An LCD is composed of a backlighted rectangular matrix of thousands of liquid crystal light valves. These light valves are liquid crystal molecules that are normally in a twisted form but can be untwisted in predictable amounts by an applied electric voltage. In the twisted form they can conduct light through two perpendicular light-polarizing panels. When they are completely untwisted, no light can pass through. Completely twisted, then, yields a white pixel; completely untwisted yields a black pixel. Varying amounts of twisting yield various gray levels. Color displays have groups of three valves with red, green, and blue filters on them. Because these groups are tiny, the individual colors are not seen but merge together to form the resulting observed color.

Various colors are presented on displays by combining what are called primary colors, that is, red, green, and blue, or RGB. Zero amounts of all three yield no light, that is, black. Equal amounts of the three colors produce grays of various brightnesses depending on the amounts. If an image memory can store numbers from 0 to 255 (8-bit memory) for each color and if the stored value for each color is 255, the brightest gray (i.e., white) that the display is capable of producing is displayed. If the stored values are all zero, then the darkest gray is shown (i.e., black).

If equal values of 128 are stored, a midlevel gray will be displayed (i.e., 50% brightness). If equal values of red and green are stored with zero blue, then yellow is displayed. If equal values of red and blue are stored with zero green, then magenta is displayed. And if equal values of green and blue are stored with zero red, then cyan is displayed. With 256 possible levels for each color, the number of possible color tints that can be displayed is 256^3, or 16,777,216.

Luminance is the intensity of light, that is, the radiant power per unit area. Brightness is the human visual perception of luminance, as loudness is the human aural perception of sound intensity. The contrast ratio of a display is the ratio of the maximum to minimum luminance values that it can display. The contrast ratio of typical displays is about 27 dB, that is, a contrast ratio of about 500 to 1.

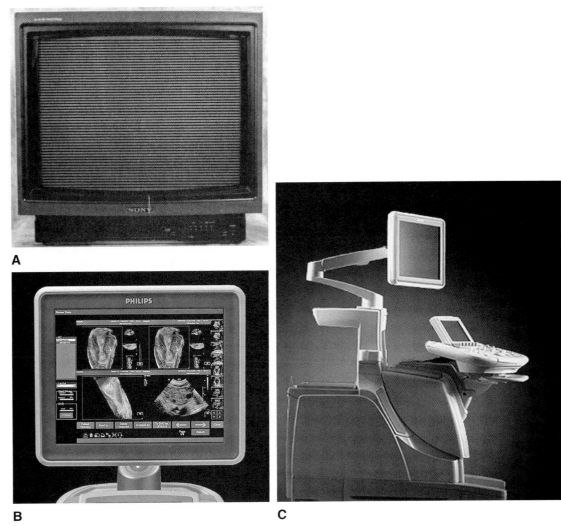

■ **FIGURE 4-45** **A,** The electron beam (and the spot of light it produces) is scanned from left to right, top to bottom in computer monitors. **B** and **C,** Flat-panel displays.

Temporal Resolution

Sonographic instruments store several frames of echo information in image memory per second. The number of sonographic images stored per second is called the frame rate. This is the rate at which the sound beam is scanned through the tissue cross section by the transducer. A rapid sequence of frames yields what appears to be a continuously changing image. The effective frame rate observed on the display is limited by the refresh rate. For example, the echo information may be entering image memory at a frame rate of 100 Hz, but if the refresh rate is 75 Hz, echo information is retrieved from memory 75 times per second, and only 75 images per second are being viewed on the display. However, there is an advantage to storing a frame rate that is higher than the refresh rate. When a frozen cine loop

is displayed, the individual frames retain the temporal resolution achieved with the frame rate.

When the freeze-frame mode is activated, ultrasound beam scanning and echo data entry into memory are halted and the last frame entered is shown continuously on the display. Although the display continues to present what is in memory at the refresh rate, it is the same image every time and so it appears as a static, unchanging image.

Real-time imaging affords rapid and convenient acquisition of the desired image (with the display changing continuously as the scan plane is moved through the tissues) and two-dimensional imaging of the motion of moving structures (with the display changing continuously as the structures move). Temporal resolution is the ability of a display to distinguish closely spaced events in time and to present rapidly

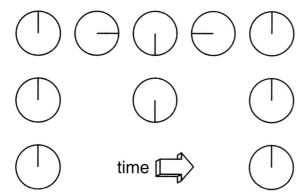

■ **FIGURE 4-46** *Temporal resolution improves with frame rate. (Top row)* A wheel is rotated in a clockwise direction. Four images are taken during one revolution; thus the frame rate is four per revolution. *(Middle row)* With a frame rate of two per revolution, it can be seen that the wheel is rotating, but the direction is ambiguous: it could be clockwise or counterclockwise. *(Bottom row)* The frame rate is one per revolution. The motion of the wheel is not observed; indeed, it appears to be stationary. A similar result would occur in echocardiography if one frame per cardiac cycle were acquired. The heart would appear to be inactive.

moving structures correctly. Temporal resolution is expressed in milliseconds, which is the time from the beginning of one frame to the beginning of the next one. This is also the time required to generate one complete frame. Temporal resolution improves as the frame rate increases (Figure 4-46) because less time elapses from one frame to the next.

Each frame is made of many scan lines. For each focus on each scan line in each frame, a pulse is required. The PRF required, therefore, is determined by the required number of foci *(n)*, lines per frame *(LPF)*, and the frame rate *(FR)* in frames per second, that is, hertz.

For each focus on each scan line in each frame, a pulse is required.

Indeed, the PRF is equal to these three quantities multiplied together.

$$PRF \text{ (Hz)} = n \times LPF \times FR \text{ (Hz)}$$

To increase the number of foci, the PRF must increase.

To increase the number of lines per frame, the PRF must increase.

To increase the frame rate, the PRF must increase.

However, time is required for echoes to return as a pulse travels into the tissue. The greater the penetration, the longer it takes for all the echoes to return (remember the 13 µs/cm rule). To avoid misplacement of echoes on the display because of late arrival, all echoes from one pulse must be received before the next pulse is emitted. To accomplish this, the PRF must decrease as penetration increases.

If penetration increases, the PRF must decrease.

That is, if a lower operating frequency is used, penetration is increased and PRF must decrease to avoid echo misplacement. This will occur as a frame rate reduction (Figure 4-47) for lower operating frequencies. Frame rate decreases when displayed depth is increased (Figure 4-47, *C* and *D*). Likewise, wider images (requiring more scan lines) and multiple foci also reduce frame rate (Figure 4-48) because in both cases, more time is required to generate each frame. The relationship between these competing variables is as follows:

$$\text{pen (cm)} \times n \times LPF \times FR \text{ (Hz)} \leq 77{,}000 \text{ cm/s}$$

If penetration increases, frame rate decreases.

If the number of foci increases, frame rate decreases.

If the lines per frame increases, frame rate decreases.

The symbol ≤ means "less than or equal to." That is, when penetration is multiplied by the number of foci, the number of scan lines per frame, and the frame rate, the result must not exceed 77,000. Otherwise, the PRF required would not allow return of all echoes before emission of the next pulse (resulting in echo misplacement).

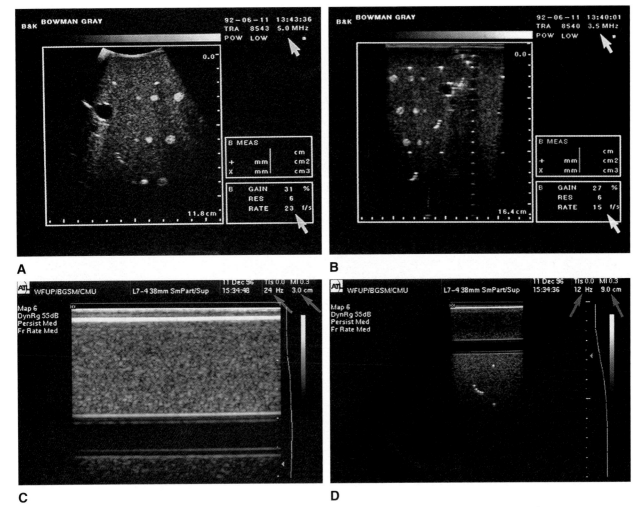

■ **FIGURE 4-47** A lower operating frequency allows greater penetration, thereby necessitating longer echo arrival time, which slows down the frame rate. **A,** 5 MHz, penetration of 9 cm, 23 frames per second. **B,** 3.5 MHz, penetration of 13 cm, 15 frames per second. **C,** With a displayed depth of 3 cm, the frame rate is 24 frames per second (hertz; *arrow*). **D,** A displayed depth increase to 9 cm reduces the frame rate to 12 Hz. At first this seems surprising, because the operating frequency (5.5 MHz) and therefore the penetration, is the same in both cases. However, the effective penetration is reduced with the reduced displayed depth in **C** by increasing the pulse repetition frequency. The echoes from beyond the displayed depth are weaker because of attenuation. When the next pulse is sent, the amplifier gain drops with the restarting of the time gain control. Thus the deeper echoes are not amplified enough to be seen (in incorrect locations, that is, range ambiguity artifact).

ADVANCED CONCEPTS

Previously in this chapter we saw that

$$pen \ (cm) \times PRF \ (kHz) \leq 77 \ (cm/ms)$$

This equation is equivalent to

$$pen \ (cm) \times PRF \ (Hz) \leq 77,000 \ (cm/s)$$

and because

$$PRF = n \times LPF \times FR$$

we have

$$pen \ (cm) \times n \times LPF \times FR \ (Hz) \leq 77,000 \ (cm/s)$$

The number 77,000 is one half the average speed of ultrasound in tissues (154,000 cm/s). The one half results because the penetration (expressed in centimeters) is only half the round-trip distance the sound must travel for the deepest echoes.

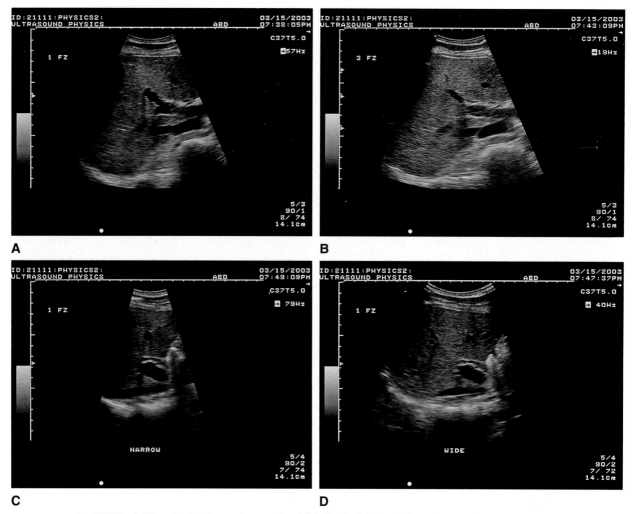

■ **FIGURE 4-48** **A,** One focus; frame rate of 57. **B,** Multiple foci (3) reduce the frame rate to 19. **C,** Frame rate of 79. **D,** An increased frame width (doubling the number of scan lines) reduces the frame rate to 40.

Table 4-6 lists the allowable PRFs and frame rates for various penetration and lines-per-frame values. Multiple foci reduce permitted frame rates inversely (e.g., two foci with a penetration of 20 cm and 100 lines per frame are equivalent to $^{1}/_{2} \times 38$, or 19 frames per second).

Temporal resolution is the ability to follow moving structures in temporal detail. Temporal resolution depends on frame rate, which depends on depth, lines per frame, and number of foci.

For measurement purposes, displays include range marker dots and calipers (Figure 4-49). Marker dots are presented as a series of dots in a line with a given separation (e.g., 1 cm). Calipers are two plus signs (or some other symbol) that can be placed anywhere on the display. The instrument calculates the distance between them and shows it on the display.

TABLE 4-6 Pulse Repetition Frequencies (PRF) and Frame Rates (FR) Permitted for Various Single-Focus Imaging Depths (Penetration) and 100 or 200 Scan Lines per Frame

Penetration (cm)	PRF (Hz)	FR 100 Lines	200 Lines
20	3,850	38	19
15	5,133	51	25
10	7,700	77	38
5	15,400	154	77

M Mode and A Mode

Another common display mode (M mode) is used to show the motion of cardiac structures (Figure 4-50). M mode is a display form that presents depth (vertical

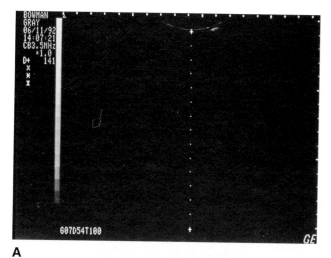

A

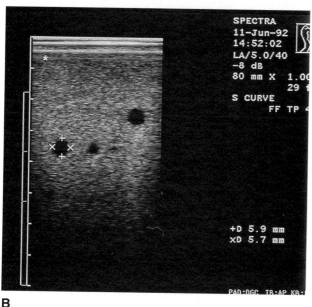

B

■ **FIGURE 4-49** **A,** Range marker dots. **B,** Calipers with 5.7-mm (×) and 5.9-mm (+) separations.

axis) versus time (horizontal). An uncommon display, except in ophthalmologic sonography, shows the amplitudes of echoes and is called A mode. A mode is a depth (vertical) versus amplitude (horizontal) display. Temporal resolution in M and A modes is equal to the pulse repetition period because each pulse produces a new line of echo information on these displays. The sound beam is stationary in these presentations. Ultrasound pulses travel down the same path over and over. In the M mode display the vertical scan lines are written next to each other across the horizontal time axis.

Television Monitor

External television monitors (Figure 4-51) sometimes are connected to video output connectors on sonographic instruments. A television monitor is a CRT in which a particular electron beam-scanning format is used. As with any CRT, the electron beam current is changed continually as the beam is scanned to provide varying brightness of the spot, thus providing a gray-scale image. Color television monitors use triple cathodes and phosphor-dot triplets. The television-scanning format consists of a left-to-right, top-to-bottom scanning pattern consisting of 525 horizontal display scan lines that produce one television frame of a real-time image. This picture is updated 30 times each second. Such a slow frame rate has a displeasing flicker characteristic. Therefore the television picture is scanned in alternating odd and even line fields on the display to reduce the flicker. The field rate is 60 per second (two fields make up one image frame).

Television monitors present images at a rate of 30 per second using 525 horizontal lines interlaced as odd and even line fields.

Output Devices

External recording devices (Figure 4-52) often are provided to allow videotaping of real-time scanning or to produce hard copy of frozen images. These devices include VCRs, color printers, and multiformat film cameras, although they are being phased out in favor of digital devices. Figure 4-53 shows a diagram of the instrument with input and output devices. An internal magneto-optical hard disk commonly is included in the instrument on which images can be stored in digital form. They also can be sent to a computer via a CD (Figure 4-52, *D*) or a USB line. Various standard protocols are used for communicating and storing digital images (e.g., JPEG and TIFF) and video clips (e.g., AVI and MPG). Quality depends on the number of pixels per image and the amount of compression used (image compression is a process that reduces digital file size while retaining data essential to acceptable image quality). Because sonographic images are not collections of random echo data, their repeating patterns allow shortened coding, called lossless compression, to reduce file size. Lossless compression reduces file size to

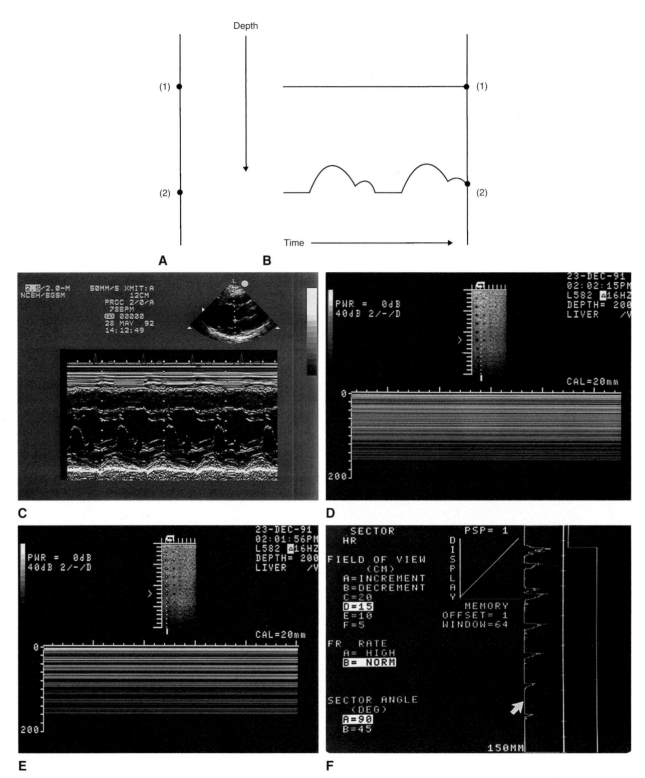

■ **FIGURE 4-50** **A,** B mode presentation of echo depth with echoes from both a stationary structure *(1)* and a moving one *(2)*. **B,** If pulses are sent down the same path repeatedly, and vertical scan lines are placed next to each other, a display of depth-versus-time results. The pattern of motion of moving structures *(2)* is traced out on the display for evaluation. This is called an M mode display. **C,** M mode presentation of a moving structure (mitral valve) in the adult heart. Time increases to the right. The two-dimensional real-time anatomic cross-sectional image also is shown *(upper right)*. **D,** Stationary structures appear on M mode display as straight horizontal lines because there is no motion. **E,** The echo-free regions in the cyst phantom are seen as stationary, horizontal, dark regions on the M mode display. **F,** A series of eight echoes is shown in A mode form *(arrow)*.

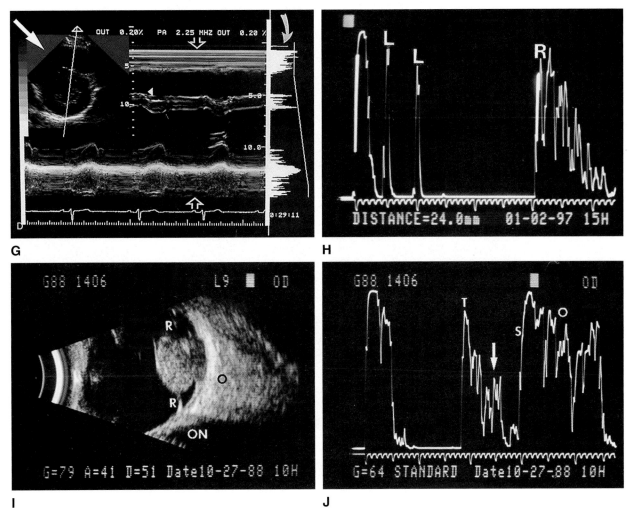

■ FIGURE 4-50, cont'd   G, An echocardiogram, including B scan *(straight arrow),* M mode *(open arrows),* and A mode *(curved arrow)* presentations. **H,** A normal ophthalmologic A mode presentation where *L* represents lens echoes and *R* represents the retina. A longitudinal B scan **(I)** and standardized A mode presentation **(J)** demonstrate the typical acoustic appearance of a choroidal melanoma. The B scan shows a mushroom-shaped mass with exudative retinal detachment *(R)* at the tumor margins *(O,* orbital fat; *ON,* optic nerve). The A mode scan demonstrates a high spike from the tumor surface *(T)* and low to medium echogenicity within the lesion *(arrow) (S,* sclera; *O,* orbital fat).

about half without altering the image. Lossy compression involves visually similar, but not identical, images. The JPEG file is a compressed image file (file extension .jpg). File size is a trade-off with quality. The TIFF file (file extension .tif) has better quality than JPEG but has larger files. The same is true for MPEG (file extension .mpg) compared with AVI (file extension .avi). A single 8-bit (1 byte; 256 shade) uncompressed gray scale image with 1024 × 768 pixels requires 768 kilobytes (kB) of memory for the image data. Including the remaining data for proper handling of the image, the TIFF file size is 779 kB. A moderately compressed JPEG file size for the same image is 83 kB. A comparable color image would have TIFF file size of 2.26 megabytes (MB) (3 times the gray-scale file because data on three primary colors

[red, green, blue] is stored rather than just one color, i.e., gray). The compressed JPEG color file size is 95 kB. Communicating an uncompressed 256 gray-shade video clip of 30, 1024 × 768 pixel frames per second requires data transfer at 189 Mb/s (megabits/second) or 24 MB/s (megabytes/second). Compression such as MPEG reduces this requirement to a more manageable value.

Picture Archiving and Communications Systems

Picture archiving and communications systems provide means for electronically communicating images and associated information to workstations (Figure 4-52, *E*) and devices external to the sonographic instrument, the

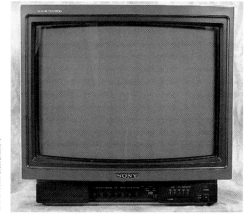

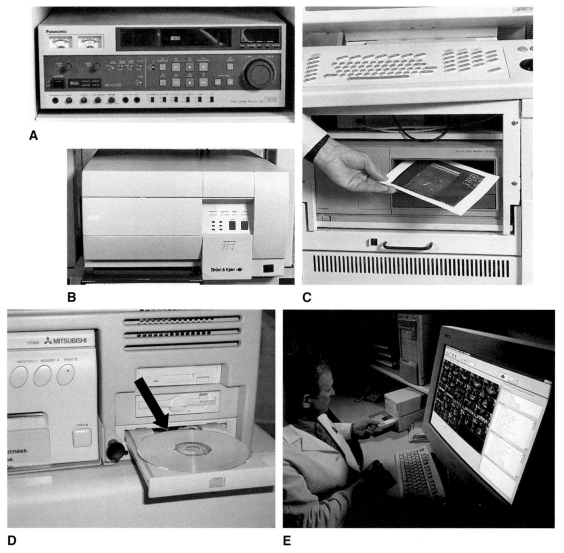

■ **FIGURE 4-51** **A,** The television display format has 525 horizontal display scan lines, which are written out in $\frac{1}{30}$ of a second. Half of these *(alternate, odd, solid lines)* are written first, followed by the remaining ones *(alternate, even, dashed lines)*. Each of these sets of lines (solid or dashed in this illustration) makes up a field. Two fields make a frame. Writing each frame in the format of an odd and an even field reduces flicker. **B,** A television monitor.

■ **FIGURE 4-52** Videocassette recording of real-time scanning **(A)**. Film **(B)** and print recording **(C)** of frozen images. **D,** CD burner in a sonographic instrument (arrow indicates CD in tray). **E,** Picture archiving and communications system workstation.

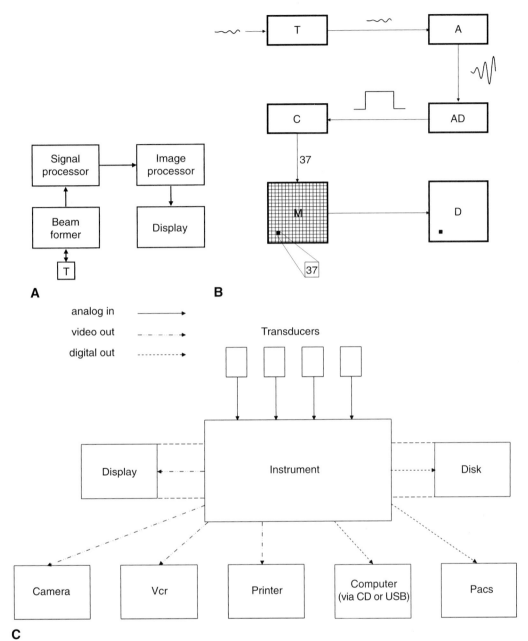

■ **FIGURE 4-53** **A,** Components of a sonographic instrument. **B,** The chain of events as an echo signal travels through the instrument. The transducer *(T)* converts the echo pressure variation to a voltage variation. The amplifier *(A)* increases the amplitude of the echo voltage. The amplitude detector *(AD)* converts the echo voltage from radio frequency to video (amplitude) form.The analog to digital convertor *(C)* digitizes the echo voltage amplitude. The echo amplitude is stored in image memory *(M)*. The echo is presented on the display *(D)*. **C,** Echo information enters the instrument from the transducers in analog form. Image information flows in video form to the internal display and externally to a film camera, VCR, and printer. Image information flows in digital form (numbers) to an internal magneto-optical disk and externally to a computer (via a CD or USB connection) and picture archiving and communications system *(PACS)* to be stored in digital format, just as it is in the image memory of the instrument. Such storage involves no loss of quality and allows postprocessing, measurements, and any other function that can be applied to a stored (frozen) image in the instrument memory.

examining room, and even the building in which the scanning is done. Indeed, through the Internet, these files can be transmitted to virtually anywhere in the world. Picture archiving and communications systems are used with all digital imaging modes, including ultrasound. The protocols for communicating images and associated information between imaging devices and workstations have been standardized in the Digital Imaging and Communications in Medicine (DICOM) standard.[13] This standard specifies a hardware interface, a minimum set of software commands, and a consistent set of data formats. The standard promotes communication of information, regardless of manufacturers of the linked devices, including the sonographic instrument, the picture archiving and communications systems reading station, and other hospital/clinic information systems. The standard also enables the creation of diagnostic information bases that can be interrogated by a wide variety of devices geographically distributed.

REVIEW

The key points presented in this chapter are the following:

■ Sonographic instruments are of the pulse-echo type.
■ These instruments use the strength, direction, and arrival time of received echoes to generate A, B, and M mode displays.
■ Sonographic instruments include a beam former, signal processor, image processor, and display, and often are attached to peripheral recording and display devices.
■ The beam former is responsible for directing, focusing, and optimizing the ultrasound beam on transmission and reception. The beam former also amplifies the echo voltages, compensates for attenuation using TGC, and digitizes the voltages.
■ The signal processor filters, detects, and compresses the echo signal.
■ The scan converter converts the echo data in scan line format to image format for storage and display.
■ A mode presents an echo versus amplitude display.
■ B and M modes use a brightness display echo strength as brightness.
■ M mode shows reflector motion in time. M mode is a presentation of echo depth versus time.
■ B mode scans show anatomic cross sections through the scanning plane.
■ Image memories store echo intensity information as binary numbers in memory elements.
■ Contrast resolution improves with increasing bits per pixel.
■ Real-time imaging is the rapid sequential display of ultrasound images (frames), resulting in a moving presentation.

■ Real-time imaging requires rapid, repeatable, sequential scanning of the sound beam through the tissue. This is accomplished with electronic transducer arrays.
■ Increasing frame rate improves temporal resolution.

EXERCISES

1. The ultrasound pulse repetition frequency is equal to the voltage _____ repetition frequency of the pulser.
2. Increased voltage amplitude produced by the pulser increases the _____ and _____ of ultrasound pulses produced by the transducer.
3. If a 6-MHz transducer images to a depth of 10 cm, to avoid range ambiguity, the maximum pulse repetition frequency permitted is
   a. 7.7 kHz.
   b. 6.0 kHz.
   c. 10.0 kHz.
   d. 1.54 MHz.
   e. 13.0 MHz.
4. Functions performed by the signal processor include _____, _____, and _____.
5. Match the following functions with what they accomplish:
   a. Amplification: _____
   b. Compensation: _____
   c. Filtering: _____
   d. Detection: _____
   e. Compression: _____

   1. Converts pulses from radio frequency to video form
   2. Increases all amplitudes
   3. Decreases dynamic range
   4. Corrects for tissue attenuation
   5. Reduces noise
6. If the input voltage to an amplifier is 1 mV and the output voltage is 10 mV, the voltage amplification ratio is _____. The power ratio is _____. The gain is _____ dB.
7. An amplifier with a gain of 60 dB has 1 μW of power applied to the input. The output power is _____ W.
8. An amplifier with a gain of 60 dB has 10 μV of voltage applied to the input. The output voltage is _____ mV.
9. Time gain compensation is accomplished in the
   a. pulser.
   b. beam former.
   c. signal processor.
   d. scan converter.
   e. image processor.
10. Compensation takes into account reflector _____

11. Compensation amplifies echoes differently, according to their arrival _____.
12. Compression decreases the _____ range to a range that the _____ and human _____ can handle.
13. If a display has a dynamic range of 20 dB and the smallest voltage it can handle is 200 mV, then the largest voltage it can handle is _____ V.
14. Detection converts voltage pulses from _____ form to _____ form.
15. Filtering widens bandwidth. True or false?
16. Filtering is accomplished in the
    a. pulser.
    b. beam former.
    c. signal processor.
    d. scan converter.
    e. image processor.
17. The compression or dynamic range control reduces the range of echo amplitudes displayed by reducing the weakest to _____ and/or the strongest ones to the _____ value and assigning the others to increasing _____. This produces a _____ contrast image with elimination of _____ and maximizing of _____ echoes.
18. An amplifier has a power output of 100 mW when the input power is 0.1 mW. The amplifier gain is _____ dB.
19. If the beam-former output to the transducer is reduced by 3, 6, and 9 dB, the ultrasound pulse output intensity is reduced by _____%, _____%, and _____%, respectively.
20. One watt is _____ dB below 100 W.
21. One watt is _____ dB above 100 mW.
22. If the input power is 1 mW and the output is 10,000 mW, the gain is _____ dB.
23. If an amplifier has a gain of 15 dB, the ratio of output power to input power is _____. (Use Table 4-1.)
24. If the output of a 22-dB gain amplifier is connected to the input of a 23-dB gain amplifier, the total gain is _____ dB. The overall power ratio is _____. (Use Table 4-1.)
25. If a 17-dB electric attenuator is connected to a 15-dB amplifier, the net gain is _____ dB. The net attenuation is _____ dB. For a 1-W input, the output is _____ W. (Use Table 2-3.)
26. For the digital memory shown in Figure 4-54, enter the number stored in each pixel location:
    a. Lower right: _____
    b. Middle right: _____
    c. Upper right: _____
    d. Upper middle: _____
    e. Upper left: _____

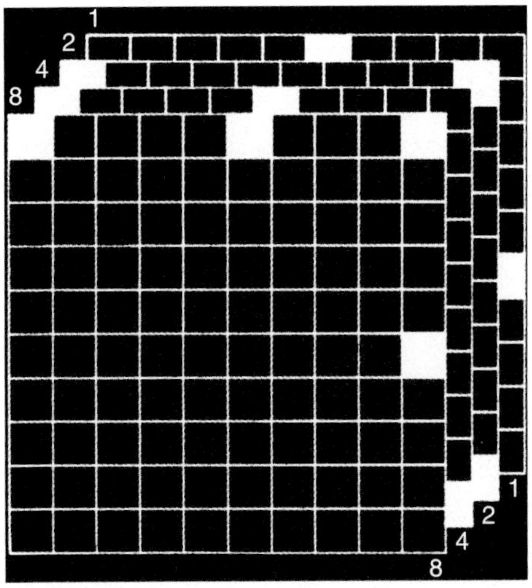

■ **FIGURE 4-54** Digital memory description to accompany Exercise 26. The white indicates that the memory device is on.

27. The contrast resolution for an instrument that has an echo dynamic range of 43 dB and 32 shades is _____ dB per shade.
    a. 1.3
    b. 3.2
    c. 4.3
    d. 32
    e. 43
28. The contrast resolution for an instrument that has a 6-bit memory and a 45-dB echo dynamic range is _____ dB per shade.
    a. 0.3
    b. 0.5
    c. 0.7
    d. 0.9
    e. 6
29. Match the following:
    a. Analog: _____   1. Picture element
    b. Digital: _____   2. Assignment of stored numbers
    c. Preprocessing: 3. Discrete
    _____   4. Binary digit
    d. Postprocessing: 5. Proportional
    _____   6. Assignment of displayed brightness
    e. Pixel: _____
    f. Bit: _____
30. Typical image pixel dimensions are _____.
    a. 640 × 128
    b. 16 × 64
    c. 100 × 100
    d. 512 × 1540
    e. 512 × 384
31. How many bits per pixel are required for each number of shades?

a. 16: _____
b. 32: _____
c. 64: _____
d. 128: _____
e. 256: _____

32. _____ total memory elements are required for a 100×100-pixel, 5-bit digital memory.

33. Memories of _____ bits per pixel are common in ultrasound today.
    a. 4-8
    b. 4-6
    c. 6-8
    d. 5-7
    e. 4-5

34. Digital memories store _____.
    a. Logarithms
    b. Electric magnetism
    c. Electric current
    d. Electric charge
    e. Numbers

35. _____ is commonly controllable by the operator.
    a. Postprocessing
    b. Pixel matrix
    c. Bits per pixel
    d. Digitization
    e. All of the above

36. In binary numbers, how many symbols are used?

37. The term *binary digit* commonly is shortened into the single word _____.

38. Each binary digit in a binary number is represented in memory by a memory element, which at any time is in one of _____ states that are _____ or _____.

39. Match the following:
    Column in an 8-bit binary number hgfedcba:
    Decimal number represented by a 1 in the column:
    a. _____   1. 64
    b. _____   2. 32
    c. _____   3. 1
    d. _____   4. 16
    e. _____   5. 8
    f. _____   6. 128
    g. _____   7. 2
    h. _____   8. 4

40. The binary number 10110 represents zero 1s, one 2, one 4, zero 8s, and one 16; that is, the decimal number $0 + 2 + 4 + 0 + 16 = 22$. What decimal number does the binary number 11001 represent?

41. The decimal number 13 is made up of one 1, zero 2s, one 4, and one 8 $(8 + 4 + 0 + 1 = 13)$. The number therefore is represented by the binary number _____.

42. Match the following:
Decimal Number	Binary Number
a. 1 _____	1. 0001111
b. 5 _____	2. 0011001
c. 10 _____	3. 0001010
d. 15 _____	4. 0110010
e. 20 _____	5. 0000001
f. 25 _____	6. 1100100
g. 30 _____	7. 0101000
h. 40 _____	8. 0011110
i. 50 _____	9. 0010100
j. 100 _____	10. 0000101

43. How many binary digits are required in the binary numbers representing the following decimal numbers?
    a. 0 _____
    b. 1 _____
    c. 5 _____
    d. 10 _____
    e. 25 _____
    f. 30 _____
    g. 63 _____
    h. 64 _____
    i. 75 _____
    j. 100 _____

44. How many bits are required to represent each decimal number in binary form?
    a. 7 _____
    b. 15 _____
    c. 3 _____
    d. 511 _____
    e. 1023 _____
    f. 63 _____
    g. 255 _____
    h. 1 _____
    i. 127 _____
    j. 31 _____

45. How many bits are required to store numbers representing each number of different gray shades?
    a. 2 _____
    b. 4 _____
    c. 8 _____
    d. 15 _____
    e. 16 _____
    f. 25 _____
    g. 32 _____
    h. 64 _____
    i. 65 _____
    j. 128 _____

46. The primary formats of image presentation are called _____ mode, _____ mode, and _____ mode. They are used in _____, _____, and _____ types of clinical imaging, respectively.

47. Match the following display modes with the appropriate statements (answers may be used more than once):
    a. B mode:

    _____,
    _____,
    _____

    b. M mode:

    _____,
    _____,
    _____,

    1. Cross-sectional display (two spatial dimensions)
    2. Dot brightened by increasing echo strength
    3. A depth-versus-time display
    4. Requires the beam to be scanned to develop the image
    5. Not a cross-sectional display

48. The display device used in each mode is either a _____-_____ tube, also called a _____, or a _____ _____ display.

49. The spot on a cathode-ray tube may be moved by applying voltage to the _____ coils.

50. Electron beam strength controls the _____ of echoes.

51. _____ mode is used for studying the motion of a structure such as a heart valve.

52. A B scan presents a cross section through the _____ plane.

53. A display that shows various echo strengths as different brightnesses is called a _____-_____ or _____ display.

54. The _____ _____ stores the gray-scale image and allows it to be displayed on a computer monitor.

55. Television monitors produce _____ images per second.
    a. 10
    b. 15
    c. 30
    d. 60
    e. 100

56. How many horizontal lines are used to produce a picture on a television monitor?
    a. 60
    b. 100
    c. 256
    d. 525
    e. 1024

57. It takes _____ ms to produce a single frame on a television monitor using the television scan format.

58. It takes _____ µs to write one horizontal line of information on a television monitor.

59. Match the following:

    Transducer
    a. Linear array _____
    b. Convex array _____
    c. Phased array _____
    d. Vector array _____

    Display
    1. Rectangular
    2. Sector

60. If the pulse repetition frequency of an instrument is 1 kHz and it displays (single focus) 25 frames per second, there are _____ lines per frame.

61. The pulse repetition frequency is _____ Hz if 30 frames (40 lines each) are displayed per second (single focus).

62. Imaging involving 10-cm penetration, a single focus, 100 scan lines per frame, and 30 frames per second can be accomplished without range ambiguity. True or false?

63. The maximum frame rate permitted for 15-cm penetration, three foci, and 200 scan lines per frame is
    a. 3.0
    b. 5.5
    c. 8.5
    d. 15
    e. 30

64. The primary components of a diagnostic ultrasound imaging system are the _____, _____ _____, _____ _____, _____ _____, and _____.

65. Match each component with a function:
    a. Beam former:

    _____

    b. Transducer:

    _____

    c. Signal processor:

    _____

    d. Image processor:

    _____

    e. Display: _____

    1. Produces ultrasound pulses
    2. Processes voltages received from the beam former
    3. Converts image information from electrical to visual form
    4. Sends electric pulses to the transducer
    5. Sends electric information to the display

66. Match the following ultrasound parameters with the instrument components that determine them (answers may be used more than once):
    a. Frequency: _____,

    _____

    b. Period: _____,

    _____

    c. Wavelength:

    _____,
    _____,
    _____

    1. Pulser
    2. Transducer
    3. Tissue

d. Propagation speed:

_____

e. Pulse repetition frequency: _____

f. Pulse repetition period: _____

g. Pulse duration:

_____, _____

h. Duty factor:

_____, _____

i. Spatial pulse length:

_____, _____,

_____

j. Axial resolution:

_____, _____,

_____

k. Amplitude: _____,

_____

l. Intensity: _____,

_____

m. Attenuation:

_____, _____,

_____

n. Imaging depth:

_____, _____,

_____

o. Beam width:

_____, _____

p. Lateral resolution:

_____, _____

67. The information that can be obtained from an M mode display includes
   a. distance and motion pattern.
   b. transducer frequency, reflection coefficient, and distance.
   c. acoustic impedances, attenuation, and motion pattern.
   d. none of the above.

68. The time gain compensation control compensates for
   a. machine instability in the warm-up time.
   b. attenuation.
   c. transducer aging.
   d. the ambient light in the examining area.
   e. patient examination time.

69. A gray-scale display shows
   a. gray color on a white background.
   b. echoes with one brightness level.
   c. a white color on a gray background.
   d. a range of echo amplitudes.

70. The dynamic range of an ultrasound system is
   a. the speed with which ultrasound examination can be performed.
   b. the range over which the transducer can be manipulated while performing an examination.

c. the ratio of the maximum amplitude to the minimum echo strength that can be displayed.
   d. the range of voltages applied to the transducer.

71. A _____ _____ formats scan line data to image form.

72. Which of the following is not performed by a signal processor?
   a. Detection
   b. Filtering
   c. Digital-to-analog conversion
   d. Radio frequency–to–video conversion
   e. Compression

73. Commercial television displays produce _____ frames per second with _____ lines in each.
   a. 30, 60
   b. 30, 525
   c. 60, 512
   d. 512, 512
   e. 60, 120

74. In a digital memory, echo intensity is represented by
   a. positive charge distribution.
   b. a number stored in memory.
   c. electron density of the scan converter writing beam.
   d. a and c.
   e. all of the above.

75. If there were no attenuation in tissue, _____ would not be needed.
   a. Filtering
   b. Compression
   c. Detection
   d. Time gain compensation

76. The television scanning format uses _____ fields per frame so that there are _____ fields presented on the monitor per second.

77. Which of the following are capable of displaying gray-scale information?
   a. Computer monitor
   b. Television monitor
   c. Demodulator
   d. a and b
   e. None of the above

78. Echo imaging includes ultrasound generation, propagation and reflection in tissues, and reception of returning _____.

79. The diagnostic ultrasound systems in common clinical use today are of the _____-_____ type.

80. Gray-scale instruments show echo amplitude as _____ on the display.

81. Pulse-echo instruments look for three things: the _____, _____, and arrival _____ of echoes returning from tissues.

82. An image memory stores image information in the form of _____ numbers.
    a. Electric charge
    b. Binary
    c. Decimal
    d. Impedance
    e. None of the above
83. Imaging systems produce a visual _____ from the electric _____ received from the transducer.
84. The transducer is connected to the signal processor through the _____ _____.
85. The transducer receives voltages from the _____ _____ in pulse-echo systems.
86. The _____ _____ receives digitized echo voltages from the beam former.
87. Increasing gain generally produces the same effect as
    a. decreasing attenuation.
    b. increasing attenuation.
    c. increasing compression.
    d. increasing rectification.
    e. b and c.
88. The digital-to-analog converter is part of the
    a. beam former.
    b. signal processor.
    c. image processor.
    d. display.
    e. a and b.
    f. c and e.
89. Voltage pulses from the pulser are applied through delays to the _____.
90. Detection is a function of the
    a. beam former.
    b. signal processor.
    c. image processor.
    d. display.
    e. a and b.
91. If gain is reduced by one half with input power unchanged, the output power is _____ what it was before.
    a. Equal to
    b. Twice
    c. One half
    d. None of the above
92. If gain is 30 dB and output power is reduced by one half, the new gain is _____ dB.
    a. 15
    b. 60
    c. 33
    d. 27
    e. None of the above
93. If four shades of gray are shown on a display, each twice the brightness of the preceding one, the brightest shade is _____ times the brightness of the dimmest shade.

    a. 2
    b. 4
    c. 8
    d. 16
    e. 32
94. The dynamic range displayed in Exercise 93 is _____ dB.
    a. 10
    b. 9
    c. 5
    d. 2
    e. 0
95. Gain and attenuation are usually expressed in which units?
    a. dB
    b. dB/cm
    c. cm
    d. cm/3 dB
    e. None of the above
96. Time gain compensation makes up for the fact that reflections from deeper reflectors arrive at the transducer with greater amplitude. True or false?
97. The modes that show one-dimensional (depth) real-time images are _____ and _____ mode.
98. The mode that shows two-dimensional real-time images is _____ mode.
99. A real-time B mode display may be produced by rapid _____ scanning of a transducer array.
100. Each complete scan of the sound beam produces an image on the display that is called a _____.
101. For a single focus, the number of lines in each frame is equal to the number of times the transducer is _____ while the frame is produced; that is, while the sound beam is scanned.
102. In real-time scanning, the pulse repetition frequency depends on the number of _____ per frame and the _____ rate.
103. Increasing the number of foci reduces _____ _____.
104. To correct for attenuation, time gain compensation must _____ the gain for increasing depth.
105. If a higher frequency is used, resolution is _____, imaging depth _____, and the time gain compensation slope must be _____.
106. For pixel dimensions 256 × 512 or 512 × 512, calculate the number of image pixels.
107. Which type of array gives a wide view close to the transducer? _____ Which of the following produce(s) a sector format image? _____
    a. Vector
    b. Linear

c. Phased
d. Convex
e. More than one of the above

108. If a single-focus ultrasound instrument produces 1000 pulses per second and 20 frames per second, how many scan lines make up each frame?

109. In Figure 4-55, if two foci were used, the frame rate would be _____.
    a. 33
    b. 22
    c. 11
    d. 6
    e. 1

110. What is adjusted improperly in Figure 4-56?
    a. Gain
    b. Time gain compensation
    c. Compression

d. Frame rate
e. Rejection

111. The *decreasing* gain of the time gain compensation curve *(arrows)* in Figure 4-57 is caused by _____.
    a. Weak attenuation
    b. Refraction
    c. Strong attenuation
    d. Beam broadening
    e. Beam narrowing

112. In the linear amplifier of Figure 4-58, the gain is _____ dB.
    a. 1000
    b. 300
    c. 100
    d. 60
    e. 10

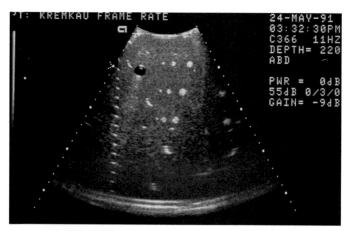

■ **FIGURE 4-55**   Illustration to accompany Exercise 109.

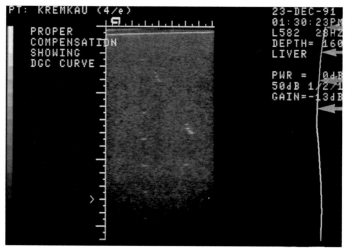

■ **FIGURE 4-57**   Illustration to accompany Exercise 111.

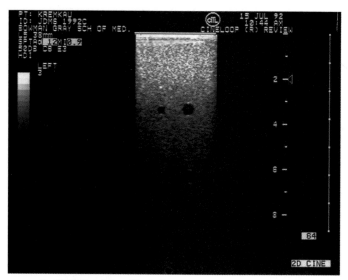

■ **FIGURE 4-56**   Illustration to accompany Exercise 110.

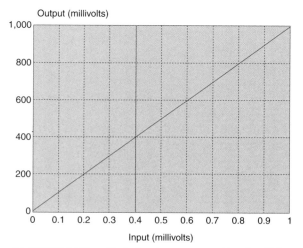

■ **FIGURE 4-58**   Illustration to accompany Exercise 112.

113. Compression is a function of the
    a. beam former.
    b. signal processor.
    c. image processor.
    d. scan converter.
    f. image memory.

114. The scan converter is part of the _____ _____.

115. Presentation of echo strength in color improves _____ resolution.

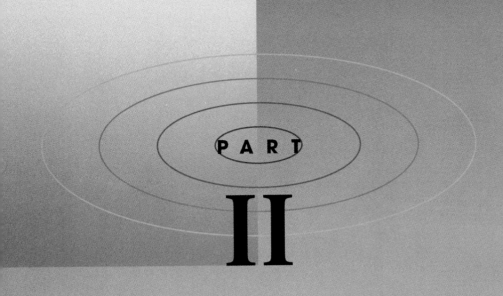

Doppler Principles

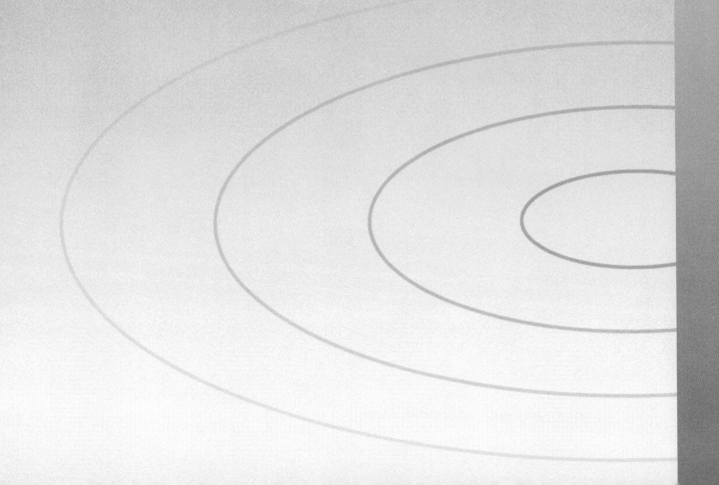

CHAPTER 5

Doppler Effect*

LEARNING OBJECTIVES

After reading this chapter, the student should be able to do the following:

- Define the terms fluid, pressure, and resistance.
- Describe how pressure and resistance affect flow.
- List and compare the various kinds of flow encountered in blood circulation.
- Explain how a stenosis affects flow.
- Define and discuss the Doppler effect, the Doppler shift, and the Doppler angle.
- Describe how the Doppler shift for a moving reflector depends on frequency and reflector motion.

KEY TERMS

The following terms are introduced in this chapter:

Bernoulli effect
Compliance
Cosine
Critical Reynolds number
Disturbed flow
Doppler angle
Doppler effect
Doppler equation
Doppler shift

Eddies
Flow
Fluid
Inertia
Laminar flow
Mass
Parabolic flow
Plug flow
Poise

Poiseuille's equation
Pulsatile flow
Resistance (flow)
Reynolds number
Stenosis
Streamline
Turbulence
Viscosity
Volumetric flow rate

The word *hemodynamics* is derived from two Greek words meaning blood and power. The word refers to the forces and motion of blood flow and the study of blood circulation. Doppler ultrasound is used primarily to detect and evaluate blood flow in the body. The sonographer must understand the principles of blood flow so as to be able to use ultrasound as an effective diagnostic tool.

The circulatory system consists of the heart, arteries, arterioles, capillaries, venules, and veins, altogether containing about 5 liters (L) of blood. The heart is the pump that produces blood flow through the circulatory system. The heart is a contracting and relaxing muscle (the myocardium) with four chambers: two atria and two ventricles. Flow is from the superior and inferior

---

*NOTE: Appendix I provides a condensed version of the material in Chapters 5 to 7 for readers who need less depth and breadth of coverage on Doppler topics. Because of the importance of blood flow and Doppler techniques in echocardiography and vascular ultrasound, the complete coverage in Chapters 5 to 7 is recommended for persons working in those fields.

vena cava and pulmonary veins into the right and left atria, respectively, and from there into the ventricles. From the left and right ventricles, flow is into the aorta and pulmonary artery, respectively. When the heart contracts, the intended result is forward flow into the aorta and pulmonary artery. Valves are present in the heart to permit forward flow and prevent reverse flow. Malfunctioning valves can restrict forward flow by not opening sufficiently (stenotic valve) or allow reverse flow by not closing completely (insufficiency or regurgitation). Doppler ultrasound is useful for detecting both of these conditions.

Body orientation and respiration affect hemodynamics. For example, because of the pull of gravity (called hydrostatic pressure) on the blood in the abdomen and thorax, venous pressure in the lower limbs is greater when a person is erect than when prone or supine. Venous valves and leg muscular action assist the return of blood to the heart against this pressure. The descent of the diaphragm during inspiration decreases intrathoracic pressure and increases intraabdominal pressure, decreasing venous return flow from the legs. With expiration, flow increases from the legs to the abdomen but decreases from the abdomen to the thorax. Such fluctuations in venous flow can be observed with Doppler ultrasound. Liquids are essentially incompressible so that variations in pressure have little effect on blood volume. However, vessels are normally distensible so that the distribution of the volume of blood in the circulatory system can be modified by pressure and flow conditions.

Flow in the heart, arteries, and veins can be detected with Doppler ultrasound. The capillaries are the tiniest vessels, measuring a few micrometers in diameter. The human body has about 1 billion capillaries. Across the walls of capillaries the exchange of gases, nutrients, and waste products takes place with the cells, sustaining their life (this is the reason for the existence of the circulatory system). In this chapter we consider the characteristics of **fluids,** such as blood, and their behavior when they flow through tubes, such as blood vessels, in steady and **pulsatile flow** forms.[14-16]

The **Doppler effect** is a change in frequency (and wavelength) caused by motion of a sound source, receiver, or reflector. If the source is moving toward the receiver, or the receiver is moving toward the source, or the reflector is moving toward the source and receiver, the received wave has a higher frequency than would be experienced without the motion. Conversely, if the motion is away (receding), the received wave has a lower frequency. The amount of increase or decrease in the frequency depends on the speed of motion, the angle between the wave propagation direction and the motion direction, and the frequency of the wave emitted by the source.

FLOW
Fluid

Matter generally is classified into three categories: gas, liquid, and solid. Gases and liquids are fluids; that is, they are substances that **flow** and conform to the shape of their containers. To flow is to move in a stream, continually changing position and, possibly, direction. Rivers flow downstream. Water flows through a garden hose. Air flows through a fan. Blood flows through the heart, arteries, capillaries, and veins.

Gases and liquids are materials that flow.

Blood

Blood is a liquid the function of which is to supply nutrients and oxygen to the cells of the body and to remove their waste products. Blood is comprised of plasma, erythrocytes (red cells), leukocytes (white cells), and platelets. Plasma is primarily water (about 90%) and proteins. About 40% of blood volume is cells. This percentage is called the hematocrit. Erythrocytes are the dominant cells in circulation, constituting about 99% of all the blood cells in the body. Erythrocytes contain hemoglobin, which is responsible for the transport of oxygen. Leukocytes are larger than erythrocytes but are less numerous in the blood. Their chief function is to protect the body against disease organisms. Platelets are smaller than erythrocytes and are important in blood clotting.

Blood supplies body cells with nutrients and removes waste products.

Two important characteristics of fluids are density and **viscosity**. The density of a fluid is its mass per unit volume, commonly expressed in grams per milliliter (g/mL). Mass is a measure of the resistance of an object to acceleration. This resistance is called **inertia**. The greater the mass, the greater the inertia. If two different masses are to be accelerated at the same rate, more force must be applied to the greater mass. The density of blood (1.05 g/mL) is slightly greater than that of water (1 g/mL) because of the presence of proteins and cells. Viscosity is the **resistance** to flow offered by a fluid in motion. Viscosity is given in units of **poise** or kilograms per meter-second (kg/m-s). One poise is 1 g/cm-s or 0.1 kg/m-s. Water has a relatively low viscosity compared with, for example, molasses, which has a high viscosity.

The viscosity of blood plasma is about 50% greater than that of water. The viscosity of normal blood is 0.035 poise at 37°C, approximately 55 times that of water. Blood viscosity can vary from about 0.02 (with anemia) to about 0.10 (with polycythemia). Blood viscosity also varies with flow speed.

Density is the mass per unit volume of a fluid. Viscosity is the resistance of a fluid to flow.

Pressure, Resistance, and Volumetric Flow Rate

Pressure is the driving force behind fluid flow. Pressure is force per unit area. Pressure is distributed equally throughout a static fluid and exerts its force in all directions (Figure 5-1). A pressure *difference* is required for flow to occur. Equal pressures applied at both ends of a liquid-filled tube will result in no flow. If the pressure is greater at one end than at the other, the liquid will flow from the higher-pressure end to the lower-pressure end. This pressure difference can be generated by a pump (e.g., the heart in the circulatory system) or by the force of gravity (i.e., by raising one end of a tube above the other). (Because this is the situation in the lower extremity veins in a standing person, these vessels have valves in them to prevent reverse flow.) The greater the pressure difference, the greater the flow rate will be. This pressure difference sometimes is called a pressure gradient, although strictly defined, pressure gradient is the pressure difference *divided by the distance between the two pressure locations*. The term *gradient* comes from the Latin *gradus* and refers to the upward or downward sloping of something. As the pressure drops from one end of the tube to the other, this decrease can be

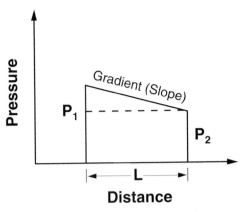

The pressure gradient or slope is the pressure difference ($P_1 - P_2$) divided by the separation (*L*) between the two pressure locations.

thought of as a slope (i.e., the pressure difference divided by the distance over which the pressure drop occurs; Figure 5-2). A constant driving pressure produces steady (unchanging with time) flow. The driving pressure produced by the heart varies with time. This will be considered later in this section.

Fluid flows in a tube in response to a pressure difference at the ends.

The **volumetric flow rate** (*Q*) (sometimes simply called flow, although that term also is used in other ways) is the volume of blood passing a point per unit of time. This rate usually is expressed in milliliters (mL) per minute or per second. The total adult blood flow rate (cardiac output) is about 5000 mL/min (i.e., the total blood volume circulates in about 1 minute). The volumetric flow rate in a long straight tube is determined not only by the pressure difference (ΔP) but also by the resistance (*R*) to flow.

$$Q \ (\text{mL/s}) = \frac{\Delta P \ (\text{dyne/cm}^2)}{R \ (\text{poise})}$$

If pressure difference increases, volumetric flow rate increases.

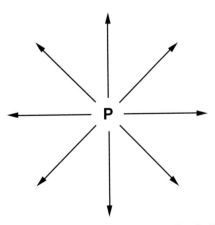

■ **FIGURE 5-1** Pressure (*P*) is distributed uniformly throughout a static fluid and exerts its force in all directions.

If flow resistance increases, volumetric flow rate decreases.

The flow resistance in a long, straight tube depends on the fluid viscosity (η) and the tube length (L) and radius (r) as follows:

$$R \ (g/cm^4\text{-}s) = 8 \times L \ (cm) \times \frac{\eta \ (poise)}{\pi \times [r^4 \ (cm^4)]}$$

If tube length increases, flow resistance increases.

If tube radius increases, flow resistance decreases.

If viscosity increases, flow resistance increases.

As expected, an increase in viscosity or tube length increases the resistance, whereas an increase in the size (radius or diameter) of the tube decreases the resistance. The latter effect is particularly strong, with the resistance depending on the radius to the fourth power. Thus doubling the radius of a tube decreases its resistance to one sixteenth its original value. By experience, we know that a longer or smaller-diameter garden hose reduces water flow rate. And we could guess that if we tried to force molasses through the hose, we would not get nearly the flow rate we get with water.

Poiseuille's Equation

Substituting the equation for flow resistance into the flow-rate equation and using tube diameter (d) rather than radius yields **Poiseuille's equation** for volumetric flow rate:

$$Q \ (mL/s) = \frac{\Delta P \ (dyne/cm^2) \times \pi \times d^4 \ (cm^4)}{128 \times L \ (cm) \times \eta \ (poise)}$$

Recall that this equation is for steady flow in long straight tubes. Thus the equation serves only to provide a rough approximation of the conditions in blood circulation. The equation is useful, however, in making qualitative conclusions and predictions as follows:

If pressure difference increases, flow rate increases.

If diameter increases, flow rate increases.

If length increases, flow rate decreases.

If viscosity increases, flow rate decreases.

The resistance of the arterioles accounts for about half the total resistance in the systemic circulation.[14] The muscular walls of the arterioles can constrict or relax, producing dramatic changes in flow resistance. Arterioles thus can control blood flow to specific tissues and organs in response to their needs.

The volumetric flow rate in a tube depends on the pressure difference, the length and diameter of the tube, and the viscosity of the fluid.

Types of Flow

Flow can be divided into five spatial categories: plug, laminar, parabolic, disturbed, and turbulent. At the entrance to a tube, the speed of the fluid is essentially constant across the tube (Figure 5-3). This is called **plug flow** because it is similar to the motion of a solid object (a plug, for example) that does not flow but moves as a unit. As the fluid flows down the tube, laminar (from the Latin term for layer) flow develops. **Laminar flow** is a flow condition in which **streamlines** (which describe the motion of fluid particles) are straight and parallel to each other. The fluid has a maximum flow speed at the center of the tube and minimum or zero flow at the tube walls. A decreasing profile of flow speeds from center to wall exists. Successive layers of fluid slide on each other with relative motion. The pressure difference at each end of the tube overcomes the viscous resistance of the layers sliding over each other, maintaining the laminar flow through the tube. Steady flow in a long, straight tube results in a **parabolic flow** profile (Figure 5-4). This is a particular pattern of laminar flow in which varying flow speeds across the tube are described by a parabola (the curved dashed line in Figure 5-4). For parabolic flow, the average flow speed across the vessel is equal to one half the maximum flow speed (at the center). Parabolic flow commonly is not seen in blood

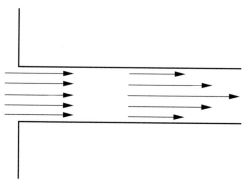

■ **FIGURE 5-3**   At the entrance to a tube or vessel, plug flow exists. After some distance, laminar flow is achieved.

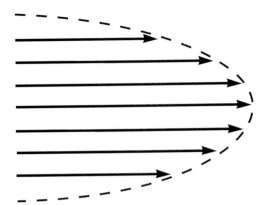

■ **FIGURE 5-4** Parabolic flow profile. The dashed line is a parabola.

circulation because the vessels generally are not long and straight. However, nonparabolic laminar flow commonly is seen; indeed, its absence is often an indicator of abnormal flow conditions at a site where there is vascular or cardiac valvular disease.

Laminar flow is flow in which layers of fluid slide over each other.

Various flow profiles are seen in normal flow in various vessels and at different points in the cardiac cycle.[15] For example, a profile approximating a parabolic shape is seen in the common carotid artery at systole (Figure 5-5, A). A blunted profile approximating plug flow is observed in diastole (Figure 5-5, B). Even the twisting type of flow called helical is likely to be present in vessels.[16-20]

Disturbed flow occurs when the parallel streamlines describing the flow (Figure 5-3) are altered from their straight form (Figure 5-6). This occurs, for example, in the region of stenoses or at a bifurcation (the point at which a vessel splits into two). In disturbed flow, particles of fluid still flow in the forward direction. Parabolic and disturbed flows are forms of laminar flow.

In the final category, turbulent flow or **turbulence,** the flow pattern is random and chaotic, with particles moving at different speeds in many directions, even in circles called **eddies,** yet with forward net flow maintained (Figure 5-7). As flow speed increases in a tube, turbulent flow will eventually occur (Figure 5-7, A). The flow speed at which turbulent flow occurs depends on the density and viscosity of the fluid and the diameter of the tube. The **Reynolds number** (R_e) predicts the onset of turbulent flow as it depends on average flow speed (v_a), vessel diameter, density (ρ), and viscosity.

$$R_e = \frac{v_a \ (cm/s) \times d \ (cm) \times \rho \ (g/mL)}{\eta \ (poise)}$$

If flow speed increases, the Reynolds number increases.

If diameter increases, the Reynolds number increases.

If density increases, the Reynolds number increases.

If viscosity increases, the Reynolds number decreases.

For example, blood flow in a long, straight tube becomes turbulent at a Reynolds number of about 2000. This is called the **critical Reynolds number.** With the exception of the heart and proximal aorta, turbulent flow is not likely in normal human circulation. Turbulent flow can occur more easily beyond an obstruction (Figure 5-7, B and C), such as a **stenosis,** particularly in systole.

Disturbed flow is a form of laminar flow in which streamlines are not straight. Turbulent flow is nonlaminar flow with random and chaotic speeds and directions.

Pulsatile Flow

Thus far we have considered steady flow in which pressures, flow speeds, and flow patterns do not change with time. This is generally the situation on the venous side of the circulatory system, although cardiac pulsations or respiratory cycles can influence venous flow in some locations. However, in the heart and the arterial circulation, flow is pulsatile, directly experiencing the effects of the beating heart with pulsatile variations of increasing and decreasing pressure and flow speed. For steady flow, volumetric flow rate simply is related to pressure difference and flow resistance. With pulsatile flow, the relationship between the varying pressure and flow rate depends on the flow impedance, which includes the resistance formerly considered, the inertia of the fluid as it accelerates and decelerates, and the **compliance** (expansion and contraction) of the non-rigid vessel walls. The mathematical analysis is complicated and is not presented here. Two dominant characteristics of interest in this type of flow are the Windkessel effect and flow reversal. When the pressure pulse forces a fluid into a compliant vessel, such as the

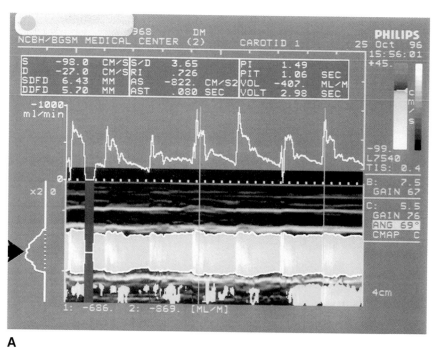

A

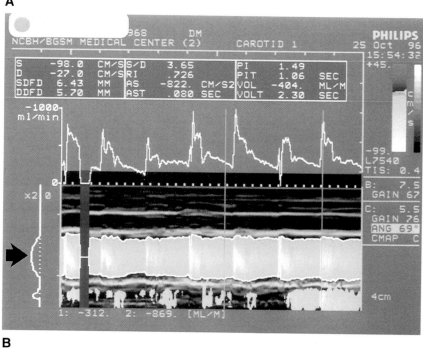

B

■ **FIGURE 5-5** Common carotid flow profiles *(arrows)* are approximately parabolic at systole **(A)** and plug in diastole **(B)**.

aorta, it expands and increases the volume within it. (This is why you can feel your pulse on your wrist or neck.) Later in the cycle, when the driving pressure is reduced, the compliant vessel can contract, producing extended flow later in the pressure cycle. This is known as the Windkessel effect. In the aorta this effect results in continued flow in the forward direction, because aortic valve closure prevents flow back into the heart. In the distal circulation, expansion of the distensible vessels results in the reversal of flow in diastole as the pressure

decreases and the distended vessels contract. Where there are no valves to prevent it, flow reversal occurs (Figure 5-8). This is a normal observation in these locations. Pulsatile flow in compliant vessels thus includes added forward flow and/or flow reversal in diastole, depending on location within arterial circulation. Arterial diastolic flow (absence, presence, direction, quantity) reveals much concerning the state of downstream arterioles, in which flow cannot be measured directly with ultrasound.

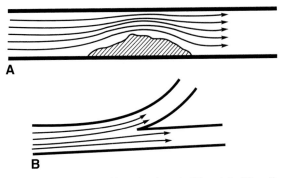

A

B

■ **FIGURE 5-6**   Disturbed flow at a stenosis **(A)** and at a bifurcation **(B).**

Pulsatile flow is nonsteady flow, with acceleration and deceleration over the cardiac cycle.

Pulsatile flow in distensible vessels includes added forward flow and/or flow reversal over the cardiac cycle in some locations in circulation.

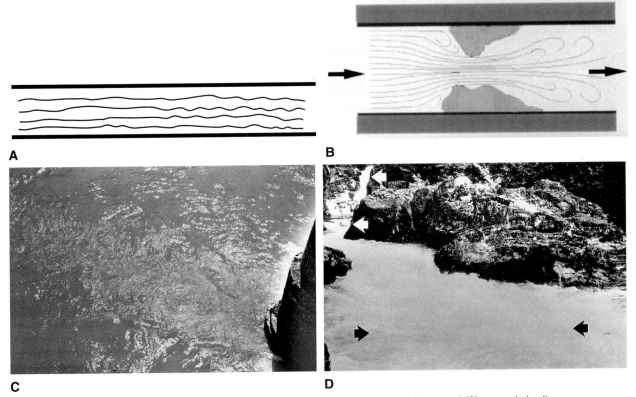

■ **FIGURE 5-7**   Turbulent flow in a vessel may result from too great a flow speed **(A)** or an obstruction **(B). C,** Turbulent flow in a river beyond an obstruction (bridge pier). **D,** In a narrow gorge ("stenosis"; *white arrows*), flow speeds are high. Beyond the narrow region (*black arrows*) there is abundant turbulence.

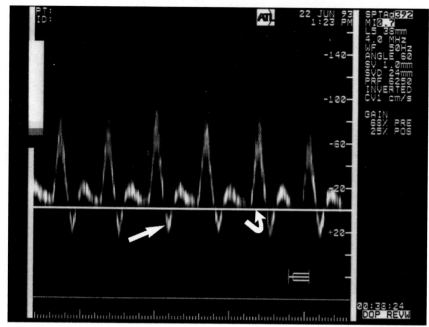

■ FIGURE 5-8 Flow reversal *(straight arrow)* below the baseline *(curved arrow)* is seen in the superficial femoral artery in diastole.

STENOSES

Continuity Rule

A narrowing of the lumen of a vessel, or stenosis, produces disturbed (Figure 5-6, *A*) and possibly turbulent flow (Figure 5-7, *B* and *D*). The average flow speed in the stenosis must be greater than that proximal and distal to it so that the volumetric flow rate is constant throughout the vessel. Examples of increased flow speed at a stenosis and turbulence beyond it are given in the next chapter. Volumetric flow rate must be constant for the three regions: proximal to, at, and distal to the stenosis. This is true because blood is neither created nor destroyed as it flows through the vessel. This is called the continuity rule. Volumetric flow rate is equal to the average flow speed across the vessel multiplied by the cross-sectional area of vessel. Therefore if the stenosis has an area measuring one half that of the proximal and distal vessel, the average flow speed within the stenosis is twice that proximal and distal to it. An analogy to this is traffic flow on a multilane highway (Figure 5-9). To maintain constant flow rate (number of vehicles past a point per unit of time), the vehicles must travel faster in the narrow region. If a stenosis has a diameter that is one half of that adjacent to it, the area at the stenosis is one fourth that adjacent to it, so the average flow speed in the stenosis must quadruple.

Flow speed increases at a stenosis, and turbulence can occur distal to it.

Poiseuille's law converted to average flow speed, rather than volumetric flow rate, is as follows:

$$v_a \text{ (cm/s)} = \frac{[\Delta p \text{ (dyne/cm}^2) \times d^2 \text{ (cm}^2)]}{[32 \times L \text{ (cm)} \times \eta \text{ (poise)}]}$$

This form of the pressure flow relationship is particularly useful because **Doppler shift** is directly related to flow speed, not volumetric flow rate. Volumetric flow rate must be calculated from Doppler flow speed measurements. We see that flow speed, and therefore Doppler shift, increases with tube diameter squared. In summary, volumetric flow rate depends on diameter to the fourth power, whereas flow speed depends on diameter squared.

The seeming contradiction between Poiseuille's law and the continuity rule for a stenosis sometimes puzzles students. One states that flow speed decreases with smaller diameters (Poiseuille's law), whereas the other says that flow speed increases with smaller diameters (continuity rule). How can this be so? The answer is that the two situations are different. Poiseuille's law deals with a long, straight vessel with no stenosis. The diameter in Poiseuille's law is that for the *entire* vessel. By contrast, the diameter in the continuity rule is that for a *short portion* of a vessel (the stenosis). If the diameter of the entire vessel is reduced (as in vasoconstriction), flow speed *is* reduced. If the diameter of only a short segment of a vessel is reduced (stenosis), the flow speed in the vessel is unaffected except at the stenosis, where it is increased. This is true because the stenosis has little effect on the overall flow resistance of the entire vessel if the stenosis length is small compared with the vessel length and if the lumen in the stenosis is not too small (does not approach occlusion). Figure 5-10 shows the

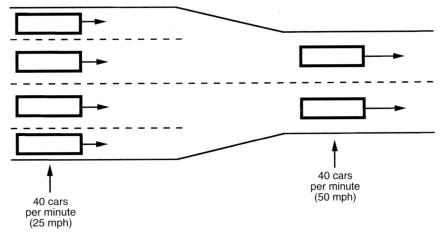

■ **FIGURE 5-9** Highway traffic flow is analogous to fluid volumetric flow. In the four-lane portion of the highway, 40 cars pass by each minute at a speed of 25 miles per hour. In the two-lane region, to maintain the flow rate of 40 cars per minute, a speed of 50 miles per hour is required. In this case, the speed times the number of lanes must be constant (100 lane-miles/hr). This is analogous to fluid volumetric flow, in which tube cross-sectional area multiplied by flow speed must be constant.

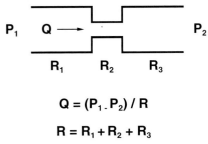

$$Q = (P_1 - P_2) / R$$

$$R = R_1 + R_2 + R_3$$

■ **FIGURE 5-10** The overall flow resistance (R) for a vessel with a stenosis is equal to the sum of the resistances of the three parts (proximal (R_1), stenosis (R_2), and distal (R_3)). Volumetric flow rate (Q) is equal to the pressure difference at the ends of the vessel ($P_1 - P_2$) divided by the total resistance.

situation for a stenosis, indicating that the overall flow resistance for the vessel is the sum of the resistances of the three parts (proximal, stenosis, distal). If the length of segment 2 (stenosis) is not too large and its radius is not too small, there will be a negligible effect on the overall resistance and therefore on the proximal and distal flow. However, the flow speed must increase in the stenosis to maintain volumetric flow rate continuity. These dependencies[21] of volumetric flow rate and flow speed at the stenosis with increasing stenosis are seen in Figure 5-11. The maximum normal flow speed in circulation is about 100 cm/s. However, in stenotic regions, flow speeds can increase to a few meters per second. Doppler ultrasound is useful for detecting flow speed increases associated with vascular disease.

The increased flow speed within a stenosis can cause turbulence distal to it. Sounds produced by turbulence, which can be heard with a stethoscope, are called bruits.

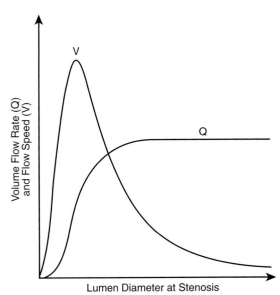

■ **FIGURE 5-11** As the diameter of the stenosis is reduced (moving to the left on the horizontal axis; tighter stenosis), volumetric flow rate (Q) is unaffected initially because the stenosis does not contribute substantially to the total vessel resistance. As the diameter continues to decrease, however, the vessel resistance increases, reducing the volumetric flow rate (eventually to zero at occlusion). Volume rate and thus distal pressure begin to drop significantly beyond a diameter reduction of about 50% (area reduction of 75%). As the diameter of the stenosis decreases, flow speed increases (because of the flow continuity requirement), reaches a maximum, and then decreases to zero as the increasing flow resistance effect dominates. (Modified from Spencer MP, Reid JM: *Stroke* 10:326-330, 1979. Reprinted with permission. Copyright 1979 American Heart Association.)

The ultimate stenosis is called an occlusion, where the vessel is blocked and there is no flow. Using our garden hose analogy again, we can compress the hose (not near the nozzle) and see little effect on the flow at the nozzle until the hose is compressed to near occlusion. At that point turbulence may occur and vibration can be felt at the surface of the hose.

Bernoulli Effect

ADVANCED CONCEPTS

At a stenosis the pressure is less than it is proximal and distal to the stenotic area (Figure 5-12). This is necessary to allow the fluid to accelerate into the stenosis and decelerate out of it and to maintain energy balance. (Pressure energy is converted to flow energy upon entry, and then vice versa upon exit.) This decreased pressure in regions of high flow speed is known as the **Bernoulli effect** and is described by Bernoulli's equation, a description of the constant energy of the fluid flow through a stenosis, ignoring viscous loss. As flow energy increases, pressure energy decreases. The magnitude of the decrease in pressure that results from the increasing flow speed at the stenosis can be found from a modified form of Bernoulli's equation:

$$\Delta P = \tfrac{1}{2} \times \rho \times (v)^2$$

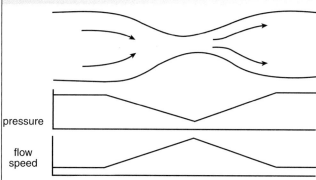

■ FIGURE 5-12 To maintain flow continuity, flow speed must increase through a stenosis. In conjunction with this, the pressure drops (the Bernoulli effect) in the stenosis. (From Kremkau FW: *J Vasc Technol* 17:153-154, 1993. Reprinted with permission.)

> If flow speed increases, the magnitude of the pressure decreases.

In this simplified equation the flow speed proximal to the stenosis is assumed to be small enough, compared with the flow speed in the stenosis, to be ignored. Pressure drop from a stenotic heart valve can reduce cardiac output. For calculating pressure drop across a stenotic

valve, the following form of the equation is used in Doppler echocardiography:

$$\Delta P = 4(v_2)^2$$

In this equation, v_2 is the flow speed (meters per second) in the jet and ΔP (millimeters of mercury) is the pressure drop across the valve. For example, if the flow speed in the jet is 5 m/s, the pressure drop is 100 mm Hg. Thus pressure drop can be calculated from a measurement of flow speed at the stenotic valve using Doppler ultrasound.

> The Bernoulli effect is a drop in pressure associated with high flow speed at a stenosis.

DOPPLER EQUATION

The Doppler effect occurs for any kind of wave, but it commonly is experienced in life with sound. The reason is that speeds of motion commonly experienced can be a significant fraction (a few percent) of the speed of sound, causing the Doppler effect to be large enough to be heard. With light, this is not true, because the speed of light is so much greater than that of sound. Thus the Doppler effect with light is not large enough to be seen with the speeds of motion that we encounter on Earth. Astronomic motions, however, provide speeds great enough to produce an observable Doppler effect with light.

> The Doppler effect is a change in frequency caused by motion of a sound source, receiver, or reflector.

A qualitative description of the Doppler effect is presented in the introduction to this chapter. A quantitative description of the Doppler effect is provided by the **Doppler equation**. The equation can deal with three situations: moving source, moving receiver, or moving reflector. The moving reflector result is the relevant situation of interest for diagnostic Doppler ultrasound.

For a moving receiver (Figure 5-13) approaching a stationary source, more cycles of a wave will be encountered in 1 second than would be if the receiver were stationary. The speed of receiver motion divided by the wavelength yields the increase in the number of cycles encountered per second (the increase in received frequency). For a moving source approaching a stationary receiver, the cycles are compressed in front of the source as it moves into its own wave (Figure 5-14). The source motion shortens the wavelength ahead of it. This

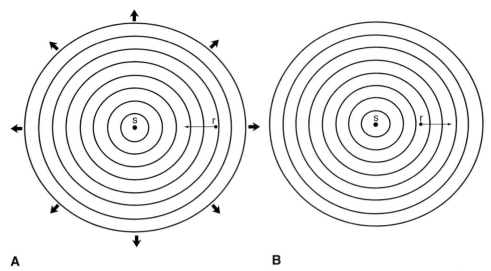

■ **FIGURE 5-13** **A,** A receiver *(r)* moving toward the source *(s)* experiences a higher frequency (more cycles per second) than a stationary one would. **B,** A receiver moving away from the source experiences a lower frequency than a stationary one would.

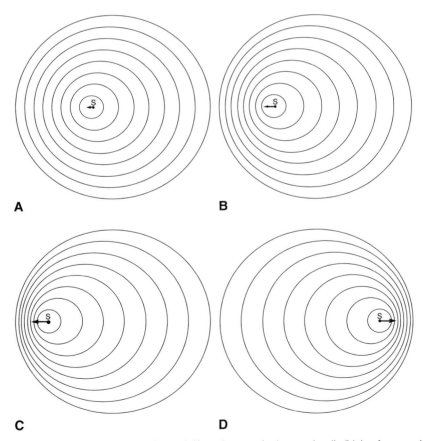

■ **FIGURE 5-14** A moving source of sound *(s)* produces a shorter wavelength (higher frequency) ahead of it and a longer wavelength (lower frequency) behind it compared with the wavelengths at the sides, which are the same as for a stationary source. **A,** Slow speed. **B,** Medium speed. **C,** High speed. **D,** High-speed movement in the opposite direction.

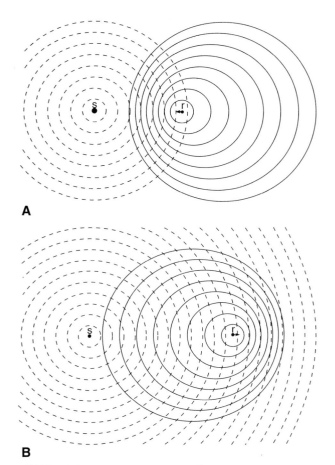

A

B

■ **FIGURE 5-15** A moving reflector (r) returns a higher frequency echo if it is approaching the source (s) and receiver (s) **(A)** and a lower frequency echo if it is moving away from the source and receiver **(B)**.

decreased wavelength results in an increased frequency observed by a stationary receiver in front of the approaching source. A moving reflector (Figure 5-15) or scatterer of a wave is a combination of a moving receiver and moving source.

Doppler Shift

The *change* in frequency caused by motion is called the Doppler shift frequency or, more commonly, just the Doppler shift (f_D). Doppler shift is equal to the received frequency (f_R) minus the source frequency (f_T). For an approaching reflector (scatterer), Doppler shift is positive; that is, the received frequency is greater than the source frequency. For a receding reflector, Doppler shift is negative; that is, the received frequency is smaller than the source frequency. The relationship between the Doppler shift and the reflector speed (v) is given by the Doppler equation:

$$f_D \text{ (kHz)} = f_R \text{ (kHz)} - f_T \text{ (kHz)} = f_o \text{ (kHz)} \times \frac{[2 \times v \text{ (cm/s)}]}{c \text{ (cm/s)}}$$

where f_o is operating frequency and c is propagation speed.

If scatterer speed increases, Doppler shift increases. If source frequency increases, Doppler shift increases.

The Doppler shift is the difference between the emitted frequency and the echo frequency returning from moving scatterers.

Take, for example, a source frequency of 5 MHz, a scatterer speed of 50 cm/s (0.5 m/s), and a propagation (sound) speed of 1540 m/s. The scatterer is approaching the source, so the received frequency is greater than the source frequency, with a positive Doppler shift of 0.0032 MHz or 3.2 kHz. For a scatterer moving away from a receiver, the Doppler shift is −3.2 kHz. Table 5-1 gives other examples using various source frequencies and scatterer speeds.

ADVANCED CONCEPTS

The Doppler effect occurs for a moving source (Figure 5-14) or receiver (detector) (Figure 5-13). The Doppler equation for a source moving at speed v_s is

$$f_D = f_o \left(\frac{v_s}{c - v_s} \right)$$

And the equation for a receiver moving at speed v_r is

$$f_D = f_o \left(\frac{v_r}{c} \right)$$

A moving reflector (Figure 5-15) is a combined moving receiver *and* source. For a reflector moving at speed v, the Doppler equation is

$$f_D = f_o \left(\frac{2v}{c - v} \right)$$

As an example, let $f_o = 5$ MHz, $v = 5$ m/s (500 cm/s), and $c = 1540$ m/s. The Doppler shift f_D is then 0.032 MHz (32 kHz).

Physiologic blood flow speeds, even in extreme cases, are less than 1% of the speed of sound in tissues. Because blood flow speed is small compared with sound speed, it may be ignored in the denominator of the foregoing Doppler equation, yielding the commonly used form of the Doppler equation for a moving reflector. Using the same values as in the foregoing example, $f_D = 32$ kHz again.

The factor of two in the Doppler equation (for a moving reflector or scatterer) is the result of two Doppler shifts: (1) the Doppler shift that occurs when a moving receiver (the scatterer) encounters the wave, and (2) the Doppler shift that occurs when the moving emitter (the scatterer again) reradiates the wave. Another way to view the factor of two is to consider the transducer to be the source and receiver of sound separated by the round-trip sound path distance, which is twice the distance from the transducer to the reflector. As the reflector approaches or recedes from the transducer, this round-trip distance is reduced at a rate that is double the speed of the reflector.

The Doppler shift is what the instruments described in the next two chapters detect. However, we are interested in the speed of tissue motion or blood flow, not the Doppler shift itself. To facilitate this, the Doppler equation is rearranged to place the speed of motion alone on the left side of the equation. Substituting the speed of sound in tissues (154,000 cm/s) and using units as indicated for the various quantities yields the equation in the following form:

$$v \text{ (cm/s)} = \frac{77 \text{ (cm/ms)} \times f_D \text{ (kHz)}}{f_0 \text{ (MHz)}}$$

ADVANCED CONCEPTS

The speed of sound used in this equation is the average speed of sound in soft tissues: 1540 m/s or 1.54 mm/μs. Use of the speed of sound in blood[22] (1570 to 1575 m/s) is tempting. Strictly speaking, however, this is not appropriate[23-25] because the scatterers (blood cells) are not moving through their medium (blood plasma) but along with it; that is, there is no relative motion between the cells and their suspending medium to produce a Doppler shift. Where then *does* the Doppler shift occur? Doppler shift occurs where the relative motion exists; that is, at the blood-intima boundary for plug flow, in which case the tissue sound speed is relevant. For other types of flow (laminar, disturbed, and turbulent), relative motion occurs between flow layers (laminae), and some (unknown) combination of sound speeds for tissue and blood would be appropriate. Fortunately, this level of accuracy is not required for Doppler techniques to be useful.

The Doppler equation relates the Doppler shift to the flow speed and the frequency.

The fact that the Doppler shift is proportional to the blood flow speed explains why the Doppler effect is so useful in medical diagnosis. Doppler instruments measure the Doppler shift. However, the blood flow is what interests us. The measured shifts are proportional to flow speed, which is the information we seek.

The Doppler equation indicates not only that the Doppler shift is proportional to the speed of the moving reflector but, more specifically, that it is proportional to the ratio of that speed to the propagation speed. In other words, to get a Doppler shift that is 2% of the operating frequency, the reflector speed must be 1% of the propagation speed. With sound, this is reasonable to accomplish. However, as mentioned previously, the Doppler effect with light is not experienced in daily life because the speed of light is about 1 million times that of sound.

Doppler Applications

Using electromagnetic microwaves, Doppler radar has been applied in weather forecasting, aviation safety, and in the familiar application of police radar detection of vehicle speeds on highways. They are examples of detected Doppler shifts resulting from reflections from moving objects. Ultrasonic door openers and burglar alarms (see Figure 1-12) are common in public buildings and homes. They also use the Doppler shift resulting from a moving reflector (person in motion). These systems operate at around 25 kHz, emitting ultrasound into and receiving it from the air. A person walking at one step per second generates a Doppler shift of about 65 Hz in such a system.[26] A long-standing application of Doppler ultrasound in medicine is in monitoring the fetal heartbeat during labor and delivery. Instruments that perform this function (Figure 5-16) can be less sophisticated and

TABLE 5-1 Doppler Frequency Shifts for Various Scatterer Speeds toward* the Sound Source at a Zero Doppler Angle

Incident Frequency (MHz)	Scatterer Speed (cm/s)	Reflected Frequency (MHz)	Doppler Shift (kHz)
2	50	2.0013	1.3
5	50	5.0032	3.2
10	50	10.0065	6.5
2	200	2.0052	5.2
5	200	5.013	13.0
10	200	10.026	26.0

*Motion away from the source would yield negative Doppler shifts.

less sensitive than blood flow measurement systems because the echoes from the beating fetal heart are much stronger than those emanating from flowing blood.

Doppler Ultrasound

With diagnostic medical ultrasound, stationary transducers are used to emit and receive the ultrasound. The Doppler effect is a result of the motion of blood, the flow of which we wish to measure, or the motion of tissue that we wish to evaluate. Physiologic flow speeds, even in highly stenotic jets, do not exceed a few meters per second. Table 5-1 gives Doppler shifts resulting from typical physiologic flow speeds. Figure 5-17 illustrates the proportional dependence of Doppler shift on scatterer speed. The intensity of the returning Doppler-shifted echoes is not affected by the flow speed.[27] The minimum detectable blood flow speed with Doppler ultrasound is a few millimeters per second. The maximum is determined by aliasing (discussed later).

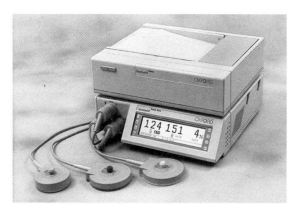

FIGURE 5-16 A Doppler antepartum fetal monitor.

Doppler shift is proportional to flow speed.

Operating Frequency

For a given flow in a vessel, the Doppler shift measured by an instrument is proportional to the operating frequency of the instrument (Figure 5-18 and Table 5-1). Thus measurement of Doppler shifts from flow in the same vessel using two transducers operating at 2 MHz and 4 MHz will yield two Doppler shifts. The higher-frequency transducer will have a Doppler shift that is twice that of the lower-frequency transducer. When comparing Doppler shifts, therefore, one must consider the frequency of the devices.[28] In the calculation of flow speed, the operating frequency is incorporated. Thus comparisons of flow speeds between different instruments have taken this variable into account.

Doppler shift is proportional to operating frequency.

Doppler frequencies used in vascular studies are slightly less than those used for anatomic imaging because echoes from blood are weaker than those from soft tissues.

Doppler Angle

If the direction of sound propagation is exactly opposite the flow direction, the maximum positive Doppler shift is obtained. If the flow speed and propagation speed directions are the same (parallel), the maximum nega-

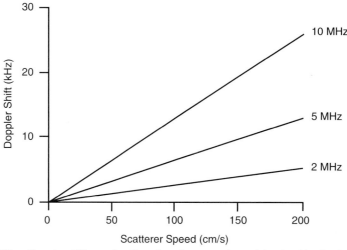

■ FIGURE 5-17 Doppler shift as a function of scatterer speed, as determined by the Doppler equation for three incident frequencies (at a zero Doppler angle).

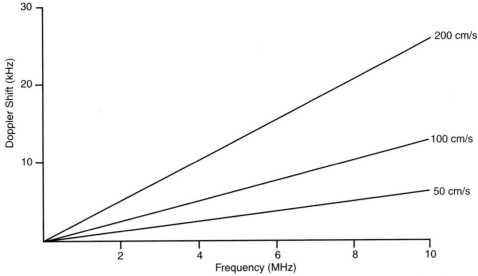

■ **FIGURE 5-18** Doppler shift as a function of operating frequency, as determined by the Doppler equation for various flow speeds (at a zero Doppler angle).

tive Doppler shift is obtained. If the angle between these two directions (Figure 5-19) is not zero, lesser Doppler shifts will occur. The Doppler shift depends on the **cosine** of the **Doppler angle.**

$$f_D \text{ (kHz)} = \frac{[f_o \text{ (kHz)} \times 2 \times v \text{ (cm/s)} \times (\cos \theta)]}{c \text{ (cm/s)}}$$

$$v \text{ (cm/s)} = \frac{[77 \text{ (cm/ms)} \times f_D \text{ (kHz)}]}{[f_o \text{ (MHz)} \times \cos \theta]}$$

Table 5-2 gives cosine values for various angles. Only the portion of the motion direction that is parallel to the sound beam contributes to the Doppler effect. The cosine gives the component of the flow velocity vector that is parallel to the sound beam (Figure 5-20). For a given flow, the larger the Doppler angle, the less the Doppler shift (Figure 5-19, *B* and *C*). Table 5-3 lists examples of Doppler shifts for various angles.

If Doppler shift increases, calculated scatterer speed increases.
If source frequency increases, calculated scatterer speed decreases.
If cosine increases, calculated scatterer speed decreases.
If Doppler angle increases, calculated scatterer speed increases.

TABLE 5-2	Cosines for Various Angles
Angle A (degrees)	**cos A**
0	1.00
5	0.996
10	0.98
15	0.97
20	0.94
25	0.91
30	0.87
35	0.82
40	0.77
45	0.71
50	0.64
55	0.57
60	0.50
65	0.42
70	0.34
75	0.26
80	0.17
85	0.09
90	0.00

Angle Accuracy

Flow speed calculations based on Doppler shift measurements can be accomplished correctly only with proper Doppler angle incorporation. They are therefore only as good as the accuracy of the measurement, estimate, or guess of that angle. Estimation of the angle normally is

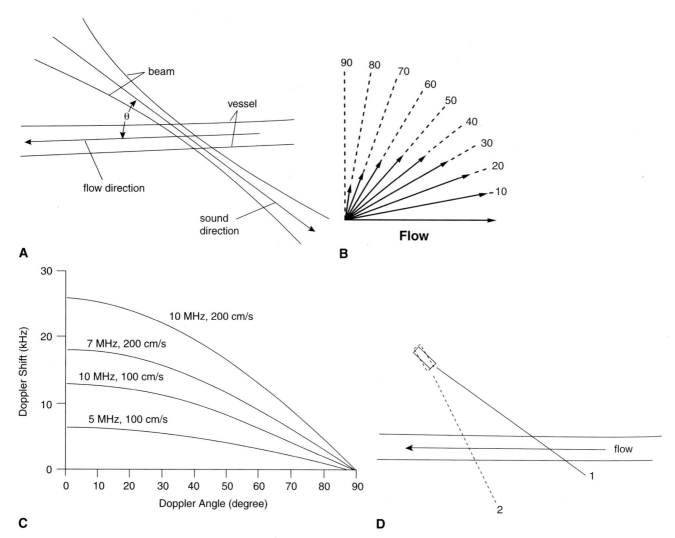

■ **FIGURE 5-19** **A,** Doppler angle θ is the angle between the direction of flow and the sound propagation direction. **B,** With constant flow, as the Doppler angle increases, echo Doppler shift frequency decreases. The direction of the arrows indicates the beam direction. The length of the arrows indicates the magnitude of the Doppler shift. **C,** Doppler shift as a function of angle, as determined by the Doppler equation for various incident frequencies and scatterer speeds. **D,** The same flow in a vessel, viewed at different angles, yields different Doppler shifts.

TABLE 5-3   Doppler Frequency Shifts for Various Angles and Scatterer Speeds toward the Sound Source of Frequency 5 MHz

Scatterer Speed (cm/s)	Angle (degrees)	Doppler Shift (kHz)
100	0	6.5
100	30	5.6
100	60	3.2
100	90	0.0
300	0	19.0
300	30	17.0
300	60	9.7
300	90	0.0

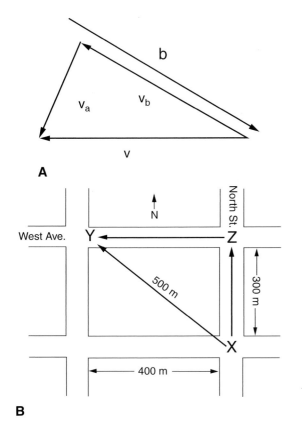

A

B

■ **FIGURE 5-20**   **A,** The flow velocity vector (v) can be broken into two components: one (v_b) that is parallel to the sound beam (b) direction and one (v_a) that is perpendicular to the sound beam direction. Only the component parallel to the beam contributes to the Doppler effect. **B,** A city block can be used as an analogy to the vector components in **A.** To get from point X to point Y, one could walk diagonally across the block, a distance of 500 m. However, if buildings blocked that path, an alternate route would be 300 m north on North Street and then 400 m west on West Avenue. The 500-m northwest vector from X to Y is equivalent to a 300-m north vector plus a 400-m west vector (i.e., the result is the same: depart from X and arrive at Y). In this example, the component of the XY vector parallel to North Street is the XZ vector and the component parallel to West Avenue is the ZY vector.

done by orienting an indicator line on the anatomic display so that it is parallel to the presumed direction of flow (e.g., parallel to the vessel wall for a straight vessel with no flow obstruction). This is a subjective operation performed by the instrument operator. Error in this estimation of the Doppler angle is more critical at large angles than at small ones because the cosine changes rapidly at large angles. Table 5-4 gives error values for various angles. For example, if the correct Doppler angle is 60 degrees but the estimation is 5 degrees in error (the angle estimate is 55 or 65 degrees), the error in the cosine value is about 15%, yielding a calculated speed that is in error by about 18%. Figure 5-21 shows how the error in calculated flow speed increases with angle. For this reason and because Doppler shift frequencies become very small at large angles, thereby reducing the system sensitivity, Doppler measurements (and particularly calculated flow speeds) are not achieved reliably at Doppler angles greater than about 60 degrees. In principle, if angle is incorporated correctly, the calculated flow speed in the vessel should be the same, regardless of what the Doppler angle is; that is, the actual flow speed is certainly not altered by the Doppler angle used in detecting it (Table 5-5). Not surprisingly, however, inaccuracies in angle estimation *are* experienced. Also, flow is often not parallel to vessel walls, even in unobstructed vessels.[15-20]

At Doppler angles less than about 30 degrees, the sound no longer enters the blood at all but is reflected totally at the wall-blood boundary.[29] Success is obtained, then, generally at angles greater than this. However, in Doppler echocardiography, Doppler angles of nearly zero *are* useful, and zero commonly is assumed (i.e., angle correction is not incorporated in this application like it is in vascular work). In this application, the angle between the beam and the heart wall is large, thereby avoiding the total reflection problem (Figure 5-22).

TABLE 5-4   Cosine and Calculated-Speed Errors for Angle Errors of 2 and 5 Degrees

True Angle (degrees)	Cosine Error (%)		Speed Error (%)	
	+2 Degrees	+5 Degrees	+2 Degrees	+5 Degrees
0	−0.1	−0.4	+0.1	+0.4
10	−0.7	−1.9	+0.7	+2.0
20	−1.3	−3.6	+1.3	+3.7
30	−2.1	−5.4	+2.1	+5.7
40	−3.0	−7.7	+3.1	+8.3
50	−4.2	−10.8	+4.4	+12.1
60	−6.1	−15.5	+6.5	+18.3
70	−9.6	−24.3	+10.7	+32.1
80	−19.9	−49.8	+24.8	+99.2

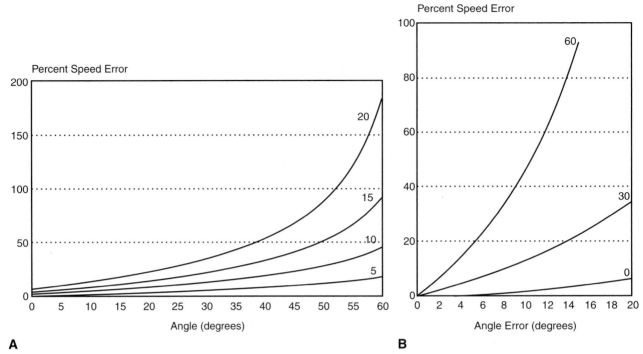

■ **FIGURE 5-21** **A,** Percent calculated speed error versus correct Doppler angle for 5-, 10-, 15-, and 20-degree angle errors. **B,** Percent calculated speed error versus angle error for three values (0, 30, and 60 degrees) of the correct Doppler angle.

TABLE 5-5   Doppler Shifts (for 4 MHz) at Various Doppler Angles for the Same Flow Yielding a Consistent Calculated Flow Speed

Doppler Shift (kHz)	Angle (degrees)	Calculated Flow Speed (cm/s)
2.25	30	50
1.99	40	50
1.84	45	50
1.67	50	50
1.30	60	50

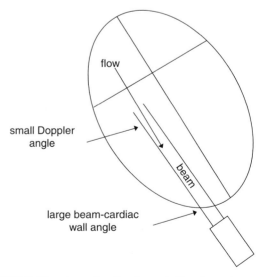

■ **FIGURE 5-22** In cardiac Doppler work, Doppler angles are usually small, whereas the angle between the beam and the cardiac wall is usually large.

In conclusion, one must emphasize that to proceed from a measurement of Doppler shift frequency to a correct calculation of flow speed, Doppler angle must be incorporated correctly; otherwise, an incorrect flow speed calculation will result. Seldom is angle estimation accomplished with no error. But even so, Doppler calculations are useful because errors in most cases are acceptable for Doppler angles less than about 60 degrees. Table 5-6 gives examples of Doppler shifts for various frequencies, angles, and speeds.

We have considered in this discussion the Doppler angle in the scan plane only. One must remember that the flow may not be parallel to the imaging scan plane, which includes the Doppler beam, so that there may be a component of Doppler angle between the flow direction and the scan plane. Thus one must keep in mind the three-dimensional character of the components involved in the process (vessel anatomy, flow, and ultrasound image scan plane).

REVIEW

The key points presented in this chapter are the following:

- Fluids (gases and liquids) are substances that flow.
- Blood is a liquid that flows through the vascular system.
- The heart provides the pulsatile pressure necessary to produce blood flow.
- Volumetric flow rate is proportional to pressure difference at the ends of a tube.
- Volumetric flow rate is inversely proportional to flow resistance.
- Flow resistance increases with viscosity and tube length and decreases greatly with increasing tube diameter.
- Flow classifications include steady, pulsatile, plug, laminar, parabolic, disturbed, and turbulent.
- In a stenosis, flow speeds up, pressure drops (Bernoulli effect), and flow is disturbed.
- If flow speed exceeds a critical value, as described by the Reynolds number, turbulence occurs.
- Pulsatile flow is common in arterial circulation.
- Diastolic flow and/or flow reversal occur in some locations within the arterial system.
- Fluid inertia and vessel compliance are characteristics that are important in determining flow with pulsatile driving pressure.
- The Doppler effect is a change in frequency resulting from motion.
- In medical ultrasound applications, blood flow and tissue motion are the sources of the Doppler effect.
- The change in frequency of the returning echoes with respect to the emitted frequency is called the Doppler shift.
- For flow toward the transducer, the Doppler shift is positive.
- For flow away from the transducer, the Doppler shift is negative.
- The Doppler shift depends on the speed of the scatterers of sound, the Doppler angle, and the operating frequency of the Doppler system.
- Reporting of a Doppler shift frequency without specifying the operating frequency and Doppler angle is incomplete reporting.
- A moving scatterer of sound produces a double Doppler shift.
- Greater flow speeds and smaller Doppler angles produce larger Doppler shifts, but not stronger Doppler-shifted echoes.

TABLE 5-6 Doppler Shifts for Various Frequencies, Angles, and Speeds			
Frequency (MHz)	Angle (degrees)	Speed (cm/s)	Shift (kHz)
2	0	10	0.26
2	0	50	1.30
2	0	100	2.60
2	30	10	0.22
2	30	50	1.12
2	30	100	2.25
2	45	10	0.18
2	45	50	0.92
2	45	100	1.84
2	60	10	0.13
2	60	50	0.65
2	60	100	1.30
5	0	10	0.65
5	0	50	3.25
5	0	100	6.49
5	30	10	0.56
5	30	50	2.81
5	30	100	5.62
5	45	10	0.46
5	45	50	2.30
5	45	100	4.59
5	60	10	0.32
5	60	50	1.62
5	60	100	3.25
10	0	10	1.30
10	0	50	6.49
10	0	100	13.0
10	30	10	1.12
10	30	50	5.62
10	30	100	11.2
10	45	10	0.92
10	45	50	4.59
10	45	100	9.18
10	60	10	0.65
10	60	50	3.25
10	60	100	6.49

- Higher operating frequencies produce larger Doppler shifts.
- Typical ranges of flow speeds (10 to 100 cm/s), Doppler angles (30 to 60 degrees), and operating frequencies (2 to 10 MHz) yield Doppler shifts in the range of 100 Hz to 11 kHz for vascular studies.
- In Doppler echocardiography, in which zero angle and speeds of a few meters per second can be encountered, Doppler shifts can be as high as 30 kHz.

EXERCISES

1. Which of the following are parts of the circulatory system? (more than one correct answer)
   a. Heart
   b. Cerebral ventricle
   c. Artery
   d. Arteriole
   e. Capillary
   f. Bile duct
   g. Venule
   h. Vein
2. The _____ are the tiniest vessels in the circulatory system.
3. Doppler ultrasound can detect flow in which of the following? (more than one correct answer)
   a. Heart
   b. Arteries
   c. Arterioles
   d. Capillaries
   e. Venules
   f. Veins
4. Which of the following are fluids?
   a. Gas
   b. Liquid
   c. Solid
   d. a and b
   e. a, b, and c
5. Which of the following do (does) not flow?
   a. Gas
   b. Liquid
   c. Solid
   d. a and b
   e. a, b, and c
6. To flow is to move in a _____.
7. Blood is made up of _____, _____, leukocytes, and platelets. Plasma is primarily _____.
8. A normal hematocrit is about _____%.
   a. 10
   b. 20
   c. 30
   d. 40
   e. 50

9. Which are the dominant cells in blood?
   a. Erythrocytes
   b. Lymphocytes
   c. Monocytes
   d. Leukocytes
   e. Platelets
10. The mass per unit volume of a fluid is called its
    a. resistance.
    b. viscosity.
    c. inertia.
    d. impedance.
    e. density.
11. The characteristic of a fluid that offers resistance to flow is called
    a. resistance.
    b. viscosity.
    c. inertia.
    d. impedance.
    e. density.
12. Resistance to acceleration is called
    a. resistance.
    b. viscosity.
    c. inertia.
    d. impedance.
    e. density.
13. Poise is a unit of _____.
14. Kilograms per liter (kg/L) is a unit of _____.
15. Grams per milliliter (g/mL) is a unit of _____.
16. Give the normal values for blood for the following:
    Density _____
    Viscosity _____
17. Pressure is _____ per unit area.
18. Pressure is
    a. nondirectional.
    b. unidirectional.
    c. omnidirectional.
    d. all of the above.
    e. none of the above.
19. Flow is a response to pressure _____ or _____.
20. If the pressure is greater at one end of a liquid-filled tube or vessel than it is at the other, the liquid will flow from the _____ pressure end to the _____ pressure end.
    a. Higher, lower
    b. Lower, higher
    c. Depends on the liquid
    d. All of the above
    e. None of the above
21. A pressure difference can be generated by a _____ or by _____.
22. Pressure gradient is pressure _____ divided by _____ between the two pressure locations.
23. The volumetric flow rate in a tube is determined by _____ difference and _____.

24. If the following is increased, flow increases.
    a. Pressure difference
    b. Pressure gradient
    c. Resistance
    d. a and b
    e. All of the above
25. As flow resistance increases, volumetric flow rate _____.
26. If pressure difference is doubled, volumetric flow rate is
    a. unchanged.
    b. quartered.
    c. halved.
    d. doubled.
    e. quadrupled.
27. If flow resistance is doubled, volumetric flow rate is
    a. unchanged.
    b. quartered.
    c. halved.
    d. doubled.
    e. quadrupled.
28. Tubes that carry blood in the circulatory system are called _____.
29. The largest vessels are
    a. arteries.
    b. veins.
    c. arterioles and venules.
    d. capillaries.
    e. a and b.
30. The smallest vessels are
    a. arteries.
    b. veins.
    c. arterioles and venules.
    d. capillaries.
    e. a and b.
31. Flow resistance in a vessel depends on
    a. vessel length.
    b. vessel radius.
    c. blood viscosity.
    d. all of the above.
    e. none of the above.
32. Flow resistance decreases with an increase in which of the following?
    a. Vessel length
    b. Vessel radius
    c. Blood viscosity
    d. All of the above
    e. None of the above
33. Flow resistance depends most strongly on which of the following?
    a. Vessel length
    b. Vessel radius
    c. Blood viscosity
    d. All of the above
    e. None of the above

34. Doubling the radius of a vessel decreases its resistance to _____ of the original value.
    a. One half
    b. One fourth
    c. One eighth
    d. One sixteenth
    e. One thirty-second
35. Volumetric flow rate decreases with an increase in which of the following?
    a. Pressure difference
    b. Vessel radius
    c. Vessel length
    d. Blood viscosity
    e. c and d
36. When the speed of a fluid is constant across a vessel, the flow is called _____ flow.
    a. Volume
    b. Parabolic
    c. Laminar
    d. Viscous
    e. Plug
37. The type of flow (approximately) seen in Figure 5-23, *A*, is _____.
    a. Volume
    b. Steady
    c. Parabolic
    d. Viscous
    e. Plug
38. The type of flow seen in Figure 5-23, *B*, is _____.
    a. Volume
    b. Steady
    c. Parabolic
    d. Viscous
    e. Plug
39. _____ flow occurs when straight parallel streamlines describing the flow are altered.
40. _____ flow involves random and chaotic flow patterns, with particles flowing in all directions.
41. Turbulent flow occurs in a vessel when the _____ number exceeds about 2000.
42. A narrowing of the lumen of a tube is called a _____.
43. Proximal to, at, and distal to a stenosis, _____ must be constant.
    a. Laminar flow
    b. Disturbed flow
    c. Turbulent flow
    d. Volumetric flow rate
    e. None of the above
44. For the answer to Exercise 43 to be true, flow speed at the stenosis must be _____ that proximal and distal to it.
    a. Greater than
    b. Less than

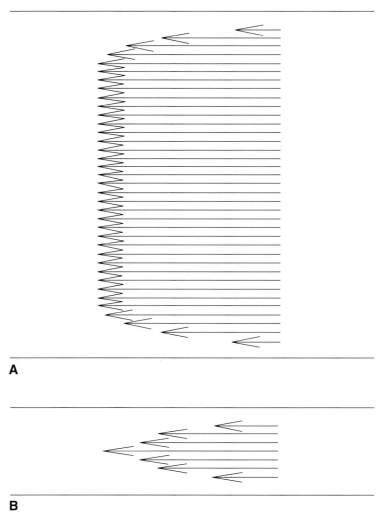

A

B

■ **FIGURE 5-23**   Two types of flow patterns (to accompany Exercises 37 and 38).

c. Less turbulent than
d. Less disturbed than
e. None of the above

45. Poiseuille's equation predicts a(n) _____ in flow speed with a decrease in vessel radius.

46. The continuity rule predicts a(n) _____ in flow speed with a localized decrease (stenosis) in vessel diameter.

47. The volumetric flow rate out of the heart into the aorta is about
a. 1 L/min.
b. 2 L/min.
c. 3 L/min.
d. 4 L/min.
e. 5 L/min.

48. Maximum flow speed encountered in stenotic jets is about
a. 100 cm/s.
b. 200 cm/s.
c. 300 cm/s.
d. 400 cm/s.
e. 5000 cm/s.

49. In a stenosis, the pressure is _____ the proximal and distal values.
a. Less than
b. Equal to
c. Greater than
d. Depends on the fluid
e. None of the above

50. Added forward flow and flow reversal in diastole can occur with _____ flow.
a. Volume
b. Turbulent
c. Laminar
d. Disturbed
e. Pulsatile

51. Calculate the flow speed above which turbulent blood flow should occur in the aorta. Assume a diameter of 2 cm and a Reynolds number of 2000.

52. For the stenosis shown in Figure 5-10, vessel diameters are $d_1 = 2$ cm, $d_2 = 1$ cm, and $d_3 = 2$ cm. For blood flowing through the stenosis at a rate of 50 mL/s, find the average flow speeds and the Reynolds numbers proximal to, at, and distal to the stenosis.

53. Turbulence generally occurs when the Reynolds number exceeds
    a. 100.
    b. 200.
    c. 1000.
    d. 2000.
    e. a and b.

54. As stenosis diameter decreases, the following pass(es) through a maximum.
    a. Flow speed at the stenosis
    b. Flow speed proximal to the stenosis
    c. Volumetric flow rate
    d. Doppler shift at the stenosis
    e. a and d

55. In Figure 5-24, at which point is pressure lowest?
    a. P
    b. S
    c. D
    d. P and D
    e. None of the above

56. In Figure 5-24, at which point is flow speed the lowest?
    a. P
    b. S
    c. D
    d. P and D
    e. None of the above

57. In Figure 5-24, at which point is volumetric flow rate the lowest?
    a. P
    b. S
    c. D
    d. P and D
    e. None of the above

58. In Figure 5-24, at which point is flow energy the greatest?
    a. P
    b. S
    c. D
    d. P and D
    e. None of the above

59. In Figure 5-24, at which point is pressure energy the greatest?
    a. P
    b. S
    c. D
    d. P and D
    e. None of the above

60. In Figure 5-24, at which point is viscosity the greatest?
    a. P
    b. S
    c. D
    d. P and D
    e. None of the above

61. The _____ effect is used to detect and measure _____ in vessels.

62. Motion of an echo-generating structure causes an echo to have a different _____ than the emitted pulse.

63. The Doppler effect is a change in reflected _____ caused by reflector _____.

64. If the reflector is moving toward the source, the reflected frequency is _____ than the incident frequency.

65. If the reflector is moving away from the source, the reflected frequency is _____ than the incident frequency.

66. If the reflector is stationary with respect to the source, the reflected frequency is _____ the incident frequency.

67. Measurement of Doppler shift yields information about reflector _____.

68. If the incident frequency is 1 MHz, the propagation speed is 1600 m/s, and the reflector speed is 16 m/s toward the source, the Doppler shift is _____ MHz, and the reflected frequency is _____ MHz.

69. If 2-MHz ultrasound is reflected from a soft tissue boundary moving at 10 m/s toward the source, the Doppler shift is _____ MHz.

70. If 2-MHz ultrasound is reflected from a soft tissue boundary moving at 10 m/s away from the source, the Doppler shift is _____ MHz.

71. Doppler shift is the difference between _____ and _____ frequencies.

72. When incident sound direction and reflector motion are not parallel, calculation of the reflected frequency involves the _____ of the angle between these directions.

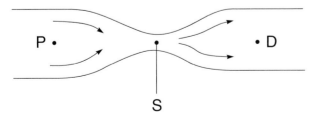

■ **FIGURE 5-24**   Proximal to *(P)*, at *(S)*, and distal to *(D)* a stenosis. (Illustration to accompany Exercises 55 to 60.) (From Kremkau FW: *J Vasc Technol* 17:153-154, 1993. Reproduced with permission.)

73. If the angle between incident sound direction and reflector motion is 60 degrees, the Doppler shift and reflected frequency in Exercise 68 are _____MHz and _____ MHz.

74. If the angle between incident sound direction and reflector motion is 90 degrees, the cosine of the angle is _____, and the reflected frequency in Exercise 68 is _____ MHz.

75. A policeman in a Doppler radar–equipped patrol car detects the speed of an automobile to be 55 mph. If the angle between the radar beam and the direction of the automobile is 60 degrees, the actual speed of the automobile is _____ mph.

76. Fill in the missing values in the following table below.

f (MHz)	v (cm/s)	θ (degrees)	f_D (kHz)
2.5	50	0	(a)
5	50	(b)	3.25
7.5	(c)	0	4.87
(d)	100	0	3.25
5	100	0	(e)
7.5	100	(f)	9.74
2.5	(g)	0	4.87
(h)	150	0	9.74
7.5	150	0	(i)
5	50	30	(j)
5	50	(k)	1.62
5	50	(l)	0
5	(m)	30	5.62
5	100	60	(n)
5	(o)	90	0
5	150	(p)	8.44
(q)	150	60	4.87
5	150	90	(r)

77. The maximum normal flow speed encountered in the circulatory system is approximately
   a. 1 mm/s.
   b. 1 cm/s.
   c. 100 cm/s.
   d. 100 m/s.
   e. 1 km/s.

78. For an operating frequency of 2 MHz, a flow speed of 10 cm/s, and a Doppler angle of 0, calculate the Doppler shift.

79. For an operating frequency of 4 MHz, a flow speed of 10 cm/s, and a Doppler angle of 30 degrees, calculate the Doppler shift.

80. For an operating frequency of 6 MHz, a flow speed of 50 cm/s, and a Doppler angle of 60 degrees, calculate the Doppler shift.

81. For an operating frequency of 5 MHz, a Doppler angle of 45 degrees, and a Doppler shift of 4.60 kHz, calculate the flow speed.

82. For an operating frequency of 6 MHz, a Doppler angle of 60 degrees, and a Doppler shift of 1.95 kHz, calculate the flow speed.

83. If the propagation speed in blood is greater than that in the surrounding tissue, does the effect of refraction increase or decrease the Doppler angle?

84. Does the result in Exercise 83 increase or decrease the Doppler shift frequency?

85. What is the Doppler shift if a reflector is moving toward a 5-MHz source at a speed of 10 cm/s?

86. If a reflector is moving away from a 5-MHz source at 100 cm/s, what is the Doppler shift?

87. In Exercise 86, what frequency does the transducer receive?

88. At 10 MHz, with 50 cm/s flow speed, and at a Doppler angle of 60 degrees, what is the Doppler shift?

89. At 10 MHz, with 50 cm/s flow speed, and at a Doppler angle of 30 degrees, what is the Doppler shift?

90. The Doppler shifts for a moving source, a moving receiver, or a moving reflector (all moving at the same speed) are the same. True or false?

91. For blood flowing in a vessel with a plug flow profile, the Doppler shift is _____ across the vessel.

92. What is the role of blood cells in Doppler ultrasound?

93. Physiologic flow speeds can be as much as _____ % of the propagation speed in soft tissues.
   a. 0.01
   b. 0.3
   c. 5
   d. 10
   e. 50

94. Which Doppler angle yields the greatest Doppler shift?
   a. −90
   b. −45
   c. 0
   d. 45
   e. 90

95. To proceed from a measurement of Doppler shift frequency to a calculation of flow speed, _____ _____ must be known or assumed.

96. The intensity of returning Doppler-shifted echoes is not affected by _____ or _____.

97. Doppler shift frequency does not depend on
   a. amplitude.
   b. flow speed.
   c. operating frequency.
   d. Doppler angle.
   e. propagation speed.

98. If operating frequency is doubled, Doppler shift is _____.

99. If flow speed is doubled, Doppler shift is _____.

100. If Doppler angle is doubled, Doppler shift is _____.

101. Calculate the 5-MHz Doppler shift for a reflector moving at 100 m/s.

102. In Figure 5-18, what are the operating frequencies, assuming a 60-degree angle?

103. In Figure 5-19, what is the Doppler angle if the flow speeds are 282, 141, and 70?

104. A 4-MHz, 500 cm/s curve would be identical to which curve in Figure 5-20, C?

105. A 2-MHz, 250 cm/s curve would be identical to which curve in Figure 5-20, C?

106. For a Doppler angle of 60 degrees, a flow speed of 1.5 m/s, and an operating frequency of 5 MHz, the Doppler shift is _____ kHz, which is _____ % of the operating frequency.

107. In Figure 5-25, which angle is the incidence angle? Which angle is the Doppler angle? Which angle is the transmission angle? If there is no refraction, which angle is equal to the transmission angle? With no refraction, which angle is equal to the Doppler angle? Incidence angle plus Doppler angle (no refraction) equals what?

108. The cosine of an angle can be no greater than
    a. π
    b. 1
    c. 0
    d. −1
    e. −π

109. The cosine of an angle can be no less than
    a. 10.
    b. 1.
    c. 0.
    d. −1.
    e. −10.

110. The difference between the Doppler shift for a moving receiver and a moving source is negligible if the speed of movement is _____ enough.

111. As a reflector approaches a transducer at 50 cm/s, the round-trip distance between them is reduced at the rate of _____ cm/s.

112. As a reflector recedes from a transducer at 50 cm/s, the round-trip distance between them is increased at the rate of _____ cm/s.

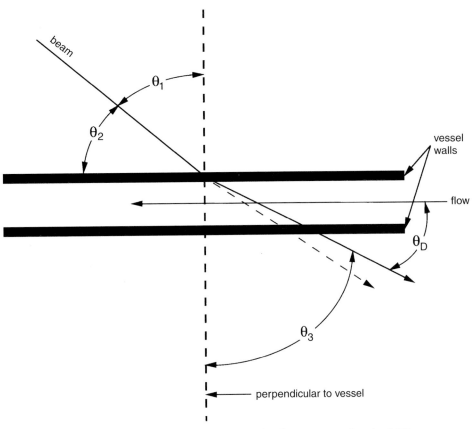

■ **FIGURE 5-25** Diagram of various angles (to accompany Exercise 107).

113. Exercises 111 and 112 present one reason why there is a factor of _____ in the Doppler equation for a reflector.

114. Figure 5-26 shows a police radar unit *(P)* using the Doppler effect to determine the speed of an automobile *(A)*. What happens to the Doppler shift as the vehicle travels down the highway at constant speed?

115. In Figure 5-20, *D*, which viewing angle *(1* or *2)* gives the greatest Doppler angle? Which gives the greatest Doppler shift?

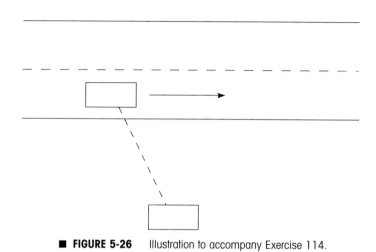

■ **FIGURE 5-26**   Illustration to accompany Exercise 114.

Color Doppler Instruments*

*NOTE: Appendix I provides a condensed version of the material in Chapters 5 to 7 for readers who need less depth and breadth of coverage on Doppler topics. Because of the importance of blood flow and Doppler techniques in echocardiography and vascular ultrasound, the complete coverage in Chapters 5 to 7 is recommended for persons working in those fields.

LEARNING OBJECTIVES

After reading this chapter, the student should be able to do the following:

- Describe the technique used to determine two-dimensional Doppler information rapidly.
- Explain how two-dimensional flow information is color-encoded on a sonographic display.
- List the types of flow information that are presented on such displays.
- Compare Doppler-shift and Doppler-power displays.

KEY TERMS

The following terms are introduced in this chapter:

Autocorrelation
Clutter
Color Doppler display
Doppler-power display

Ensemble length
Hue
Luminance
Priority

Saturation
Variance
Wall filter

Doppler instruments present information on the presence, direction, speed, and character of blood flow (Box 6-1) and on the presence, direction, and speed of tissue motion. This information is present in audible, color Doppler, and spectral Doppler forms (Box 6-2). Color Doppler imaging[30-39] presents two-dimensional, cross-sectional, real-time blood flow or tissue motion information along with two-dimensional, cross-sectional, gray-scale anatomic imaging. Two-dimensional real-time presentations of flow information allow the observer to locate regions of abnormal flow readily for further evaluation using spectral analysis. The direction of flow is appreciated readily, and disturbed or turbulent flow is presented dramatically in two-dimensional form. Color Doppler instruments present anatomic information in the conventional gray-scale form but also rapidly detect Doppler-shift frequencies at several locations along each scan line, presenting them in color at appropriate locations in the cross-sectional image.

COLOR DOPPLER PRINCIPLE

Color Doppler imaging (sometimes called color flow imaging) extends the use of the pulse-echo imaging principle to include Doppler-shifted echoes that indicate blood flow or tissue motion. Echoes returning from stationary tissues are detected and presented in gray

---

BOX 6-1   Types of Flow Information Provided by Doppler Ultrasound

Presence of flow
- Yes
- No

Direction of flow
- ←
- →

Speed of flow
- Slow
- Fast

Character of flow
- Laminar
- Turbulent

BOX 6-2   Various Forms of Presentation of Doppler Information

Audible sounds
Strip-chart recording
Spectral display
Color Doppler display

---

scale in appropriate locations along scan lines. Depth is determined by echo arrival time, and brightness is determined by echo intensity. If a returning echo has a different frequency than what was emitted, a Doppler shift has occurred because the echo-generating object was moving. Depending on whether the motion is toward or away from the transducer, the Doppler shift is positive or negative. At locations along scan lines where Doppler shifts are detected, appropriate colors are assigned to the display pixels.

Color Doppler imaging is an extension of conventional gray-scale sonography that shows regions of blood flow or tissue motion in color.

Doppler-shifted echoes can be recorded and presented in color at many locations along each scan line (Figure 6-1, *A* and *B* [see Color Plate 4]). As in all sonography, many such scan lines make up one cross-sectional image (Figure 6-1, *C* and *D* [see Color Plate 4]). Several of these images (frames) are presented each second, yielding real-time color Doppler sonography.

Linear array presentation of color Doppler information is sometimes inadequate when the vessel runs parallel to the skin surface. The pulses (and scan lines) run perpendicular to the transducer surface (and therefore to the skin surface), resulting in a 90-degree

Doppler angle at which the pulses intersect the flow in the vessel. If the flow is parallel to the vessel walls, the 90-degree Doppler angle would yield no Doppler shift, and hence no color within the vessel. To solve this problem, phasing is used to steer each emitted pulse from the array in a given direction (e.g., 20 degrees away from perpendicular). All the color pulses and color scan lines are steered at the same angle, resulting in a parallelogram presentation of color Doppler information on the display (Figure 6-2 [see Color Plate 5]).

Components of Color

The three components of a color, as seen on a display, include **hue, saturation,** and **luminance** (Figure 6-3 [see Color Plate 5]). Hue is the color that is perceived by the viewer. Hue represents the frequency of the light, an electromagnetic wave. The range of frequencies detectable by the human eye includes from the lowest (red) to the highest (violet), with increasing frequency progression through orange, yellow, green, and blue in between. The visible light frequency range is about 400,000,000 to 800,000,000 MHz. Saturation is the amount of hue present in a mix with white (which is a combination of all visible hues). This is comparable to mixing a deep-color paint with white to produce a pale color (e.g., mixing red with white to yield pink). The less white that is present, the greater the saturation. The more white that is present, the less the saturation (red is more saturated than pink). Luminance is the brightness of the hue and saturation presented. In conventional gray-scale anatomic imaging, saturation is zero (there is no hue), and luminance represents echo intensity. This yields gray-scale imaging, ranging from black to white through various shades of gray. In color Doppler imaging, various combinations of hue, saturation, and luminance are used to indicate the sign, magnitude of the mean, and sometimes the power or the **variance** of the Doppler shifts found at each location. The mean and variance are encountered because Doppler shift, representing flow within each sample volume, is not the result of a single moving reflector (such as an erythrocyte) but of millions of moving cells which, even in normal flow, are not all moving at the same speed and direction. The instrument detects the mean of these many Doppler shifts at each location and, in some cases, the variance (which is a measure of the spread around the mean, and therefore an indicator of the extent of flow disturbance or turbulence).

Hue, saturation, and luminance are the three characteristics of color that are used to indicate the nature of the Doppler-shifted echoes encountered, that is, their mean Doppler shift, sign, power, and variance.

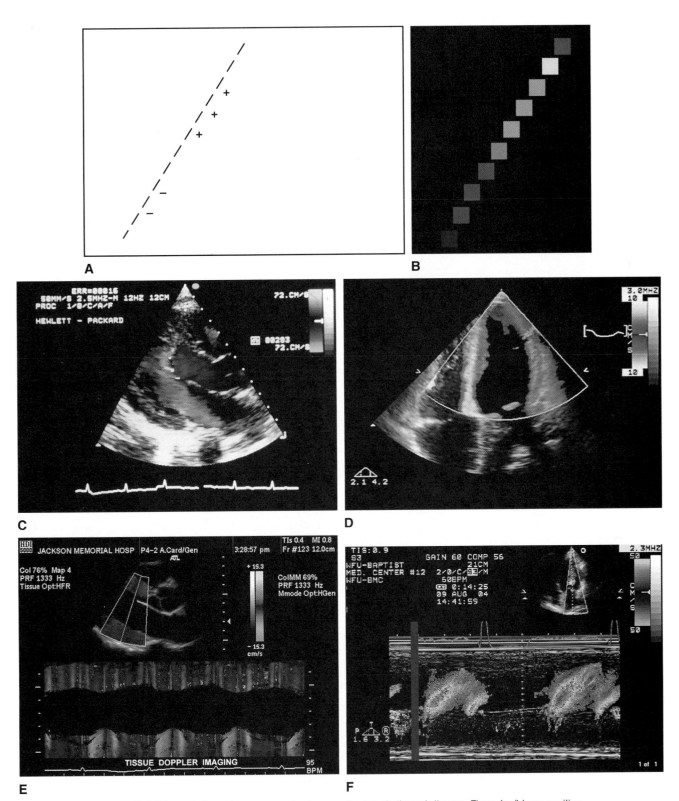

■ **FIGURE 6-1** **A,** Ten echoes are received as a pulse travels through tissues. Three *(red)* have positive Doppler shifts and two *(blue)* have negative shifts. **B,** These echoes are shown as red and blue pixels, respectively, on the color Doppler display. As in gray-scale sonography, a two-dimensional cross-sectional image is made up of many scan lines. **C,** A parasternal long-axis image of normal mitral valve blood flow. **D,** Tissue Doppler imaging of myocardial motion. **E,** Color Doppler M mode display with tissue motion detected. **F,** Color Doppler M mode display with blood flow detected. (See Color Plate 4.)

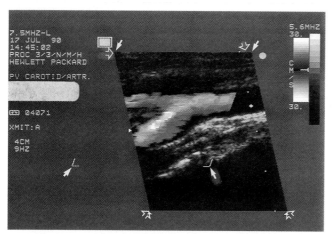

■ **FIGURE 6-2** A perpendicular Doppler angle is avoided in this image by electronically steering the color-producing Doppler pulses to the left of vertical. The corners of the resulting parallelogram in which color can be displayed are shown by the solid arrows. Note that on this instrument, the gray-scale anatomic imaging pulses also can be steered (in this case, to the right of vertical). The corners of the resulting gray-scale parallelogram are shown by the open arrows. (See Color Plate 5.) (From Kremkau FW: Principles and pitfalls of real-time color-flow imaging. In Bernstein EF, editor: *Vascular diagnosis*, ed 4, St Louis, 1993, Mosby.)

INSTRUMENTS

The color Doppler instrument has the same block diagram as the gray-scale sonographic instrument (see Figure 4-1, *A*). The beam former, signal processor, image processor, and display perform the same functions as they do in the sonographic instrument. But in addition, the signal processor must include the ability to detect Doppler shifts, and the display must be capable of presenting echoes in color.

Color Doppler instruments are conventional sonographic instruments that have the ability to detect Doppler shifts and present them on the display in color.

Doppler-Shift Detection

The signal processor receives the digitized voltages from the beam former that represent the echoes returning from tissue. Non–Doppler-shifted echoes are processed conventionally, as in any sonographic instrument. Doppler-shifted echoes commonly are detected in the signal processor using a mathematical technique, called **autocorrelation,** that rapidly determines the mean and variance of the Doppler-shift signal (Figure 6-4) at each location along the scan line (at each selected echo arrival time during pulse travel). The autocorrelation

technique[40] is a mathematical process that yields the Doppler-shift information for each sample time (and corresponding depth down the scan line) following pulse emission. The sign, mean, and variance of the Doppler signal are stored at appropriate locations in the memory corresponding to anatomic sites where the Doppler shifts have been found. A **color Doppler display** typically shows 100 to 400 Doppler samples (locations) per scan line. Depending on the depth and width of the color presentation, the display typically shows 5 to 50 frames per second. Recall that for gray-scale sonography, a single pulse produces one scan line. For multiple foci, multiple pulses per scan line are required. In color Doppler instruments, multiple pulses are involved in all images because they are required in the autocorrelation process. One pair of pulses yields a phase (discussed in the next chapter) difference determination. Two phase determinations yield a Doppler shift (flow speed) estimate. Therefore a three-pulse minimum is required for one speed estimate. More pulses are required for improved accuracy of the estimates, for variance determinations, or to improve detection of lower-frequency mean Doppler shifts (slower flows).

Autocorrelation is the mathematical process commonly used to detect Doppler shifts in color Doppler instruments.

ADVANCED CONCEPTS

Autocorrelation is a mathematical process that compares a function with itself, in this case signal phase at different times. Autocorrelation is a measure of similarity (or nonrandomness) of the function at the different times. Autocorrelation is the cross-correlation of the signal with a time-delayed version of itself. Autocorrelation is useful for finding repeating patterns in a signal, such as determining the presence of a periodic signal that has been buried under noise. For our purpose, autocorrelation can determine the phase shift that has occurred over some short time interval. This phase shift is a measure of the Doppler shift and an indicator of the motion of a reflector over the time interval.

Color Controls

Color controls (Figure 6-5) include color window location, width and depth, gain, steering angle, color inversion, **wall filter, priority,** baseline shift, velocity range (pulse repetition frequency [PRF]), color map selection, variance, smoothing, and **ensemble length.** Steering angle control permits avoidance of 90-degree angles

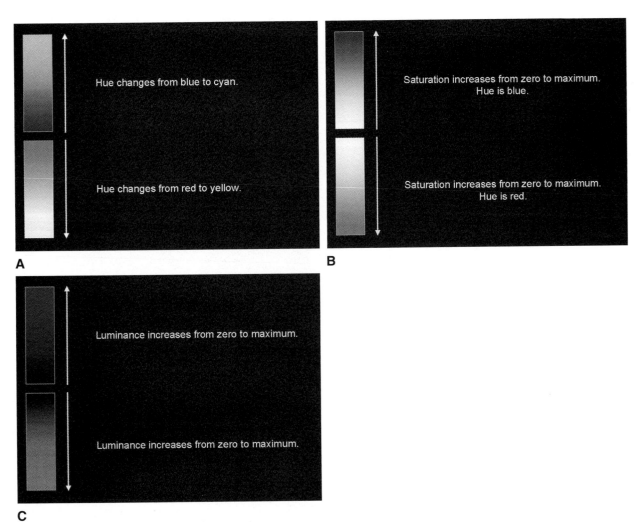

■ **FIGURE 6-3** **A,** Hue is the color that is perceived by the viewer. **B,** Saturation is the amount of hue present in a mix with white. **C,** Luminance is the brightness of the hue and saturation presented. (See Color Plate 5.)

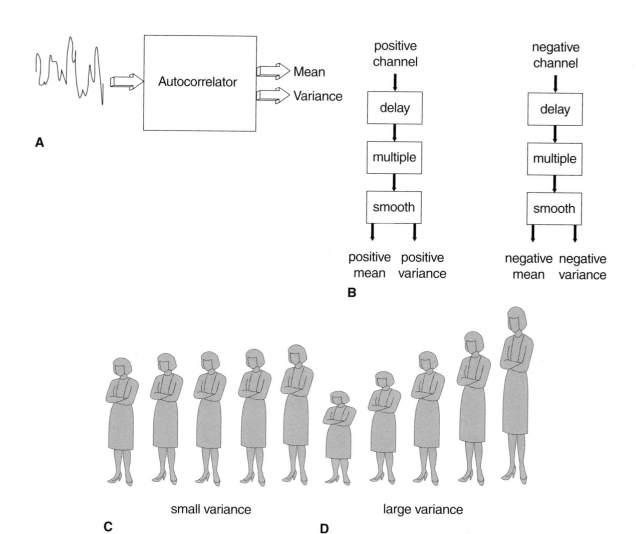

■ **FIGURE 6-4** **A,** The autocorrelator rapidly performs Doppler demodulation on the complicated echo signal *(entering at left)*. The outputs of the autocorrelator yield the magnitude of the mean and the variance of the Doppler shifts at each location in the scanned cross section. These items of information are stored in each pixel location in the memory. Color assignments are selected appropriately to indicate these items of information two-dimensionally on the display. **B,** After division of the Doppler signal into positive and negative Doppler-shift channels, each signal is multiplied by a version of itself delayed by one pulse repetition period. High-frequency variations are filtered out (smoothed) to yield the mean and variance of the Doppler shifts. Variance is a measure of data spread around a mean. Variance is equal to the standard deviation squared. **C** and **D,** Two groups of women with equal mean heights but unequal variances.

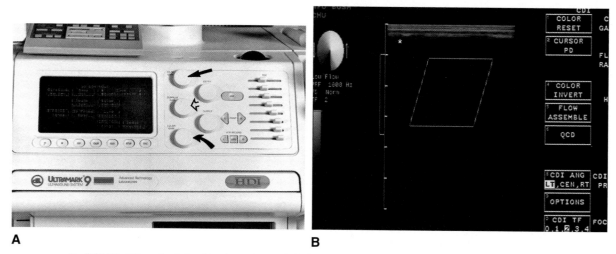

■ **FIGURE 6-5** **A,** Color Doppler gain control *(curved arrow)*. The gray-scale *(straight arrow)* and spectral Doppler *(open arrow)* gain controls also are indicated. **B,** Software panel controls for color Doppler functions.

(Figure 6-6 [see Color Plates 6 to 8]). Color inversion alternates the color assignments on either side of the baseline on the color map (Figure 6-6, *D* and *E* [see Color Plate 7]). The wall filter allows elimination of **clutter** caused by tissue and wall motion (Figure 6-7 [see Color Plates 9 and 10]). However, one must take care not to set the wall filter too high, or slower blood flow signals will be removed (Figure 6-7, *C* [see Color Plate 9]). The operator of a gray-scale sonographic instrument does not have direct control of the PRF. But in Doppler instruments the operator does control the PRF with the scale control. This control sets the PRF and the limit at the color bar extremes. Decreasing the value permits observation of slower flows (smaller Doppler shifts) but increases the probability of aliasing for faster flows (aliasing is described in Chapter 8). Priority selects the gray-scale echo strength below which color will be shown instead of gray level at each pixel location (Figure 6-8 [see Color Plate 11]). Baseline control allows shifting the baseline up or down to eliminate aliasing. Smoothing (also called persistence) provides frame-to-frame averaging to reduce noise (Figure 6-9 [see Color Plates 12 and 13]). Ensemble length is the number of pulses used for each color scan line. The minimum is 3, with 10 to 20 being common. Greater ensemble lengths provide more accurate estimates of mean Doppler shift, improved detection of slow flows, and complete representation of flow within a vessel but at the expense of longer time per frame and therefore lower frame rates (see Figure 6-9 [see Color Plates 12 and 13]). Wider color windows (viewing areas) also reduce frame rates because more scan lines are required for each frame (Figure 6-10 [see Color Plate 14]).

Autocorrelation requires several pulses per scan line for Doppler detection. The number of pulses per scan line is called ensemble length.

Color Doppler Limitations

Several aspects of color Doppler imaging by their nature are limiting. They include angle dependence, lower frame rates, and lack of detailed spectral information. Spectral Doppler presents the entire range of Doppler shift frequencies received as they change over the cardiac cycle. Color Doppler displays present only a statistical representation of the complete spectrum at each pixel location on the display. The sign, mean value, and, if chosen, the power or the variance of the spectrum are color-coded into combinations of hue, saturation, and luminance, which are presented at each display pixel location. Some Doppler instruments have the capability of reading the quantitative digital values for mean Doppler shift (sometimes converted to angle-

corrected equivalent flow speed) at chosen pixel locations (Figure 6-11 [see Color Plate 15]). One must realize that these are mean values that must be compared carefully with the peak systolic values that are used commonly to evaluate spectral displays. Because color Doppler techniques require several pulses per scan line (as opposed to one pulse per scan line for single-focus, gray-scale anatomic imaging), frame rates are lower than those for gray-scale anatomic imaging. Therefore multiple foci are not used in color Doppler. The relationship between penetration, line density, and frame rate is the same as presented in Chapter 4 except that ensemble length (*n*) replaces number of focuses. The maximum permissible frame rate (*FR_m*) is as follows:

$$FR_m \text{ (Hz)} = \frac{77,000 \text{ (cm/s)}}{\text{pen (cm)} \times \text{LPF} \times n}$$

If ensemble length increases, frame rate decreases.

If the frame rate is low enough, a significant portion of the cardiac cycle is represented across the color image from left to right. In Figure 6-12 (see Color Plate 16) the time across the color window represents about 20% of the cardiac cycle. The bright portion represents the largest Doppler shifts. However, they are not a result of a region where the Doppler angle is the smallest (because the Doppler angle is approximately constant across the color window in this example) or where there is vessel narrowing (there is none in this example). The bright region represents the largest Doppler shifts at peak systole, with the darker red to the left representing late diastole and early systole and that on the right representing early diastole. In such a case, it would be a mistake to consider the single frame being viewed as a representation of the flow at an instant in time. In fact, the frame represents flow at various instants in time over a significant portion of the cardiac cycle, with time progressing from left to right across the color window.

Frame rates are lower in color Doppler imaging than in gray-scale sonography because of the ensemble length.

DOPPLER-SHIFT DISPLAYS

Where Doppler-shifted echoes have been stored, hue, saturation, and luminance appropriate to the shift information are presented according to a choice of schemes, the one selected being presented on the display as a color map (Figure 6-13 [see Color Plates 17 and 18]). The map allows the observer to interpret what the hue,

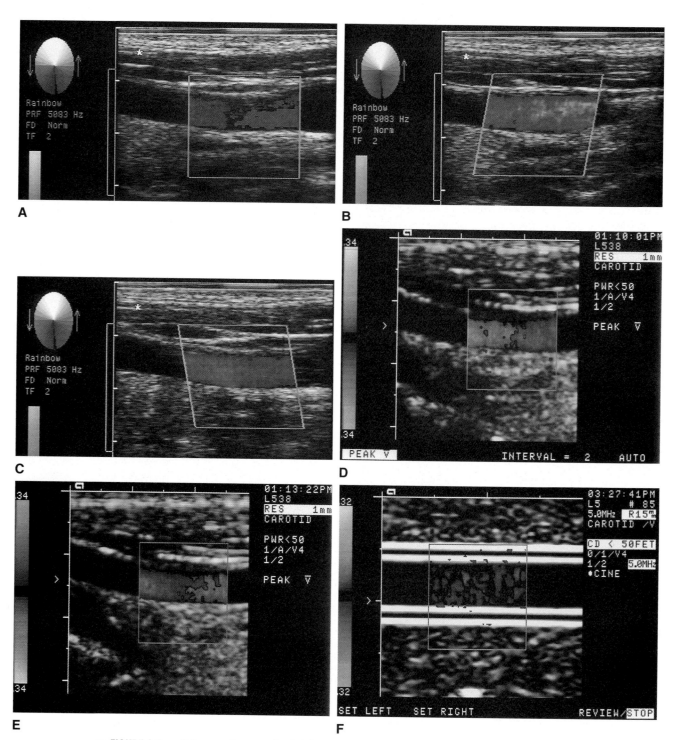

■ **FIGURE 6-6** Color scan lines are directed down vertically **(A),** to the left of vertical **(B),** and to the right of vertical **(C).** Flow is from left to right, producing positive or negative Doppler shifts, depending on the relationship between scan lines and flow. **D,** In this hue map, red and blue are assigned to positive and negative Doppler shifts, respectively, progressing to yellow and cyan (by the addition of green) at the Nyquist limits. **E,** In this map the color assignments are reversed from those presented in **D** (i.e., blue and red are assigned to positive and negative Doppler shifts, respectively). Note the color change occurring within each color window. This is caused by vessel curvature. **F,** With flow in a straight tube, positive and negative Doppler shifts are distributed equally throughout the color window with a Doppler angle of 90 degrees.

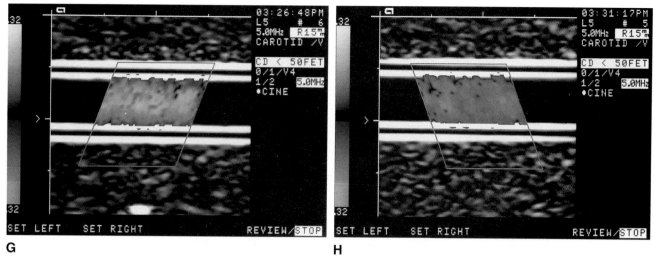

■ **FIGURE 6-6, cont'd**   **G,** Uniform positive Doppler shifts are observed with the color window steered 20 degrees to the left (70-degree Doppler angle). **H,** Uniform negative Doppler shifts are observed with the color window steered to the right. (See Color Plates 6 to 8.) (**A** to **C** from Kremkau FW: *Semin Roentgenol* 27:6-16, 1992; **D** and **E** from Kremkau FW: Principles and pitfalls of real-time color-flow imaging. In Bernstein EF, editor: *Vascular diagnosis,* ed 4, St Louis, 1993, Mosby.)

saturation, and luminance mean at each location in terms of sign, magnitude, and variance of the Doppler shifts. Hue indicates Doppler-shift sign. Changes in hue, saturation, or luminance up or down the map from the center indicate increasing Doppler-shift magnitude. When selected, variance is shown as a change in hue from left to right across the map.

The color map, always shown on the display, is the key to understanding how the image colors are related to the Doppler characteristics.

Angle

As with any Doppler technique, angle is important. Figure 6-14 (see Color Plates 19 and 20) shows convex array and linear array views of vascular flow. Note that the images are similar in appearance, with red on the left and blue on the right. But note that the relative position of the color bars is inverted. How is this inconsistency explained? In fact, why does the color change at all, considering there is no reason not to expect unidirectional flow in these vessels? The color changes in the vessel in part *A* because, with the sector image format, pulses and scan lines travel in different directions away from the transducer. They thus have different Doppler angles with the flow in a straight vessel. Some pulses view the flow upstream and some downstream. At the 90-degree Doppler angle point, the color changes because the situation changes from upstream to downstream. However, in part *C*, this is not the case. All the pulses travel in the same direction (straight down) from this linear array transducer. If the color change is not due to changing scan line directions, then it must be due to changing flow direction. Careful inspection of part *C* reveals that the vessel is not perfectly straight but curves up. Flow is from right to left in the vessel, so that flow is away from the transducer on the right (negative Doppler shift is blue on this map) and toward the transducer on the left (positive Doppler shift is red) (Figure 6-14, *D*). A view farther to the left reveals a second color change caused by the curve downward (Figure 6-14, *E*). Figure 6-14, *F,* shows an example of lack of color in a vessel. This lack of Doppler shift could be caused by lack of flow or flow viewed with a 90-degree Doppler angle. With an acceptable angle (Figure 6-14, *G*), flow is revealed.

Changing Doppler angle in an image produces various colors in different locations.

Figure 6-15, *A* (see Color Plate 21), shows various Doppler shifts as Doppler angle changes across the display in the sector format. Yellow corresponds to a large positive shift, red to a small positive shift, black to a zero shift, blue to a small negative shift, and cyan to a large negative shift. Flow is from left to right. Parts *B* to *F* confirm all this by spectral displays, which are discussed in the next chapter.

Text continued on p. 199.

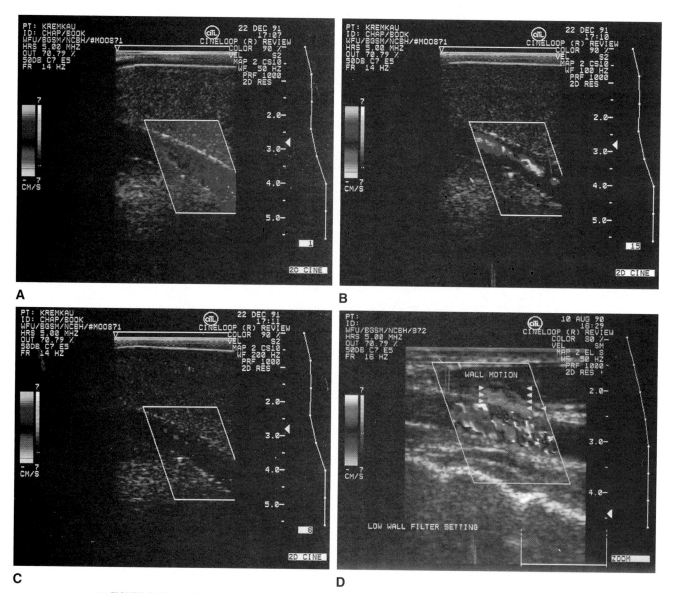

■ **FIGURE 6-7**   **A,** Tissue motion causes clutter, obscuring the flow in the vessel and clouding the gray-scale tissue with color Doppler information. **B,** Wall filter has been increased to 100 Hz, thereby eliminating the color clutter. **C,** Wall filter has been increased (too much) to 200 Hz, eliminating virtually all the color Doppler information derived from the vessel. **D,** With a low wall filter setting (50 Hz), wall motion appears in color on the image.

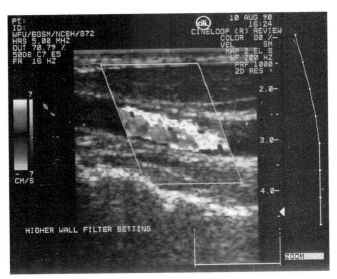

E

■ **FIGURE 6-7, cont'd** **E,** With a higher wall filter setting (200 Hz), this motion no longer appears in color. (See Color Plates 9 and 10.) (**A** to **C** from Kremkau FW: Principles and pitfalls of real-time color-flow imaging. In Bernstein EF, editor: *Vascular diagnosis,* ed 4, St Louis, 1993, Mosby; **D** and **E** from Kremkau FW: Principles and instrumentation. In Merritt CRB, editor: *Doppler color imaging,* New York, 1992, Churchill Livingstone.)

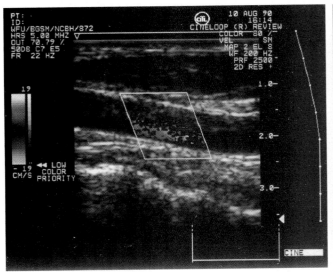

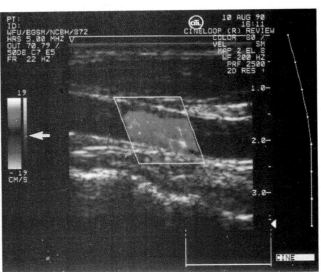

A

B

■ **FIGURE 6-8** **A,** With the color priority set low (at the bottom of the gray bar), weak, non–Doppler-shifted reverberation and off-axis echoes within the vessel take precedence over the Doppler-shifted echoes, and little color is displayed. **B,** With a higher color priority setting (halfway up the gray bar *(arrow)*), the Doppler-shifted echoes *(color)* take precedence over the weaker gray-scale echoes. (See Color Plate 11.) (From Kremkau FW: Principles and instrumentation. In Merritt CRB, editor: *Doppler color imaging,* New York, 1992, Churchill Livingstone.)

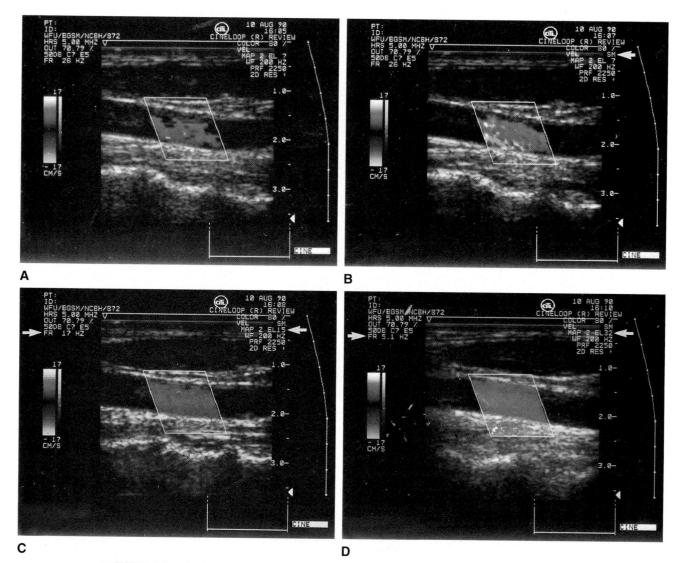

■ FIGURE 6-9 **A,** With no smoothing (persistence), only the Doppler-shifted echoes received from the pulses generating an individual frame are shown. **B,** With smoothing, consecutive frames are averaged, filling gaps in the presentation and presenting a smoother but less detailed representation of flow. **C** and **D,** More accurate and complete detection of flow information is obtained with increasing ensemble lengths. The ensemble lengths shown are 7 **(B),** 15 **(C),** and 32 **(D).** Note the decrease in frame rate from 26 to 17 to 5.1 frames per second. (See Color Plates 12 and 13.) (From Kremkau FW: Principles and instrumentation. In Merritt CRB, editor: *Doppler color imaging,* New York, 1992, Churchill Livingstone.)

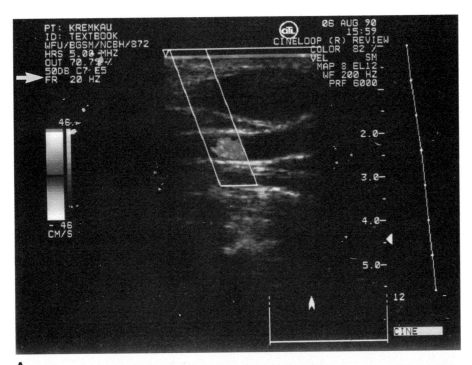

A

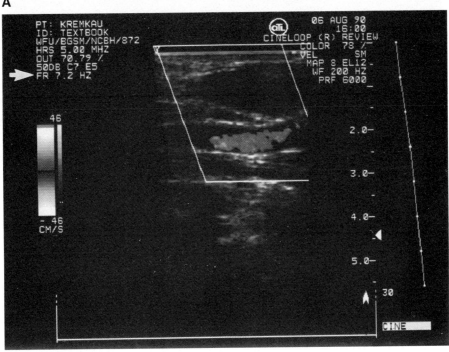

B

■ **FIGURE 6-10** Tripling the color window width decreases the frame rate from 20 Hz **(A)** to 7.2 Hz **(B).** (See Color Plate 14.) (From Kremkau FW: Principles and instrumentation. In Merritt CRB, editor: *Doppler color imaging,* New York, 1992, Churchill Livingstone.)

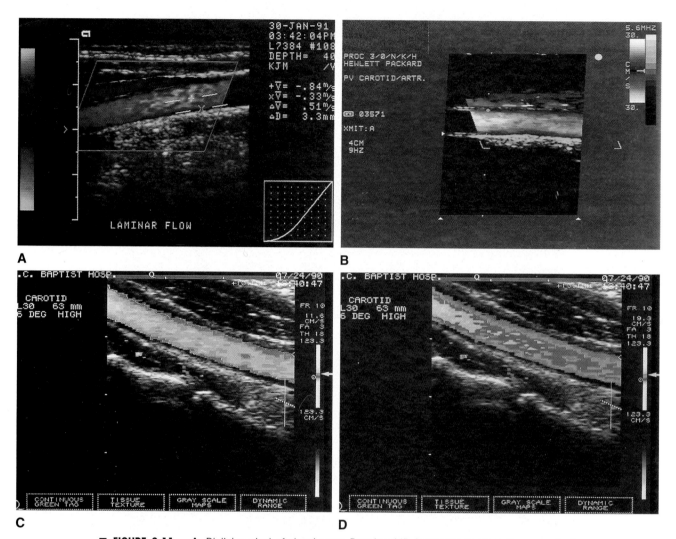

■ **FIGURE 6-11** **A,** Digital readout of stored mean Doppler shift (converted to mean flow speed) at specific pixel locations. Conversion to speed requires angle correction, just as in spectral Doppler techniques. The value at the vessel center (84 cm/s) is greater than at the edge (33 cm/s), as expected for laminar flow. **B,** Laminar flow. The color bar used in this scan progresses from dark red and dark blue to bright white (indicating decreasing saturation and increasing luminance). The regions near the vessel wall are dark, with progressive brightening and decreasing saturation to white at the center left. This corresponds to the low flow speeds at the vessel wall and high flow speeds at the vessel center that are characteristic of laminar flow. **C,** The green tag is set at a specific level (11.6; *arrow*) on an angle-corrected, calibrated color bar. The green region on the display, therefore, indicates areas where that specific flow speed exists. **D,** The green tag is set at 19.3. As the set flow speed value increases, the indicated region *(green)* moves to the center, where higher speeds are expected. (See Color Plate 15.) (**A** from Kremkau FW: *Semin Roentgenol* 27:6-16, 1992; **B** to **D** from Kremkau FW: Principles and instrumentation. In Merritt CRB, editor: *Doppler color imaging*, New York, 1992, Churchill Livingstone.)

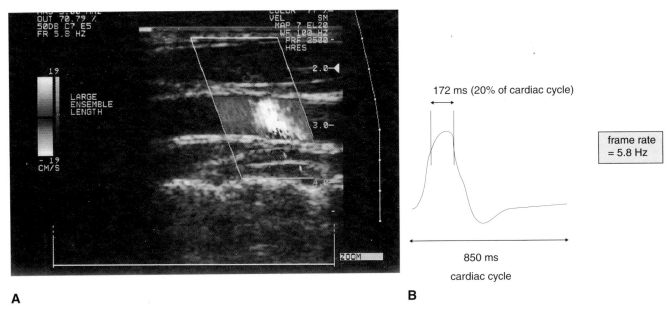

A   **B**

■ **FIGURE 6-12** **A,** In this scan a large ensemble length (20 pulses per color scan line) is used. This yields accurate Doppler-shift determination at each location with color filling in to the vessel walls in the region of slow flow. However, this is done at the expense of frame rate, which in this example is less than 6 Hz. (See Color Plate 16.) **B,** Thus **A** represents not an instant in time but about 20% of the cardiac cycle, with the left and right edges of the color window, respectively, at times before and after the systolic peak. At a frame rate of 5.8 Hz, 172 ms are required to generate one color frame. (**A** from Kremkau FW: *J Vasc Technol* 15:104-111, 1991.)

In Figure 6-16 (see Color Plate 22), some interesting questions arise. First, in part *A,* what is the blood flow direction? According to the color map in the upper left-hand corner of the figure, negative Doppler shifts are coded in red and yellow, whereas positive Doppler shifts are coded in blue and cyan. The color scan lines (and pulses) are steered to the left, and negative Doppler shifts (red and yellow) are received from the blood flowing within the vessel in the upper and lower portions of the figure. If we are looking to the left and seeing blood flowing away from us (negative Doppler shifts), the blood must be flowing from right to left in the upper and lower horizontal portions of the vessel. What about the central portion of the vessel? Clearly, the blood would have to be flowing from left to right there, but why are negative Doppler shifts also seen in this portion? The answer is that this portion of the vessel is not horizontal but is angled down, so that even though the blood is flowing from left to right, it is also flowing away from the transducer because of the downward direction (more precisely, it is flowing from upper left to lower right). Thus negative Doppler shifts are found throughout the vessel in this scan. Another way to say this is that the flow direction gets close to but never crosses the perpendicular to the scan lines (Figure 6-16, *B*).

Another intriguing question arises concerning Figure 6-16, *A:* Does the yellow region in the bend at the upper left indicate where the blood flows fastest? According to the color map, this region is where the highest negative Doppler shifts are generated. Does that mean, however, that this is where the highest flow speeds are encountered? The answer in this case is no. The highest negative Doppler shifts are found in this region because the smallest Doppler angles are encountered there, not because high flow speeds are found there. In this region the flow is approximately parallel to the scan lines (Figure 6-16, *B*), yielding Doppler angles of around zero. No evidence of vessel narrowing exists to explain increased flow speed. The increased Doppler shift can be explained purely on the grounds of angle.

In Figure 6-16, *C,* the region shown in cyan (aqua or blue-green) indicates positive Doppler shifts according to the color map, whereas the blood flow in the rest of the vessel is generating negative Doppler shifts (red and yellow). Again, the scan lines are steered to the left, so that negative Doppler shifts indicate that we are looking downstream, seeing flow away from the transducer. Therefore blood flow is from right to left in this carotid artery, with the head oriented to the left as usual. How then can we explain the positive Doppler shifts found in the upper left-hand portion of the vessel? Possibilities

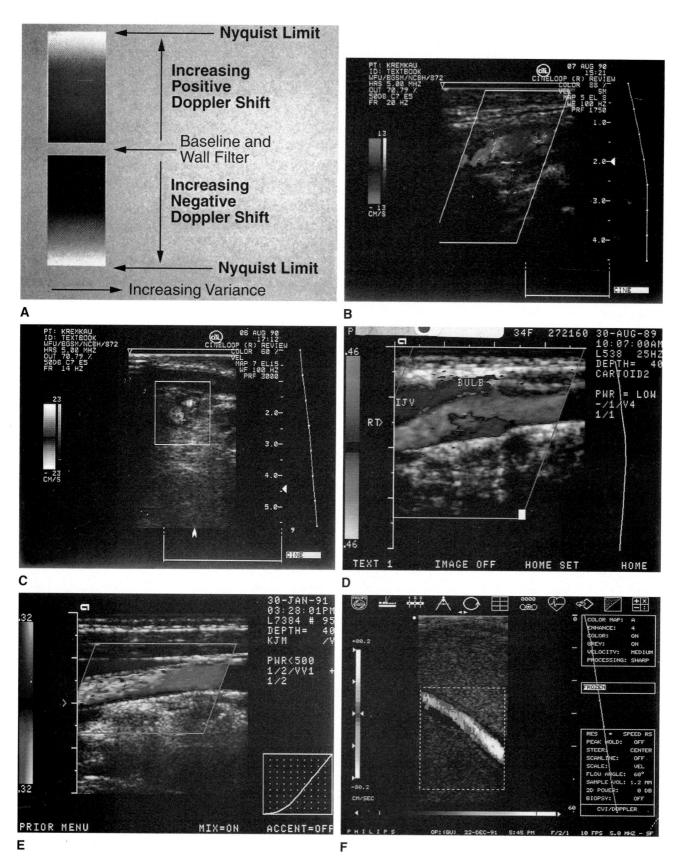

■ FIGURE 6-13   See legend on opposite page.

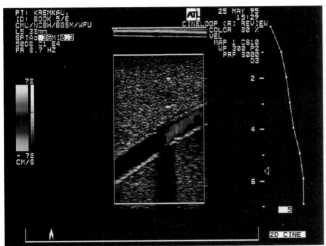

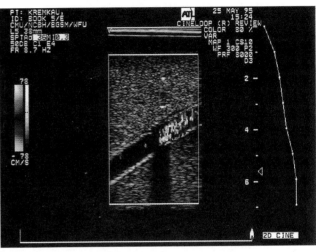

G   H

■ **FIGURE 6-13**   Color map information. **A,** Diagram describing the information contained in a color map or color bar. The color wheel type of map is shown in Figure 6-6, *A,* and has the baseline at the bottom and the Nyquist limits joined at the top. **B,** A luminance map. Increasing luminance of red or blue indicates, respectively, increasing positive or negative mean Doppler shifts. **C,** A saturation map is used to show flow transversely in two vessels. Flow in the upper vessel is toward the transducer, yielding positive Doppler shifts *(red).* Flow in the lower vessel is away from the transducer, yielding negative Doppler shifts *(blue).* On this color map, red and blue progress to white (decreasing saturation, increasing luminance) with increasing positive and negative Doppler shift means, respectively. **D,** A hue map showing flow in the carotid artery (with reversal in the bulb) and jugular vein. Increasingly positive Doppler shifts progress from dark blue to bright cyan (blue plus green). Increasingly negative Doppler shifts progress from dark red to bright yellow (red plus green). **E,** A luminance (dark blue and red to bright blue and red) map with variance included. Increasing variance adds green to red or blue (producing yellow or cyan), progressing from left to right across the map. **F,** A saturation map. Red and blue progress toward white. **G,** A stenosis in a tube *(located at the shadow)* increases the flow speed. Proximal to *(left of)* the stenosis, flow speed is too slow to be detected, whereas distal to *(right of)* the stenosis, positive Doppler shifts are seen. **H,** The variance map shows spectral broadening *(green)* in the turbulent flow region distal to the stenosis. (See Color Plates 17 and 18.) (**A** from Kremkau FW: Principles and instrumentation. In Merritt CRB, editor: *Doppler color imaging,* New York, 1992, Churchill Livingstone; **B** to **F** from Kremkau FW: *J Vasc Technol* 15:104-111, 1991.)

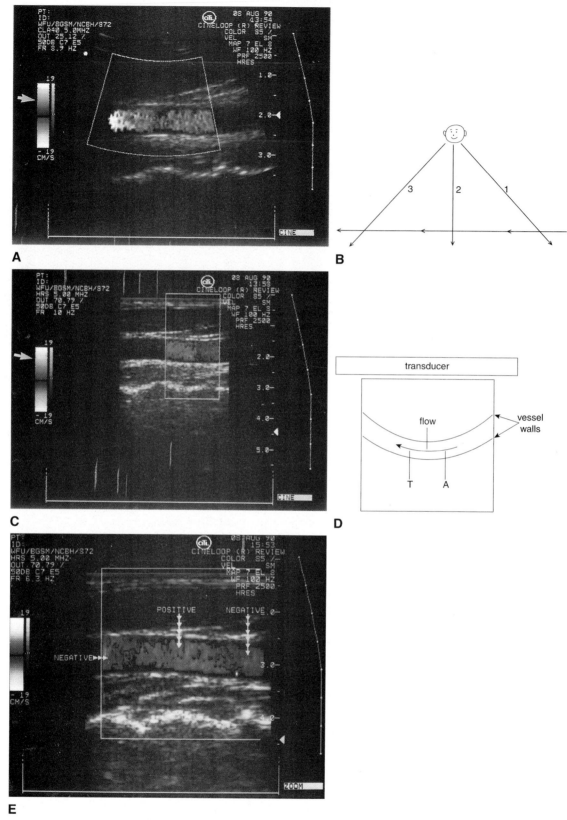

■ **FIGURE 6-14**   **A,** In this saturation map, blue and red are assigned to positive and negative Doppler shifts, respectively, progressing to white at the extremes. **B,** With flow moving from right to left, an observer looking to the right (1) is looking upstream; when looking to the left (3), the observer has a downstream view. The perpendicular view (2) is neither upstream nor downstream. **C,** In this map the color assignments are reversed from those in **A** (i.e., red and blue are assigned to positive and negative Doppler shifts, respectively). **D,** Exaggerated representation of the image in **C** in which point A represents flow away from the transducer and point T represents flow toward the transducer. **E,** Extension to the left of the color box in **C** reveals another color change caused by vessel curvature (concave-down).

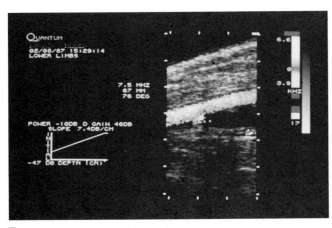
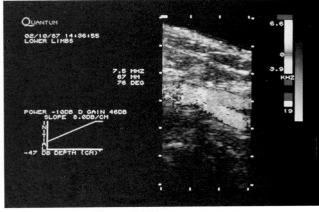

F   **G**

■ **FIGURE 6-14, cont'd**   **F,** The profunda branch off the femoral artery appears to have no flow (no color within it). **G,** This view of the profunda shows color within it. The 90-degree Doppler angle in **F** causes no Doppler shift, and therefore color is lacking. (See Color Plates 19 and 20.) (**A** and **C** from Kremkau FW: *J Vasc Technol* 15:104-111, 1991; **E** from Kremkau FW: *J Vasc Technol* 15:265-266, 1991.)

include turbulent flow, flow reversal, and flow speed exceeding 32 cm/s in this region, producing aliasing. Flow reversal and turbulent flow can be eliminated because the region between the negative (red and yellow) and positive (cyan) Doppler shift regions contains no dark or black region (baseline indicating flow reversal). One can distinguish easily between true flow reversal (which involves dark regions, as shown around the baseline of the color bar) (Figure 6-16, *D*) and aliasing, which involves bright colors, as indicated at the bar extremes. Thus the aqua region is a region of flow away from the transducer that has exceeded the negative aliasing limit of 32 cm/s and has become an aliased positive Doppler shift (cyan).

Does this mean that the flow speed in the aliased aqua region exceeds 32 cm/s? In this case the answer is no. The aliasing limit, which is one half the PRF, has been exceeded. This aliasing limit has been converted, using the Doppler equation, to an equivalent flow speed of 32 cm/s, as indicated at the map extremes. However, because there is no angle correction in this scan, an angle of zero was assumed in the conversion from Doppler shift to flow speed. Therefore aliased flow exceeds 32 cm/s only when it is parallel to the scan lines. Because the Doppler angle in this example is approximately 60 degrees, the Doppler shifts are only about one half what they would be at 0 degrees. Therefore the flow in the aliased region has exceeded approximately 64 cm/s. One must exercise care in estimating flow speeds with tagging (Figure 6-11, *C* and *D*) or aliasing limits that are converted to flow speed units without correcting for angle.

Proper understanding of the effects of angle on Doppler shift and of how color is related to Doppler shift is necessary to interpret complicated images properly.

Transverse Views

Figure 6-17 (see Color Plate 23) shows a transverse view through the external and internal carotid arteries. The external artery, according to the color map on the left, contains negative Doppler-shifted echoes (red and yellow) around its periphery and positive Doppler-shifted echoes (cyan and blue) in its central core. What is the direction of blood flow in this vessel: toward or away from the observer? Are the flow directions in the central core and periphery opposite? With the help of Figure 6-18 (see Color Plate 24), we can conclude that Figure 6-17 is a downstream view in the periphery and an upstream view in the central core. However, the flow directions in these two regions are not likely to be opposite. A better explanation needs to be found. Because the region between the dark red and the blue in the vessel corresponds to the bright yellow and cyan color bar extremes, aliasing is indicated. Now we can interpret the colors in Figure 6-17 correctly. The slower flows (and smaller Doppler shifts) in the periphery indicate a downstream view; that is, the negative Doppler shifts tell us that the flow is moving through the vessel, away from the observer and transducer, in this transverse view. In progressing from the vessel edge

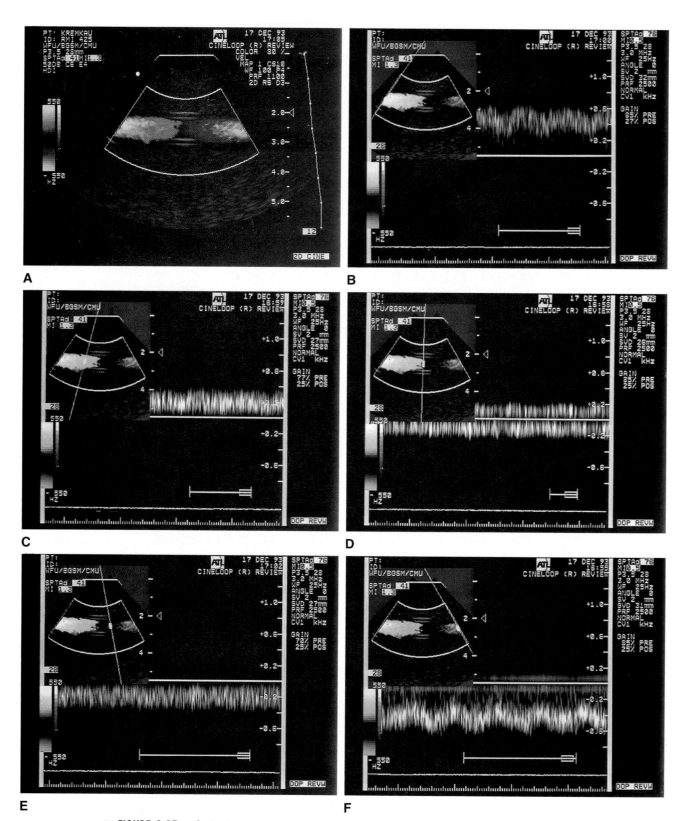

■ **FIGURE 6-15** Sector format, color Doppler presentation of flow from left to right in a straight tube. **A,** Approximate Doppler shifts (from the color map) are yellow (500 Hz), red (200 Hz), black (0 Hz), blue (−200 Hz), and cyan (−500 Hz). (See Color Plate 21.) Spectra from these five regions, shown in **B** to **F,** confirm these estimates. Doppler shifts decrease as Doppler angles increase toward the center of the color window.

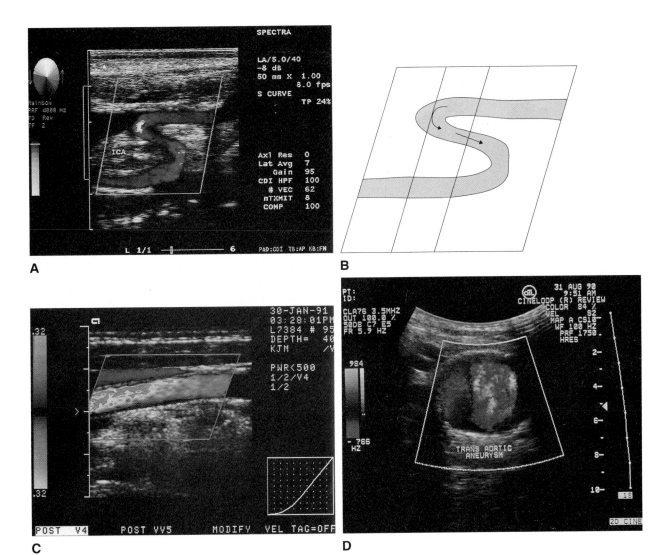

■ **FIGURE 6-16** **A,** A tortuous artery. **B,** This drawing shows the angle relationships depicted in **A.** **C,** A (nearly) straight artery. **D,** Circular flow in an aneurysm. The black area between the red and blue areas indicates true flow reversal. (See Color Plate 22.) (**A** and **C** from Kremkau FW: *J Vasc Technol* 16:215-216, 1992.)

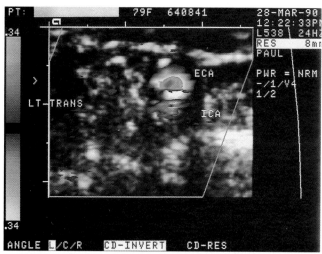

■ FIGURE 6-17 Transverse view of external and internal carotid arteries. (See Color Plate 23.) (From Kremkau FW: *J Vasc Technol* 16:309-310, 1992.)

toward the center, we find increasing Doppler shifts consistent with laminar flow (dark red progressing to bright yellow). Where the yellow changes to cyan, the negative aliasing limit has been exceeded and positive Doppler shifts result. Continuing toward the center of the vessel, the cyan changes to blue as the positive Doppler shift decreases down the bar. The aliased Doppler shifts are a result of the fastest flow speeds away from the transducer that exceed the aliasing limit of 0.34. Does this mean that, at the point where yellow changes to cyan, the flow speed is 34 cm/s? No, because the aliasing limits on the color bar are not angle-corrected and therefore are correct only if the flow is parallel to the scan lines (i.e., parallel to the scan plane), which it clearly is not in this transverse view.

Transverse views show colors that depend on whether the view is upstream or downstream, that is, how the scan plane is angled in the transverse view.

DOPPLER-POWER DISPLAYS

Doppler-shift displays encode mean Doppler *shifts* in a two-dimensional matrix according to the color map selected. Doppler-power displays present two-dimensional Doppler information by color-encoding the strength of the Doppler shifts. This approach is free of aliasing and angle dependence and is more sensitive to slow flow and flow in small or deep vessels. Names applied to this technique include color power Doppler, ultrasound angio, color Doppler energy, and color power angio. Rather than assigning various hue, satu-

ration, and luminance values to mean Doppler-shift frequency values, as in Doppler-shift displays, this technique assigns these values to Doppler-shift power values. The power of the Doppler shifts is determined by the concentration of moving scatterers producing the Doppler shifts and is independent of Doppler-shift frequency (and thus independent of Doppler angle). In addition to the colors already encountered, magenta (a combination of red and blue) is used on some Doppler-power maps.

Doppler-power displays color-encode Doppler-shift power values on the display.

ADVANCED CONCEPTS

In **Doppler-power displays** a cross-correlation calculation yields the integral of power density with respect to time. Noise is less of a problem in Doppler-power displays compared with Doppler-shift displays because noise is spread over all frequencies and thus interferes with all aspects of a Doppler-shift display. However, noise is not spread over all amplitudes but mostly at the weaker levels. Thus the stronger Doppler-shifted echoes are lifted out of the noise and are assigned colors different from the background noise. The result is that Doppler-power displays are more sensitive and can show flow in slower-flow, deeper-vessel, and smaller-vessel situations than Doppler-shift display can. However, directional, speed, and flow character information is not presented. Conventional Doppler-shift displays are still useful for presentation of that information dynamically over cardiac cycle. Because Doppler-power displays show only the presence of flow (and not dynamic changes over cardiac cycle), integration of signal over time also improves signal-to-noise ratio.

Advantages and Disadvantages

The Doppler detector in color Doppler imaging instruments yields the sign, mean, variance, and amplitude and power of the Doppler spectrum (Figure 6-19, *A*) at each of hundreds of sample volume locations in an anatomic cross section. Traditionally, in color Doppler imaging, sign and mean Doppler shift, and sometimes variance (usually in cardiac applications), are color-encoded and displayed. These parameters depend on Doppler angle and are subject to aliasing (Figure 6-20, *A* [see Color Plate 25]). Power Doppler integrates the area under the spectrum (Figure 6-19, *B*). This area is independent of angle and aliasing, displaying the effects of neither (Figure 6-20, *B* [see Color Plate 25]). Thus

PLATE 1

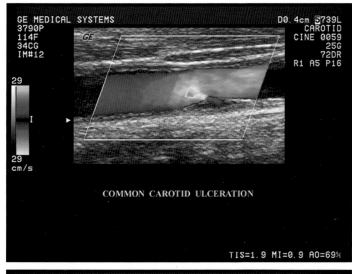

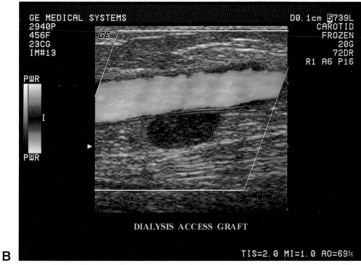

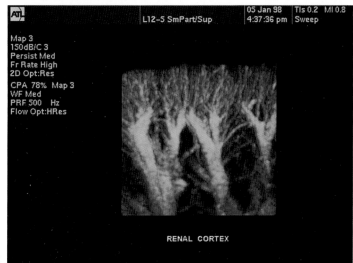

■ **FIGURE 1-13** Color Doppler displays of blood flow presented in forms called **(A)** color Doppler-shift, **(B)** color Doppler-power, and **(C)** 3D color Doppler-power displays.

PLATE 2

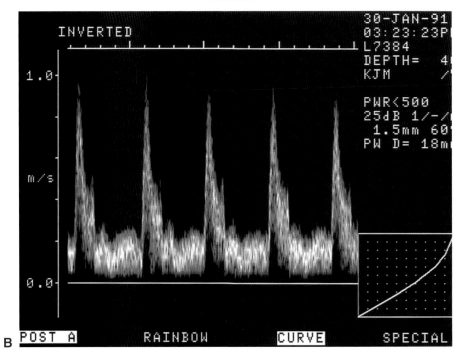

■ **FIGURE 1-14**   **B,** Display of Doppler information (in a form called a spectral display) from common carotid arterial blood flow.

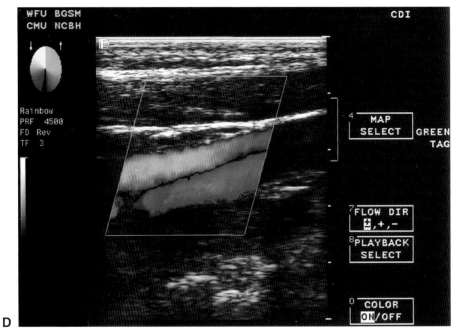

■ **FIGURE 3-27**   **D,** A phased linear array producing a parallelogram-shaped color Doppler display.

PLATE 3

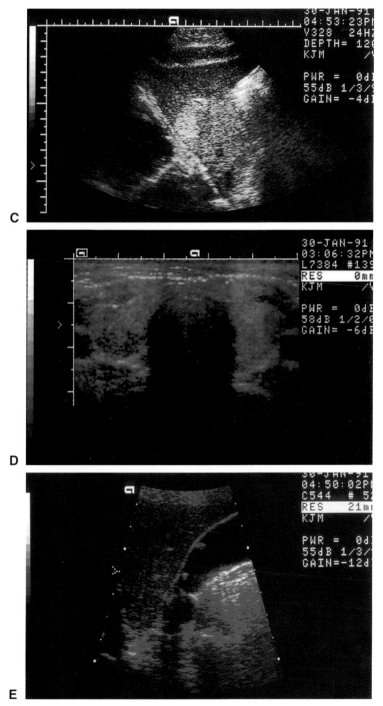

■ **FIGURE 4-41** **C** to **E,** Color displays of a hemangioma (**C;** compare with Figure 4-41, *A* and *B*), thyroid **(D),** and gallbladder **(E).** Color assignments, shown in the color bars on the left, are designated as follows: **(C)** temperature (increasing intensity assigned dark orange through yellow to white), **(D)** magenta (dark magenta through light magenta to white), and **(E)** rainbow (dark violet through various colors to white).

PLATE 4

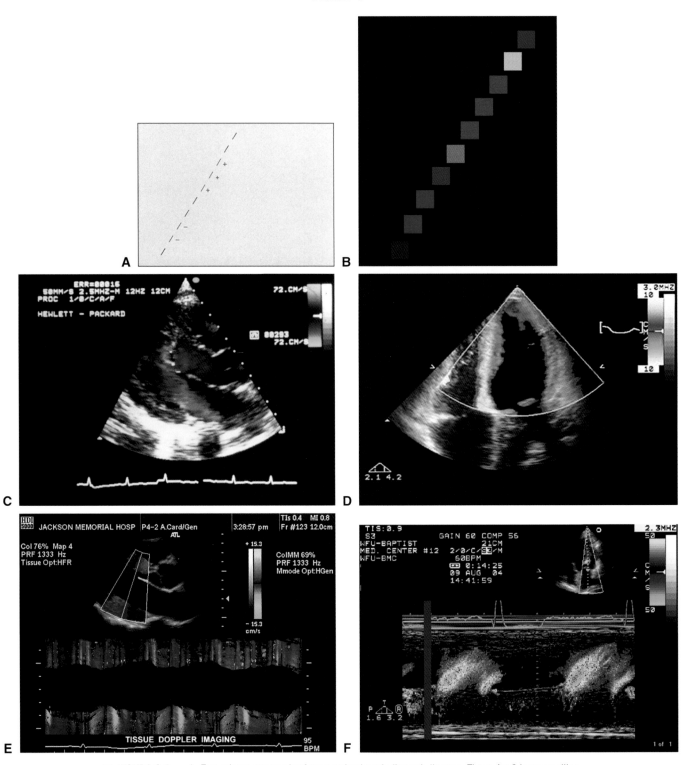

■ **FIGURE 6-1** **A,** Ten echoes are received as a pulse travels through tissues. Three *(red)* have positive Doppler shifts and two *(blue)* have negative shifts. **B,** These echoes are shown as red and blue pixels, respectively, on the color Doppler display. As in gray-scale sonography, a two-dimensional cross-sectional image is made up of many scan lines. **C,** A parasternal long-axis image of normal mitral valve blood flow. **D,** Tissue Doppler imaging of myocardial motion. **E,** Color Doppler M mode display with tissue motion detected. **F,** Color Doppler M mode display with blood flow detected.

PLATE 5

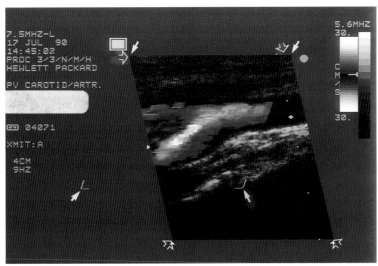

■ **FIGURE 6-2** A perpendicular Doppler angle is avoided in this image by electronically steering the color-producing Doppler pulses to the left of vertical. The corners of the resulting parallelogram in which color can be displayed are shown by the solid arrows. Note that on this instrument, the gray-scale anatomic imaging pulses also can be steered (in this case, to the right of vertical). The corners of the resulting gray-scale parallelogram are shown by the open arrows. (From Kremkau FW: Principles and pitfalls of real-time color-flow imaging. In Bernstein EF, editor: *Vascular diagnosis,* ed 4, St Louis, 1993, Mosby.)

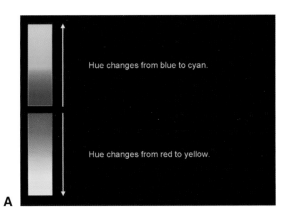

A

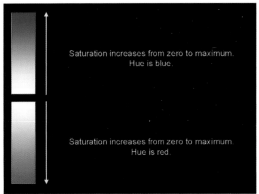

B

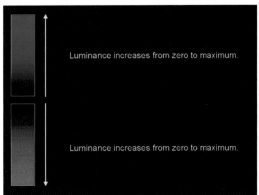

C

■ **FIGURE 6-3** **A,** Hue is the color that is perceived by the viewer. **B,** Saturation is the amount of hue present in a mix with white. **C,** Luminance is the brightness of the hue and saturation presented.

PLATE 6

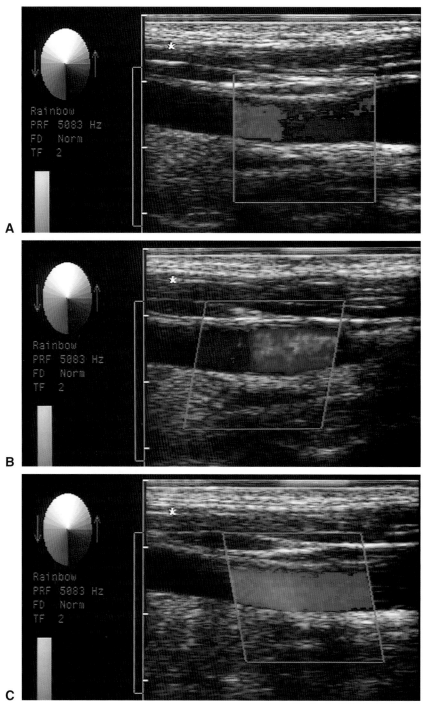

■ **FIGURE 6-6**   Color scan lines are directed down vertically **(A),** to the left of vertical **(B),** and to the right of vertical **(C).** Flow is from left to right, producing positive or negative Doppler shifts, depending on the relationship between scan lines and flow.

PLATE 7

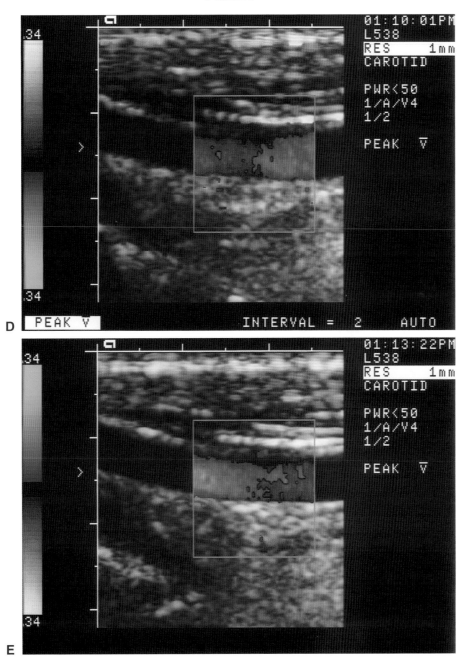

■ **FIGURE 6-6, cont'd** **D,** In this hue map, red and blue are assigned to positive and negative Doppler shifts, respectively, progressing to yellow and cyan (by the addition of green) at the Nyquist limits. **E,** In this map the color assignments are reversed from those presented in **D** (i.e., blue and red are assigned to positive and negative Doppler shifts, respectively). Note the color change occurring within each color window. This is caused by vessel curvature.

Continued.

PLATE 8

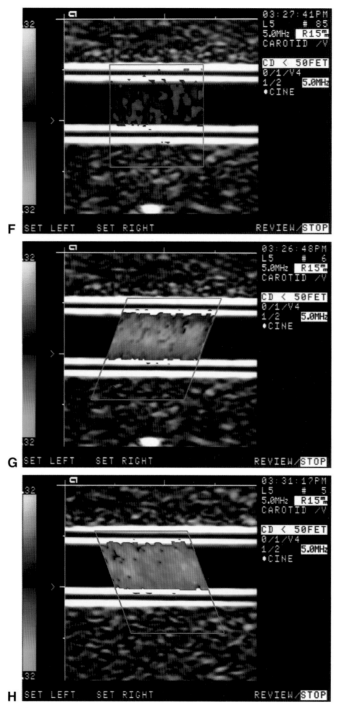

■ **FIGURE 6-6, cont'd**   **F,** With flow in a straight tube, positive and negative Doppler shifts are distributed equally throughout the color window with a Doppler angle of 90 degrees. **G,** Uniform positive Doppler shifts are observed with the color window steered 20 degrees to the left (70-degree Doppler angle). **H,** Uniform negative Doppler shifts are observed with the color window steered to the right. (**A** to **C** from Kremkau FW: *Semin Roentgenol* 27:6-16, 1992; **D** and **E** from Kremkau FW: Principles and pitfalls of real-time color-flow imaging. In Bernstein EF, editor: *Vascular diagnosis,* ed 4, St Louis, 1993, Mosby.)

PLATE 9

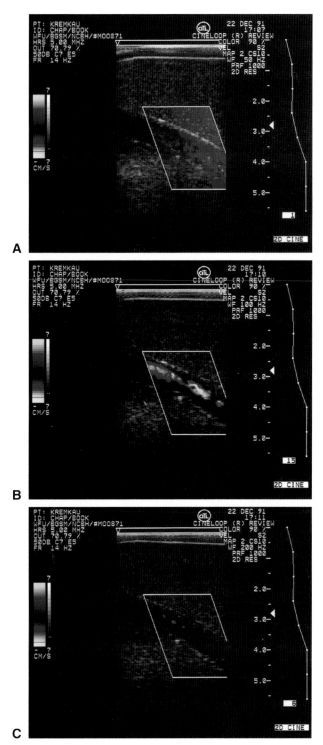

■ **FIGURE 6-7**   **A,** Tissue motion causes clutter, obscuring the flow in the vessel and clouding the gray-scale tissue with color Doppler information. **B,** Wall filter has been increased to 100 Hz, thereby eliminating the color clutter. **C,** Wall filter has been increased (too much) to 200 Hz, eliminating virtually all the color Doppler information derived from the vessel.

Continued.

PLATE 10

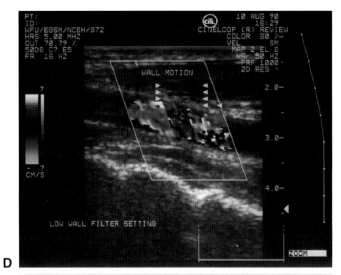

D

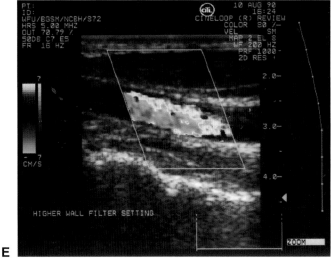

E

■ **FIGURE 6-7, cont'd**   **D,** With a low wall filter setting (50 Hz), wall motion appears in color on the image. **E,** With a higher wall filter setting (200 Hz), this motion no longer appears in color. (**A** to **C** from Kremkau FW: Principles and pitfalls of real-time color-flow imaging. In Bernstein EF, editor: *Vascular diagnosis,* ed 4, St Louis, 1993, Mosby; **D** and **E** from Kremkau FW: Principles and instrumentation. In Merritt CRB, editor: *Doppler color imaging,* New York, 1992, Churchill Livingstone.)

PLATE 11

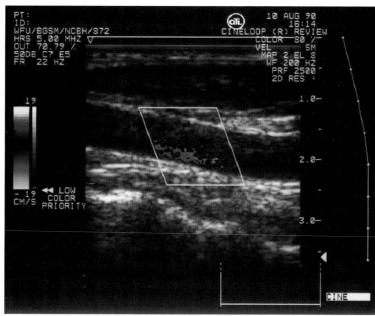

A

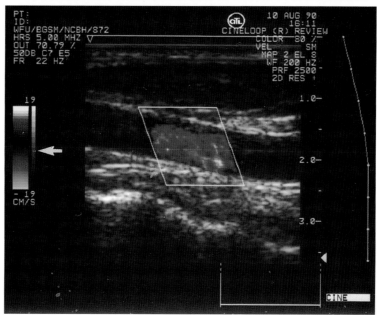

B

■ FIGURE 6-8   A, With the color priority set low (at the bottom of the gray bar), weak, non–Doppler-shifted reverberation and off-axis echoes within the vessel take precedence over the Doppler-shifted echoes, and little color is displayed. **B,** With a higher color priority setting (halfway up the gray bar *(arrow)*), the Doppler-shifted echoes *(color)* take precedence over the weaker gray-scale echoes. (From Kremkau FW: Principles and instrumentation. In Merritt CRB, editor: *Doppler color imaging*, New York, 1992, Churchill Livingstone.)

PLATE 12

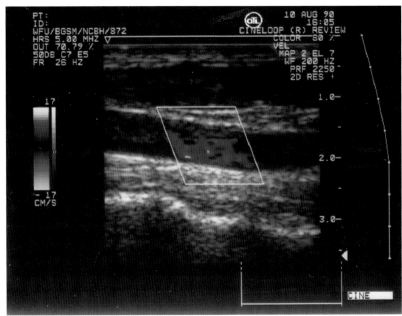

A

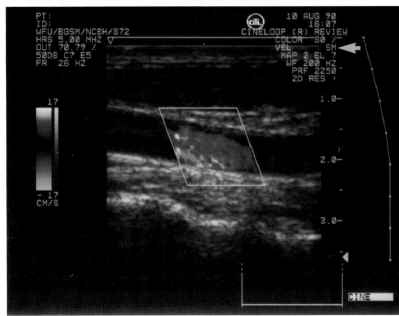

B

■ **FIGURE 6-9** **A,** With no smoothing (persistence), only the Doppler-shifted echoes received from the pulses generating an individual frame are shown. **B,** With smoothing, consecutive frames are averaged, filling gaps in the presentation and presenting a smoother but less detailed representation of flow.

PLATE 13

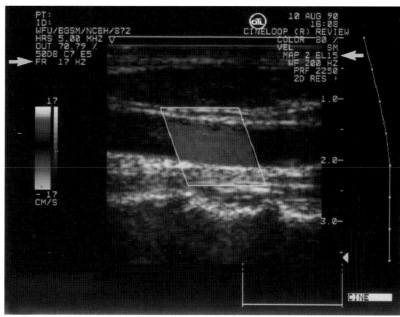

C

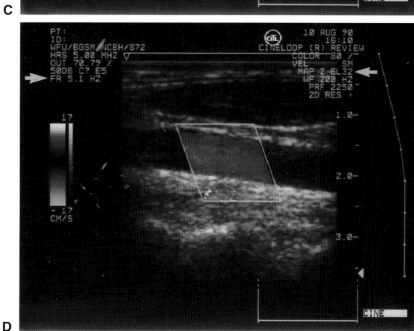

D

■ **FIGURE 6-9, cont'd** **C** and **D,** More accurate and complete detection of flow information is obtained with increasing ensemble lengths. The ensemble lengths shown are 7 **(B),** 15 **(C),** and 32 **(D).** Note the decrease in frame rate from 26 to 17 to 5.1 frames per second. (From Kremkau FW: Principles and instrumentation. In Merritt CRB, editor: *Doppler color imaging,* New York, 1992, Churchill Livingstone.)

PLATE 14

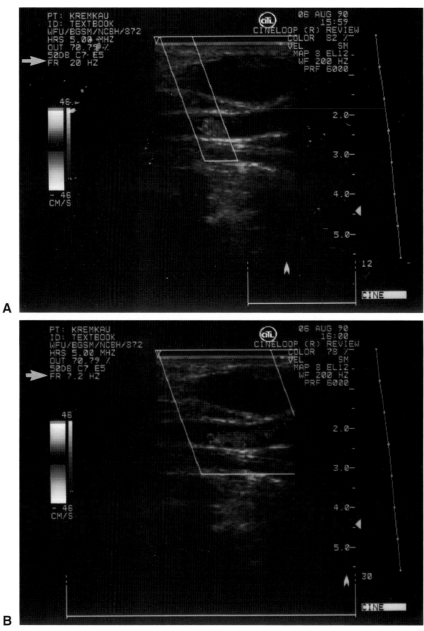

■ **FIGURE 6-10**   Tripling the color window width decreases the frame rate from 20 Hz **(A)** to 7.2 Hz **(B).**
(From Kremkau FW: Principles and instrumentation. In Merritt CRB, editor: *Doppler color imaging,* New York, 1992, Churchill Livingstone.)

PLATE 15

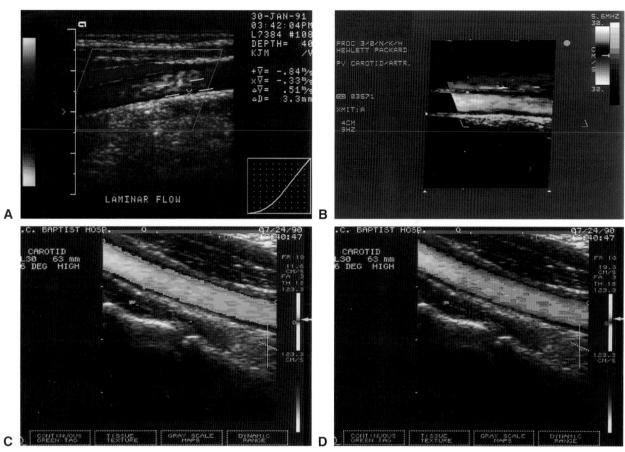

■ **FIGURE 6-11** **A,** Digital readout of stored mean Doppler shift (converted to mean flow speed) at specific pixel locations. Conversion to speed requires angle correction, just as in spectral Doppler techniques. The value at the vessel center (84 cm/s) is greater than at the edge (33 cm/s), as expected for laminar flow. **B,** Laminar flow. The color bar used in this scan progresses from dark red and dark blue to bright white (indicating decreasing saturation and increasing luminance). The regions near the vessel wall are dark, with progressive brightening and decreasing saturation to white at the center left. This corresponds to the low flow speeds at the vessel wall and high flow speeds at the vessel center that are characteristic of laminar flow. **C,** The green tag is set at a specific level (11.6; *arrow*) on an angle-corrected, calibrated color bar. The green region on the display therefore indicates areas where that specific flow speed exists. **D,** The green tag is set at 19.3. As the set flow speed value increases, the indicated region *(green)* moves to the center, where higher speeds are expected. (**A** from Kremkau FW: *Semin Roentgenol* 27:6-16, 1992; **B** to **D** from Kremkau FW: Principles and instrumentation. In Merritt CRB, editor: *Doppler color imaging,* New York, 1992, Churchill Livingstone.)

PLATE 16

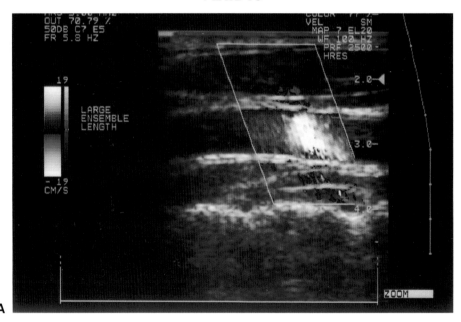

A

■ **FIGURE 6-12** **A,** In this scan a large ensemble length (20 pulses per color scan line) is used. This yields accurate Doppler-shift determination at each location with color filling in to the vessel walls in the region of slow flow. However, this is done at the expense of frame rate, which in this example is less than 6 Hz. (**A** from Kremkau FW: *J Vasc Technol* 15:104-111, 1991.)

PLATE 17

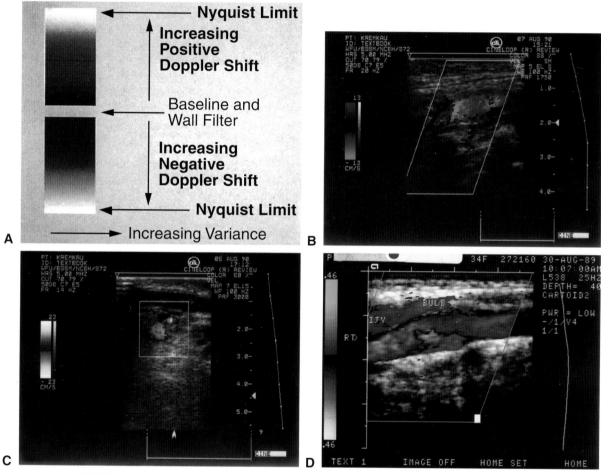

■ **FIGURE 6-13** Color map information. **A,** Diagram describing the information contained in a color map or color bar. The color wheel type of map is shown in Figure 6-6, *A,* and has the baseline at the bottom and the Nyquist limits joined at the top. **B,** A luminance map. Increasing luminance of red or blue indicates, respectively, increasing positive or negative mean Doppler shifts. **C,** A saturation map is used to show flow transversely in two vessels. Flow in the upper vessel is toward the transducer, yielding positive Doppler shifts *(red).* Flow in the lower vessel is away from the transducer, yielding negative Doppler shifts *(blue).* On this color map, red and blue progress to white (decreasing saturation, increasing luminance) with increasing positive and negative Doppler shift means, respectively. **D,** A hue map showing flow in the carotid artery (with reversal in the bulb) and jugular vein. Increasingly positive Doppler shifts progress from dark blue to bright cyan (blue plus green). Increasingly negative Doppler shifts progress from dark red to bright yellow (red plus green).

Continued.

PLATE 18

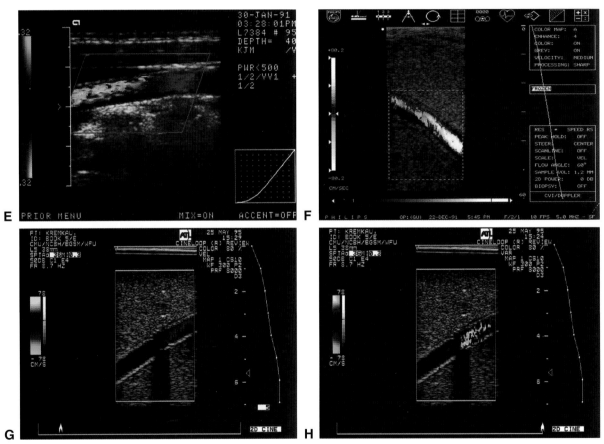

■ **FIGURE 6-13, cont'd**   **E,** A luminance (dark blue and red to bright blue and red) map with variance included. Increasing variance adds green to red or blue (producing yellow or cyan), progressing from left to right across the map. **F,** A saturation map. Red and blue progress toward white. **G,** A stenosis in a tube *(located at the shadow)* increases the flow speed. Proximal to *(left of)* the stenosis, flow speed is too slow to be detected, whereas distal to *(right of)* the stenosis, positive Doppler shifts are seen. **H,** The variance map shows spectral broadening *(green)* in the turbulent flow region distal to the stenosis. (**A** from Kremkau FW: Principles and instrumentation. In Merritt CRB, editor: *Doppler color imaging,* New York, 1992, Churchill Livingstone; **B** to **F** from Kremkau FW: *J Vasc Technol* 15:104-111, 1991.)

PLATE 19

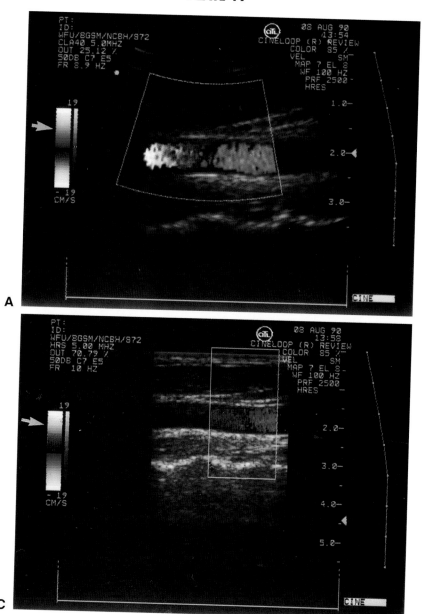

■ FIGURE 6-14 **A,** In this saturation map, blue and red are assigned to positive and negative Doppler shifts, respectively, progressing to white at the extremes. **C,** In this map the color assignments are reversed from those in **A** (i.e., red and blue are assigned to positive and negative Doppler shifts, respectively).

Continued.

PLATE 20

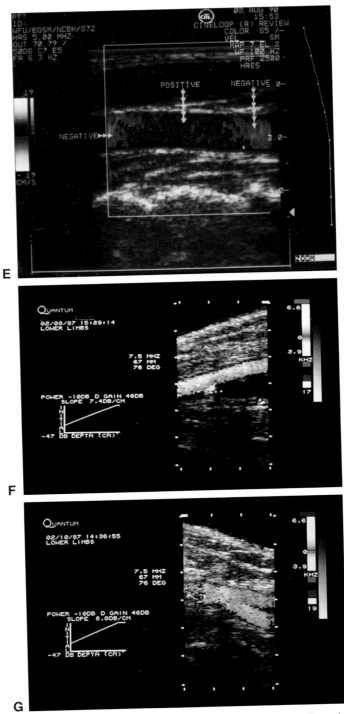

■ FIGURE 6-14, cont'd   E, Extension to the left of the color box in **C** reveals another color change caused by vessel curvature (concave-down). **F,** The profunda branch off the femoral artery appears to have no flow (no color within it). **G,** This view of the profunda shows color within it. The 90-degree Doppler angle in **F** causes no Doppler shift, and therefore color is lacking. (**A** and **C** from Kremkau FW: *J Vasc Technol* 15: 104-111, 1991; **E** from Kremkau FW: *J Vasc Technol* 15:265-266, 1991.)

PLATE 21

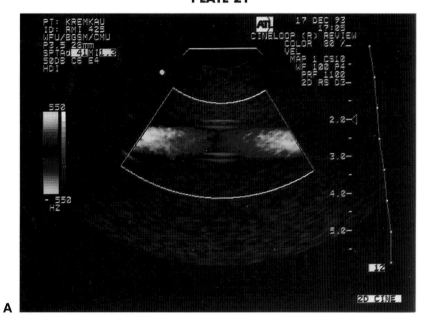

■ FIGURE 6-15 Sector format, color Doppler presentation of flow from left to right in a straight tube. **A,** Approximate Doppler shifts (from the color map) are yellow (500 Hz), red (200 Hz), black (0 Hz), blue (–200 Hz), and cyan (–500 Hz).

PLATE 22

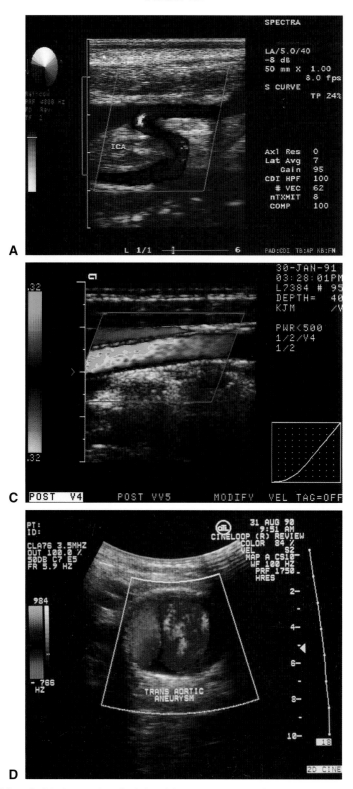

■ **FIGURE 6-16** **A,** A tortuous artery. **C,** A (nearly) straight artery. **D,** Circular flow in an aneurysm. The black area between the red and blue areas indicates true flow reversal. (**A** and **C** from Kremkau FW: *J Vasc Technol* 16:215-216, 1992.)

PLATE 23

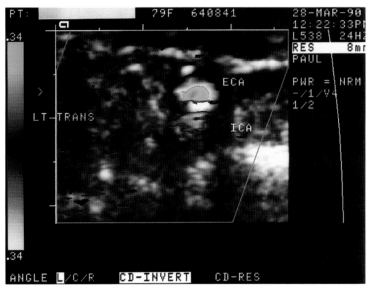

■ **FIGURE 6-17**   Transverse view of external and internal carotid arteries. (From Kremkau FW: *J Vasc Technol* 16:309-310, 1992.)

PLATE 24

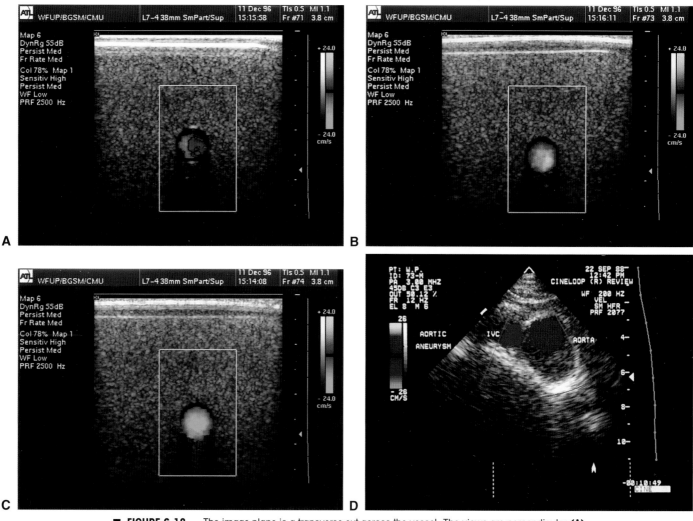

■ **FIGURE 6-18**   The image plane is a transverse cut across the vessel. The views are perpendicular **(A)**, upstream **(B)**, and downstream **(C)**. The Doppler shifts obtained are **(A)** zero (or weakly positive and negative because of beam spreading), **(B)** positive, and **(C)** negative. The image plane is being viewed edge-on in the line drawings. **D,** A transverse view upstream (positive Doppler shift) in the aorta (the scan plane is angled toward the heart) and downstream (negative Doppler shift) in the inferior vena cava. **(A** to **C** from Kremkau FW: *J Vascular Technol* 16:309-310, 1992.)

PLATE 25

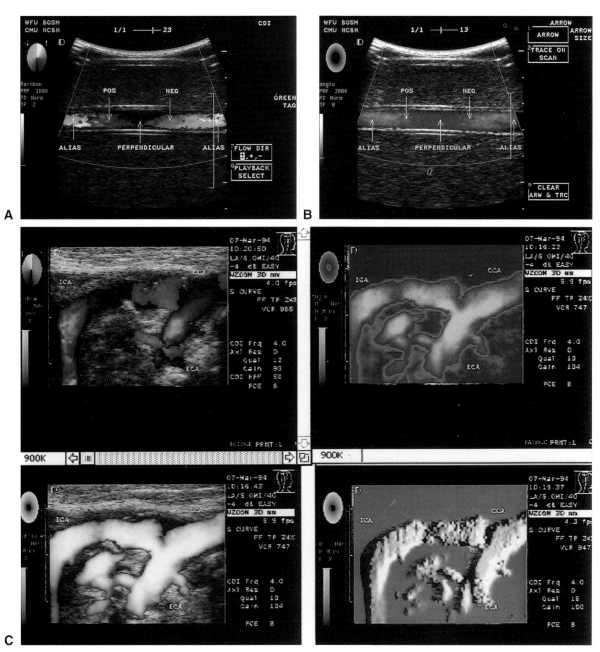

■ **FIGURE 6-20** **A,** A color Doppler-shift image of flow in a straight tube, acquired in sector format. The varying Doppler angle from left to right yields aliasing and positive, negative, and zero Doppler-shift regions. **B,** A Doppler-power presentation of the situation shown in **A** yields a uniform image, free of angle dependence and aliasing. However, it contains no directional, speed, or dynamic information. **C,** Angle independence is seen in the Doppler-power images of the carotid artery; compare them to the Doppler-shift display *(upper left)*. Doppler-power imaging is shown in color, topographic, and gray-scale forms *(clockwise from upper right)*. (See also Figure 1-13, *B,* and Color Plate 1.)

PLATE 26

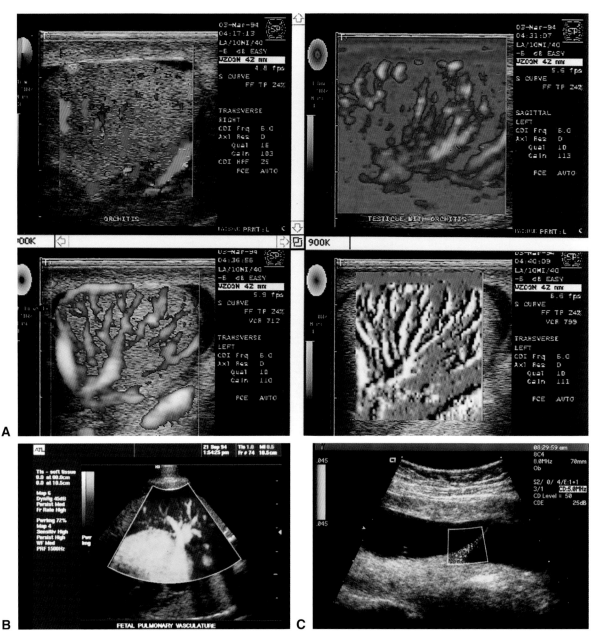

■ **FIGURE 6-21** **A,** Improved sensitivity to testicular flow compared with Doppler-shift imaging *(upper left).* Small vessel flow is imaged in fetal pulmonary vasculature **(B)** and within the membrane separating a twin gestation **(C).**

PLATE 27

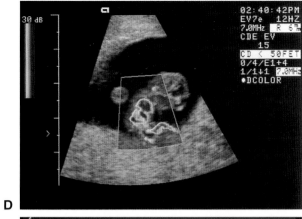

D

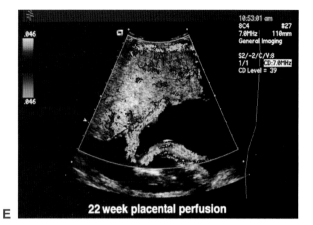

E

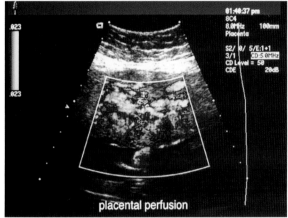

F

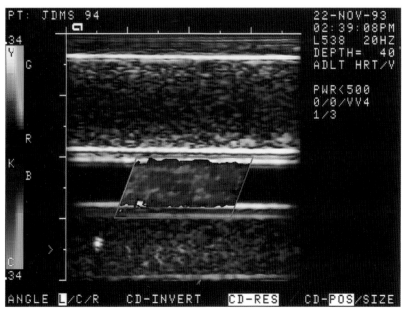

■ **FIGURE 6-21, cont'd** **D,** First trimester fetal circulation. A comparison of placental Doppler-shift imaging **(E)** and Doppler-power imaging **(F)** reveals improved flow detection with the latter.

■ **FIGURE 6-22** Display to accompany Exercises 51 to 54.

PLATE 28

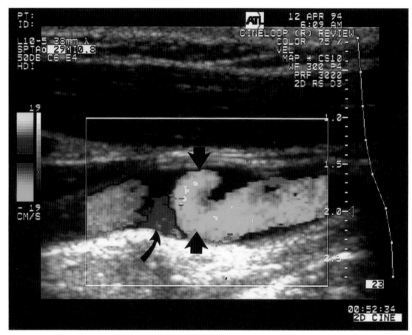

■ **FIGURE 6-23**   Display to accompany Exercises 55 and 56.

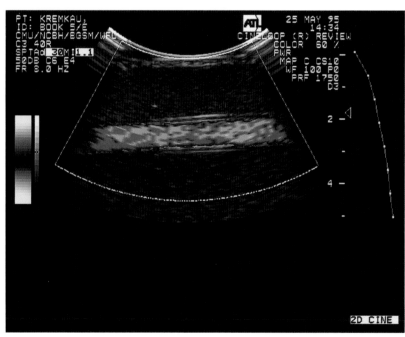

■ **FIGURE 6-24**   Display to accompany Exercise 60.

PLATE 29

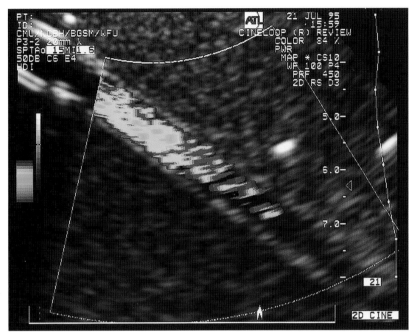

■ **FIGURE 6-25** Display to accompany Exercises 61 and 62.

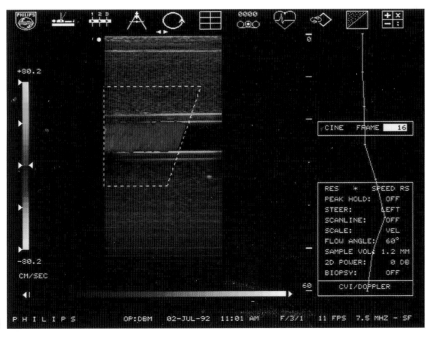

C

■ **FIGURE 9-11** **C,** Color Doppler image from a flow phantom.

PLATE 30

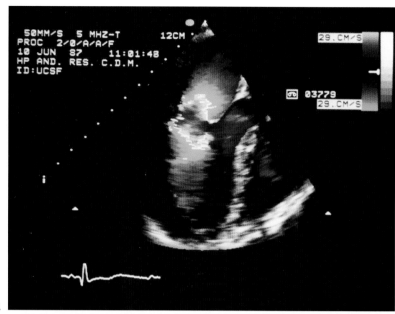

A

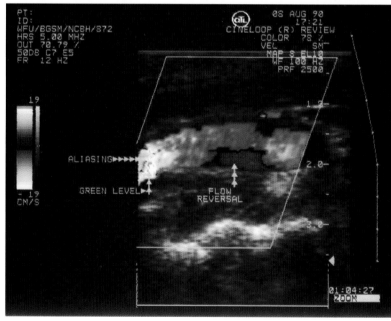

B

■ **FIGURE 8-33** **A,** A transesophageal cardiac color Doppler image of the long axis in diastole. The blue colors in the left atrium *(upper)* and left ventricle *(lower)* represent blood traveling away from the transducer, but where the flow speeds exceed the Nyquist limit (29 cm/s), aliasing occurs and the yellow and orange colors have replaced the blue colors. **B,** Color Doppler presentation of common carotid artery flow, including flow reversal and aliasing. The two can be distinguished because the boundary between the different directions with flow reversal passes through the baseline *(black)*, whereas the aliasing boundary passes through the upper and lower extremes of the color bar *(white)*. In this particular color bar assignment, the maximum positive Doppler shifts are assigned the color green, so that a thin green region shows the exact boundary where aliasing occurs. The aliasing occurs in the distal portion of the vessel because it is curving down, reducing the Doppler angle between the flow and the scan lines.

PLATE 31

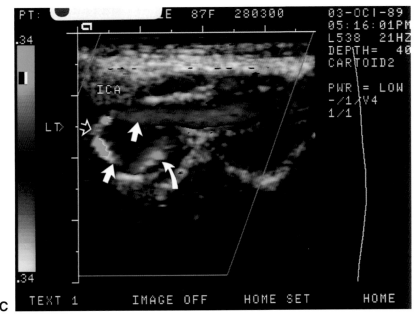

■ FIGURE 8-33, cont'd   **C,** In a tortuous internal carotid artery, negative Doppler shifts are indicated in the red regions *(solid straight arrows)*. Two regions of positive Doppler shifts *(blue)* are seen *(open arrow and curved arrow)*. In the latter, legitimate flow toward the transducer is indicated. In the former the flow away from the transducer has yielded high Doppler shifts (because of a small Doppler angle; i.e., flow is approximately parallel to scan lines), which produces a color shift to the opposite side of the map because of aliasing. The boundaries from and to normal negative Doppler shifts into and out of the aliased region are bright yellow and cyan from the ends of the color bars. The transition from unaliased negative Doppler shift into unaliased positive Doppler shift *(near bottom)* is black, representing the baseline of the color bar. (**B** from Kremkau FW: *Semin Roentgenol* 27:6-16, 1992; **C** from Kremkau FW: *J Vasc Technol* 15:265-266, 1991.)

PLATE 32

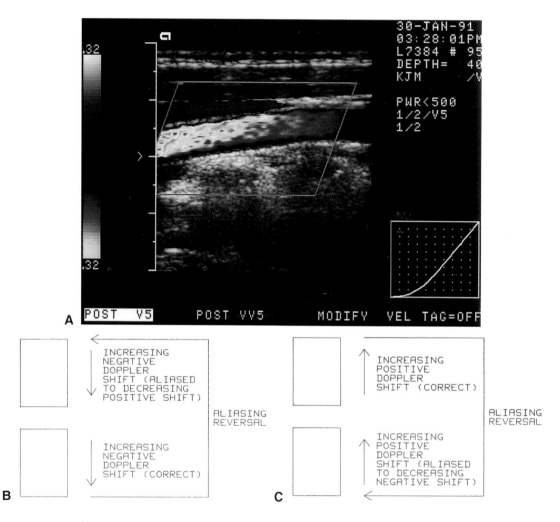

■ **FIGURE 8-34** **A,** Positive *(blue)* Doppler shifts are shown in the arterial flow in this image. These are actually negative Doppler shifts that have exceeded the lower Nyquist limit (converted here to the equivalent flow speed: −0.32 m/s) and are wrapped around to the positive portion of the color bar **(B).** Positive shifts that exceed the +0.32 m/s limit would alias to the negative side **(C).** (From Kremkau FW: Principles and pitfalls of real-time color-flow imaging. In Bernstein EF, editor: *Vascular diagnosis,* ed 4, St Louis, 1993, Mosby.)

PLATE 33

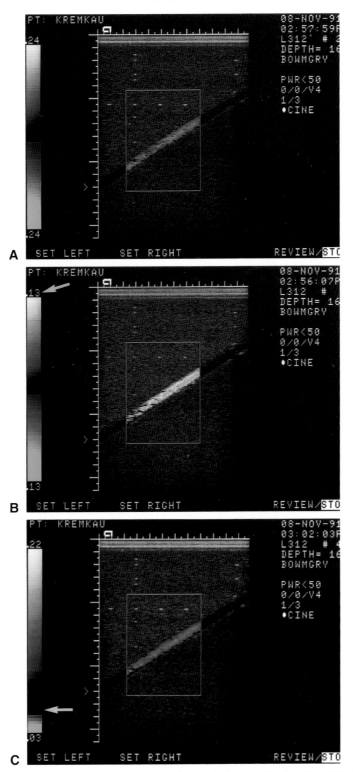

■ FIGURE 8-35 **A,** Flow is toward the upper right, producing positive Doppler shifts. **B,** The pulse repetition frequency and Nyquist limit (0.13) are too low, resulting in aliasing (negative Doppler shifts) at the center of the flow in the vessel (see Figure 8-34, *C*). **C,** With the same pulse repetition frequency setting as in **B,** the aliasing has been eliminated by shifting the base line *(arrow)* down 10 cm/s below the center of the color bar.

Continued.

PLATE 34

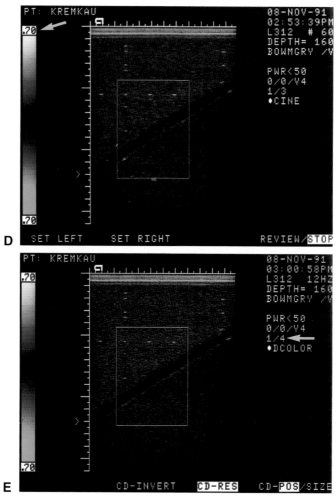

■ **FIGURE 8-35, cont'd** **D,** The Nyquist limit setting (0.70) is too high, causing the detected Doppler shifts to be well down the positive scale, producing a dark red appearance. **E,** With the Nyquist limit set as in **D,** an increase in the wall filter setting *(arrow)* eliminates what little color flow information there was in **D.** (From Kremkau FW: Principles and pitfalls of real-time color-flow imaging. In Bernstein EF, editor: *Vascular diagnosis,* ed 4, St Louis, 1993, Mosby.)

PLATE 35

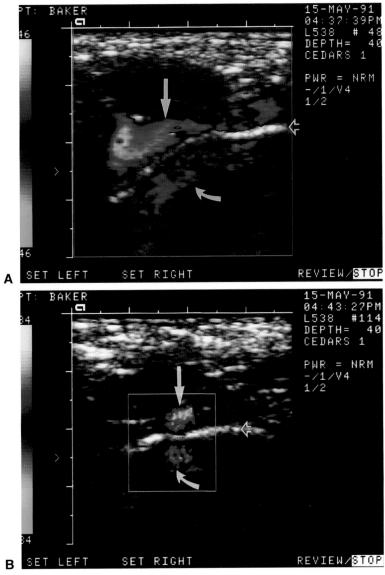

■ FIGURE 8-36 Color Doppler imaging of the subclavian artery *(straight arrow)* in longitudinal **(A)** and transverse **(B)** views. The pleura *(open arrow)* causes the mirror image *(curved arrow)*. The diagram in Figure 8-29, *D,* shows how this artifact occurs.

PLATE 36

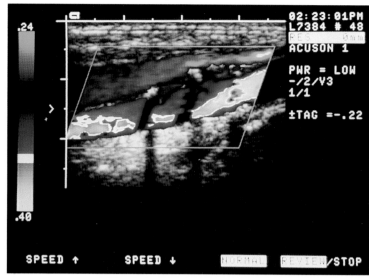

■ **FIGURE 8-37**   Shadowing from calcified plaque follows the gray-scale scan lines straight down while following the angled color scan lines parallel to the sides of the parallelogram. (From Kremkau FW: Principles and instrumentation. In Merritt CRB, editor: Doppler color imaging, New York, 1992, Churchill Livingstone.)

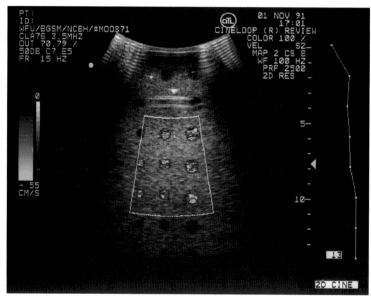

■ **FIGURE 8-39**   Color appears in echo-free (cystic) regions of a tissue-equivalent phantom. The color gain has been increased sufficiently to produce this effect. The instrument tends to write color information preferentially in areas where non–Doppler-shifted echoes are weak or absent. (From Kremkau FW: Principles and pitfalls of real-time color-flow imaging. In Bernstein EF, editor: *Vascular diagnosis,* ed 4, St Louis, 1993, Mosby.)

PLATE 37

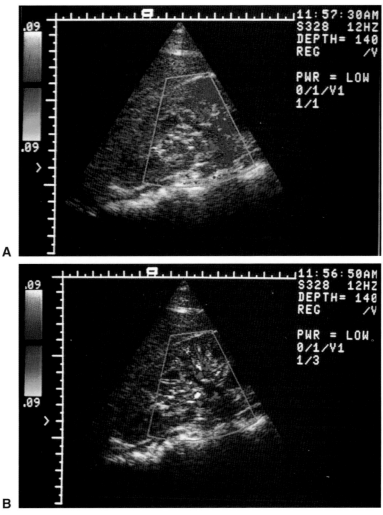

■ FIGURE 8-38 **A,** Clutter from tissue motion (caused by respiration) obscures underlying blood flow in the renal vasculature. **B,** An increased wall filter setting removes the clutter revealing the underlying flow.

PLATE 38

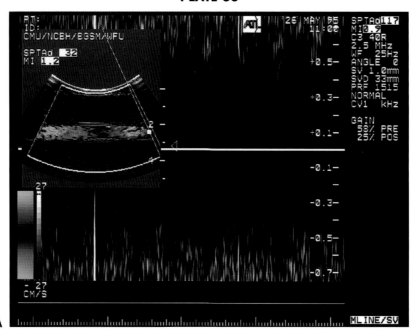

■ **FIGURE 8-45**   **A,** Illustration to accompany Exercise 47.

PLATE 37

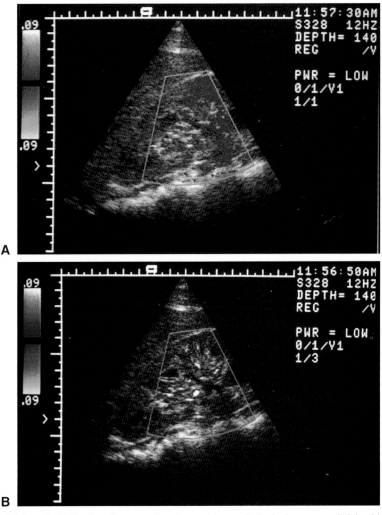

■ **FIGURE 8-38** **A,** Clutter from tissue motion (caused by respiration) obscures underlying blood flow in the renal vasculature. **B,** An increased wall filter setting removes the clutter revealing the underlying flow.

PLATE 38

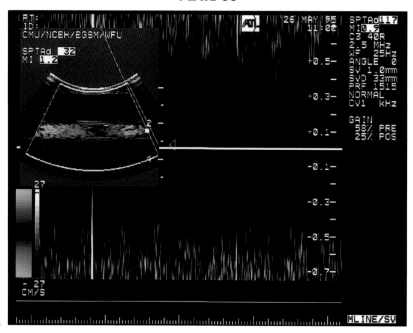

■ **FIGURE 8-45**   **A,** Illustration to accompany Exercise 47.

PLATE 39

A

B

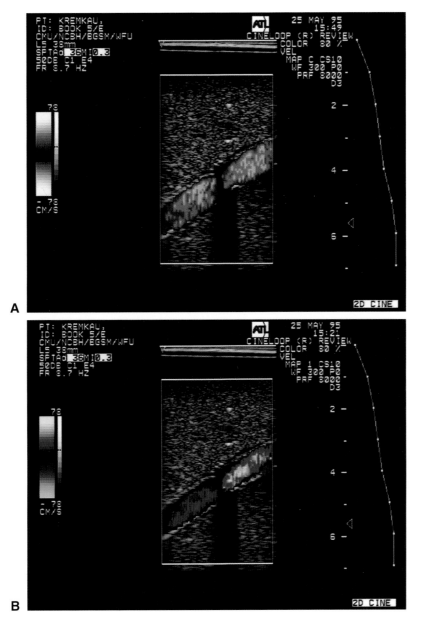

■ **FIGURE 8-46** **A** to **D,** Illustrations to accompany Exercises 48 to 50.

Continued.

PLATE 40

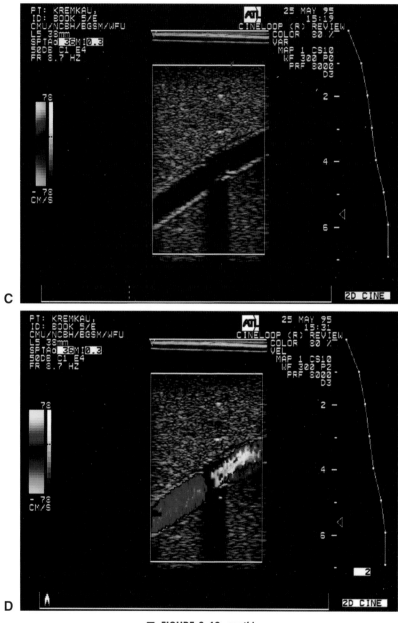

■ FIGURE 8-46, cont'd

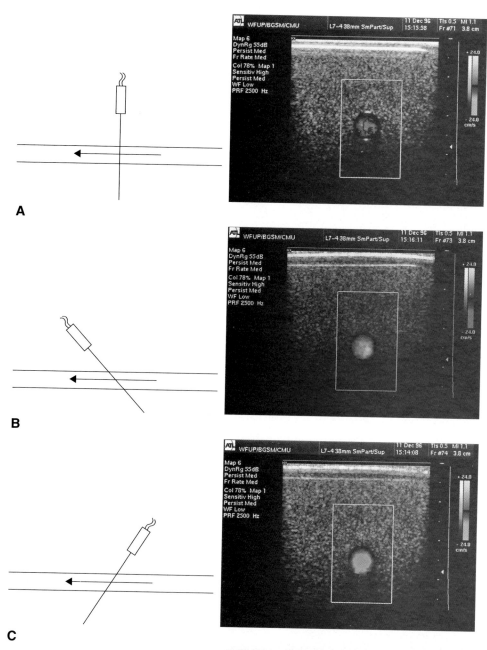

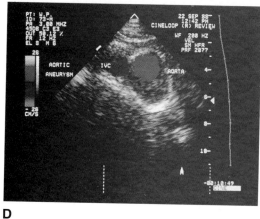

■ **FIGURE 6-18** The image plane is a transverse cut across the vessel. The views are perpendicular **(A)**, upstream **(B)**, and downstream **(C)**. The Doppler shifts obtained are **(A)** zero (or weakly positive and negative because of beam spreading), **(B)** positive, and **(C)** negative. The image plane is being viewed edge-on in the line drawings. **D,** A transverse view upstream (positive Doppler shift) in the aorta (the scan plane is angled toward the heart) and downstream (negative Doppler shift) in the inferior vena cava. (See Color Plate 24.) (**A** to **C** from Kremkau FW: *J Vascular Technol* 16:309-310, 1992.)

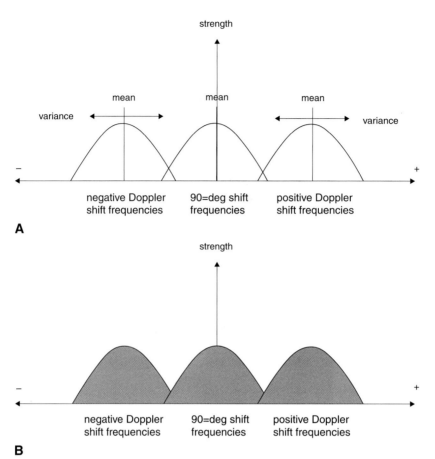

■ **FIGURE 6-19**   **A,** Spectra for flow toward (*positive*) and away from (*negative*) the transducer and perpendicular (90 degrees) to the sound beam. Conventional color Doppler imaging determines and displays, in color-coded form, the sign and mean (and sometimes the variance) of the Doppler-shift frequency spectrum. **B,** Power Doppler determines and displays, in color-coded form, the size of the area under the spectral curve. The axes of the spectral graph represent strength (amplitude, power, energy, or intensity) versus frequency.

an advantage of power Doppler is the uniform (angle-independent and alias-free) presentation of flow information, although this is accomplished with a loss in direction, speed, and flow character information. This extends even through regions of 90-degree Doppler angle (Figure 6-20, *B* and *C* [see Color Plate 25]) because the Doppler shift spectrum there has a nonzero area (Figure 6-19, *B*), even though its mean is zero, yielding a black region in color Doppler imaging displays (Figure 6-20, *A* and *C* [see Color Plate 25]). Power Doppler is also essentially free of variations in flow speed (as in the cardiac cycle) and thus can be frame-averaged to improve the signal-to-noise ratio and sensitivity substantially (Figure 6-21 [see Color Plates 26 and 27]). Because aliasing is not a problem in power Doppler, lower PRFs can be used to detect slow flows.

Box 6-3 lists the advantages and disadvantages of Doppler-power displays. In general, Doppler ultrasound can determine the presence or absence of flow, the direction and speed of flow, and the character of flow. Power Doppler is superior in terms of the first, but at the expense of the other three. Table 6-1 compares the color Doppler displays.

Doppler-power displays do not have direction, speed, or flow character information included and are insensitive to angle effects and aliasing. They are more sensitive than Doppler-shift displays in that they can present slower flows and flow in deeper or tinier vessels.

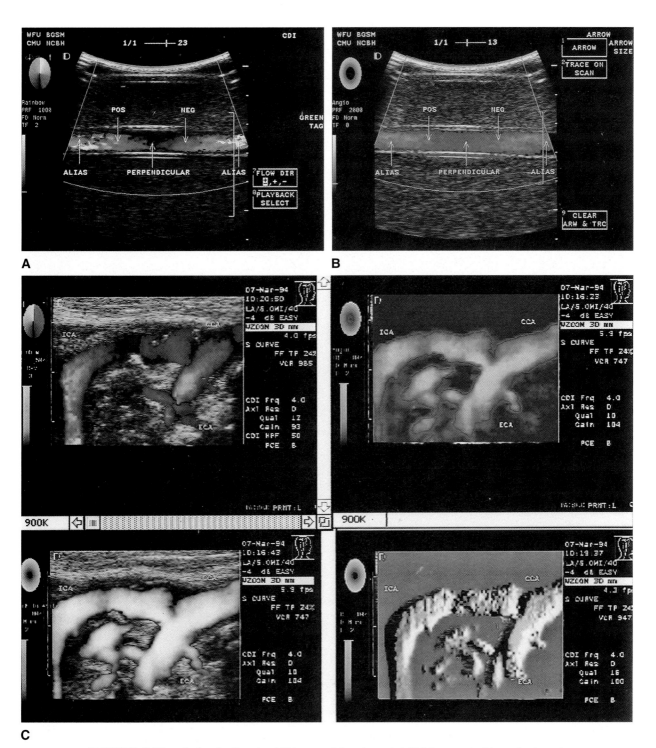

■ **FIGURE 6-20**   **A,** A color Doppler-shift image of flow in a straight tube, acquired in sector format. The varying Doppler angle from left to right yields aliasing and positive, negative, and zero Doppler-shift regions. **B,** A Doppler-power presentation of the situation shown in **A** yields a uniform image, free of angle dependence and aliasing. However, it contains no directional, speed, or dynamic information. **C,** Angle independence is seen in the Doppler-power images of the carotid artery; compare them to the Doppler-shift display *(upper left)*. Doppler-power imaging is shown in color, topographic, and gray-scale forms *(clockwise from upper right).* (See also Figure 1-13, *B,* and Color Plates 1 and 25.)

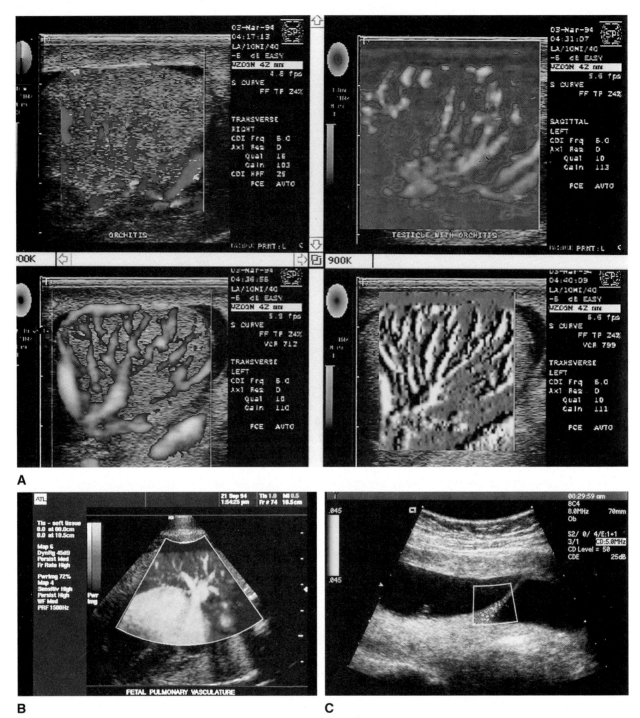

■ **FIGURE 6-21** **A,** Improved sensitivity to testicular flow compared with Doppler-shift imaging *(upper left)*. Small vessel flow is imaged in fetal pulmonary vasculature **(B)** and within the membrane separating a twin gestation **(C).**

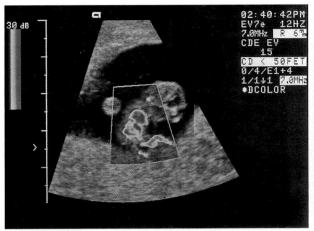

D

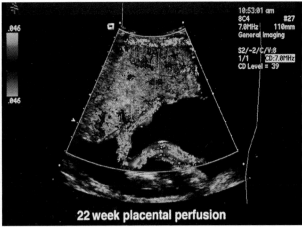

E

F

■ **FIGURE 6-21, cont'd** **D,** First trimester fetal circulation. A comparison of placental Doppler-shift imaging **(E)** and Doppler-power imaging **(F)** reveals improved flow detection with the latter. (See Color Plates 26 and 27.)

BOX 6-3 **Advantages and Disadvantages of Doppler-Power Displays with Respect to Doppler-Shift Displays**

ADVANTAGES
Angle independence
No aliasing
Improved sensitivity (deeper penetration, smaller vessels, slower flows)

DISADVANTAGES
No directional information
No flow speed information
No flow character information

TABLE 6-1 **Comparison of Doppler-Shift and Doppler-Power Displays**

	Doppler-Shift Display	Doppler-Power Display
Quantitative	No	No
Global	Yes	Yes
Perfusion	No	Yes

REVIEW

The key points presented in this chapter are the following:

■ Color Doppler imaging acquires Doppler-shifted echoes from a two-dimensional cross section of tissue scanned by an ultrasound beam.

■ Doppler-shifted echoes are presented in color and are superimposed on the gray-scale anatomic image of nonshifted echoes that were received during the scan.

■ Flow echoes are assigned colors according to the color map chosen.

■ Several pulses (the number is called the ensemble length) are needed to generate a color scan line.

■ Color controls include gain, map selection, variance on/off, persistence, ensemble length, color/gray priority, scale (PRF), baseline shift, wall filter, and color window angle, location, and size.

■ Doppler-shift displays are subject to Doppler angle dependence and aliasing.

■ Doppler-power displays color-encode Doppler-shift strengths into angle-independent, aliasing-independent, more sensitive presentations of flow information.

EXERCISES

1. What colors are used on color Doppler maps?
   a. Red and blue
   b. Yellow and cyan
   c. Black and white
   d. Green and magenta
   e. More than one of the above

2. Multiple focus is not used in color Doppler imaging because
   a. it would not improve the image.
   b. Doppler transducers cannot focus.
   c. of the ensemble length.
   d. frame rates would be too low.
   e. more than one of the above.

3. In Figure 6-16, A (see Color Plate 22), red and yellow indicate negative Doppler shifts. Therefore flow in this vessel is
   a. from upper right to lower left.
   b. rom lower left to upper right.

4. In the bend at the upper left of Figure 6-16, A (see Color Plate 22), there is a yellow region in the center of the vessel. This indicates the region in the image where blood flow speed is the greatest. True or false?

5. In Figure 6-16, C (see Color Plate 22), the region shown in cyan (aqua or blue-green) indicates
   a. turbulent flow.
   b. flow reversal.

   c. flow speed exceeding 32 cm/s.
   d. all of the above.
   e. none of the above.

6. Color Doppler instruments present two-dimensional, color-coded images representing _____ that are superimposed on gray-scale images representing _____.

7. Which of the following on a color Doppler display is (are) presented in real time?
   a. Gray-scale anatomy
   b. Flow direction
   c. Doppler spectrum
   d. a and b
   e. All of the above

8. If red represents flow toward the transducer and blue represents flow away, what color would be seen for normal flow toward the transducer? What color would be seen for aliasing flow toward the transducer? What color would be seen for normal flow away from the transducer? For aliasing flow away from the transducer? What color is representative of a positive Doppler shift? What color represents a negative shift? What color represents power?

9. Color Doppler instruments use an _____ technique to yield Doppler information in real time.

10. The information in Exercise 9 includes _____ Doppler shift, _____, _____, and _____.

11. The angle dependencies of Doppler-shift and Doppler-power displays are different. True or false?

12. The autocorrelation technique requires an ensemble length of at least _____.
    a. 1
    b. 2
    c. 3
    d. 4
    e. 5

13. Do the different colors appearing in Figure 6-14, A and C (see Color Plate 19), indicate that flow is going in two different directions in the vessel?

14. In color Doppler instruments, color is used only to represent flow direction. True or false?

15. In practice, approximately _____ pulses are required to obtain one line of color Doppler information.
    a. 1
    b. 10
    c. 100
    d. 1000
    e. 1,000,000

16. There are approximately _____ samples per line in a color Doppler display.
    a. 2
    b. 20

c. 200

d. 2000

e. 2,000,000

17. About _____ frames per second are produced by a color Doppler instrument.

    a. 10

    b. 20

    c. 40

    d. 80

    e. More than one of the above

18. Doppler-shift displays are not dependent on Doppler angle. True or false?

19. If two colors are shown in the same vessel using a color Doppler instrument, it always means flow is occurring in opposite directions in the vessel. True or false?

20. A region of bright color on a Doppler-shift display always indicates the highest flow speeds. True or false?

21. Increasing the ensemble length _____ the frame rate.

22. The _____ technique commonly is used to detect echo Doppler shifts in color Doppler instruments.

23. Widening the color box on the display _____ the frame rate.

24. The autocorrelation technique yields

    a. mean Doppler shift.

    b. power of the Doppler shift.

    c. spread around the mean (variance).

    d. all of the above.

    e. none of the above.

25. Which of the following reduce the frame rate of a color Doppler image? (more than one correct answer)

    a. Wider color window

    b. Longer color window

    c. Increased ensemble length

    d. Higher transducer frequency

    e. Higher priority setting

20. Lack of color in a vessel containing blood flow may be attributable to (more than one correct answer)

    a. low color gain.

    b. a high wall filter setting.

    c. a low priority setting.

    d. baseline shift.

    e. aliasing.

27. Increasing ensemble length _____ color sensitivity and accuracy and _____ frame rate.

    a. Improves, increases

    b. Degrades, increases

    c. Degrades, decreases

    d. Improves, decreases

    e. None of the above

28. Which controls can be used to deal with aliasing? (more than one correct answer)

    a. Wall filter

    b. Gain

    c. Baseline shift

    d. Pulse repetition frequency

    e. Smoothing

29. Pink, as compared with red, is an example of

    a. hue.

    b. luminance.

    c. saturation.

    d. b and c.

    e. none of the above.

30. Yellow is the combination of

    a. red and green.

    b. red and blue.

    c. blue and green.

    d. red, green, and blue.

31. Cyan is the combination of

    a. red and green.

    b. red and blue.

    c. blue and green.

    d. red, green, and blue.

32. White is the combination of equal amounts of

    a. red and green.

    b. red and blue.

    c. blue and green.

    d. red, green, and blue.

33. Which control can be used to help with clutter?

    a. Wall filter

    b. Gain

    c. Baseline shift

    d. Pulse repetition frequency

    e. Smoothing

34. Color map baselines are always represented by

    a. white.

    b. black.

    c. red.

    d. blue.

    e. cyan.

35. Autocorrelation is a modified form of variance. True or false?

36. Autocorrelation is used only in Doppler-power displays. True or false?

37. If a green tag indicates that flow speed is 50 cm/s, but the Doppler angle is 60 degrees and no angle correction is used, the flow speed is actually _____ cm/s.

38. Doubling the width of a color window produces a(n) _____ frame rate.

    a. Doubled

    b. Quadrupled

    c. Unchanged

    d. Halved

    e. Quartered

39. Steering the color window to the right or left produces a(n) _____ frame rate.
    a. Doubled
    b. Quadrupled
    c. Unchanged
    d. Halved
    e. Quartered

40. Autocorrelation produces (more than one correct answer)
    a. the color of Doppler shift.
    b. the mean value of Doppler shift.
    c. variance.
    d. spectrum.
    e. peak Doppler shift.

41. If the heart rate is 60 beats/min and the frame rate is 10 Hz, one edge of the color display lags the other by what fraction of the cardiac cycle?
    a. One sixtieth
    b. One thirtieth
    c. One tenth
    d. One sixth
    e. One third

42. Steering the color window to the right or left changes
    a. frame rate.
    b. pulse repetition frequency.
    c. Doppler angle.
    d. Doppler shift.
    e. more than one of the above.

43. Color Doppler frame rates are _____ gray-scale rates.
    a. Equal to
    b. Less than
    c. More than
    d. Depends on color map
    e. Depends on priority

44. In a single frame, color can change in a vessel because of
    a. vessel curvature.
    b. sector format.
    c. helical flow.
    d. diastolic flow reversal.
    e. all of the above.

45. Angle is not important in transverse color Doppler views through vessels. True or false?

46. In Figure 6-6, D (see Color Plate 7), match the following:
    a. Zero Doppler shift _____   1. Yellow
    b. Small positive shift _____   2. Red
    c. Large positive shift _____   3. Black
    d. Small negative shift _____   4. Blue
    e. Large negative shift _____   5. Cyan

47. In Figure 6-7, C (see Color Plate 9), the mean Doppler shifts in the vessel are less than _____ Hz.

    a. 10
    b. 25
    c. 50
    d. 100
    e. 200

48. What is the direction of flow indicated by red in the vessel in Figure 6-11, B (see Color Plate 15)?

49. The flow in the aneurysm shown in Figure 6-16, D (see Color Plate 22), is _____
    a. Clockwise
    b. Counterclockwise
    c. Left to right
    d. Top to bottom
    e. Right to left

50. The dark red and blue colors in Figure 6-18, D (see Color Plate 24), show that flow in the vessels is at speeds of less than 26 cm/s. True or false?

51. In Figure 6-22 (see Color Plate 27), match the color map colors with what they indicate.
    a. Black (K) _____   1. Large positive shift
    b. Yellow (Y) _____,   2. Large negative shift
       _____   3. Zero shift
    c. Cyan (C) _____,   4. Large variance
       _____   5. Zero variance
    d. Red (R) _____   6. Small positive shift
    e. Blue (B) _____   7. Small negative shift
    f. Green (G) _____,
       _____
    g. Green (G) _____,
       _____

52. What is the direction of flow in Figure 6-22?

53. What color would be displayed if the color window were steered to the right in Figure 6-22 (see Color Plate 27)?

54. For the color map in Figure 6-22 (see Color Plate 27), green would indicate _____ _____.

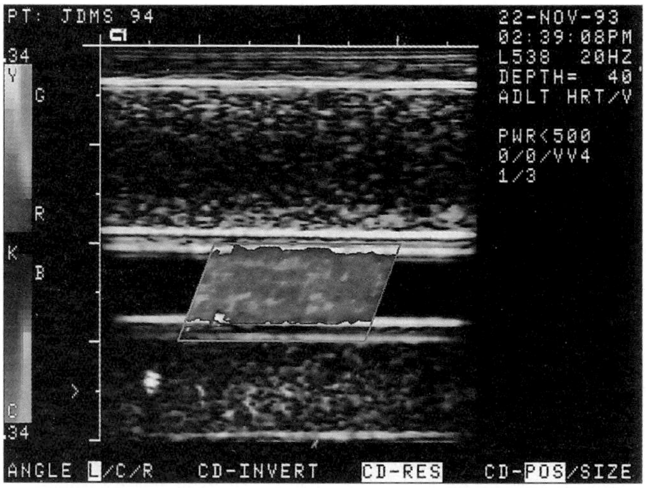

■ **FIGURE 6-22** Display to accompany Exercises 51 to 54. (See Color Plate 27.)

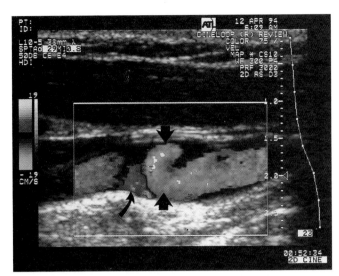

■ **FIGURE 6-23** Display to accompany Exercises 55 and 56. (See Color Plate 28.)

55. In Figure 6-23 (see Color Plate 28), the red region (curved arrow) indicates
    a. plaque.
    b. clot.
    c. down flow.
    d. up flow.
    e. turbulent flow.
56. In the curved blue region (straight arrows) in Figure 6-23 (see Color Plate 28), the flow is
    a. up.
    b. down.
    c. turbulent.
    d. an eddy current.
    e. circular.
57. Compared with Doppler shift imaging, Doppler-power imaging is
    a. more sensitive.
    b. angle-independent.
    c. aliasing-independent.
    d. speed-independent.
    e. all of the above.
58. Doppler-power imaging indicates (with color) the _____ of flow.
    a. Presence
    b. Direction
    c. Speed
    d. Character
    e. More than one of the above
59. Doppler shift imaging indicates (with color) the _____ of flow.
    a. Presence
    b. Direction
    c. Speed
    d. Character
    e. More than one of the above

60. In Figure 6-24 (see Color Plate 28), what is the flow direction?
61. For the color map in Figure 6-25 (see Color Plate 29), match the following
    a. High power _____   1. Black
    b. Medium power _____   2. Red
    c. Low power _____   3. Orange
    d. Zero power _____   4. Green
                                     5. Blue
62. In Figure 6-25 (see Color Plate 29), the change from green to red with increasing depth is caused by _____.

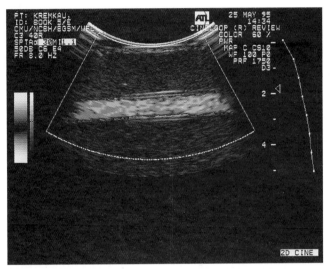

■ **FIGURE 6-24** Display to accompany Exercise 60. (See Color Plate 28.)

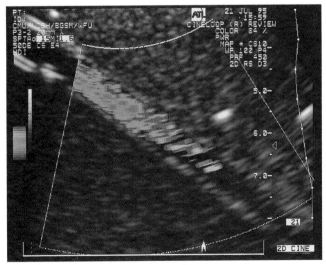

■ **FIGURE 6-25** Display to accompany Exercises 61 and 62. (See Color Plate 29.)

63. Doppler-shift imaging is good for
    a. indicating flow direction.
    b. indicating flow speed.
    c. indicating flow character.
    d. indicating flow in small or deep vessels.
    e. more than one of the above.
64. Doppler-power imaging is good for
    a. indicating flow direction.
    b. indicating flow speed.
    c. indicating flow character.
    d. indicating flow in small or deep vessels.
    e. more than one of the above.
65. Color Doppler instruments use
    a. continuous wave Doppler.
    b. pulsed Doppler.
    c. compressed Doppler.
    d. all of the above.
    e. none of the above.

CHAPTER 7

Spectral Doppler Instruments*

*NOTE: Appendix I provides a condensed version of the material in Chapters 5 to 7 for readers who need less depth and breadth of coverage on Doppler topics. Because of the importance of blood flow and Doppler techniques in echocardiography and vascular ultrasound, the complete coverage in Chapters 5 to 7 is recommended for persons working in those fields.

LEARNING OBJECTIVES

After reading this chapter, the student should be able to do the following:

- List the ways in which Doppler information is presented.
- Explain how flow detection is localized to a specific site in tissue using pulsed Doppler techniques.
- Describe spectral analysis.
- Discuss examples of how spectral analysis is applied to evaluate flow conditions at the site of measurement and elsewhere.
- Compare continuous wave and pulsed wave Doppler spectral instruments.

KEY TERMS

The following terms are introduced in this chapter:

Bidirectional	Frequency spectrum	Spectral analysis
Clutter	Gate	Spectral broadening
Continuous wave Doppler	Phase	Spectral display
Doppler spectrum	Phase quadrature	Spectrum analyzer
Duplex instrument	Pulsatility index	Wall filter
Fast Fourier transform	Pulsed Doppler	Window
Filter	Range gating	Zero-crossing detector
Fourier transform	Sample volume	

n addition to color Doppler instruments, two types of spectral Doppler instruments are used for Doppler detection of flow in the heart and blood vessels: continuous wave (CW) and pulsed wave (PW). All three often are combined into one multipurpose instrument (Figure 7-1). The CW instrument detects Doppler-shifted echoes in the region of overlap between the beams of the transmitting and receiving transducer elements. A difference between other transducers and those designed exclusively for CW Doppler use is that the latter are not damped. The PW Doppler instrument emits ultrasound pulses and receives echoes using a single element transducer or an array. Because of the required Doppler frequency shift detection, the pulses are longer than those used in imaging. Through **range gating**, PW Doppler has the ability to select information from a particular depth along the beam. To use PW Doppler effectively, it commonly is combined with gray-scale sonography in one instrument. Such instru-

217

ments are called duplex scanners because of their dual functions (anatomic imaging *and* flow measurement). Continuous wave and pulsed wave instruments present Doppler shift information in audible form and as a visual display.

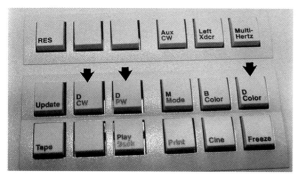

■ FIGURE 7-1   Continuous wave (CW), pulsed wave (PW), and color Doppler instruments can be combined in one device, with each mode selectable from the control panel *(arrows)*.

CONTINUOUS WAVE INSTRUMENTS

Spectral Doppler instruments provide continuous or pulsed voltages to the transducer and convert echo voltages received from the transducer to audible and visual information corresponding to scatterer motion. If an instrument distinguishes between positive and negative Doppler shifts, it is called **bidirectional. Continuous wave Doppler** instruments include a CW oscillator and a Doppler detector that detects the changes in frequency (Doppler shifts) resulting from scatterer motion for presentation as audible sounds and as a visual presentation corresponding to the motion.

Components of a Continuous Wave Doppler System

A diagram of the components of a CW Doppler system is presented in Figure 7-2, *A*. The oscillator produces a continuously alternating voltage with a 2- to 10-MHz frequency, which is applied to the source transducer ele-

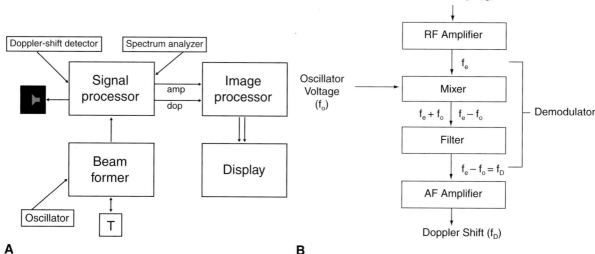

■ FIGURE 7-2   A, Block diagram of a sonographic instrument functioning as a continuous wave Doppler instrument. The oscillator (part of the beam former) produces a continuously alternating voltage that drives the source transducer element *(T)*. The receiving transducer element *(T)* produces a continuous voltage in response to echoes it continuously is receiving. The signal processor includes a Doppler-shift detector that detects differences in frequency between the voltages produced by the oscillator and by the receiving element. The Doppler shifts produce voltages that drive loudspeakers and a visual display. The frequency of the audible sound is equal to the Doppler shift and is proportional to the reflector speed and to the cosine of the angle between the sound propagation direction and the boundary motion. **B,** Block diagram of a continuous wave Doppler detector. The radio frequency *(RF)* amplifier increases the echo voltage amplitude. The frequency of the echo voltage is f_e. In the mixer, this frequency is combined with the oscillator voltage, the frequency of which is f_o. The mixer yields the sum and difference of these two frequency inputs ($f_e + f_o$ and $f_e - f_o$). The low-pass (high-frequency rejection) filter removes $f_e + f_o$, leaving $f_e - f_o$, which is the Doppler-shift frequency (f_D). This frequency then is strengthened in the audio frequency *(AF)* amplifier. The mixer and filter together constitute the Doppler demodulator.

ment. The ultrasound frequency is determined by the oscillator. The oscillator frequency is set to equal the operating frequency of the transducer. In the transducer assembly a separate receiving transducer element produces voltages with frequencies equal to the frequencies of the returning echoes. If there is scatterer motion, the reflected ultrasound and the ultrasound produced by the source transducer will have different frequencies. The Doppler detector detects the difference between these two frequencies, which is the Doppler shift, and drives a loudspeaker at this frequency. Doppler shifts are typically one thousandth of the operating frequency, which puts them in the audible range. The Doppler shifts also commonly are sent through a **spectrum analyzer** to a **spectral display** for visual observation and evaluation.

The detector (Figure 7-2, *B*) amplifies the echo voltages it receives from the receiving element, detects the Doppler shift information in the returning echoes, and usually determines motion direction from the sign of the Doppler shift. Doppler shifts are determined by mixing the returning voltages with the CW voltage from the oscillator. This produces the sum and difference of the oscillator and echo frequencies (Figure 7-2, *B*). The difference is the desired Doppler shift. The sum is a much higher frequency (approximately double the operating frequency) and is filtered out easily. The difference is zero for echoes returning from stationary structures. For echoes from moving structures or flowing blood, this difference is the Doppler shift, which provides information about motion and flow.

The Doppler detector detects Doppler shifts and determines their sign.

Positive and negative shifts indicate motion toward and away from the transducer, respectively. The detector shown in Figure 7-2, *B*, does not provide this directional information. Determining direction and separating Doppler shift voltages into separate forward and reverse channels is accomplished by the **phase quadrature** detector (Figure 7-3).

ADVANCED CONCEPTS

In the phase quadrature detector, two voltages from the oscillator (one leading by one quarter of a cycle [Figure 7-4], i.e., "quad") are mixed with the returning echo voltages to yield the difference, which is the Doppler shift. The echo voltages contain the Doppler shifts representing flow toward (f_t) and away from (f_a) the transducer. The **filter** outputs of the direct channel and

the delayed (quadrature) channel are the Doppler shifts from the echo voltage input. If the Doppler shift is positive, the shift in the direct channel lags behind that in the quadrature channel by one quarter of a cycle (90 degrees). If the Doppler shift is negative, the shift in the quadrature channel lags behind that in the direct channel by one quarter of a cycle. The Doppler shifts in both of these channels are next shifted by a quarter cycle. A negative Doppler shift in the direct channel at that point leads the one in the quadrature channel (before the additional 90-degree shift) by half a cycle. When added, these two voltages cancel (Figure 7-5), yielding no output. Positive Doppler shifts in these two channels are in **phase** (no lead or lag), yielding output from the direct channel adder. Positive shifts in the quadrature channel lead those in the direct channel by half a cycle, whereas negative shifts in the two channels are in phase. Thus the negative shifts are the output of the quadrature channel adder. The outputs of the two adders are sent to separate loudspeakers so that forward and reverse Doppler shifts can be heard separately. The outputs are also sent to a visual display to show positive and negative Doppler shifts above and below the display baseline, which represents zero Doppler shift.

The forward and reverse channel signals are sent to separate loudspeakers so that forward and reverse Doppler shifts can be heard separately. The signals are also sent to a visual display to show positive and negative Doppler shifts above and below the display baseline, which represents zero Doppler shift (Figure 7-6).

Simpler instruments, such as a handheld, nondirectional device, yield only an audible output. Analog **zero-crossing detector** devices (Figure 7-7) provide an instantaneous-average Doppler shift that varies over cardiac cycle. This is fed to a strip-chart recorder that produces a hard copy of the average Doppler shift versus time. The zero-crossing detector gets its name from the fact that it counts how often the Doppler shift voltage changes from negative to positive or vice versa per second. The higher the count, the higher the frequency. This count is presented on the vertical axis of a two-dimensional graph in which the horizontal axis represents time (Figure 7-7, *C*). More sophisticated systems have spectral displays, as shown in Figure 7-6. The average Doppler shift yielded by the zero-crossing approach favors lower frequencies because the higher ones often do not cross the baseline (Figure 7-7, *A*).

Zero-crossing detectors present mean Doppler shift on a strip-chart recorder.

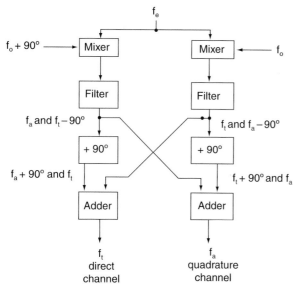

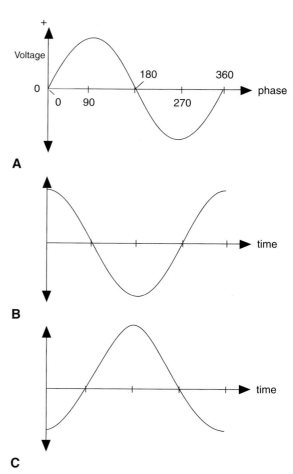

■ **FIGURE 7-3** The phase quadrature detector detects the positive (f_t) and negative (f_a) Doppler shifts contained in the incoming echo voltage (f_e) and separates them into separate channels for delivery to loud-speakers and visual display. These channels are designated as direct and quadrature (on the left and right, respectively). Detection proceeds as described in the following. The echo voltage is mixed with the oscillator voltage (f_o) in two mixers. The oscillator voltage in the direct channel leads that in the quadrature channel by one-quarter cycle (90 degrees; Figure 7-4). The frequency sum $(f_e + f_o)$ is filtered out, as in Figure 7-2, B, yielding the Doppler shift f_D, which is $f_e - f_o$. The Doppler shift may be positive $(f_t$, for flow toward the transducer) or negative $(f_a$, for flow away from the transducer). Because of the oscillator-voltage phase difference $(f_o + 90$ degrees versus $f_o)$, the two filter outputs are different. Positive shifts in the direct channel lag those in the quadrature channel by 90 degrees (Figure 7-5, A). Negative shifts in the quadrature channel lag those in the direct channel by 90 degrees (Figure 7-5, B). Next, another 90-degree phase shift results in the separation of the positive and negative shifts into separate channels—direct and quadrature, respectively—as follows. The phase-shifted positive Doppler shifts in the direct channel are now in phase with the unshifted ones in the quadrature channel (Figure 7-5, C), whereas the negative shifts are 180 degrees out of phase (Figure 7-5, D). When added together, the negative shifts will cancel (Figure 7-4, B and C), yielding positive shifts as the output voltage in the direct channel. A similar process in the quadrature channel yields the negative shifts as output.

■ **FIGURE 7-4** Phase. **A,** One complete variation (cycle) of alternating voltage may be thought of as traveling around a 360-degree circle. One quarter of a cycle is 90 degrees of phase angle. Phase is a description of progression through a cycle (analogous to the phase of the moon). One quarter of a cycle is 90 degrees, and one half of a cycle is 180 degrees. The completion of a cycle occurs at 360 degrees, but this is also the 0-degree phase of the next cycle. **B,** This voltage leads that in **A** by 90 degrees (one-quarter cycle). **C,** This voltage lags that in **A** by 90 degrees and lags that in **B** by 180 degrees. If the voltages in **B** and **C** are added together, a zero voltage results. (The two voltages are equal and opposite, so they cancel each other when summed.)

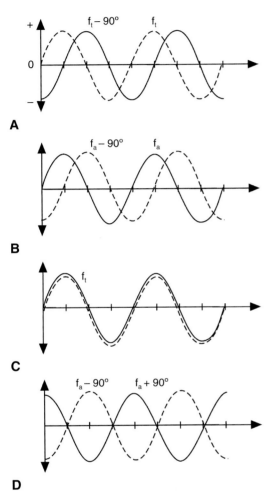

■ **FIGURE 7-5** The solid curves refer to the direct channel, whereas the dashed curves refer to quadrature. The vertical axis represents voltage and the horizontal one represents time. **A,** Positive Doppler shifts (f_t) at the output of the direct channel filter lag those in the quadrature channel by 90 degrees. **B,** Negative Doppler shifts (f_a) at the output of the quadrature channel lag those in the direct channel by 90 degrees. **C,** Positive Doppler shifts at the input to the direct channel adder are in phase (0-degree phase difference), yielding an f_t output. **D,** Negative Doppler shifts at the input to the direct channel adder are 180 degrees out of phase, yielding a zero f_a output.

Continuous Wave Sample Volume

A CW instrument detects flow that occurs anywhere within the intersection of the transmitting and receiving beams of the dual-transducer assembly (Figure 7-7, *D*). The **sample volume** is the region from which Doppler-shifted echoes return and are presented audibly or visually. In this case, the sample volume is the overlapping region of the transmitting and receiving beams. Because the sample volume is rather large, CW Doppler systems can give complicated and confusing presentations if two or more different motions or flows are included in the sample volume (e.g., two blood vessels being viewed simultaneously). **Pulsed Doppler** systems solve this problem by detecting motion or flow at a selected depth with a relatively small sample volume. However, the large sample volume of a CW system is helpful when searching for a Doppler maximum associated with a vascular or valvular stenosis.

Because a distribution of flow velocities is encountered by the beam as it traverses a vessel, a distribution of many Doppler-shifted frequencies returns to the transducer and the instrument. In arterial circulation or in the heart, these Doppler shifts are changing continually over the cardiac cycle and are displayed as a function of time with appropriate real-time frequency-spectrum processing (Figure 7-8). These displays provide quantitative data for evaluating Doppler-shifted echoes. The display device is again the cathode-ray tube or flat-panel display. The displayed Doppler information is stored in digital memory before display so that it can be frozen and backed up over the last few seconds of information before freezing.

Angle Incorporation or Correction

To convert a display correctly from Doppler shift versus time to flow speed versus time, the Doppler angle must be incorporated accurately into the calculation process (Figure 7-9). Angle incorporation commonly is called "angle correction." Either term is appropriate because lack of angle incorporation leaves the instrument to assume that the Doppler angle is zero, which is incorrect unless the angle is in fact zero. Figure 7-9, *B* and *C*, illustrate the importance of accurate angle correction. Figure 7-9, *C* to *F*, show errors encountered when the Doppler angle is handled incorrectly. Recall that as angle increases, Doppler shift decreases. Thus when the angle indicator on the instrument is set at 60 degrees, the instrument responds by doubling the calculated flow speed from what it would have been at a Doppler angle of zero. Another way to say this is that the Doppler equation, arranged to have calculated flow speed alone on one side of the equal sign, has cosine Doppler angle in the denominator on the other side. As the angle

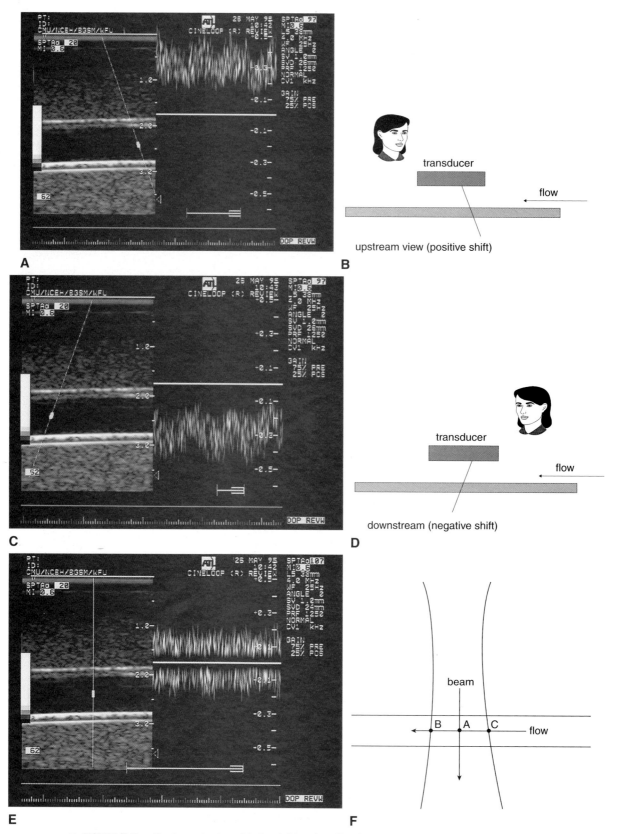

■ **FIGURE 7-6**   The beam is steered to the right and positive Doppler shifts are received **(A).** Thus this is an upstream view **(B),** and flow is from right to left. Therefore steering the beam to the left **(C)** would provide a downstream view **(D)** with negative Doppler shifts. With the beam perpendicular to the flow **(E),** Doppler shifts *are* received, positive and negative, because of beam spreading **(F);** that is, a portion of the beam views upstream while a portion views downstream. The beam axis portion (90-degree angle) yields a zero Doppler shift.

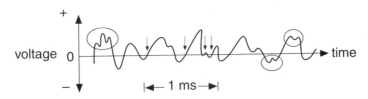

A

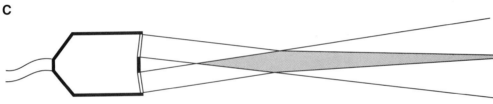

B

C

D.E. Hokanson, Inc

D

■ **FIGURE 7-7** **A,** A zero-crossing detector counts the number of zero crossings per second in the positive or negative direction. In the 1-ms period shown, four zero crossings (negative to positive) occurred *(arrows),* corresponding to a mean frequency of 4 kHz. Higher frequencies that are missed by the zero-crossing technique are circled. **B,** A zero-crossing continuous wave Doppler instrument. **C,** Chart output from a zero-crossing instrument shows an average Doppler shift. **D,** Continuous wave Doppler systems have dual-element transducer assemblies, one for transmitting and one for receiving. The region over which Doppler information can be acquired (Doppler sample volume) is the region of overlap between the transmitting and receiving beams *(shaded region).*

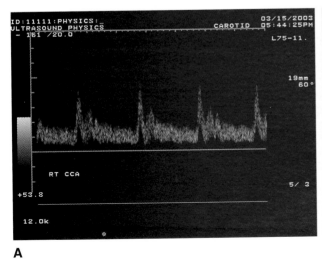

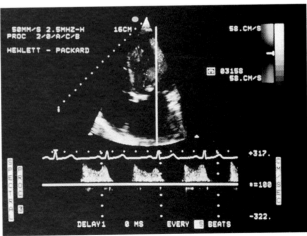

A   **B**

■ **FIGURE 7-8** **A,** A display of Doppler-shift frequencies as a function of time. This is a pulsed Doppler spectral display. **B,** A cardiac continuous wave Doppler spectral display.

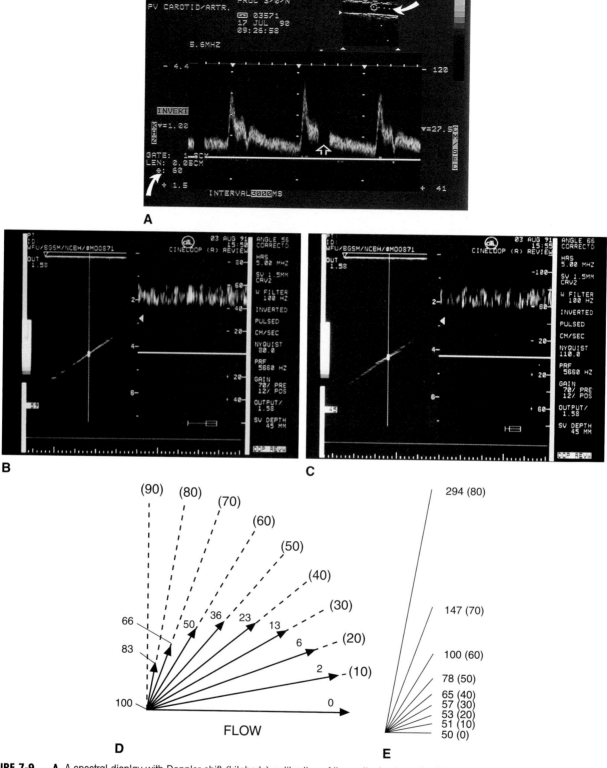

■ FIGURE 7-9   A, A spectral display with Doppler-shift (kilohertz) calibration of the vertical axis on the left and flow speed (centimeters per second) calibration on the right. Conversion from the former to the latter requires angle incorporation *(curved arrows).* The Doppler angle in this example is 60 degrees. The gap in Doppler information *(open arrow)* occurs when the instrument takes time to generate a frame of the anatomic image *(upper right).* **B** and **C,** A moving-string test object is imaged, resulting in the Doppler spectral display shown. With proper angle incorporation (56 degrees) the 50 cm/s string speed is shown correctly **(B).** With improper angle incorporation (66 degrees), an incorrect string speed of 70 cm/s is shown **(C).** This is a 40% error. **D,** If a zero Doppler angle is assumed correctly, there is zero error in the calculated flow speed. However, if the angle is actually nonzero, error results. The error in flow speed increases as the angle error *(in parentheses)* increases. For example, if the Doppler angle is 10 degrees but is assumed to be zero, the calculated flow speed will be 2% less than the correct value. At 60 and 80 degrees, the errors are 50% and 83%, respectively. At 90 degrees, there is zero Doppler shift. The calculated flow speed is zero (100% error). **E,** If the Doppler angle is zero but is assumed to be some other value, the calculated flow speeds are too large. Here the correct value is 50 cm/s. The error increases with angle *(in parentheses).* For example, at 60 and 80 degrees, the calculated values are 100 and 294 cm/s, respectively.

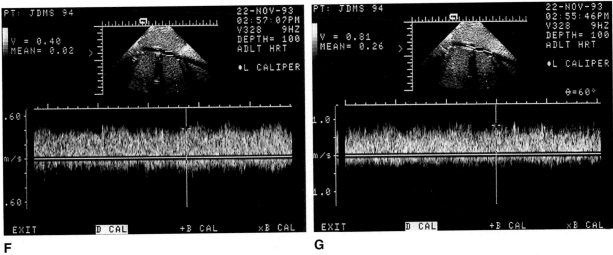

■ FIGURE 7-9, cont'd **F,** No angle correction is used in this display. The instrument assumes a Doppler angle of zero and calculates flow speed (v) at 40 cm/s. However, the Doppler angle is actually 60 degrees, yielding half the Doppler shift that a 0-degree angle would. **G,** When the cosine of 60 degrees (0.5) is incorporated into the Doppler equation, the result is 81 cm/s. (**B** and **C** from Kremkau FW: *Semin Roentgenol* 27:6-16, 1992; **F** and **G** from Kremkau FW: *J Diagn Med Sonogr* 10:337-338, 1994. Reprinted by permission of Sage Publications, Inc.)

indicator is increased, the cosine goes down, increasing the calculated speed value. This compensates for the reduction in Doppler shift cause by the Doppler angle actually involved in the ultrasound beam and flow intersection. For example, if the actual Doppler angle is 60 degrees, the Doppler shift is half what it would have been at 0 degrees. If the angle is set properly on the instrument at 60 degrees, the cosine in the denominator of the Doppler equation is set at 0.5. This doubles the calculated flow speed to the correct value.

> The Doppler sample volume of a continuous wave Doppler instrument is relatively large, being the overlapping region of the transmission and reception beams.

Wall Filter

In vascular studies, to eliminate the high-intensity, low-frequency Doppler shift echoes called **clutter** caused by heart or vessel wall or cardiac valve motion with pulsatile flow, a **wall filter** that rejects frequencies below an adjustable value is used (Figure 7-10). Sometimes called a wall-thump filter, the filter rejects these strong echoes that otherwise would overwhelm the weaker echoes from the blood. These strong echoes have low Doppler-shift frequencies because the tissue structures do not move as fast as the blood does. The upper limit of the filter is adjustable over a range of about 25 to 3200 Hz. The filter, however, can erroneously alter conclusions

regarding diastolic flow and distal flow resistance if not used properly (Figure 7-10, *I*).

> Wall filters remove clutter (low-frequency Doppler shifts from moving tissue).

PULSED WAVE INSTRUMENTS

Components of a Pulsed Wave Doppler System

A diagram of the components of a PW Doppler instrument is given in Figure 7-11, *A*. The pulser (in the beam former) is similar to that in the sonographic instrument, except that it generates pulses of several cycles of voltage that drive the transducer where ultrasound pulses are produced. Recall that imaging pulses are two or three cycles long. Pulses used in Doppler instruments, however, have pulse lengths of about 5 to 30 cycles. This length is necessary to determine the Doppler shifts of returning echoes accurately. Echo voltages from the transducer are processed in the detector, where they are amplified, their frequency is compared with the pulser frequency, and the Doppler shifts are determined. The Doppler shifts are sent to loudspeakers for audible output and to the display for visual observation. Based on their arrival time (recall the 13 μs/cm rule), echoes coming from reflectors at a given depth may be selected by the amplifier **gate.** Thus motion information may be obtained

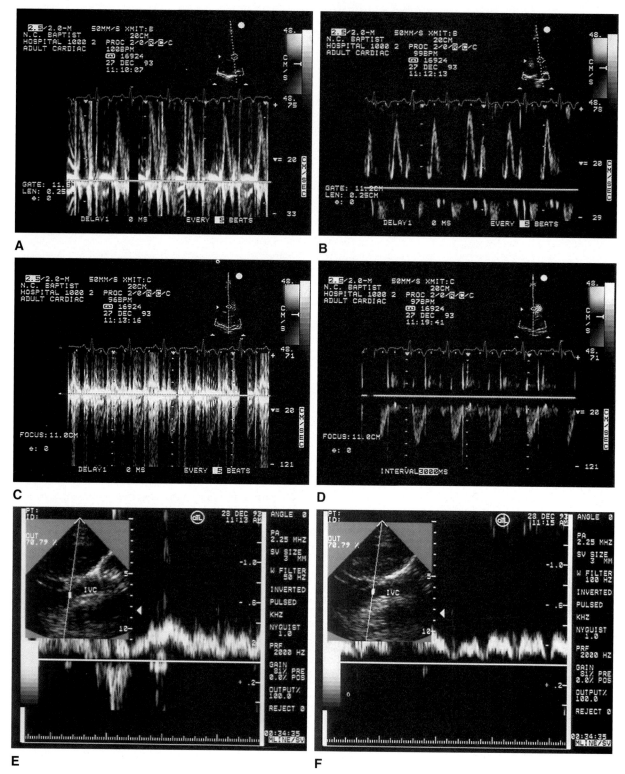

■ **FIGURE 7-10** **A,** Clutter in the spectrum of inflow at the mitral valve is shown. **B,** The clutter in **A** is removed by increasing the wall filter setting. **C,** Clutter in the spectrum of the left ventricular outflow tract. **D,** The clutter in **C** is removed with an increase in the wall filter setting. **E,** Clutter in the display of inferior vena caval flow. **F,** The clutter shown in **E** is removed by adjusting the wall filter.

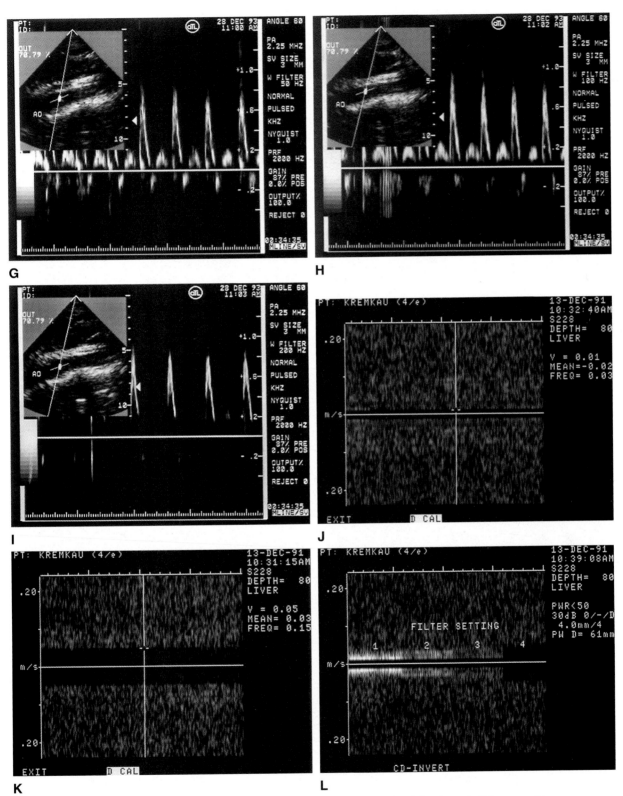

■ **FIGURE 7-10, cont'd** **G,** Clutter in the display of aortic flow. **H,** The clutter shown in **G** is removed by adjusting the wall filter. **I,** The wall filter is set too high (200 Hz), eliminating all but the peak systolic portion of the spectrum. **J,** Using electronic noise on the spectrum (with high Doppler gain), a low wall filter setting eliminates Doppler shifts corresponding to flow speeds of less than 1 cm/s. **K,** A higher setting eliminates speeds of less than 5 cm/s. **L,** Four wall filter settings reduce or eliminate frequencies as shown.

from a specific depth. This is called range gating. The operator controls the gate length and location.

Range gating enables depth selectivity and a small Doppler sample volume.

A PW Doppler instrument does not detect the complete Doppler shift as a CW instrument does but rather obtains samples of it. Because the PW instrument is a sampling system, each pulse yields a *sample* of the Doppler shift signal. The Doppler shifts are determined as described previously, except that the mixer does not receive a continuous input echo voltage but rather a sampled one. Echoes arrive from the sample volume depth in pulsed form at a rate equal to the pulse repetition frequency. Each of these returning echoes yields a sample of the Doppler shift from the Doppler detector. These samples are connected and smoothed (filtered) to yield the sampled waveform (Figure 7-11, *B* to *E*).

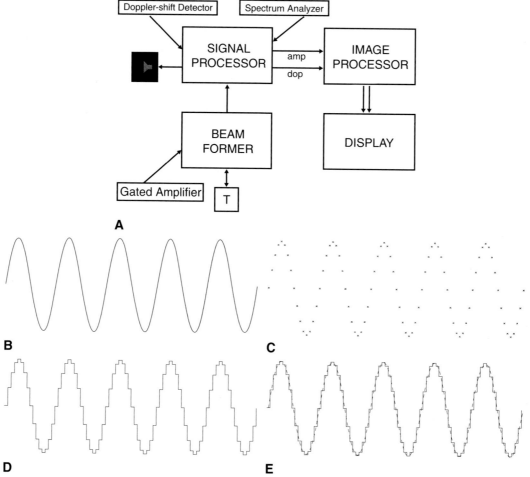

■ **FIGURE 7-11** **A,** Block diagram of a sonographic instrument functioning as a pulsed wave Doppler instrument. The beam former produces voltage pulses of several cycles each, which drive the transducer *(T)*. The signal processor includes a Doppler-shift detector, where shift frequencies are compared with the frequency of the outgoing pulses. The difference (Doppler shift) is sent to loudspeakers and, through the spectrum analyzer and image processor, to the display. The beam former also contains a gate that selects echoes from a given depth according to arrival time and thus gives motion information from a selected depth. **B,** Five cycles of a 500-Hz Doppler shift frequency occurring in 10 ms of time. **C,** In a pulsed wave Doppler instrument, each pulse yields echoes from the sample volume. These echoes, after Doppler detection, yield samples *(x)* of the Doppler shift from the sample volume. In this example, 80 samples are determined in a 10-ms time period. Therefore the pulse repetition frequency of the instrument is 8 kHz (with each pulse yielding one sample of the Doppler shift). **D,** The pulsed wave Doppler gate also is called a sample-and-hold amplifier. It samples the returning stream of echoes (resulting from one emitted pulse of ultrasound) at the appropriate time for the desired depth (Table 7-1) and holds the value until the next pulse and sample are accomplished. **E,** Low-pass filtering (which removes higher frequencies) smooths the sampled result *(solid line),* yielding the desired Doppler shift waveform *(dashed line)* comparable to that shown in **B.**

A pulsed wave Doppler system is a sampling system.

Range Gate

The gate selects the sample volume location from which returning Doppler-shifted echoes are accepted (Table 7-1 and Figures 7-12 to 7-14). The width of the sample volume is equal to the beam width. The gate has some length over which it permits reception (Table 7-2). For example (applying the 13 μs/cm rule), a gate that passes echoes arriving from 13 to 15 μs after pulse generation is listening over a depth range of 10.0 to 11.5 mm. In this case the gate is located at a depth of 10.8 mm with a length (depth range) of ±0.8 mm. Longer gate lengths are used when searching for the desired vessel and flow location and shorter gate lengths are used for **spectral analysis** and evaluation. The shorter gate length improves the quality of the spectral display.

The Doppler sample volume is determined by the beam width, the gate length, and the emitted pulse length. One half the pulse length (the same as axial resolution in sonography) is added to the gate length to yield the effective sample volume length (Table 7-3). Thus the pulse length must shorten as gate length is reduced. The sample volume width is equal to the beam width at the sample volume depth.

Volume flow rate (milliliters per second) can be calculated from spatial-mean flow speed multiplied by vessel cross-sectional area. To do this correctly, however, one must average properly the various Doppler shifts representing the cells moving at various speeds, must account properly for the angle to convert mean Doppler shift to mean speed, and must determine correctly the vessel cross-sectional area. Much can go wrong in this complicated process, yielding faulty results.[41-43]

Duplex Instrument

Including PW Doppler capability in a gray-scale sonographic instrument yields what commonly is called a **duplex instrument** (Figure 7-14, G). The instrument has the capacity to image anatomic structures and to analyze motion and flow at a known point in the anatomic field. Imaging allows intelligent positioning of the gate and angle correction in a PW Doppler system.

Duplex systems must be time-shared; that is, imaging and Doppler flow measurements cannot be done simultaneously. Electronic scanning with arrays permits rapid switching between imaging and Doppler functions (several times per second), allowing what can appear to be simultaneous acquisition of real-time image and Doppler flow information. Imaging frame rates are slowed to allow for acquisition of Doppler information between frames. Likewise, time out is taken from the spectral display to present a sonographic frame (Figure 7-9, A, open arrow).

Duplex instruments enable intelligent use of the Doppler sample volume by showing its location in the gray-scale anatomic display.

SPECTRAL ANALYSIS

The Doppler shift voltage from the detector does not go directly to the display but undergoes further processing because otherwise it would look like Figure 7-15, A. This is the visual picture of what a listener hears from the loudspeaker. Spectral analysis (Figure 7-15, B) provides a more meaningful and useful way to present the Doppler information visually. The presentation is in the form of a Doppler **frequency spectrum.**

Frequency Spectrum

The term *spectral* means relating to a spectrum. A spectrum is an array of the components of a wave, separated and arranged in order of increasing wavelength or frequency. The term *analysis* comes from a Greek word meaning to break up or to take apart. Thus spectral analysis is the breaking up of the frequency components of a complex wave or signal and spreading them out in order of increasing frequency.

Spectral analysis presents Doppler shift frequencies in frequency order.

TABLE 7-1	**Echo Arrival Time for Various Reflector Depths (Gate Locations)**
Depth (mm)	**Time (μs)**
10	13
20	26
30	39
40	52
50	65
60	78
70	91
80	104
90	117
100	130
150	195
200	260

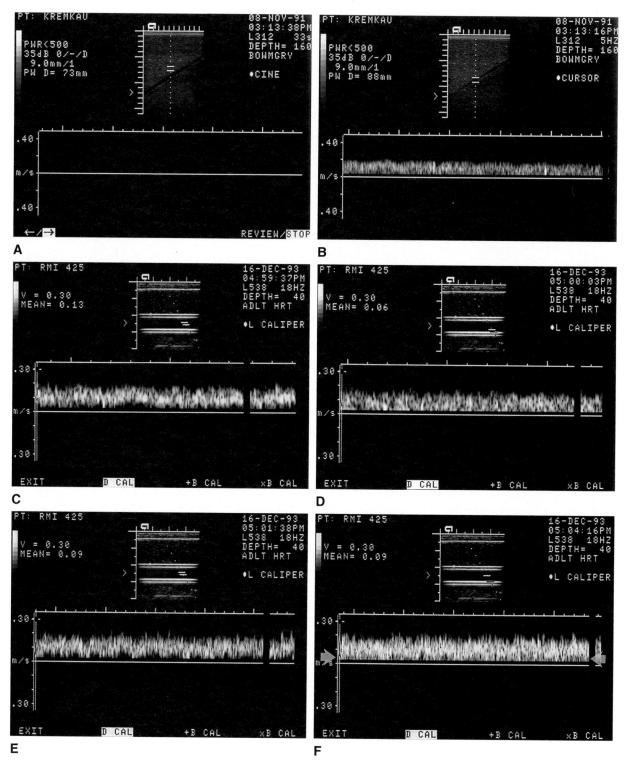

■ **FIGURE 7-12** **A,** The pulsed wave Doppler sample volume is located at 73 mm of depth (95 μs arrival time). No Doppler shift is seen on the lower display because the Doppler-shifted echoes from within the tube arrive at about 114 μs. **B,** When the gate is open later (corresponding to a depth of 88 mm), the Doppler shifts are received and displayed (indicating a constant flow rate in the tube). **C,** The gate is located in the center of the tube. **D,** The gate is located near the tube wall. Mean flow speed is 6 cm/s compared with 13 cm/s in **C.** This is the expected result with laminar flow. **E,** The gate is again located at the center of the tube. **F,** The gate length is extended to include the flow from the center, out to the tube wall. Note the strengthening of the lower flow speeds (Doppler shifts) *(arrows)* compared with **E,** where the slower flow is not included in the sample volume.

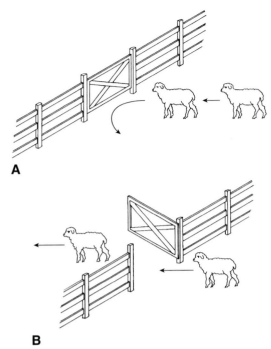

A

B

■ **FIGURE 7-13**   **A,** Two sheep arrive at a closed gate and are not received into the pen. **B,** Two sheep arrive later at the gate, when it is open, and are received into the pen. In a Doppler detector the gate accepts and rejects echoes in a similar manner.

TABLE 7-2   Spatial Gate Length for Various Temporal Gate Lengths

Length (mm)	Time (μs)
1	1.3
2	2.6
3	3.9
4	5.2
5	6.5
10	13.0
15	19.5
20	26.0

TABLE 7-3   The Amount Added to Effective Gate Length by Pulse Length for Various Cycles per Pulse and Frequencies

Amount Added (mm)	Cycles	f (MHz)
1.9	5	2
3.8	10	2
7.7	20	2
0.8	5	5
1.5	10	5
3.1	20	5
0.4	5	10
0.8	10	10
1.5	20	10

A prism does this for light. When white light passes through a prism, the light is separated into a sequence of the various colors making up the white appearance. White light is a combination of the full range of frequencies (colors) visible to the human eye. Frequency is interpreted as color by the brain, with red representing the lowest frequency and violet representing the highest. The prism breaks up these frequency components and spreads them out so that the various colors are seen in what is called a color spectrum. This spectrum of colors is also a spectrum of light frequencies. A similar process is performed electronically for the returning echoes in a Doppler system.

The human auditory system analyzes sound. The ear and brain break down the complex sounds we receive into the component frequencies contained in the sounds. Thus we can listen to a Doppler signal and recognize normal and abnormal flow sounds. Visual presentation of these sounds provides additional capability for recognition of flow characteristics and diagnosis of disease.

Various kinds of flow occur in blood vessels. Changes in vessel size, turns, and abnormalities, such as the presence of plaque or stenoses, can alter the flow character. We have seen that flow can be characterized as plug, laminar, parabolic, disturbed, and turbulent. Portions of the flowing blood within a vessel are moving at different speeds (even for normal flow) and sometimes in different directions. Thus as the ultrasound beam intersects this flow and produces echoes, many different Doppler shifts are received from the vessel by the system, even from a small sample volume. This is called the Doppler frequency spectrum. The extent of the range of generated Doppler shift frequencies depends on the character of the flow. For near-plug flow, a narrow range of Doppler shift frequencies is received. In disturbed and turbulent flow, broader and much broader ranges of Doppler shift frequencies, respectively, can be received.

Different flow conditions produce various spectral presentations.

Fast Fourier Transform

The **fast Fourier transform** (FFT) is the mathematical technique[44-46] the instrument uses to derive the **Doppler spectrum** from the returning echoes of various frequencies (Figure 7-16). Fast Fourier transform displays can show **spectral broadening,** which is widening of the Doppler shift spectrum (i.e., an increase in the

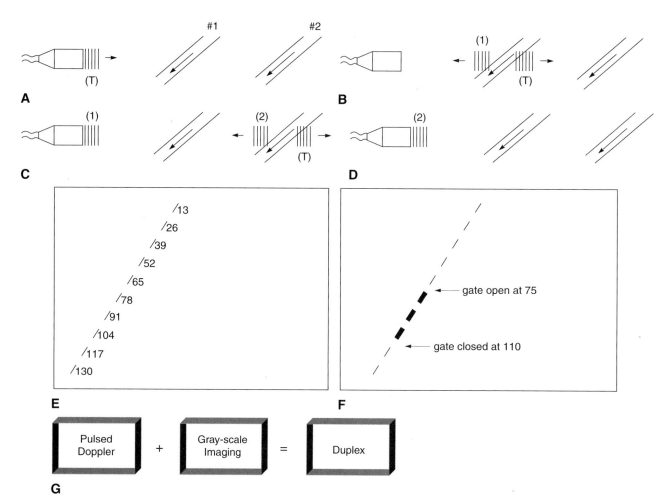

■ **FIGURE 7-14** **A,** A pulse *(T)* leaves the transducer. **B,** An echo *(1)* is generated in vessel number 1. **C,** Echo 1 arrives at the transducer. At the same time, another echo *(2)* is generated at vessel number 2. **D,** Echo 2 arrives at the transducer after echo 1. These echoes will be processed by the instrument if the gate is open when they arrive. **E,** Echoes from 1-, 2-, 3-, 4-, 5-, 6-, 7-, 8-, 9-, and 10-cm depths arrive at the times (microseconds) indicated. **F,** If the gate is open from 75 to 110 μs after pulse emission, only the echoes in **E,** arriving at 78, 91, and 104 μs, will be accepted. The others will be rejected. **G,** A duplex instrument is a sonographic instrument with pulsed wave Doppler capability incorporated.

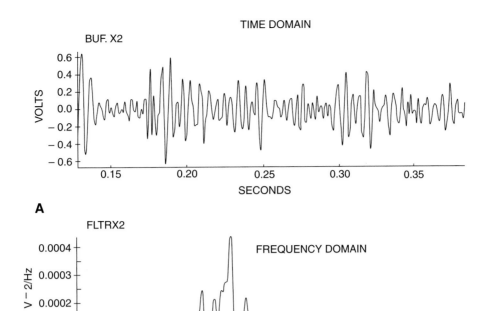

■ **FIGURE 7-15** **A,** Demodulated Doppler shift signal for microspheres flowing at nearly uniform speed. When applied to a loudspeaker, a mix of many frequencies is heard. Approximately 10 cycles occur over the time period of 0.20 to 0.25 second. Thus the fundamental period of this signal is about 50 ms, yielding a fundamental frequency of 200 Hz. **B,** After the Fourier transform is applied, a frequency spectrum is obtained. The center frequency is approximately 200 Hz. This is what was predicted in **A.** (From Burns PN: *J Clin Ultrasound* 15:567-590, 1987. Reprinted by permission of John Wiley & Sons, Inc.)

range of Doppler shift frequencies present) resulting from a broader range of flow speeds and directions encountered by the sound beam with disturbed or turbulent flow.

ADVANCED CONCEPTS

The **Fourier transform** is defined as follows:

$$F(f) = \int_{\infty}^{\infty} g(t)\,(\cos 2\pi f t - i \sin 2\pi f t)\,dt$$

where *f* is frequency, *g(t)* is the function of time to be analyzed, and *i* is the square root of −1.

The fast Fourier transform is a computation that reduces the number of mathematical operations in the evaluation of the discrete Fourier transform:

$$F(\upsilon) = (1/n) \sum_{\tau=0}^{n-1} g(t)\,(\cos 2\pi \upsilon \tau - i \sin 2\pi \upsilon \tau)$$

where υ is related to frequency and τ is related to the time interval between sample points.

The FFT process includes sampling the complicated, multifrequency Doppler signal at a rate of approximately 25,600 times per second (or higher), which is a 25.6-kHz sampling rate. A 10-ms period of time (yielding 256 samples) is sufficient to provide a useful spectrum. Thus 100 such spectra can be produced per second. Each spectrum can include the amplitudes of 128 frequencies, the lowest of which is equal to the number of FFTs per second (100 Hz in this case) and the highest of which is equal to one half the sampling rate (or 12.8 kHz in this case). This rapid sequence of FFT-generated spectra (100 per second) can be displayed visually in real time. Some current processors can calculate up to 1000 FFTs per second.

The fast Fourier transform is used to generate Doppler-shift spectral displays.

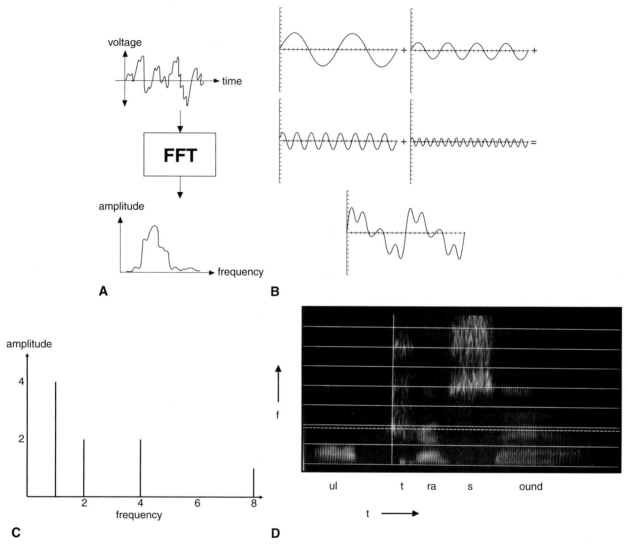

■ **FIGURE 7-16** Fast Fourier transform *(FFT)*. **A,** The Doppler shift signal (containing many frequencies) is transformed by the FFT into a spectrum. (See Figure 7-15 for an example of the Doppler signal before **[A]** and after **[B]** FFT processing.) **B,** Four voltages of different frequencies are combined to give the complicated result. **C,** The FFT analysis of this combined voltage yields this spectrum of four frequency components (a frequency of 1 with amplitude 4, two frequencies [2 and 4] with amplitude 2, and one frequency of 8 with amplitude 1). **D,** Spectral analysis of the word *ultrasound.* Time progresses to the right as the word is uttered, and about 100 FFTs are performed. The vertical axis represents frequency. The low frequencies of the *ul, ra,* and *ound* syllables are seen, along with the high frequencies of the *t* and *s* sounds.

SPECTRAL DISPLAYS

The received Doppler signal is a combination of many Doppler shift frequencies, yielding a complicated waveform (Figures 7-15, *A*, and 7-16, *B*). Using the FFT, these frequencies are separated into a spectrum that is presented on a two-dimensional display as Doppler shift frequency on the horizontal axis and power or amplitude of each frequency component on the vertical axis (Figures 7-15, *B*, and 7-16, *A* and *C*). Depending on the speed of the processor, about 100 to 1000 spectra can be generated per second. For venous flow, such a spectral display usually would be rather constant. However, for the pulsatile flow in arterial circulation, such a presentation is changing continually, shifting to the right in systole as the blood accelerates and Doppler shifts increase, shifting to the left in diastole, and changing in amplitude distribution over the cardiac cycle. The interpretation of this changing presentation is difficult, and indeed the character of the changes over the cardiac cycle could be important. Therefore presentation of this changing spectrum as a function of time is valuable and useful. Such a trace is shown in Figures 7-17 and 7-18. In these presentations the vertical axis represents Doppler shift frequency and the horizontal represents time (Figure 7-19). The amplitude or power of each Doppler shift frequency component at any instant now is presented as brightness (gray scale; Figure 7-8, *A*) or color (see Figure 1-14, *B* [Color Plate 2]). Doppler signal power is proportional to blood cell concentration (number of cells per unit volume). A bright spot on a spectral display means that a strong Doppler shift frequency component at that instant of time was received (Figure 7-8). A dark spot means that a Doppler-shift frequency component at that point in time was

weak or nonexistent. Intermediate values of gray or brightness indicate intermediate amplitudes or powers of frequency components at the given times. A strong signal at a particular frequency and time means that there are many scattering blood cells moving at speeds and directions corresponding to that Doppler shift. A weak frequency means that few cells are traveling at speeds and directions corresponding to that Doppler shift at that point in time.

> *The spectral display is a presentation of Doppler spectra versus time.*

Spectral Broadening

Spectral trace presentations provide information about flow that can be used to discern conditions at the site of measurement and distal to it.[47,48] Peak flow speeds and spectral broadening are indicative of the degree of stenosis. Spectral broadening means a vertical thickening of the spectral trace (Figure 7-20). If all the cells were moving at the same speed, the spectral trace would be a thin line (Figure 7-17, *A*). As stated previously, though, this is not the case in practice. However, narrow spectra can be observed, particularly in large vessels (Figure 7-21, *A*). The apparent narrowing of the spectrum as the blood accelerates in systole can be misinterpreted. A spectrum of consistent width appears to be thinner in a steep-rise portion of a curve (Figure 7-22). As flow is disturbed or becomes turbulent, greater variation in velocities of various portions of the flowing blood

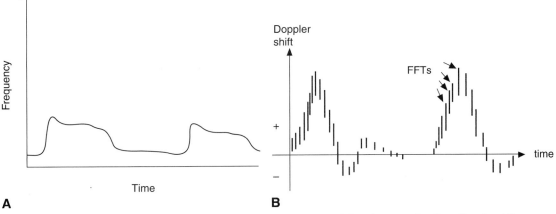

■ **FIGURE 7-17** **A,** A display of Doppler shift as a function of time for pure plug flow. Doppler-shift frequency is represented on the vertical axis. The amplitude of the Doppler-shift frequency at each instant of time is represented by gray level or color. In this example, there is only a single shift frequency at each instant of time (i.e., no spectrum). **B,** A spectral display for nonplug flow is composed of several (about 100 per second) fast Fourier transform *(FFT)* spectra arranged vertically next to each other across the time (horizontal) axis.

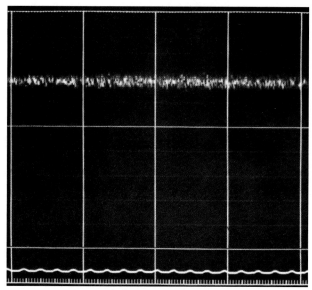

■ **FIGURE 7-18**   A spectral display of the signal shown in Figure 7-15. The flow is constant, yielding Doppler shift frequencies of approximately 200 Hz. (The horizontal markers represent 100 Hz.) (From Burns PN: *J Clin Ultrasound* 15:567-590, 1987. Reprinted by permission of John Wiley & Sons, Inc.)

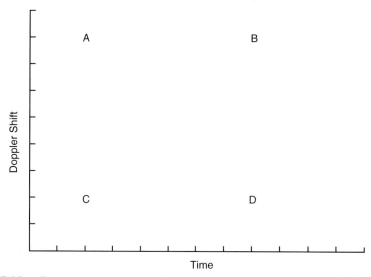

■ **FIGURE 7-19**   Four points on a spectral display. Points A and C occur at an earlier time, compared with points B and D, which occur later. Points A and B represent higher Doppler-shift frequencies than points C and D.

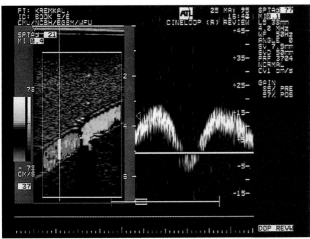

A

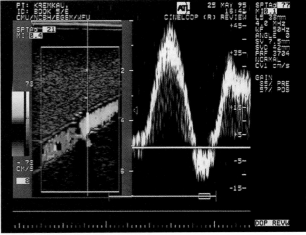

B

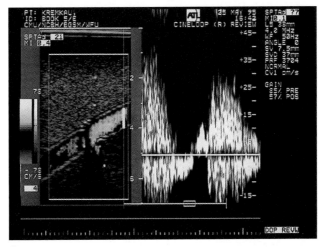

C

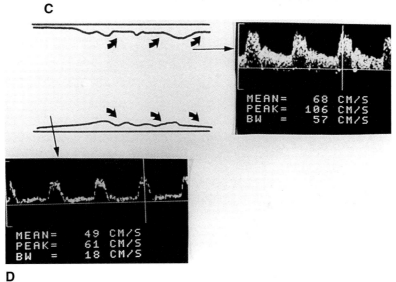

D

■ **FIGURE 7-20**   Flow *(lower left to upper right)* in a tube with a stenosis in tissue-equivalent material. **A,** Proximal to the stenosis, a narrow spectrum is observed (indicating approximately plug [i.e., blunted] flow). **B,** At the stenosis a reasonably narrow spectrum still is seen, but the Doppler shifts have tripled because of the high flow speed through the stenosis. **C,** Distal to the stenosis a broad spectrum is observed, along with negative Doppler shifts, both of which are caused by turbulent flow. Compare these observations with the flow conditions in and beyond a narrow gorge (see Figure 5-7, *D*). **D,** Spectral broadening produced by atheroma.

Continued.

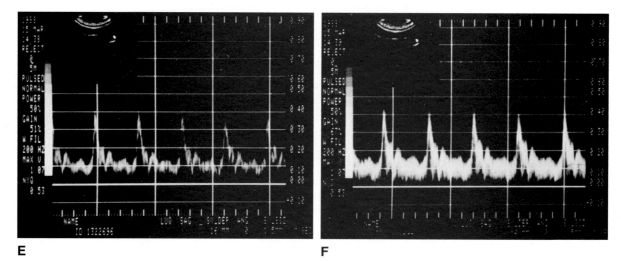

E   F

■ **FIGURE 7-20, cont'd   E,** Display produced at a correct Doppler gain setting. **F,** Apparent spectral broadening caused by excessive gain. (**D** to **F** from Taylor KJW, Holland S: *Radiology* 174:297-307, 1990.)

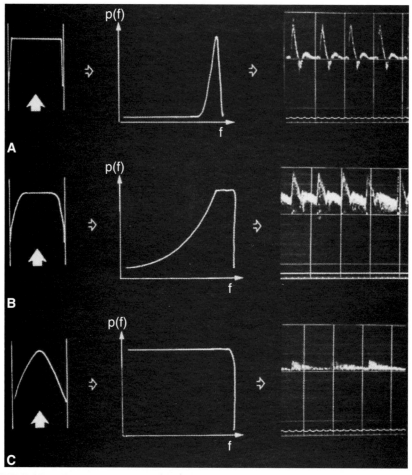

■ **FIGURE 7-21**   Flow speed profiles *(left),* Doppler spectra (power versus frequency; *center),* and spectral displays *(right)* are shown for nearly plug flow in the aorta **(A),** blunted parabolic flow in the celiac trunk **(B),** and parabolic flow in the ovarian artery **(C).** (From Burns PN: *J Clin Ultrasound* 15:567-590, 1987. Reprinted by permission of John Wiley & Sons, Inc.)

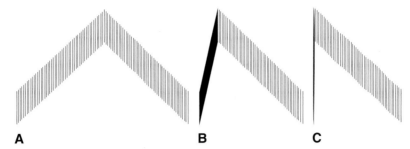

■ **FIGURE 7-22** Apparent spectral narrowing in rapidly accelerating flow. **A,** Slowly accelerating and decelerating flow shows that the spectral widths (bandwidths) are all equal. **B** and **C,** As the acceleration phase becomes steeper, the bandwidths appear to narrow. However, the vertical lines representing bandwidth in all cases are the same.

produce a greater range of Doppler-shift frequencies. This results in a broadened spectrum presented on the spectral display (Figure 7-20, *A* to *D*). Thus spectral broadening is indicative of disturbed or turbulent flow and can be related to a pathologic condition. However, spectral broadening also can be produced artificially by excessive Doppler gain (Figure 7-20, *E* and *F*), and some broadening is produced by beam spreading (Figure 7-6, *F*), particularly with wide-aperture arrays.[49,50]

ADVANCED CONCEPTS

Spectral broadening also occurs because of the finite size of the sample volume. This sometimes is called geometric spectral broadening. The shorter the gate-open time, the smaller the sample volume and shorter the time the propagating pulse has to interact with the blood flow. This shortens the returning Doppler-shifted echo, broadening its bandwidth. The effective bandwidth of the Doppler-shifted echo is a combination of the various contributions to spectral broadening: the bandwidth of the initial transmitted pulse, the range of flow speeds and angles encountered by the pulse, excessive Doppler gain, beam spreading, and geometric broadening. Effective bandwidth is the broadening resulting from flow character that is of physiologic interest in Doppler analysis.

Disturbed or turbulent flow conditions produce spectral broadening.

Another term related to spectral broadening is **window**. This term refers to the dark, anechoic area in the lower portion of the spectral trace in systole for normal flow (Figure 7-20). As flow is disturbed or becomes turbulent, spectral broadening occurs and the window is diminished or eliminated. Therefore spectral broadening and window reduction are equivalent terms.

Narrow spectra often are seen in large vessels, broad spectra in small vessels, and intermediate spectra in medium-sized vessels, as shown in Figure 7-21. This observation is partly attributable to the relationship between the minimum sample volume length and the vessel diameter. When PW Doppler is used to monitor flow at various sites inside a vessel, a narrow spectrum is expected near the center of the vessel, where the cells are moving the fastest, and a broader spectrum is expected near the walls, where viscous drag is slowing the flow (Figures 7-12, *C* to *F*, and 7-23). For example, in the approximate central two thirds of the common carotid artery, nearly plug flow is observed. Complicated flow (e.g., in the vicinity of the carotid bulb and flow divider) is not as easily predicted but is different at various sites (Figure 7-24). Turbulent flow may occur during short portions of the cardiac cycle as high enough flow speeds are achieved. Spectral broadening does not necessarily indicate turbulence. Figure 7-25 shows a broad spectrum that is probably not attributable to disturbed or turbulent flow but simply may be the result of complicated geometry; that is, a tortuous vessel causing a variety of Doppler angles and therefore a broad spectrum of Doppler-shift frequencies. A broad spectrum can be found, even in large vessels, if the sample volume length covers a large portion of the vessel diameter (Figures 7-12, *F,* and 7-26).

Downstream Conditions

Doppler flow measurements can yield information regarding downstream (distal) conditions. Flow reversal in early diastole and lack of flow in late diastole (see Figures 5-8 and 7-21, *A*) indicate high resistance to downstream flow (e.g., because of vasoconstriction of arterioles).[14] If flow resistance is reduced because of vasodilation, impressive differences in the spectral display are observed (Figure 7-27). Figure 7-28 gives a

Text continued on p. 244.

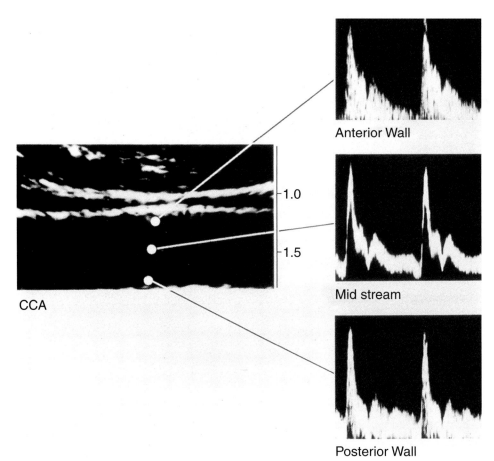

CCA

1.0

1.5

Anterior Wall

Mid stream

Posterior Wall

■ **FIGURE 7-23** Spectral traces showing increased spectral bandwidth near the vessel walls in the common carotid artery *(CCA)*. As expected, a narrower bandwidth is found at midstream. (From Taylor DC, Strandness DE: *J Clin Ultrasound* 15:635-644, 1987. Reprinted by permission of John Wiley & Sons, Inc.)

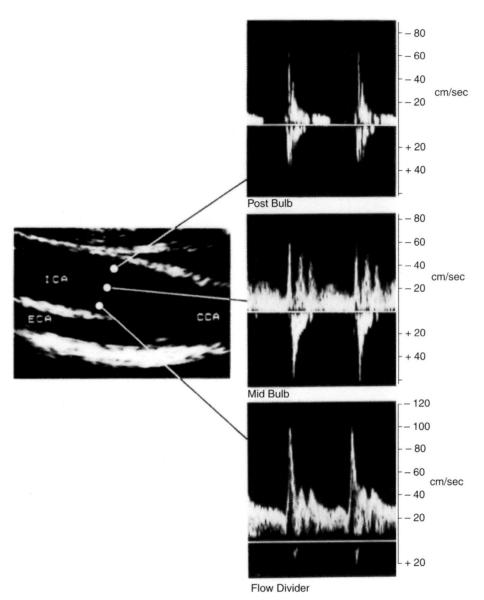

■ **FIGURE 7-24** Spectral waveforms show laminar flow with mild spectral broadening adjacent to the carotid bifurcation and areas of increasing turbulence and boundary layer separation along the outer aspect of the carotid bulb. *ICA,* Internal carotid artery; *ECA,* external carotid artery; *CCA,* common carotid artery. (From Taylor DC, Strandness DE: *J Clin Ultrasound* 15:635-644, 1987. Reprinted by permission of John Wiley & Sons, Inc.)

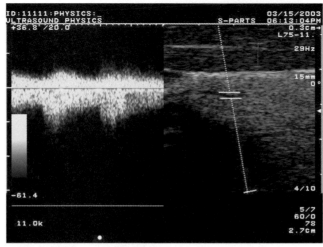

■ **FIGURE 7-25** Spectral trace from a small artery showing spectral broadening because of its tortuous nature.

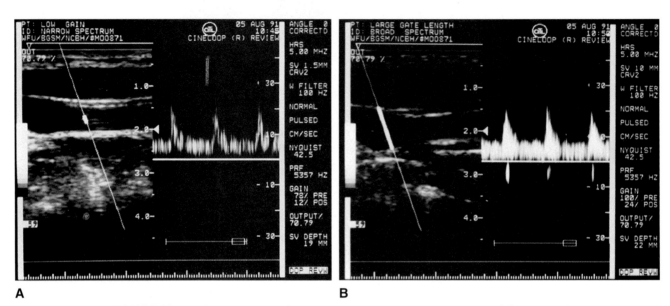

A

B

■ **FIGURE 7-26** **A,** Narrow spectral display of a common carotid artery using a small (1.5-mm) sample volume. **B,** Spectral broadening results from the inclusion of all the flow across the vessel using a large (10-mm) sample volume. (From Kremkau FW: *Semin Roentgenol* 27:6-16, 1992.)

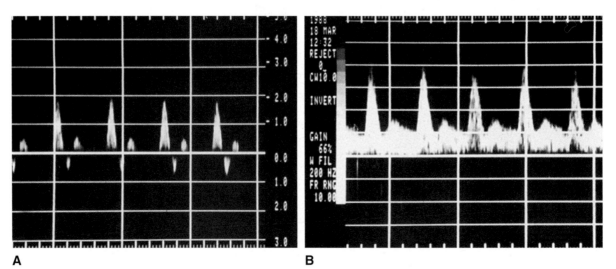

A

B

■ **FIGURE 7-27** **A,** High distal resistance flow in the popliteal artery with the patient's leg at rest. **B,** Low distal resistance flow is observed after exercise. (From Taylor KJW, Holland S: *Radiology* 174:297-307, 1990.)

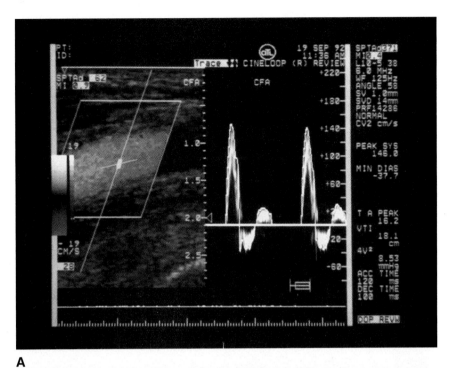

A

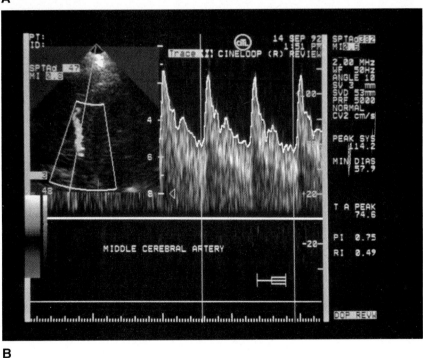

B

■ **FIGURE 7-28** **A,** High distal resistance flow is seen in the common femoral artery of the resting lower limb. **B,** Low distal resistance flow is seen in the middle cerebral artery. Although these spectral displays are very different, they are both normal for the locations and conditions given.

comparison between low-resistance and high-resistance flow spectra.

High- and low-impedance conditions downstream give rise to different spectral displays.

Normal vessels can be occluded in diastole when pressure drops below the critical value for flow.[14] When this happens, no diastolic Doppler shift is detected. Various quantitative indexes have been developed to describe differences in spectral traces indicative of downstream conditions (Figure 7-29 and Table 7-4).

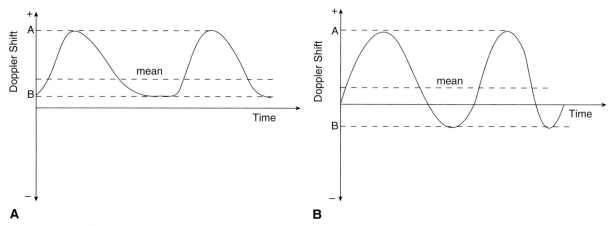

A **B**

■ **FIGURE 7-29** Spectral display of peak Doppler shift as a function of time. Point A represents the maximum value at systole, whereas point B represents the minimum value at end-diastole. **A,** Unidirectional flow. **B,** Reverse flow in diastole.

TABLE 7-4	Spectral Display Indexes	
Name	**Abbreviation**	**Expression***
Pulsatility index	PI	$\dfrac{A - B}{mean}$
Resistance index	RI	$\dfrac{A - B}{A}$
RSystolic-to-diastolic ratio	SDR	$\dfrac{A}{B}$
RB/A ratio	BAR	$\dfrac{B}{A}$

*A represents the maximum value at systole, and B represents the minimum value at end-diastole (see Figure 7-29).

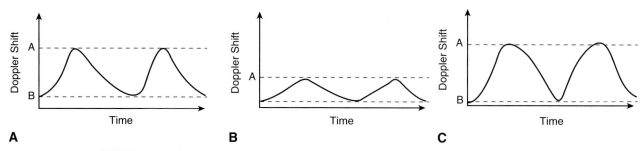

A **B** **C**

■ **FIGURE 7-30** **A,** Spectral trace for low-resistance, low-angle flow. **B,** Spectral trace for low-resistance, high-angle flow. All portions of the Doppler shift are proportionally reduced. **C,** Spectral trace for high-resistance, high-angle flow. The diastolic portions of the flow are reduced, yielding a larger pulsatility index, indicating increased distal flow resistance.

Figure 7-30 shows spectral trace shapes for high- and low-resistance flow and for high- and low-angle measurements. Changing the angle does not change the relationship between peak systolic and end-diastolic flows, but changing the distal resistance does (Figures 7-27 and 7-30). The **pulsatility index** approach works because flow impedance is not constant over the cardiac cycle with distensible vessels and pulsatile pressures. That is, impedance, rather than being constant, is greater at lower pressures and smaller at higher pressures. Recall that impedance includes flow resistance, inertia of blood, and compliance of vessel walls. One must exercise care in using the wall filter because it can affect the pulsatility index (Figures 7-31 and 7-10, *I*).

Pulsatility indexes are quantitative indicators of distal impedance.

Interpretation of spectral trace information easily can be oversimplified. In Figure 7-32, *A* may appear to represent the fastest blood flow. It is true that *A* represents the largest Doppler shift on this spectral display. However, undisturbed laminar flow is necessary for the largest spectral Doppler shift to correspond to the largest flow speed. In Figure 7-33, for example, the arrows indicate that the highest Doppler shifts correspond to the fastest flow and the lowest to the slowest. This simplified approach is true only for undisturbed and nonturbulent flow in which all portions of fluid are moving parallel to one another with a common Doppler angle. If flow is disturbed or turbulent (Figure 7-20), if the vessel is tortuous (Figure 7-25), or if flow is helical, as claimed for the carotid artery,[18,19] this assumption is not valid. In such cases the simple interpretation is incorrect. The peak Doppler shifts do not necessarily represent the fastest flow but possibly slower flow that is moving directly toward or away from the transducer (small Doppler angle, high Doppler shift). Likewise, the lowest Doppler shifts do not necessarily represent the slowest flow but possibly faster flow that is moving nearly perpendicular to the beam (large Doppler angle, low Doppler shift). Indeed, strictly speaking, spectral traces that have their vertical axes calibrated in speed units (meters per second or centimeters per second) are correctly calibrated presentations only if the Doppler angle incorporation is proper *and* if straight, parallel, laminar, undisturbed flow is being measured.

Flow velocity is a vector involving two parameters: speed and direction. A Doppler instrument detects a Doppler shift that is proportional to speed of flow

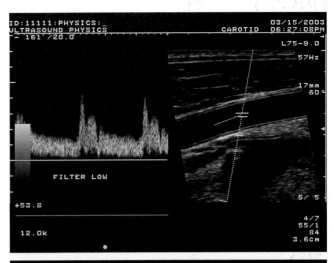

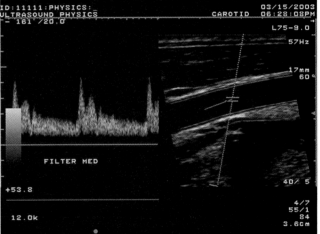

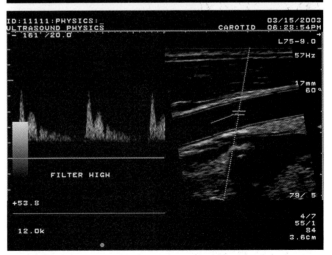

■ **FIGURE 7-31** Increasing the wall filter simulates the appearance of a high-resistance flow. If not correctly understood, this presentation can lead to misdiagnosis.

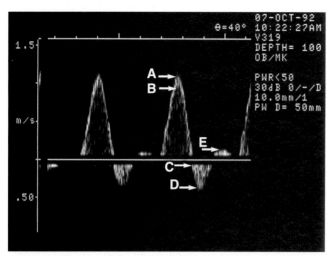

■ **FIGURE 7-32** Pulsatile Doppler spectrum from a Doppler flow phantom. Point A represents maximum Doppler shift and Point B minimum Doppler shift at peak systole. Points C and D represent minimum and maximum shifts, respectively, in early diastole. Point E represents maximum shift in late diastole. (From Kremkau FW: *J Vasc Technol* 17:321-322, 1993.)

along the sound beam direction (the magnitude of the component of the velocity vector parallel to the beam (see Figure 5-20, *A*). Thus if flow is not straight (parallel and straight streamlines), large Doppler shifts do not necessarily correspond to the fastest flow and small ones do not necessarily correspond to the slowest flow (Figure 7-34).

Table 7-5 compares the three types of Doppler displays: color Doppler shift, color Doppler power, and spectral. Figure 7-35 illustrates the Doppler controls discussed in this chapter.

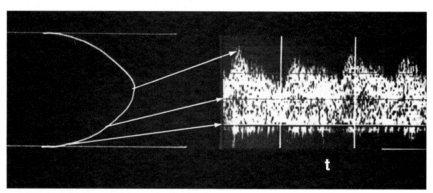

■ **FIGURE 7-33** A broad spectrum of parabolic flow is shown for a small vessel. The arrows suggest that the highest Doppler shifts correspond to the fastest flow and the lowest to the slowest. This simplified approach is true only for undisturbed and nonturbulent flow, in which all portions of fluid are flowing parallel to each other (common Doppler angle).(From Taylor KJW, Holland S: *Radiology* 174:297-307, 1990.)

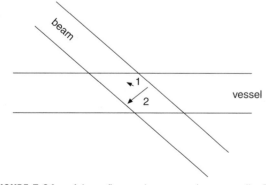

■ **FIGURE 7-34** A large flow vector can produce a smaller Doppler shift than a small flow vector if the vectors are not parallel. This small flow vector *(1)* has a larger component along the beam than the large vector *(2)*, which is nearly perpendicular to the beam. (From Kremkau FW: *J Vasc Technol* 17:321-322, 1993.)

TABLE 7-5   Comparison of Doppler-Shift, Doppler-Power, and Spectral Displays

	Color Doppler-Shift Display	Color Doppler-Power Display	Spectral Display
Quantitative	No	No	Yes
Global	Yes	Yes	No
Perfusion	No	Yes	No

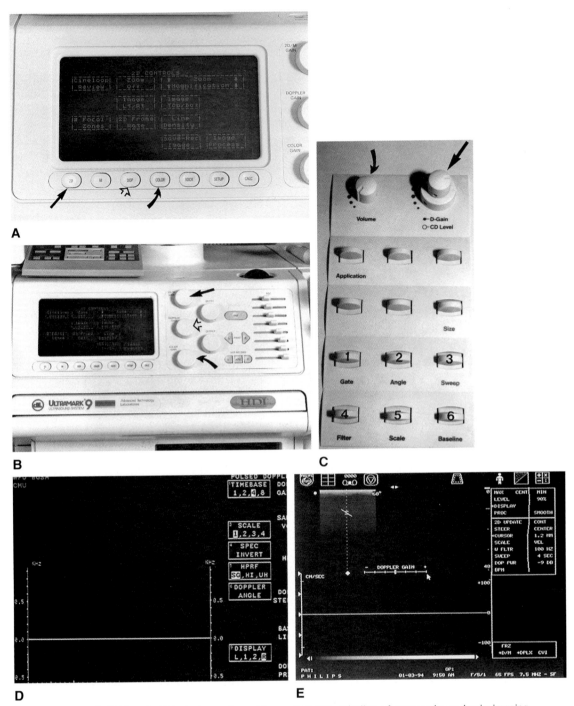

■ **FIGURE 7-35** **A,** This instrument provides push-button selection of gray-scale anatomic imaging *(straight arrow)*, spectral Doppler *(open arrow)*, color Doppler imaging *(curved arrow)*, or combinations of these operating modes. **B,** Gray-scale gain *(straight arrow)*, spectral Doppler gain *(open arrow)*, and color Doppler gain controls *(curved arrow)* are shown. **C,** Doppler controls include gain *(straight arrow)*, loudspeaker volume *(curved arrow)*, gate length *(1)*, Doppler angle adjustment *(2)*, spectral display time (horizontal) axis sweep speed *(3)*, wall filter setting *(4)*, spectral display (vertical) axis scale setting (Nyquist limit and pulse repetition frequency control) *(5)*, and baseline shift control *(6)*. **D** and **E,** Software panel controls for Doppler functions.

REVIEW

The key points presented in this chapter are the following:

- Doppler instruments make use of the Doppler shift to yield information regarding motion and flow.
- Continuous wave Doppler systems provide motion and flow information without depth selection capability.
- Pulsed wave Doppler systems provide the ability to select the depth from which Doppler information is received.
- Spectral analysis provides visual information on the distribution of Doppler-shift frequencies resulting from the distribution of the scatterer speeds and directions encountered.
- In addition to audible output, Doppler systems provide visual presentation of flow spectra.
- Duplex systems including gray-scale sonography and CW and PW Doppler are available commercially. Color Doppler capability also can be included.
- The Doppler spectrum is generated by the range of scatterer velocities encountered by the ultrasound beam.
- The spectrum is derived electronically using the FFT and is presented on the display as Doppler shift versus time, with brightness indicating power.
- Flow conditions at the site of measurement are indicated by the width of the spectrum, with spectral broadening and loss of window indicative of disturbed and turbulent flow.
- Flow conditions downstream, especially distal flow impedance, are indicated by the relationship between peak systolic and end-diastolic flow speeds.
- Various indexes for quantitatively presenting flow information have been developed.

EXERCISES

1. All Doppler instruments distinguish between positive and negative Doppler shifts. True or false?
2. Instruments that distinguish between positive and negative Doppler shifts yield motion _____ information and are called _____.
3. Continuous wave Doppler instruments use transducers similar to those used in imaging. True or false?
4. The components of a continuous wave Doppler system include _____, _____, _____, _____, _____, _____, and _____.
5. Quantitative information about the frequencies contained in returning Doppler-shifted echoes can be displayed on an _____ versus _____ plot that is continuously changing with time.
6. To display the pattern of time change of a Doppler spectrum, a display of Doppler shift _____ versus _____ can be used.
7. In Exercise 6, the amplitude of each frequency component is represented by _____ level or _____.
8. The received frequency spectrum (rather than a single frequency) exists because of the distribution of flow _____ and _____ encountered by the beam.
9. Because velocity is a measure of speed and direction, variations in either of these in the flow region monitored by the Doppler instrument contribute to the received frequency spectrum. True or false?
10. The components of a pulsed wave Doppler instrument are the same as those for a continuous wave instrument except for the _____ and _____.
11. In a duplex instrument the gated detector is part of the _____ _____.
12. The purpose of the gate is to allow selection of Doppler-shifted echoes from specific _____ according to _____.
13. Pulsed wave Doppler instruments require a two-element transducer assembly. True or false?
14. An increased gate-open time increases the length of the sample volume. True or false?
15. A later gate corresponds to a deeper gate location. True or false?
16. Pulsed wave Doppler systems are sampling systems. The sampling rate is the same as the _____.
17. Pulsed wave Doppler instruments use the _____ _____ _____ technique to present Doppler-shift spectra as a function of time.
18. The abbreviation for the technique referred to in Exercise 17 is _____.
19. In Figure 7-36, *A*, is the instrument a pulsed wave or a continuous wave device?
20. In Figure 7-36, *B*, is the instrument a pulsed wave or a continuous wave device?
21. If a sheep leaves its pen and runs to another pen 25 m distant at a speed of 50 cm/s, when must the gate to the second pen open to allow the sheep to pass through when it arrives?
22. If a sheep leaves its pen and travels to a brook and then turns around and returns to the pen, when must the gate to its pen open to allow the sheep to pass through when it returns (assuming the distance to the brook is 25 m, and the sheep travels at 50 cm/s)?
23. Transducers designed specifically for Doppler use are generally not _____. This is because they emit _____ pulses than those used in

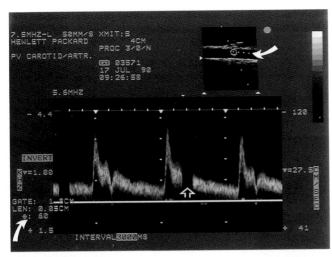

A

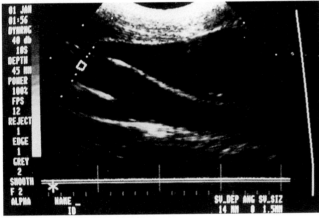

B

■ **FIGURE 7-36** **A,** Display to accompany Exercise 19. **B,** Display to accompany Exercise 20.

imaging. Undamped transducers are more _____ than damped ones.

24. For a 5-MHz instrument and 60-degree Doppler angle, a 100-Hz filter eliminates flow speeds less than
   a. 1 cm/s.
   b. 2 cm/s.
   c. 3 cm/s.
   d. 4 cm/s.
   e. 5 cm/s.

25. For a 2.5-MHz instrument and 0-degree Doppler angle, a 100-Hz filter eliminates flow speeds less than
   a. 1 cm/s.
   b. 2 cm/s.
   c. 3 cm/s.
   d. 4 cm/s.
   e. 5 cm/s.

26. The functions of a Doppler detector include which of the following?
   a. Amplification
   b. Phase quadrature detection
   c. Doppler-shift detection
   d. Sign determination
   e. All of the above

27. An earlier gate time means a _____ sample volume depth.
   a. Later
   b. Shallower
   c. Deeper
   d. Stronger
   e. None of the above

28. Name the two types of instruments used for Doppler spectral display.

29. Name the Doppler instrument the sample volume of which is the region of transmitting and receiving transducer beam overlap.

30. Name the instrument the sample volume of which is determined by the detector gate.

31. Name the instrument that combines pulsed wave Doppler with imaging.

32. Name the instrument that offers depth selectivity.

33. The _____ detects the difference between the frequencies of the emitted and received ultrasound.

34. The Doppler shift is typically _____ of the source frequency.
   a. One thousandth
   b. One hundredth
   c. One tenth
   d. 10 times
   e. 100 times

35. To convert a spectral display correctly from Doppler shift to flow speed, the _____ must be incorporated properly.

36. The Doppler spectrum is presented visually on a _____-_____ tube.

37. The high-pass filter in the signal processor is called a _____ filter or _____-_____ filter.

38. Pulsed wave Doppler instruments produce pulses that are about _____ to _____ cycles long. The length of the sample volume in a pulsed wave Doppler instrument is determined by the _____ length and the emitted _____ length.

39. The zero Doppler-shift point on a spectral display is called the _____.

40. The width of the pulsed wave Doppler sample volume is determined by the _____.

41. Which type of Doppler instrument is most likely to be used in measuring extremely high flow rates?

42. All pulsed instruments have anatomic imaging capability to allow intelligent positioning of the gate. True or false?
43. Continuous wave and pulsed wave Doppler capabilities are never provided in the same instrument. True or false?
44. Duplex instruments acquire Doppler and gray-scale information simultaneously. True or false?
45. Pulses that are two or three cycles long are used for
    a. pulsed wave Doppler.
    b. continuous wave Doppler.
    c. gray-scale imaging.
    d. color flow Doppler.
    e. all of the above.
46. Spectral analysis is the breaking up of the _____ of a complex wave or signal and spreading them out in _____.
47. Which of the following is a spectrum analyzer for light?
    a. Mirror
    b. Filter
    c. Prism
    d. Window
    e. Reflector
48. Spectral analysis is performed in a Doppler instrument _____.
    a. Electronically
    b. Mathematically
    c. Acoustically
    d. Mechanically
    e. More than one of the above
49. A Doppler spectrum is produced because many different Doppler _____ are received from the flow.
50. The statement in Exercise 49 is true because portions of the flowing fluid within the heart or a vessel are moving at different _____ and sometimes in different _____.
51. If all the blood cells in a vessel were moving in the same direction at the same speed (plug flow), a _____ Doppler shift would result at any instant in time.
52. For normal flow in a large vessel, a _____ range of Doppler-shift frequencies is often received.
    a. Narrow
    b. Broad
    c. Steady
    d. Disturbed
    e. All of the above
53. The type of flow described in Exercise 52 is called _____ flow.
    a. Turbulent
    b. Disturbed
    c. Laminar
    d. Steady
    e. Plug
54. The Doppler spectrum can be presented in two ways: as a display of _____ or _____ versus Doppler-shift frequency or as a display of Doppler-shift frequency versus _____. The latter is the common presentation in spectral Doppler instruments.
55. For pulsatile flow, in Exercise 54, which form of presentation is preferable, the first or the second?
56. Doppler-shift versus time presentations indicate the amplitude or power of each frequency component by _____ or _____.
57. Doppler signal power is proportional to
    a. volume flow rate.
    b. flow speed.
    c. Doppler angle.
    d. cell concentration.
    e. more than one of the above.
58. In Figure 7-37, point A represents
    a. early time, high Doppler shift.
    b. early time, low Doppler shift.
    c. late time, high Doppler shift.
    d. late time, low Doppler shift.
    e. none of the above.
59. In Figure 7-37, point B represents
    a. early time, high Doppler shift.
    b. early time, low Doppler shift.
    c. late time, high Doppler shift.
    d. late time, low Doppler shift.
    e. none of the above.
60. In Figure 7-37, point C represents
    a. early time, high Doppler shift.
    b. early time, low Doppler shift.
    c. late time, high Doppler shift.
    d. late time, low Doppler shift.
    e. none of the above
61. In Figure 7-37, point D represents
    a. early time, high Doppler shift.
    b. early time, low Doppler shift.
    c. late time, high Doppler shift.
    d. late time, low Doppler shift.
    e. none of the above.
62. In Figure 7-37, with a dark background, if point A is bright, it indicates that many cells are moving in such a way that a large Doppler shift occurs at an early time. True or false?
63. In Figure 7-37, with a dark background, if point D is dark, it indicates that many cells are moving in such a way as to produce low Doppler shifts at a late time. True or false?
64. In the previous six exercises, the highest Doppler shift necessarily means highest flow speed only if _____ _____ flow is assumed.

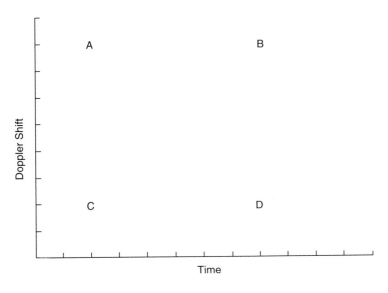

■ **FIGURE 7-37** Display to accompany Exercises 58 to 63, 65, and 66.

65. For disturbed or turbulent flow, in Figure 7-37, point A could represent
    a. high speed and large Doppler angle.
    b. high speed and small Doppler angle.
    c. low speed and small Doppler angle.
    d. low speed and large Doppler angle.
    e. more than one of the above.
66. For disturbed or turbulent flow, in Figure 7-37, point C could represent
    a. high speed and large Doppler angle.
    b. high speed and small Doppler angle.
    c. low speed and small Doppler angle.
    d. low speed and large Doppler angle.
    e. more than one of the above.
67. Doppler ultrasound provides information about flow conditions only at the site of measurement. True or false?
68. Stenosis affects
    a. peak systolic flow speed.
    b. end-diastolic flow speed.
    c. spectral broadening.
    d. window.
    e. all of the above.
69. Spectral broadening is a _____ of the spectral trace.
    a. Vertical thickening
    b. Horizontal thickening
    c. Brightening
    d. Darkening
    e. Horizontal shift
70. If all cells in a vessel were moving at the same constant speed, the spectral trace would be a _____ line.
    a. Thin horizontal
    b. Thin vertical
    c. Thick horizontal

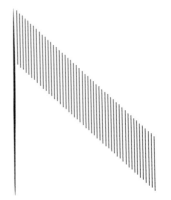

■ **FIGURE 7-38** Display to accompany Exercise 71.

    d. Thick vertical
    e. None of the above
71. In Figure 7-38, in which part of the flow cycle is spectral broadening (bandwidth) the least?
    a. Acceleration
    b. Deceleration
    c. Neither
72. Disturbed flow produces a narrower spectrum. True or false?
73. Turbulent flow produces a narrower spectrum. True or false?
74. As stenosis progresses, which of the following increase(s)?
    a. Lumen diameter
    b. Systolic Doppler shift
    c. Diastolic Doppler shift
    d. Spectral broadening
    e. More than one of the above
75. Higher flow speed always produces a higher Doppler shift on a spectral display. True or false?

76. Spectral broadening _____ the window.
    a. Increases
    b. Decreases
    c. Brightens
    d. Does not affect
77. Flow reversal in diastole indicates
    a. stenosis.
    b. aneurysm.
    c. high distal resistance.
    d. low distal resistance.
    e. more than one of the above.
78. Decreased distal resistance normally causes end-diastolic flow to
    a. increase.
    b. decrease.
    c. be disturbed.
    d. become turbulent.
    e. more than one of the above.
79. Match the following:
    a. Narrow spectra _____ 1. Small vessels
    b. Broad spectra _____ 2. Large vessels
    c. Intermediate spectra   3. Medium vessels
    _____
80. Which is expected at the center of a vessel, a narrow or broad spectrum?
81. Which is expected at the center of a vessel, a higher or lower flow speed?
82. Spectral broadening always indicates turbulence. True or false?
83. Increasing distal resistance and increasing Doppler angle have the same effect on the spectral display. True or false?
84. Which normally has the smallest end-diastolic flow?
    a. Common carotid artery
    b. Internal carotid artery
    c. External carotid artery
85. Zero flow and reverse flow in late diastole are normal findings in some locations of the circulation. True or false?
86. The pulsatility index approach works because flow impedance _____ over the cardiac cycle. This is because the vessels are _____. In this case, impedance is _____ at lower pressures and _____ at higher pressures.
87. Under what condition can a relatively high Doppler shift come from a relatively slowly moving flow?
88. Under what condition can a relatively low Doppler shift come from a relatively rapidly moving flow?

89. When the spectral trace is calibrated in flow speed (centimeters per second), the highest flow speed shown always represents the fastest cells in the vessel. True or false?
90. If a flow speed less than 125 cm/s and a Doppler shift less than 4 kHz indicate normal carotid artery flow, what operating frequency is being used if the Doppler angle is 60 degrees?
    a. 1 MHz
    b. 2 MHz
    c. 3 MHz
    d. 4 MHz
    e. 5 MHz
91. In Figure 7-39, A, if the sample volume is placed as shown and the plaque (P) is not visualized, the operator probably would place the angle correction indicator (dashed line) parallel to the vessel walls. This would result in a _____ flow speed indication.
    a. Correct
    b. High
    c. Low
92. In Figure 7-39, B, if plaque (P) were visualized, but the remainder of the plaque (shaded area) were not, the operator probably would place the angle correction indicator (dashed line) as shown. This would result in a _____ flow speed indication.
    a. Correct
    b. High
    c. Low
93. In Figure 7-39, B, if the angle correction indicator (dashed line) is placed parallel to the vessel walls, rather than as shown, the Doppler shift is _____ and the indicated flow speed is _____.
    a. Increased, unchanged
    b. Increased, increased
    c. Decreased, unchanged
    d. Decreased, decreased
    e. Unchanged, increased
94. Which control was increased where the lower Doppler shifts are missing (arrows) in Figure 7-40?
    a. Gain
    b. Angle
    c. Sweep
    d. Gate
    e. Filter
    f. Scale
    g. Baseline

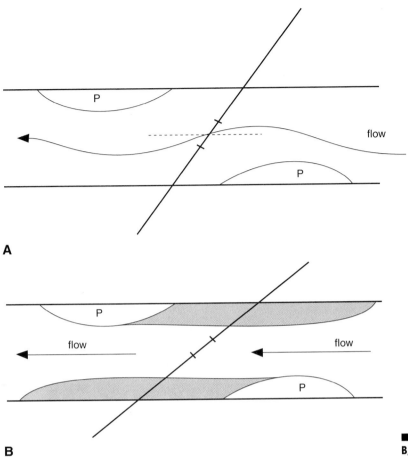

A

B

■ **FIGURE 7-39** **A,** Illustration to accompany Exercise 91. **B,** Illustration to accompany Exercises 92 and 93.

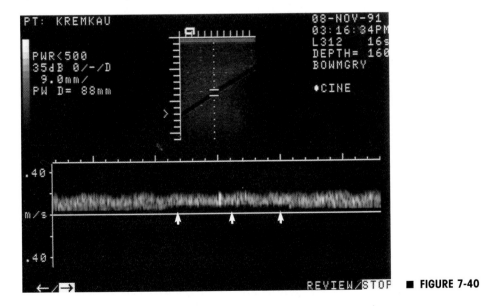

■ **FIGURE 7-40** Display to accompany Exercise 94.

95. Which control was increased between parts A and B of Figure 7-41?
    a. Gain
    b. Angle
    c. Sweep
    d. Gate
    e. Filter
    f. Scale
    g. Baseline
96. The curved arrow in Figure 7-41, B, indicates
    a. angle error.
    b. spectral broadening.
    c. high-resistance flow.
    d. low-resistance flow.
    e. stenosis.
97. The arrows in Figure 7-42 indicate
    a. aliasing.
    b. angle error.
    c. clutter.

d. turbulence.
e. stenosis.

98. To correct the problem in Exercise 97, which control should be adjusted?
    a. Gain
    b. Angle
    c. Sweep
    d. Gate
    e. Filter
    f. Scale
    g. Baseline
99. In Figure 7-43 the peak flow speed (V) is indicated as 0.51 m/s. If angle correction were not used, the indicated speed would be
    a. 0.25 m/s.
    b. 0.33 m/s.
    c. 0.51 m/s.
    d. 0.66 m/s.
    e. 1.02 m/s.

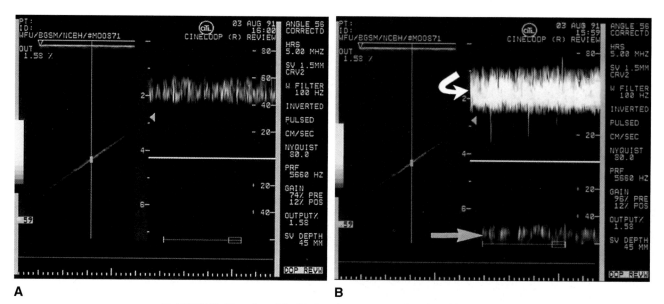

A   **B**

■ **FIGURE 7-41**   **A** and **B**, Displays to accompany Exercises 95 and 96.

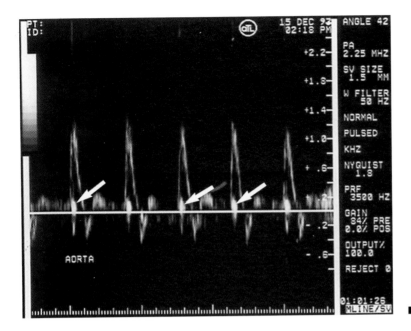

■ **FIGURE 7-42** Display to accompany Exercise 97.

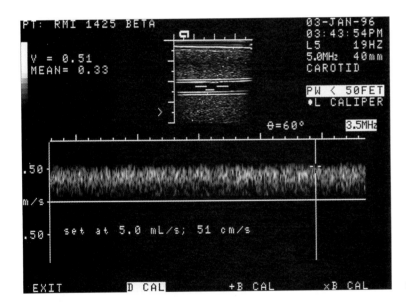

■ **FIGURE 7-43** Display to accompany Exercise 99.

100. Which part(s) of Figure 7-44 include(s) positive Doppler shifts?
101. Which part(s) of Figure 7-44 include(s) negative Doppler shifts?
102. Which part(s) of Figure 7-44 include(s) the largest Doppler shifts?
103. Which part(s) of Figure 7-44 include(s) the smallest Doppler shifts?
104. Which part(s) of Figure 7-44 include(s) the largest Doppler angle?
105. Which part(s) of Figure 7-44 include(s) the smallest Doppler angle?
106. Which part(s) of Figure 7-44 include(s) the fastest flow speed?
107. Which part(s) of Figure 7-44 include(s) the largest volume flow rate?
108. Flow in Figure 7-44 is
    a. left to right.
    b. right to left.
109. If angle correction is set at 60 degrees but should be 0 degrees, the display indicates a flow speed of 100 cm/s. The correct flow speed is _____ cm/s.
    a. 25
    b. 50
    c. 100
    d. 200
    e. 400

110. If angle correction is set at 0 degrees but should be 60 degrees, the display indicates a flow speed of 100 cm/s. The correct flow speed is _____ cm/s.
    a. 25
    b. 50
    c. 100
    d. 200
    e. 400
111. If a 5-kHz Doppler shift corresponds to 100 cm/s, then a 2.5-kHz shift corresponds to _____ cm/s.
112. In determining the answer in Exercise 111, constant _____ _____ is assumed.
113. In Exercise 111, a 2.5-kHz shift could correspond to 100 cm/s at a Doppler angle of _____ degrees if 5 kHz was for a 0-degree angle.
114. In Exercise 111, a 2.5-kHz shift could correspond to 100 cm/s at a frequency of _____ MHz if 5 kHz was for 5 MHz.
115. Which of the following is increased if Doppler angle is increased?
    a. Aliasing
    b. Doppler shift
    c. Effect of angle error
    d. b and c
    e. None of the above

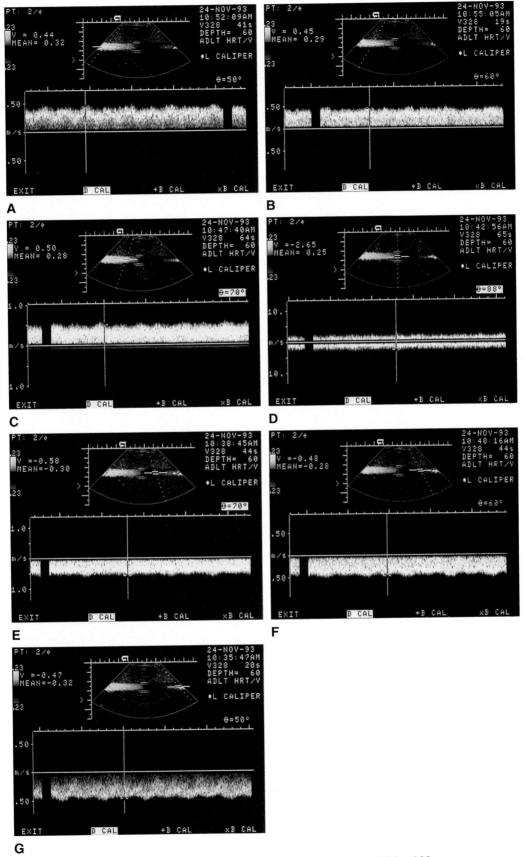

■ **FIGURE 7-44** **A** to **G,** Displays to accompany Exercises 100 to 108.

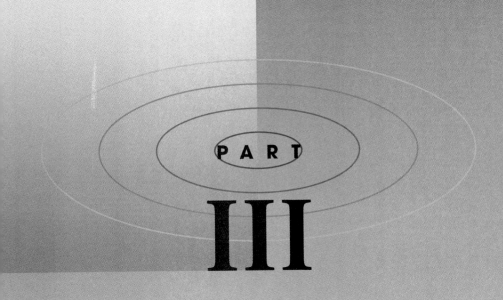

PART

III

Miscellaneous Topics

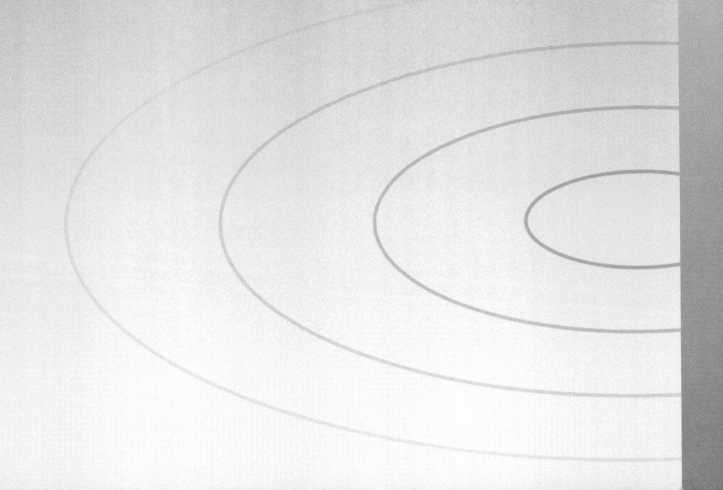

After reading this chapter, the student should be able to do the following:

- List various reasons why sonographic gray-scale images can present anatomic structures incorrectly.
- List various reasons why spectral and color Doppler displays can present motion and flow information incorrectly.
- Describe how specific artifacts can be recognized.
- Expain how various artifacts should be handled properly to avoid the pitfalls and misdiagnoses that they can cause.

KEY TERMS

The following terms are introduced in this chapter:

Aliasing
Anechoic
Baseline shift
Comet tail
Cross-talk
Enhancement

Hypoechoic
Mirror image
Multiple reflection
Nyquist limit
Range ambiguity
Resonance

Reverberation
Ring-down artifact
Section thickness
Shadowing
Speed error

In imaging, an artifact is anything that is not properly indicative of the structures or motion imaged. An artifact is caused by some problematic aspect of the imaging technique. In addition to helpful artifacts, there are several that hinder proper interpretation and diagnosis. One must avoid these artifacts or handle them properly when encountered.

Artifacts are incorrect representations of anatomy or motion.

Artifacts in sonography occur as apparent structures that are one of the following:

1. Not real
2. Missing
3. Improperly located
4. Of improper brightness, shape, or size

Some artifacts are produced by improper equipment operation or settings (e.g., incorrect gain and compensation settings). Other artifacts are inherent in the sonographic and Doppler methods and can occur even with proper equipment and technique. Artifacts that occur in sonography[51,52] are listed in Box 8-1, where they are grouped as they are considered in the following sections.

The assumptions in the design of sonographic instruments are that sound travels in straight lines, that echoes originate only from objects located on the beam axis, that the amplitude of returning echoes is related directly to the reflecting or scattering properties of distant objects, and that the distance to reflecting or scattering objects is proportional to the round-trip travel time (13 μs/cm of depth). If any of these assumptions is violated, an artifact occurs.

Several artifacts are encountered in Doppler ultrasound,[53] including incorrect presentations of Doppler flow information, either in spectral or in color Doppler form. The most common of these is **aliasing**. Others include **range ambiguity**, spectrum mirror image, location mirror image, and **speckle**.

PROPAGATION

Section Thickness

Axial and lateral resolution are artifactual because a failure to resolve means a loss of detail, and two adjacent structures may be visualized as one. The beam width perpendicular to the scan plane (the third dimension; Figure 8-1, *A*) results in **section thickness** artifacts; for example, the appearance of false debris in echo-free areas (Figure 8-1, *B*). These artifacts occur because the interrogating beam has finite thickness as it scans through the patient. Echoes are received that originate not only from the center of the beam but also from off-center. These echoes are all collapsed into a thin (zero-thickness) two-dimensional image that is composed of echoes that have come from a not-so-thin tissue volume scanned by the beam. Section thickness artifact is also called partial-volume artifact.

Beam width perpendicular to the scan plane causes section thickness artifact.

BOX 8-1	Sonographic Artifacts

PROPAGATION GROUP
Axial resolution
Comet tail
Grating lobe
Lateral resolution
Mirror image
Range ambiguity
Refraction
Reverberation
Ring-down
Section thickness
Speckle
Speed error

ATTENUATION GROUP
Enhancement
Focal enhancement
Refraction (edge) shadowing
Shadowing

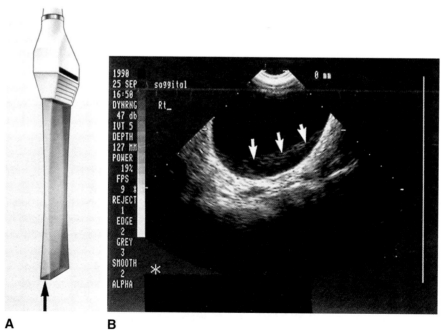

■ FIGURE 8-1   **A,** The scan "plane" through the tissue is really a three-dimensional volume. Two dimensions (axial and lateral) are in the scan plane, but there is a third dimension (called section thickness or slice thickness). The third dimension *(arrow)* is collapsed to zero thickness when the image is displayed in two-dimensional format. **B,** An ovarian cyst that should be echo-free has an echogenic region *(arrows)*. These off-axis echoes are a result of scan-plane section thickness.

Speckle

Apparent image resolution can be deceiving. The detailed echo pattern often is not related directly to the scattering properties of tissue (called tissue texture) but is a result of the interference effects of the scattered sound from the distribution of scatterers in the tissue. This phenomenon is called acoustic speckle (Figure 8-2).

Reverberation

Multiple reflection (reverberation) can occur between the transducer and a strong reflector (Figure 8-3, *A*). The multiple echoes may be sufficiently strong to be detected by the instrument and to cause confusion on the display. The process by which they are produced is shown in Figure 8-3, *B*. This results in the display of additional reflectors that are not real (Figure 8-4). The multiple reflections are placed beneath the real reflector at separation intervals equal to the separation between the transducer and the real reflector. Each subsequent reflection is weaker than prior ones, but this diminution is counteracted at least partially by the attenuation compensation (TGC) function. Reverberations can originate between two anatomic reflecting surfaces also. When closely spaced, they appear in a form called **comet tail** (Figure 8-5). Comet tail, a particular form of reverberation, is a series of closely spaced, discrete echoes.

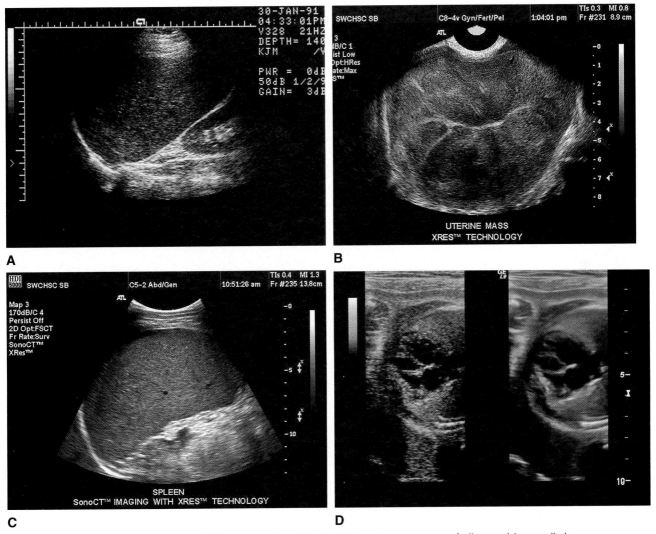

■ **FIGURE 8-2**   **A** to **C,** Three examples of the typically grainy appearance of ultrasound images that is not primarily the result of detail resolution limitations but rather of speckle. Speckle is the interference pattern resulting from constructive and destructive interference of echoes returning simultaneously from many scatterers within the propagating ultrasound pulse at any instant. **D,** Approaches to speckle reduction (*right image compared with the left*) are being implemented in modern instruments.

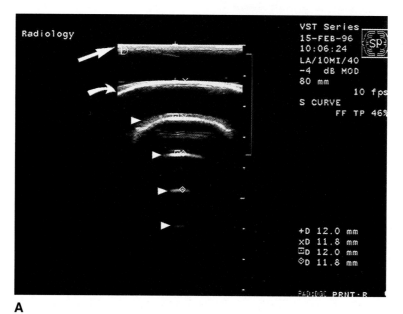

A

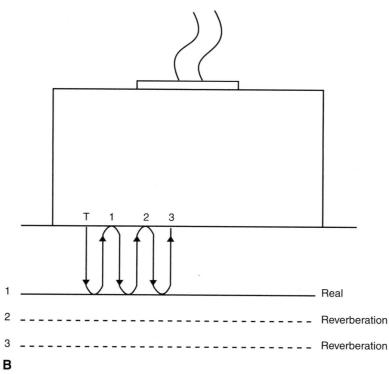

B

■ **FIGURE 8-3** **A,** Reverberation *(arrowheads)* resulting from multiple reflection through a water path between a linear array transducer *(straight arrow)* and the surface of an apple *(curved arrow).* **B,** The behavior in **A** is explained as follows: A pulse *(T)* is transmitted from the transducer. A strong echo is generated at the real reflector and is received *(1)* at the transducer, allowing correct imaging of the reflector. However, the echo is reflected partially at the transducer so that a second echo *(2)* is received, as well as a third *(3).* Because these echoes arrive later, they appear deeper on the display, where there are no reflectors. The lateral displacement of the reverberating sound path is for figure clarity. In fact, the sound travels down and back the same path repeatedly.

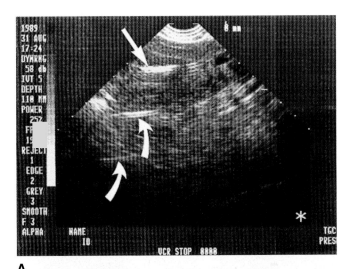

A

B

■ **FIGURE 8-4**   **A,** A chorionic villi sampling catheter *(straight arrow)* and two reverberations *(curved arrows).* **B,** A fetal scapula *(straight arrow)* and two reverberations *(curved arrows).*

Figure 8-6 shows an artifact that appears similar but is fundamentally different. Discrete echoes cannot be identified here because continuous emission of sound from the origin appears to be occurring. This continuous effect, termed **ring-down artifact,** is caused by a **resonance** phenomenon associated with the presence of a collection of gas bubbles. Resonance is the condition in which a driven mechanical vibration is of a frequency similar to a natural vibration frequency of the structure. The bubbles are stimulated into vibration by the incident ultrasound pulse. They then pulsate (expand and contract) for several cycles, acting as a source of ultrasound, producing a continuous stream of ultrasound that progresses distal to the bubble collection as the echo stream returns.

Reverberations are multiple reflections between a structure and the transducer or within a structure.

Mirror Image

The mirror-image artifact, also a form of reverberation, shows structures that exist on one side of a strong reflector as being present on the other side as well. Figure 8-7 explains how this happens and shows examples. Mirror-image artifacts are common around the diaphragm and pleura because of the total reflection from air-filled lung. They occasionally occur in other locations. Sometimes the mirrored structure is not in the unmirrored scan plane (Figure 8-7, *C*).

Mirror-image artifact duplicates a structure on the other side of a strong reflector.

Refraction

Refraction of light enables lenses to focus and distorts the presentation of objects, as shown in Figure 8-8. Refraction can cause a reflector to be positioned improperly (laterally) on a sonographic display (Figure 8-9). This is likely to occur, for example, when the transducer is placed on the abdominal midline (Figures 8-9, *C*, and 8-10), producing doubling of single objects. Beneath are the rectus abdominis muscles, which are surrounded by fat. These tissues present refracting boundaries because of their different propagation speeds.

Refraction displaces structures laterally from their correct locations.

Grating Lobes

Side lobes are beams that propagate from a single element in directions different from the primary beam. Grating lobes are additional beams emitted from an array transducer that are stronger than the side lobes of individual elements (Figure 8-11). Side and grating lobes are weaker than the primary beam and normally do not produce echoes that are imaged, particularly if they fall on a normally echogenic region of the scan. However, if grating lobes encounter a strong reflector

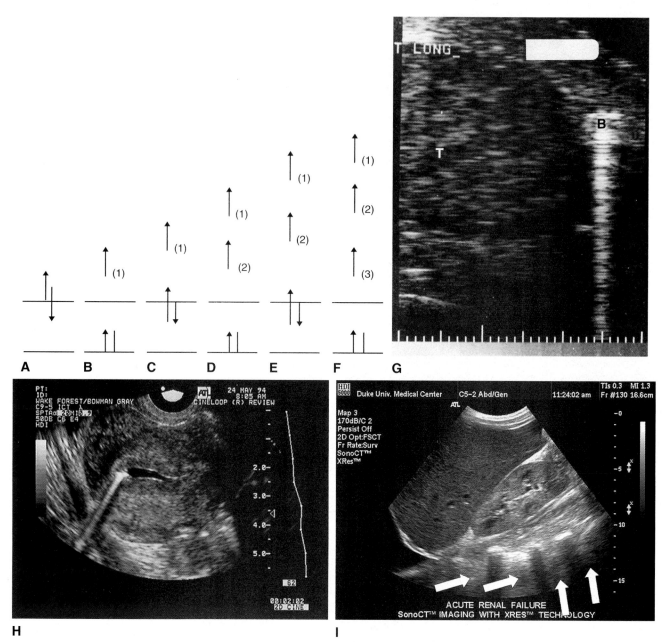

■ **FIGURE 8-5** Generation of comet-tail artifact (closely spaced reverberations). Action progresses in time from left to right. **A,** An ultrasound pulse encounters the first reflector and is reflected partially and is transmitted partially. **B,** Reflection and transmission at the first reflector are complete. Reflection at the second reflector is occurring. **C,** Reflection at the second reflector is complete. Partial transmission and partial reflection are again occurring at the first reflector as the second echo passes through. **D,** The echoes from the first *(1)* and second *(2)* reflectors are traveling toward the transducer. A second reflection (repeat of **B**) is occurring at the second reflector. **E,** Partial transmission and reflection are again occurring at the first reflector. **F,** Three echoes are now returning—the echo from the first reflector *(1)*, the echo from the second reflector *(2)*, and the echo from the second reflector *(3)*—that originated from the back side of the first reflector **(C)** and reflected again from the second reflector **(D)**. A fourth echo is being generated at the second reflector **(F). G,** Comet-tail artifact from an air rifle BB shot pellet *(B)* adjacent to the testicle *(T)*. The front and rear surface of the BB shot are the two reflecting surfaces involved in this example. **H,** Comet-tail artifact from bubbles in an intrauterine saline injection. **I,** Comet tail *(arrows)* from diaphragm. (**G** from Kremkau FW, Taylor KJW: *J Ultrasound Med* 5:227, 1986.)

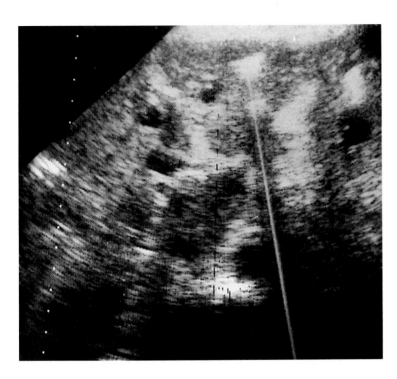

FIGURE 8-6 Ring-down artifact from air in the bile duct. (From Kremkau FW, Taylor KJW: *J Ultrasound Med* 5:227, 1986.)

(e.g., bone or gas), their echoes may well be imaged, particularly if they fall within an **anechoic** region. If so, they appear in incorrect locations (Figure 8-12).

Grating lobes duplicate structures laterally to the legitimate ones.

Speed Error

Propagation **speed error** occurs when the assumed value for propagation speed (1.54 mm/μs, leading to the 13 μs/cm rule) is incorrect. If the propagation speed that exists over a path traveled is greater than 1.54 mm/μs, the calculated distance to the reflector is too small, and the display will place the reflector too close to the transducer (Figure 8-13). This occurs because the increased speed causes the echoes to arrive sooner. If the actual speed is less than 1.54 mm/μs, the reflector will be displayed too far from the transducer (Figure 8-14) because the echoes arrive later. Refraction and propagation speed error also can cause a structure to be displayed with incorrect shape.

Propagation speed error displaces structures axially.

Range Ambiguity

In sonographic imaging, it is assumed that for each pulse all echoes are received before the next pulse is emitted. If this were not the case, error could result (Figures 8-15 and 8-16). The maximum depth imaged correctly by an instrument is determined by its pulse repetition frequency (PRF). To avoid range ambiguity, PRF automatically is reduced in deeper imaging situations. This also causes a reduction in frame rate.

The range-ambiguity artifact places structures much closer to the surface than they should be.

Sometimes two artifacts combine to present even more challenging cases. An example involving range ambiguity is shown in Figure 8-17.

ATTENUATION

Shadowing

Shadowing is the reduction in echo amplitude from reflectors that lie behind a strongly reflecting or attenuating structure. A strongly attenuating or reflecting structure weakens the sound distal to it, causing echoes from

Text continued on p. 277.

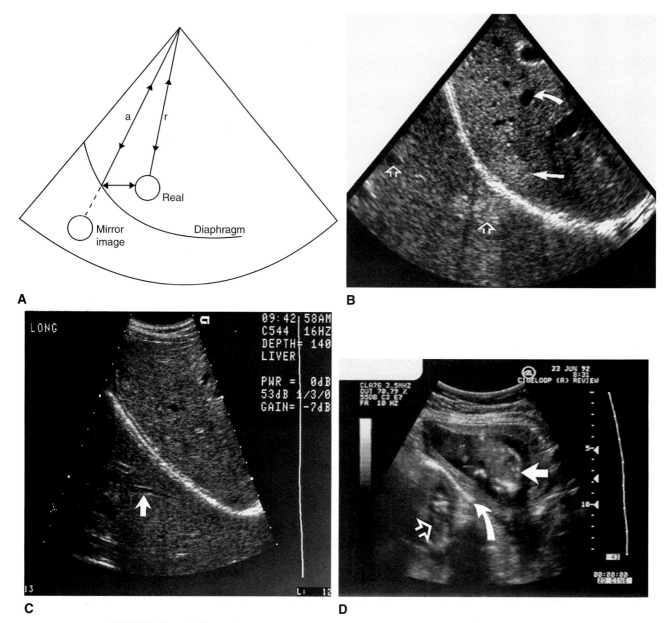

■ FIGURE 8-7   A, When pulses encounter a real hepatic structure directly *(scan line r)*, the structure is imaged correctly. If the pulse first reflects off the diaphragm *(scan line a)* and returns along the same path, the structure is displayed on the other side of the diaphragm. **B,** A hemangioma *(straight arrow)* and vessel *(curved arrow)* with their mirror images *(open arrows)*. **C,** A vessel is mirror-imaged *(arrow)* superior to the diaphragm but does not appear inferior because it is outside the unmirrored scan plane. **D,** A fetus *(straight arrow)* also appears as a mirror image *(open arrow)*. The mirror *(curved arrow)* is probably echogenic muscle.

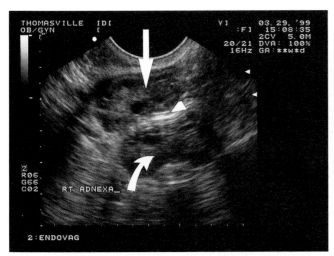

E

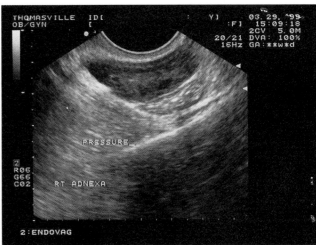

F

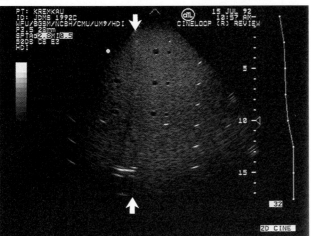

G

■ **FIGURE 8-7, cont'd**   **E,** Ovary *(arrow)* with mirror image *(curved arrow)* that could be mistaken for an adnexal mass or ectopic pregnancy. Bowel gas *(arrowhead)* is apparently the mirror in this case. **F,** Applying external abdominal pressure displaces the gas, eliminating the mirror image. **G,** Mirror image of cystic regions in a tissue-equivalent phantom. The edge of the phantom is indicated by the arrows. The image to the right of the arrows is a correct presentation. Everything to the left is mirror-image artifact.

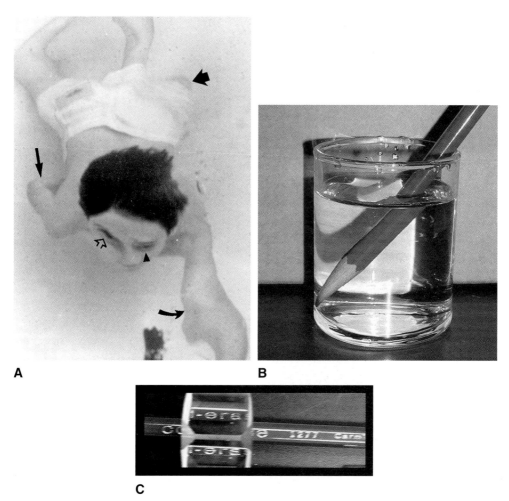

A

B

C

■ **FIGURE 8-8** **A,** Refracted light from a child in a swimming pool distorts his appearance. We see a thin arm *(straight arrow)* and a thick one *(curved arrow),* a large eye *(open arrow)* and a small one *(arrowhead),* and even a third lower limb emerging *(thick arrow).* **B,** A pencil in water appears to be broken. **C,** A pencil beneath a prism appears to be split in two.

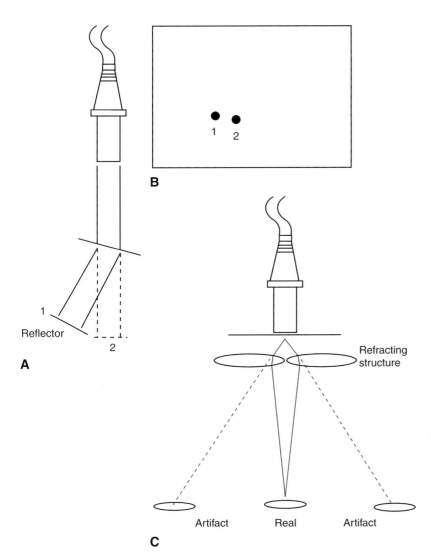

■ **FIGURE 8-9** Refraction **(A)** results in improper positioning of a reflector on the display **(B).** The system places the reflector at position 2 (because that is the direction from which the echo was received) when in fact the reflector is actually at position 1. **C,** One real structure is imaged as two artifactual objects because of the refracting structure close to the transducer. If unrefracted pulses can propagate to the real structure, a triple presentation (one correct, two artifactual) will result.

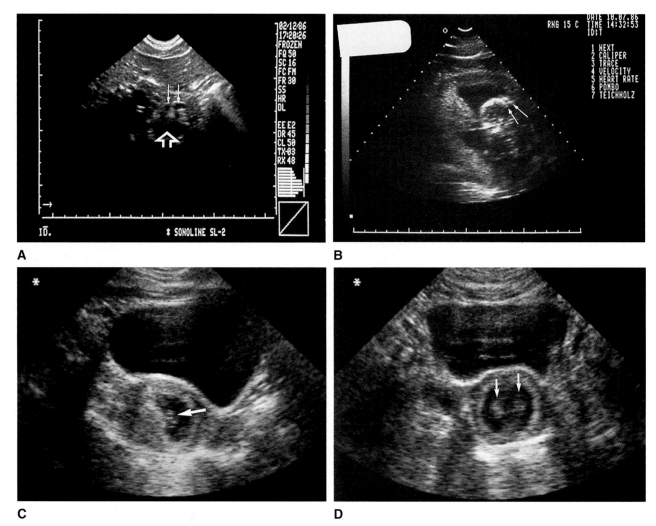

■ **FIGURE 8-10**   **A,** Refraction (probably through the rectus abdominis muscle) has widened the aorta *(open arrow)* and produced a double image of the celiac trunk *(arrows)*. **B,** Refraction has produced a double image of a fetal skull *(arrows)*. Refraction also may cause a single gestation **(C)** to appear as a double gestation **(D).**

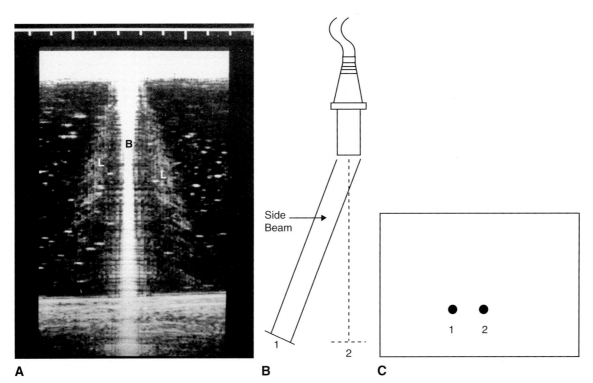

■ FIGURE 8-11 **A,** The primary beam (B) and grating lobes (L) from a linear array transducer. **B,** A side lobe or grating lobe can produce and receive a reflection from a "side view." **C,** This will be placed on the display at the proper distance from the transducer but in the wrong location (direction) because the instrument assumes that echoes originate from points along the main beam axis. The instrument shows the reflector at position 2 because that is the direction in which the main beam travels. The reflector is actually in position 1.

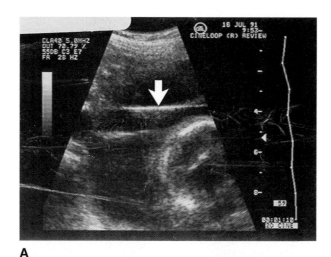

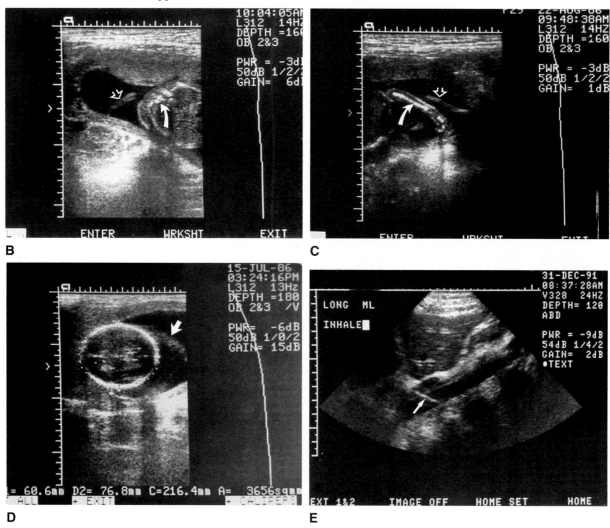

■ **FIGURE 8-12** Grating lobes in obstetric scans can produce the appearance of amniotic sheets or bands. **A,** A real amniotic sheet *(arrow).* **B** and **C,** Grating lobe duplication *(open arrows)* of fetal bones *(curved arrows)* resembles amniotic bands or sheets. **D,** Grating lobe duplication *(arrow)* of a fetal skull. **E,** Artifactual grating lobe echoes *(arrow)* cross the aorta. In these examples, we observe that the grating lobe artifact is always weaker than the correct presentation of the structure.

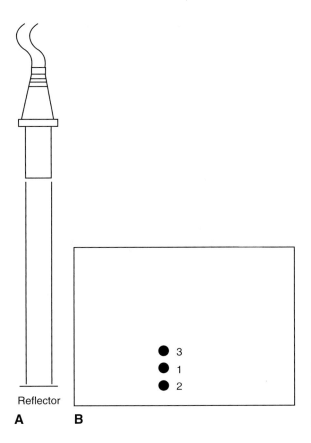

■ FIGURE 8-13 The propagation speed over the traveled path **(A)** determines the reflector position on the display **(B).** The reflector is actually in position 1. If the actual propagation speed is less than that assumed, the reflector will appear in position 2. If the actual speed is more than that assumed, the reflector will appear in position 3.

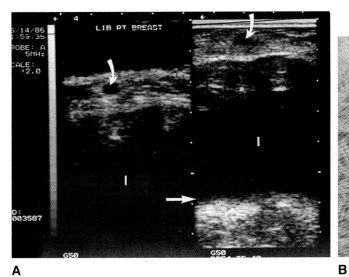

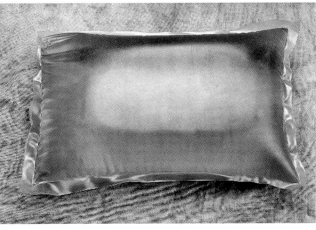

■ FIGURE 8-14 The low propagation speed in a silicone breast implant (*I*) causes the chest wall (*straight arrow*) to appear deeper than it should **(A).** Note that a cyst (*curved arrow*) is shown more clearly on the left image than on the right because a gel standoff pad **(B)** has been placed between the transducer and the breast, moving the beam focus closer to the cyst.

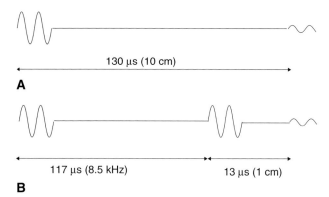

A

130 μs (10 cm)

B

117 μs (8.5 kHz)   13 μs (1 cm)

■ **FIGURE 8-15** **A,** An echo (from a 10-cm depth) arrives 130 μs after pulse emission. **B,** If the pulse repetition period were 117 μs (corresponding to a pulse repetition frequency of 8.5 kHz), the echo in **A** would arrive 13 μs after the next pulse was emitted. The instrument would place this echo at a 1-cm depth rather than the correct value. This range location error is known as the range-ambiguity artifact.

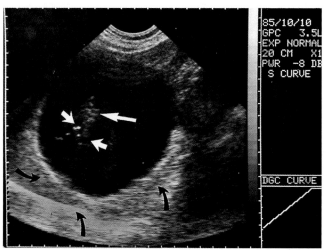

■ **FIGURE 8-16** A large renal cyst (diameter about 10 cm) has artifactual range-ambiguity echoes within it *(white arrows)*. They are generated from structure(s) below the display. These deep echoes arrive after the next pulse is emitted. Because the time from the emission of the last pulse to echo arrival is short, the echoes are placed closer to the transducer than they should be. Echoes arrive from much deeper (later) than usual in this case because the sound passes through the long, low-attenuation paths in the cyst. These echoes may have come from bone or a far body wall. Low attenuation in the cyst is indicated by the strong echoes (enhancement) below it *(curved black arrows)*.

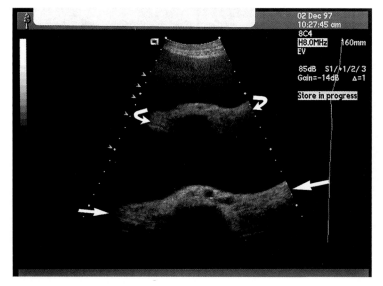

■ **FIGURE 8-17** A large pelvic cyst produces a large echo-free region in this scan. A structure is located at a depth of about 13 cm *(straight arrows)*. Located in the anechoic region at a depth of about 6 cm is a structure *(curved arrows)* shaped like that at 13 cm. How could this artifact appear closer than the actual structure, implying that these echoes arrived earlier than those from the correct location? It turns out that the artifact is actually a combination of two phenomena: reverberation and range ambiguity. The artifact seen is a reverberation from the deep structure and the transducer. But a reverberation should appear at twice the depth of the actual structure, that is, at about 26 cm. However, the arrival of the reverberation echoes occurs about 78 μs after the next pulse is emitted so that they are placed at a 6-cm depth. Single artifacts are difficult enough. Fortunately, combinations like this occur infrequently.

the distal region to be weak and thus to appear darker, like a shadow. Of course, the returning echoes also must pass through the attenuating structure, adding to the shadowing effect. Examples of shadowing structures include calcified plaque (Figure 8-18, *A*), bone (Figure 8-18, *B*), and stone (Figure 8-19, *A*). Shadowing also can occur behind the edges of objects that are not necessarily strong attenuators (Figure 8-20). In this case the cause may be the defocusing action of a refracting curved surface. Alternatively, it may be attributable to destructive interference caused by portions of an ultrasound pulse passing through tissues with different propagation speeds and subsequently getting out of phase. In either case the intensity of the beam decreases beyond the edge of the structure, causing echoes to be weakened.

Shadowing is the weakening of echoes distal to a strongly attenuating or reflecting structure or from the edges of a refracting structure.

Enhancement

Enhancement is the strengthening of echoes from reflectors that lie behind a weakly attenuating structure (Figures 8-16; 8-18, *B*; and 8-19). Shadowing and enhancement result in reflectors being placed on the image with amplitudes that are too low and too high, respectively. Brightening of echoes also can be caused by the increased intensity in the focal region of a beam because the beam is narrow there. This is called focal enhancement or focal banding (Figure 8-21). Shadowing and enhancement artifacts are often useful for determining the nature of masses and structures. Shadowing and enhancement are reduced with spatial compounding because several approaches to each anatomic site are used, allowing the beam to "get under" the attenuating or enhancing structure. This is useful with shadowing because it can uncover structures (especially pathologic ones) that were not imaged because they were located in the shadow.

Enhancement is the strengthening of echoes distal to a weakly attenuating structure.

External influences also can produce artifacts. As an example, interference from electronic equipment adds unwanted noise to the image (Figure 8-22).

SPECTRAL DOPPLER

Aliasing

Aliasing is the most common artifact encountered in Doppler ultrasound. The word *alias* comes from Middle English *elles*, Latin *alius*, and Greek *allos*, which mean "other" or "otherwise." Contemporary meanings for the word include (as an adverb) "otherwise called" or "otherwise known as" and (as a noun) "an assumed or additional name." Aliasing in its technical use indicates improper representation of information that has been sampled insufficiently. The sampling can be spatial or temporal. Inadequate spatial sampling can result in improper conclusions about the object or population sampled. For example, we could assemble 10 families, each consisting of a father, a mother, and a child, and line them up in that order—father, mother, child, father, mother, child—for all the families. If we wanted to sample the contents of these families by taking 10 photographs, we could choose to photograph one out of every three persons (e.g., the first, fourth, and seventh persons in the line). However, if we did this, we would conclude that all families are made up of three adult males, no women, and no children. In this example, spatial undersampling of one third of the population would result in an incorrect conclusion regarding the total population.

Another example of inadequate spatial sampling is shown in Figure 8-23. In *A* we see what we might call a "Doppler flower," containing 12 double-pointed petals. Each petal is made up of four lines. If we sample at the intersections of these lines, we get a 48-point dot-to-dot child's puzzle, as shown in *B*. Connecting the dots properly will yield the flower shown in *A*. In *C*, the even-numbered dots from *B* have been eliminated so that there are now 24 dots (samples). When these dots are connected, a reasonable representation of the original flower results, but it is not as good as the representation in *B*. The higher-frequency information delineating the double pointing of the petals has been lost. In *D* the even-numbered dots from *C* have been eliminated. This representation of the flower, containing 12 samples, yields a 12-sided polygon that approximates a circle and is a poor representation of the original flower. The lower-frequency information about the 12 petals has been lost. Parts *E* and *F* each eliminate half of the previous samples, yielding a hexagon and a triangle, respectively. Part *F* yields virtually no information regarding the round, double-pointed, 12-petaled flower.

In these examples, we see that inadequate spatial sampling yields an incorrect representation of the object sampled. This is similar to a disguise (false appearance or assumed identity) or alias. As the sampling was reduced, we first lost the double-pointed character of each petal, then the presence of the 12 petals, and finally

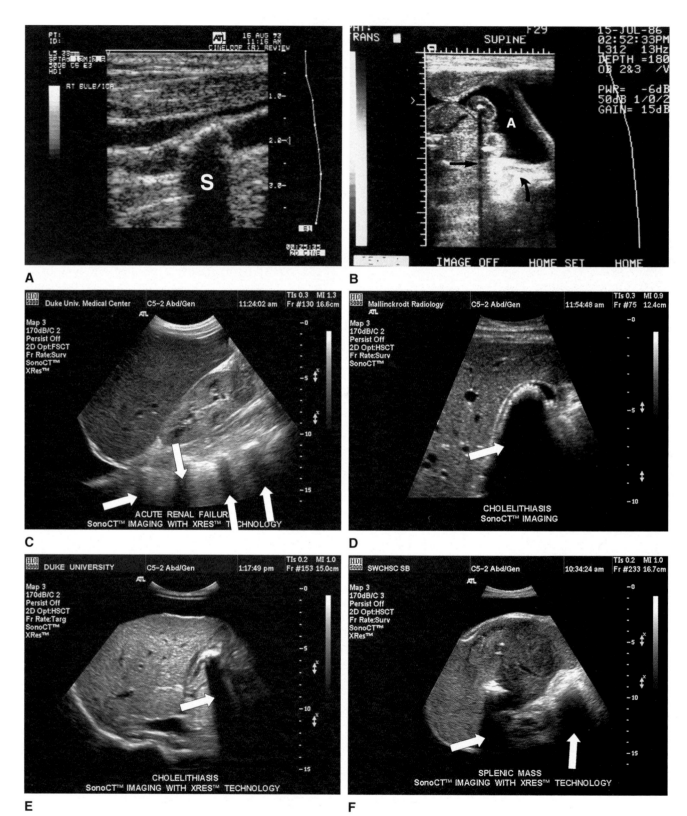

■ **FIGURE 8-18** **A,** Shadowing (*S*) from a high-attenuation calcified plaque in the common carotid artery. **B,** Shadowing (*straight arrow*) from a fetal limb bone and enhancement (*curved arrow*) caused by the low attenuation of amniotic fluid (*A*) through which the ultrasound travels. **C** to **F,** Examples of shadowing (*arrows*).

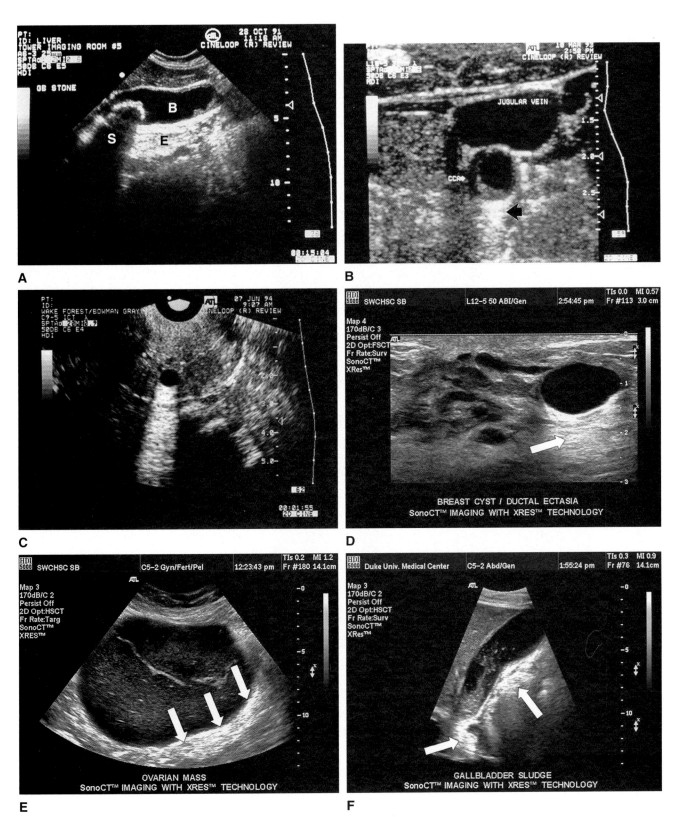

■ **FIGURE 8-19** **A,** Shadowing *(S)* from a gallstone and enhancement *(E)* caused by the low attenuation of bile *(B)*. **B,** Enhancement *(arrow)* from the low attenuation of blood in the common carotid artery *(CCA)* and jugular vein in transverse view. **C,** Enhancement beyond a cervical cyst. **D** to **F,** Examples of enhancement *(arrows)*.

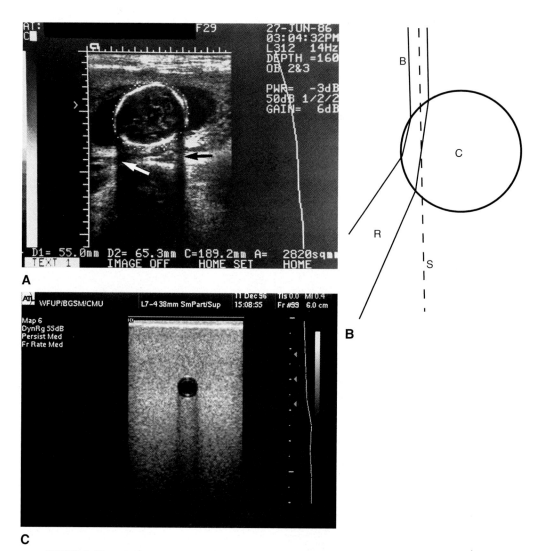

■ **FIGURE 8-20**   **A,** Edge shadows *(arrows)* from a fetal skull. **B,** As a sound beam *(B)* enters a circular region *(C)* of higher propagation speed, it is refracted, and refraction occurs again as it leaves. This causes spreading of the beam with decreased intensity. The echoes from region *R* are presented deep to the circular region in the neighborhood of the dashed line. Because of beam spreading, these echoes are weak and thus cast a shadow *(S)*. **C,** Edge shadows from a tube (shown in transverse view) are embedded in tissue-equivalent material in a flow phantom.

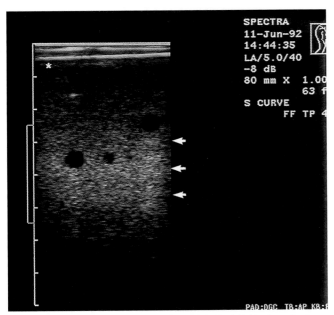

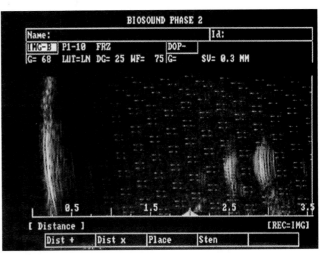

■ FIGURE 8-22 Interference *(repeating white specks)* from nearby electronic equipment.

■ FIGURE 8-21 Focal banding *(arrows)* is the brightening of echoes around the focus, where intensity is increased by the narrowing of the beam.

⊙ *Aliasing is the appearance of Doppler spectral information on the wrong side of the baseline.*

the circular nature of the flower. In each case, we were experiencing spatial aliasing. Another example of spatial aliasing is given in Figure 8-24.

An optical form of temporal aliasing occurs in motion pictures when wagon wheels appear to rotate at various speeds and in reverse direction. Similar behavior is observed when a fan is lighted with a strobe light. Depending on the flashing rate of the strobe light, the fan may appear stationary or rotating clockwise or counterclockwise at various speeds.

Nyquist Limit

Pulsed wave Doppler instruments are sampling instruments. Each emitted pulse yields a sample of the desired Doppler shift. The upper limit to Doppler shift that can be detected properly by pulsed instruments is called the **Nyquist limit** (NL). If the Doppler-shift frequency exceeds one half the PRF (which, for Doppler functions, is normally in the 5- to 30-kHz range), temporal aliasing occurs.

$$NL \text{ (kHz)} = \frac{1}{2} \times PRF \text{ (kHz)}$$

Improper Doppler shift information (improper direction and improper value) results. Higher PRFs (Table 8-1) permit higher Doppler shifts to be detected but also increase the chance of the range-ambiguity artifact occurring. Continuous wave Doppler instruments do not experience aliasing. However, recall that neither do they provide depth localization.

Figure 8-25 illustrates aliasing in the popliteal artery and in the heart of a normal subject. This figure also illustrates how aliasing can be reduced or eliminated (Box 8-2) by increasing PRF, increasing Doppler angle (which decreases the Doppler shift for a given flow), or by **baseline shift**. The latter is an electronic cut-and-paste technique that moves the misplaced aliasing peaks over to their proper location. The technique is successful as long as there are no legitimate Doppler shifts in the region of the aliasing. If there are legitimate Doppler shifts, they will get moved over to an inappropriate location along with the aliasing peaks. (This would happen if the baseline were shifted farther down in Figure 8-25, *E.*) Baseline shifting is not helpful if the desired information (e.g., peak systolic Doppler shift) is buried in another portion of the spectral display, as in Figure 8-25, *F.* Other approaches to eliminating aliasing include changing to a lower-frequency Doppler transducer (Figure 8-25, *G* and *H*) or switching to continuous wave operation. The common and convenient solutions to aliasing are shifting the baseline, increasing PRF, or doing both in extreme cases.

⊙ *Aliasing is caused by undersampling of the Doppler shifts.*

In Figure 8-25, *A*, we can see that aliasing occurs at Doppler shifts greater than 1.75 kHz. The aliased peaks

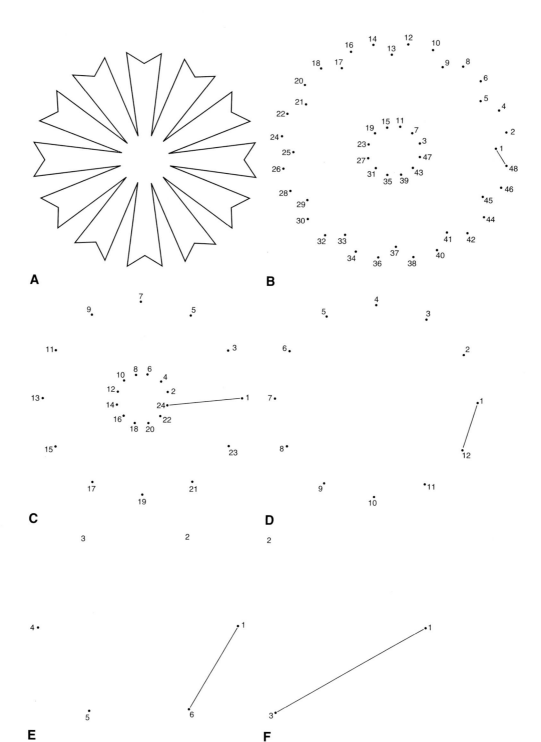

■ FIGURE 8-23   A, A "Doppler flower." **B,** Forty-eight samples. **C,** Twenty-four samples. **D,** Twelve samples. **E,** Six samples. **F** Three samples. (From Kremkau FW: *J Vasc Technol* 14:41-42, 1990.)

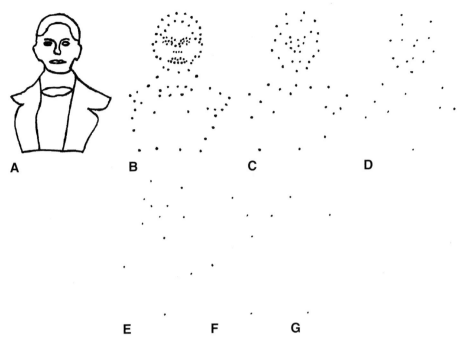

■ FIGURE 8-24 **A,** A freehand drawing of Christian Doppler. As sampling progressively decreases from 96 samples **(B)** to 48 samples **(C)**, 24 samples **(D)**, 12 samples **(E)**, 6 samples **(F)**, and 3 samples **(G)**, connecting the dots, especially in the latter three cases, yields an image that bears no resemblance to **A.** Indeed, in **G** a triangle would result. These cases are undersampled, resulting in an "aliased" image.

TABLE 8-1	**Aliasing and Range-Ambiguity Artifact Values**	
Pulse Repetition Frequency (kHz)	**Doppler Shift Above Which Aliasing Occurs (kHz)**	**Range Beyond Which Ambiguity Occurs (cm)**
5.0	2.5	15
7.5	3.7	10
10.0	5.0	7
12.5	6.2	6
15.0	7.5	5
17.5	8.7	4
20.0	10.0	3
25.0	12.5	3
30.0	15.0	2

add another 1.25 kHz of Doppler shift, so the correct peak shift is 3.0 kHz. With the higher PRF in Figure 8-25, *C*, this result is confirmed. Thus at the lower PRF, the peak shift can be determined and baseline shifting is not necessary (but is convenient). However, if the peaks were buried in other portions of the Doppler signal (as in Figure 8-25, *F*), baseline shifting would

not help, but a higher PRF, a larger Doppler angle, or a lower operating frequency would help.

Aliasing occurs with the pulsed system because it is a sampling system; that is, a pulsed system acquires samples of the desired Doppler shift frequency from which it must be synthesized (see Figure 7-11). If samples are taken often enough, the correct result is achieved. Figure 8-26 shows temporal sampling of a signal. Sufficient sampling yields the correct result. Insufficient sampling yields an incorrect result.

The Nyquist limit, or Nyquist frequency, describes the minimum number of samples required to avoid aliasing. At least two samples per cycle of the desired Doppler shift must be made for the image to be obtained correctly. For a complicated signal, such as a Doppler signal containing many frequencies, the sampling rate must be such that at least two samples occur for each cycle of the highest frequency present. To restate this rule, if the highest Doppler-shift frequency present in a signal exceeds one half the PRF, aliasing will occur (Figure 8-27).

Aliasing is corrected by shifting the baseline, increasing the pulse repetition frequency, or both.

Text continued on p. 288.

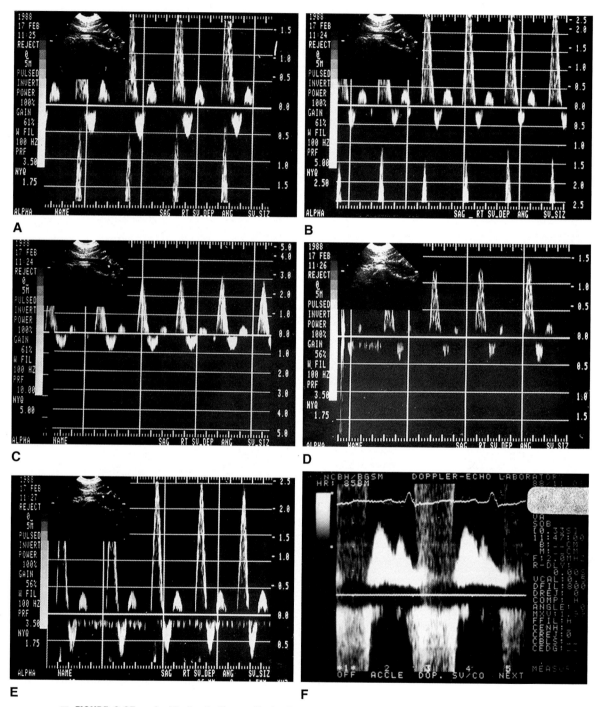

■ **FIGURE 8-25**   **A,** Aliasing in the popliteal artery. **B,** Pulse repetition frequency (PRF) is increased. **C,** The PRF is increased further. **D,** Doppler angle is increased with original PRF. **E,** Baseline is shifted down with original PRF. **F,** An example of aliasing in Doppler echocardiography.

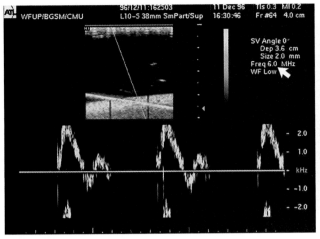

G

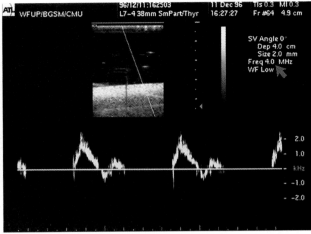

H

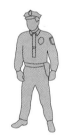

NYQUIST LIMIT

1/2 PRF

I

■ **FIGURE 8-25, cont'd** **G,** Aliasing is occurring with an operating frequency of 6 MHz *(arrow).* **H,** When operating frequency is reduced to 4 MHz, the Doppler shifts are reduced to less than the Nyquist limit, thereby eliminating the aliasing seen in **G. I,** The Nyquist limit is equal to one half the pulse repetition frequency. (**A** to **E** from Taylor KJW, Holland S: *Radiology* 174:297-307, 1990.)

BOX 8-2 Methods of Reducing or Eliminating Aliasing

1. Increase the pulse repetition frequency.
2. Increase the Doppler angle.
3. Shift the baseline.
4. Use a lower operating frequency.
5. Use a continuous wave device.

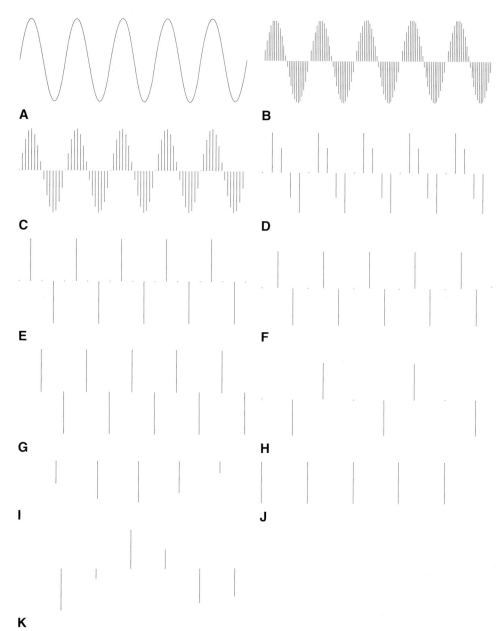

■ FIGURE 8-26   Decreasing sampling rate leads to aliasing. Sampling of a five-cycle voltage **(A)** is progressively decreased from 25 samples per cycle **(B)**, to 15 samples per cycle **(C)**, to 5 samples per cycle **(D)**, to 4 samples per cycle **(E)**, to 3 samples per cycle **(F)**, to 2 samples per cycle **(G)**, and finally to successive sampling of 1 sample per cycle **(H** to **K)**. In the last four cases, aliasing occurs.

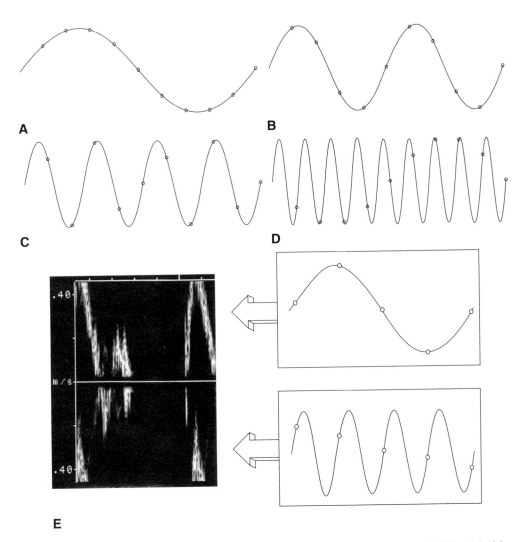

■ FIGURE 8-27 Increasing frequency leads to aliasing. Signal voltages are sampled at 10 points (o): **(A)** one cycle, **(B)** two cycles, **(C)** four cycles, and **(D)** nine cycles. As signal frequency is increased, aliasing occurs when the Nyquist limit is exceeded (in this case, beyond five cycles). Thus **D** is an example of aliasing. It can be seen that connecting the o's would yield a one-cycle representation of what is actually a nine-cycle signal voltage. **(E)** In this spectral display the presentation above the baseline is correct (unaliased, five samples per cycle), whereas the systolic peaks appear incorrectly below the baseline (aliased, one sample per cycle).

Two lessor-used correction methods are reduction of the operating frequency and switching to continuous wave operation. Operating frequency reduction reduces the Doppler shift. Continuous wave operation, because it is not pulsed, is not a sampling mode and is thus not subject to aliasing. However, it does not have range selectivity ability.

Range Ambiguity

In attempting to solve the aliasing problem by increasing the PRF, one can encounter the range-ambiguity[54] problem. This problem occurs when a pulse is emitted before all the echoes from the previous pulse have been received. When this happens, early echoes from the last pulse are received simultaneously with late echoes from the previous pulse. The instrument is unable to determine whether an echo is an early one (superficial) from the last pulse or a late one (deep) from the previous pulse (Figure 8-28). To solve this difficulty, the instrument simply assumes that all echoes are derived from the last pulse and that these echoes have originated from depths determined by the 13 μs/cm rule. As long as all echoes are received before the next pulse is sent out, this is true. However, with high PRFs, this may not be the case. Doppler flow information therefore may come from locations other than the assumed one (the gate location). In effect, multiple gates or sample volumes are operating at different depths. Table 8-1 lists, for various PRFs, the ranges beyond which ambiguity occurs. Table 8-2 lists, for various depths, the maximum Doppler-shift frequency (Nyquist limit) that avoids aliasing *and* the range-ambiguity artifact. Maximum flow speeds that avoid aliasing for given angles also are listed. Instruments sometimes increase PRF (to avoid aliasing) into a range where range ambiguity occurs. Multiple sample gates are shown on the display to indicate this condition.

High pulse repetition frequency causes Doppler range ambiguity. Multiple sample volumes appear as a result.

Mirror Image

The mirror-image artifact described previously also can occur with Doppler systems. This means that an image of a vessel and a source of Doppler-shifted echoes can be duplicated on the opposite side of a strong reflector. The duplicated vessel containing flow could be misinterpreted as an additional vessel and has a spectrum similar to that for the real vessel. Figure 8-29 shows an example of image and spectrum duplication of the sub-clavian artery. The strong reflector in this case is the air at the pleural boundary.

A **mirror image** of a Doppler spectrum can appear on the opposite side of the baseline when, indeed, flow is unidirectional and should appear only on one side of the baseline. This is an electronic duplication of the spectral information. The duplication can occur when Doppler gain is set too high (causing overloading in the amplifier and leakage, called **cross-talk,** of the signal from the proper channel into the other channel; Figure 8-30). Duplication also can occur when the Doppler angle is near 90 degrees (Figure 8-31). In this situation the duplication is usually legitimate because beams are focused and not cylindrical. Thus while the beam axis is perpendicular to the flow direction, one edge of the beam is angled upstream and the other edge downstream.[55]

Spectral mirror image is the appearance of spectral information on both sides of the baseline. It occurs at high Doppler gains.

Doppler spectra have a speckle quality[56] to them that is similar to that observed in sonography. Electromagnetic interference from nearby equipment can cloud the spectral display with lines or "snow" (Figure 8-32).

COLOR DOPPLER

Artifacts observed with color Doppler imaging[38,39,53] are two-dimensional color presentations of artifacts that are seen in gray-scale sonography and Doppler spectral displays. They are incorrect presentations of two-dimensional motion information, the most common of which is aliasing. However, others occur, including anatomic mirror image, Doppler angle effects, shadowing, and clutter.

Aliasing

Aliasing occurs when the Doppler shift exceeds the Nyquist limit (Figure 8-33 [Color Plates 30 and 31]). The result is incorrect flow direction on the color Doppler image (Figure 8-34 [Color Plate 32]). Increasing the flow speed range (which is actually an increase in PRF) can solve the problem (Figure 8-35 [Color Plates 33 and 34]). However, too high a range can cause loss of flow information, particularly if the wall filter is set high (Figure 8-35, *D* and *E*). Baseline shifting can decrease or eliminate the effect of aliasing (Figure 8-35, *C*), as in spectral displays.

Text continued on p. 297.

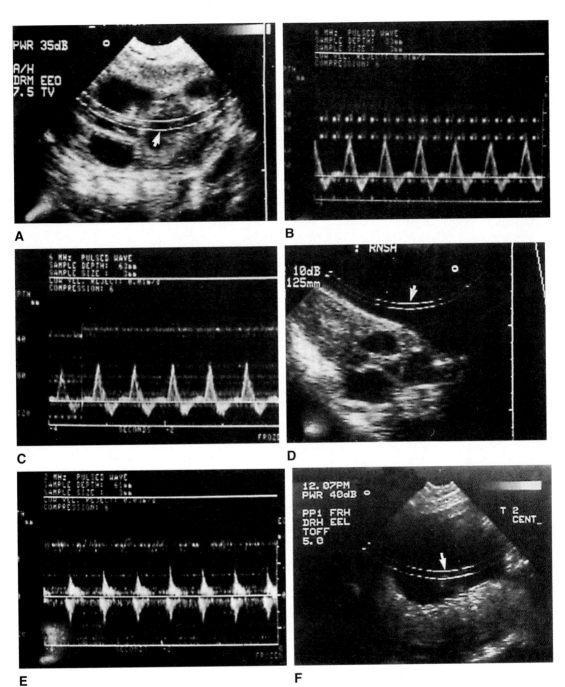

■ **FIGURE 8-28** Ambiguity is caused by sending out a pulse before all echoes from the previous pulse are received. **A,** This transvaginal image shows the pulsed Doppler range gate *(arrow)* set at 33 mm within an ovary. **B,** The resulting Doppler spectrum shows a waveform typical of the external iliac artery. **C,** A signal identical to that shown in **B** was obtained when the range was increased to 63 mm, proving that the signal actually originated from the external iliac artery at this depth. **D,** A strong arterial Doppler signal was obtained when the range gate *(arrow)* was placed within the urinary bladder at a depth of 31 mm. **E,** A signal identical to that obtained in **D** was detected when the range gate depth was increased to 61 mm, indicating that the signal actually arose from an artery at this depth. **F,** With the range gate *(arrow)* placed at a depth of 50 mm in the uterus of a pregnant woman (16 weeks' gestation), signals

Continued.

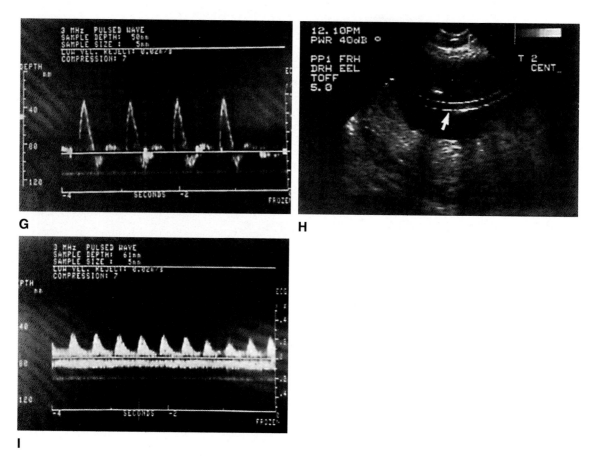

■ **FIGURE 8-28, cont'd** **(G)** typical of the external iliac artery were detected. **(H),** In the same patient a slight adjustment of the range gate *(arrow)* produced the desired umbilical artery signal **(I),** eliminating the artifactual iliac artery signal caused by range ambiguity. (From Gill RW et al: New class of pulsed Doppler US ambiguity at short ranges, *Radiology* 173:272, 1989.)

TABLE 8-2 Aliasing and Range-Ambiguity Limits*

| Depth (cm) | PRF (kHz) | Nyquist Limit (kHz) | Maximum Flow Speed (cm/s) | | |
			0	30	60
1	77.0	38.5	593	685	1186
2	38.5	19.2	296	342	593
4	19.2	9.6	148	171	296
8	9.6	4.8	74	86	148
16	4.8	2.4	37	43	74

*For various depths the maximum pulse repetition frequency (PRF) that avoids range ambiguity and the corresponding maximum Doppler shift frequency (Nyquist limit) that avoids aliasing are listed. Maximum flow speeds corresponding to the maximum Doppler shift also are listed for three Doppler angles (0, 30, and 60 degrees), assuming a 5-MHz operating frequency.

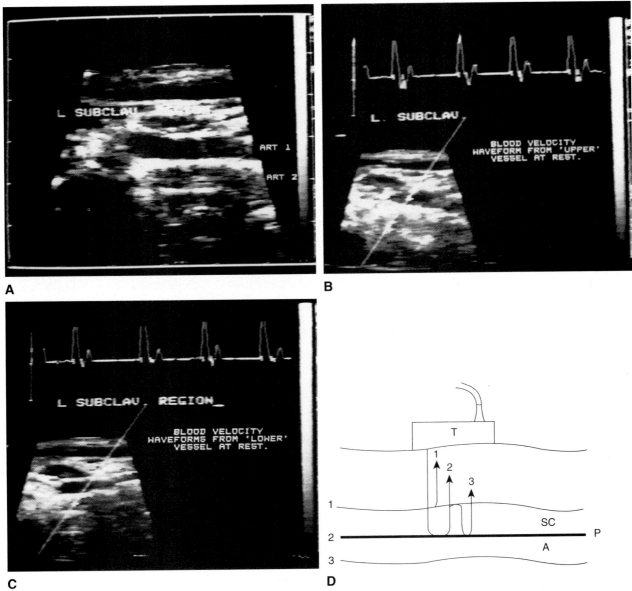

■ **FIGURE 8-29** **A,** The subclavian artery *(ART 1)* and its mirror image *(ART 2).* **B,** Flow signal from artery. **C,** Flow signal from the mirror image of the artery. **D,** Multiple reflections produce a mirror image. Paths 1 and 2 are legitimate, but path 3 arrives late, producing the artifactual deep arterial wall. *T,* Transducer; *SC,* subclavian artery; *P,* pleura; *A,* artifactual artery. (**D** from Kremkau FW: Principles and pitfalls of real-time color-flow imaging. In Bernstein EF, editor: *Vascular diagnosis,* ed 4, St Louis, 1993, Mosby.)

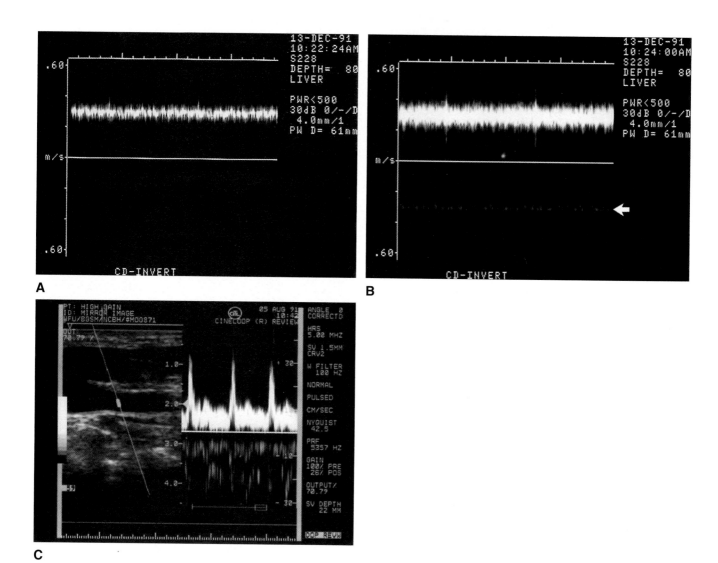

■ **FIGURE 8-30** **A,** Spectrum produced by a string moving at 30 cm/s. **B,** An increase in gain produces spectral broadening and a mirror image *(arrow).* **C,** High gain produces a mirror image of the carotid artery spectrum below the baseline. (**C** from Kremkau FW: *Semin Roentgenol* 27:6-16, 1992.)

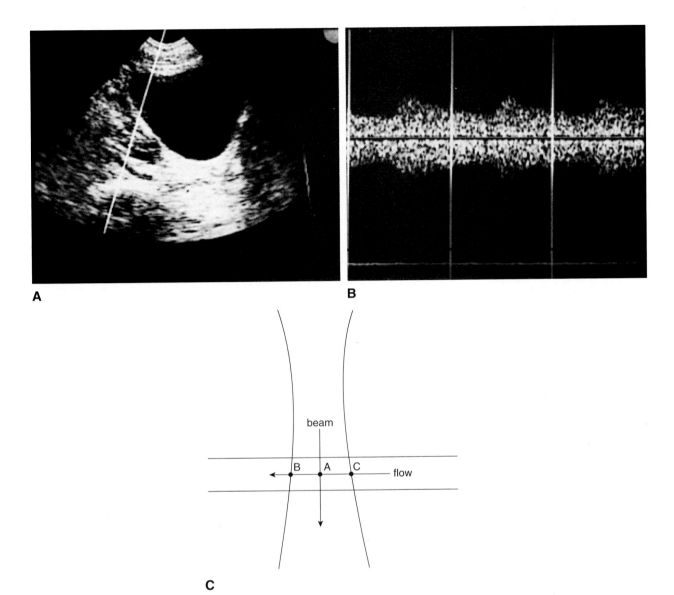

A   **B**

C

■ **FIGURE 8-31**   **A,** The Doppler angle is nearly 90 degrees at the ovarian artery. **B,** Spectral mirror image with low-resistance flow on both sides of the baseline. **C,** Because beams are focused and not cylindrical, portions of the beam *(C)* can experience flow toward the transducer, whereas other portions *(B)* can experience flow away when the beam axis intersects *(A)* the flow at 90 degrees. (**A** and **B** from Taylor KJW, Holland S: *Radiology* 174:297-307, 1990.)

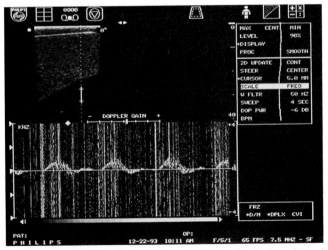

■ **FIGURE 8-32**   Interference from nearby electrical equipment clouds the spectral display with electric noise (the vertical "snow" lines).

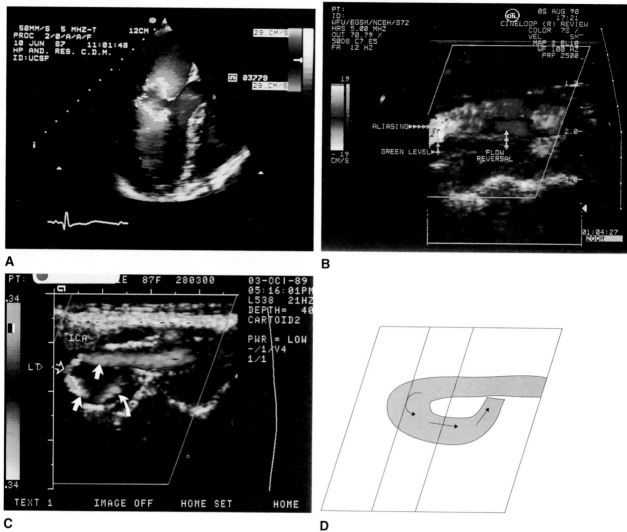

■ **FIGURE 8-33** **A,** A transesophageal cardiac color Doppler image of the long axis in diastole. The blue colors in the left atrium *(upper)* and left ventricle *(lower)* represent blood traveling away from the transducer, but where the flow speeds exceed the Nyquist limit (29 cm/s), aliasing occurs and the yellow and orange colors have replaced the blue colors. **B,** Color Doppler presentation of common carotid artery flow, including flow reversal and aliasing. The two can be distinguished because the boundary between the different directions with flow reversal passes through the baseline *(black)*, whereas the aliasing boundary passes through the upper and lower extremes of the color bar *(white)*. In this particular color bar assignment, the maximum positive Doppler shifts are assigned the color green, so that a thin green region shows the exact boundary where aliasing occurs. The aliasing occurs in the distal portion of the vessel because it is curving down, reducing the Doppler angle between the flow and the scan lines. **C,** In a tortuous internal carotid artery, negative Doppler shifts are indicated in the red regions *(solid straight arrows)*. Two regions of positive Doppler shifts *(blue)* are seen *(open arrow and curved arrow)*. In the latter, legitimate flow toward the transducer is indicated. In the former the flow away from the transducer has yielded high Doppler shifts (because of a small Doppler angle; i.e., flow is approximately parallel to scan lines), which produces a color shift to the opposite side of the map because of aliasing. The boundaries from and to normal negative Doppler shifts into and out of the aliased region are bright yellow and cyan from the ends of the color bars. The transition from unaliased negative Doppler shift into unaliased positive Doppler shift *(near bottom)* is black, representing the baseline of the color bar. **D,** Flow and scan line directions depicted in **C.** (See Color Plates 30 and 31.) (**B** from Kremkau FW: *Semin Roentgenol* 27:6-16, 1992; **C** from Kremkau FW: *J Vasc Technol* 15:265-266, 1991.)

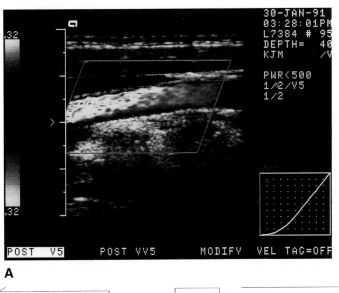

A

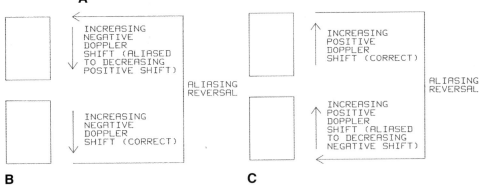

B   **C**

■ **FIGURE 8-34**   **A,** Positive *(blue)* Doppler shifts are shown in the arterial flow in this image. These are actually negative Doppler shifts that have exceeded the lower Nyquist limit (converted here to the equivalent flow speed: −0.32 m/s) and are wrapped around to the positive portion of the color bar **(B)**. Positive shifts that exceed the +0.32 m/s limit would alias to the negative side **(C)**. (See Color Plate 32.) (From Kremkau FW: Principles and pitfalls of real-time color-flow imaging. In Bernstein EF, editor: *Vascular diagnosis,* ed 4, St Louis, 1993, Mosby.)

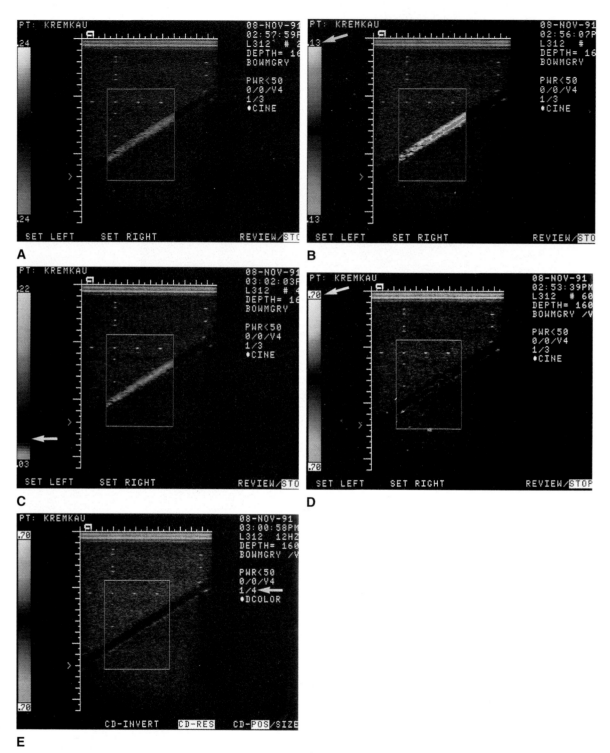

■ **FIGURE 8-35** **A,** Flow is toward the upper right, producing positive Doppler shifts. **B,** The pulse repetition frequency and Nyquist limit (0.13) are too low, resulting in aliasing (negative Doppler shifts) at the center of the flow in the vessel (see Figure 8-34, *C*). **C,** With the same pulse repetition frequency setting as in **B,** the aliasing has been eliminated by shifting the base line *(arrow)* down 10 cm/s below the center of the color bar. **D,** The Nyquist limit setting (0.70) is too high, causing the detected Doppler shifts to be well down the positive scale, producing a dark red appearance. **E,** With the Nyquist limit set as in **D,** an increase in the wall filter setting *(arrow)* eliminates what little color flow information there was in **D.** (See Color Plates 33 and 34.) (From Kremkau FW: Principles and pitfalls of real-time color-flow imaging. In Bernstein EF, editor: *Vascular diagnosis,* ed 4, St Louis, 1993, Mosby.)

Aliasing in color Doppler imaging appears as an incorrect color from the opposite side of the baseline on the color map.

Mirror Image, Shadowing, Clutter, and Noise

In the mirror (or ghost) artifact (Figure 8-36 [Color Plate 35]), an image of a vessel and source of Doppler-shifted echoes can be duplicated on the opposite side of a strong reflector (e.g., pleura or diaphragm). This is a color Doppler extension of the gray-scale and spectral mirror-image artifacts of Figure 8-29. Shadowing is the weakening or elimination of Doppler-shifted echoes beyond a shadowing object, just as occurs with non–Doppler-shifted (gray-scale) echoes (Figure 8-37 [Color Plate 36]). Clutter results from tissue, heart wall or valve, or vessel wall motion (Figure 8-38 [Color Plate 37]). Such clutter is eliminated by wall filters. Doppler angle effects include zero Doppler shift when the Doppler angle is 90 degrees (see Figure 6-14, *F*), as well as the change of color in a straight vessel viewed with a sector transducer (see Figure 6-14, *A*). Noise in the color Doppler electronics can mimic flow, particularly in **hypo-echoic** or anechoic regions[57] (Figure 8-39 [Color Plate 36]). The "twinkling" artifact has been observed at strongly reflecting scattering surfaces.[58]

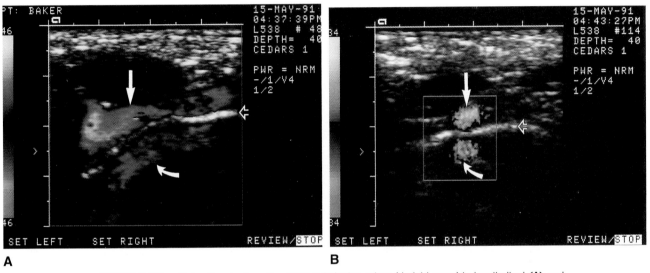

A   **B**

■ **FIGURE 8-36**   Color Doppler imaging of the subclavian artery *(straight arrow)* in longitudinal **(A)** and transverse **(B)** views. The pleura *(open arrow)* causes the mirror image *(curved arrow)*. The diagram in Figure 8-29, *D* shows how this artifact occurs. (See Color Plate 35.)

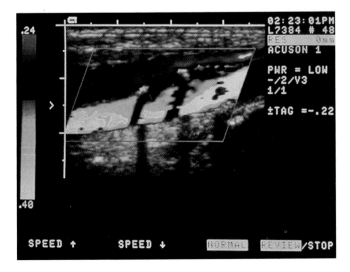

■ **FIGURE 8-37**   Shadowing from calcified plaque follows the gray-scale scan lines straight down while following the angled color scan lines parallel to the sides of the parallelogram. (See Color Plate 36.) (From Kremkau FW: Principles and instrumentation. In Merritt CRB, editor: *Doppler color imaging*, New York, 1992, Churchill Livingstone.)

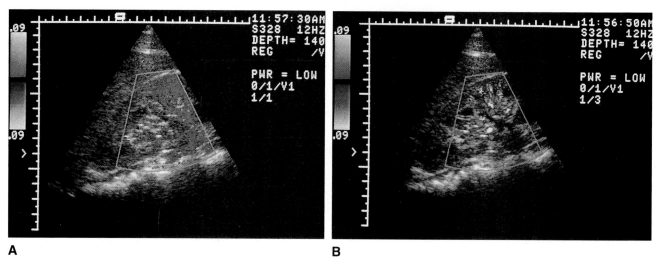

A   **B**

■ **FIGURE 8-38**   **A,** Clutter from tissue motion (caused by respiration) obscures underlying blood flow in the renal vasculature. **B,** An increased wall filter setting removes the clutter revealing the underlying flow. (See Color Plate 37.)

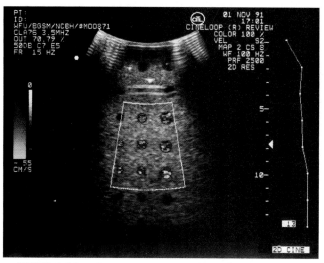

■ **FIGURE 8-39**   Color appears in echo-free (cystic) regions of a tissue-equivalent phantom. The color gain has been increased sufficiently to produce this effect. The instrument tends to write color information preferentially in areas where non–Doppler-shifted echoes are weak or absent. (See Color Plate 36.) (From Kremkau FW: Principles and pitfalls of real-time color-flow imaging. In Bernstein EF, editor: *Vascular diagnosis,* ed 4, St Louis, 1993, Mosby.)

TABLE 8-3   Artifacts and Their Causes

Artifact	Cause
Axial resolution	Pulse length
Comet tail	Reverberation
Grating lobe	Grating lobe
Lateral resolution	Pulse width
Mirror image	Multiple reflection
Refraction	Refraction
Reverberation	Multiple reflection
Ring down	Resonance
Section thickness	Pulse width
Speckle	Interference
Speed error	Speed error
Range ambiguity	High pulse repetition frequency
Shadowing	High attenuation
Edge shadowing	Refraction or interference
Enhancement	Low attenuation
Focal enhancement	Focusing
Aliasing	Low pulse repetition frequency
Spectrum mirror	High Doppler gain

This chapter has discussed several ultrasound imaging and flow artifacts, all of which are listed in Table 8-3, along with their causes. In some cases the names of the artifacts are identical to their causes. Shadowing and enhancement are useful in interpretation and diagnosis. Other artifacts can cause confusion and error. Artifacts seen in two-dimensional imaging are evidenced in three-dimensional imaging also, some-times in unusual ways.[59] All of these artifacts can hinder proper interpretation and diagnosis and so must be avoided or handled properly when encountered. A proper understanding of artifacts and how to deal with them when they are encountered enables sonographers and sonologists to use them to advantage while avoiding the pitfalls that they can cause.

REVIEW

The key points presented in this chapter are the following:

■ Axial resolution is determined by spatial pulse length.
■ Lateral resolution is determined by beam width.
■ The beam width perpendicular to the scan plane causes section thickness artifacts.
■ Apparent resolution close to the transducer is not related directly to tissue texture but is a result of interference effects from a distribution of scatterers in the tissue (speckle).
■ Reverberation produces a set of equally spaced artifactual echoes distal to the real reflector.
■ In the mirror-image artifact, objects that are present on one side of a strong reflector are displayed on the other side as well.
■ Refraction displaces echoes laterally.
■ Propagation speed error and refraction can cause objects to be displayed in improper locations or incorrect sizes or both.
■ Shadowing is caused by high-attenuation objects in the sound path.
■ Refraction also can cause edge shadowing.
■ Enhancement results from low-attenuation objects in the sound path.
■ Aliasing occurs when the Doppler shift frequency exceeds one half the PRF.
■ Aliasing can be reduced or eliminated by increasing the PRF or Doppler angle, using baseline shift, reducing operating frequency, or using a continuous wave instrument.

EXERCISES

1. The pulser of an instrument automatically reduces the pulse repetition frequency for deeper imaging to avoid the _____ _____ artifact.
2. If an echo arrives 143 μs after the pulse that produced it was emitted, it should be located at a depth of _____ cm. If a second pulse was emitted 13 μs before the arrival of this echo, it will be placed incorrectly at a depth of _____ cm.
3. If the propagation speed in a soft tissue path is 1.60 mm/μs, a diagnostic instrument assumes a propagation speed too _____ and will show reflectors too _____ the transducer.
   a. High, close to
   b. High, far from
   c. Low, close to
   d. Low, far from
4. Mirror image can occur with only one reflector. True or false?

5. The most common artifact encountered in Doppler ultrasound is
   a. aliasing.
   b. range ambiguity.
   c. spectrum mirror image.
   d. location mirror image.
   e. electromagnetic interference.
6. Which of the following can reduce or eliminate aliasing?
   a. Increased pulse repetition frequency
   b. Increased Doppler angle
   c. Increased operating frequency
   d. Use of continuous wave mode
   e. More than one of the above
7. The fine texture in the region near the transducer indicates the excellent resolution that actually exists in that region. True or false?
8. The fact that a beam, as it scans through tissue, has some nonzero width perpendicular to the scan plane results in the _____ artifact.
9. Which of the following can cause improper location of objects on a display? (more than one correct answer)
   a. Shadowing
   b. Enhancement
   c. Speed error
   d. Mirror image
   e. Refraction
   f. Grating lobe
10. Refraction can cause shadowing. True or false?
11. The transducer face is one of the reflectors involved in reverberations in which illustration, Figure 8-40, A or B?
12. Match these artifact causes with their result:
    a. Reverberation: _____
    b. Shadowing: _____, _____
    c. Enhancement: _____
    d. Propagation speed error: _____, _____
    e. Refraction: _____, _____
    1. Unreal structure displayed
    2. Structure missing on the display
    3. Structure displayed with improper brightness
    4. Structure improperly positioned
    5. Structure improperly shaped
13. Reverberation results in added reflectors being imaged with equal _____.
14. In reverberation, subsequent reflections are _____ than previous ones.
15. Enhancement is caused by a
    a. strongly reflecting structure.
    b. weakly attenuating structure.
    c. strongly attenuating structure.

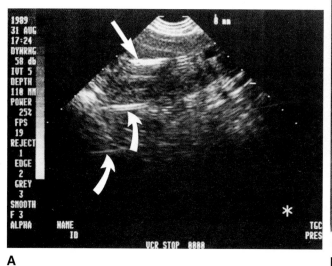

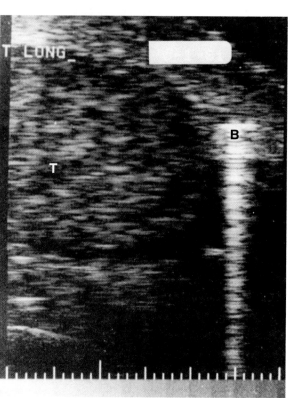

A
B

■ **FIGURE 8-40** **A** and **B,** Illustrations to accompany Exercise 11.

d. refracting boundary.

e. propagation speed error.

16. Which of the following can decrease or eliminate aliasing?
   a. Decreased pulse repetition frequency
   b. Decreased Doppler angle
   c. Increased operating frequency
   d. Baseline shifting
   e. More than one of the above

17. Shadowing results in decreased echo amplitudes. True or false?

18. Propagation speed error results in improper _____ position of a reflector on the display.
   a. Lateral
   b. Axial

19. To avoid aliasing, a signal voltage must be sampled at least _____ time(s) per cycle.
   a. 1
   b. 2
   c. 3
   d. 4
   e. 5

20. If the highest Doppler-shift frequency present in a signal exceeds _____ the pulse repetition frequency, aliasing will occur.
   a. One tenth
   b. One half

   c. 2 times
   d. 5 times
   e. 10 times

21. When Doppler gain is set too high, which artifact is likely to occur?
   a. Aliasing
   b. Range ambiguity
   c. Spectrum mirror image
   d. Location mirror image
   e. Speckle

22. Which artifact should be suspected if one observes twin gestational sacs when scanning through the rectus abdominis muscle?

23. Range ambiguity can occur in which of the following?
   a. Imaging instruments
   b. Duplex instruments
   c. Pulsed wave Doppler instruments
   d. Color flow instruments
   e. All of the above

24. If the pulse repetition frequency is 4 kHz, which of the following Doppler shifts will cause aliasing?
   a. 1 kHz
   b. 2 kHz
   c. 3 kHz
   d. 4 kHz
   e. More than one of the above

25. If the pulse repetition frequency is 10 kHz, which of the following Doppler shifts will cause aliasing?
    a. 1 kHz
    b. 2 kHz
    c. 3 kHz
    d. 4 kHz
    e. None of the above
26. There is no problem with aliasing as long as the Doppler shifts are _____ half the pulse repetition frequency.
    a. Less than
    b. Approximately equal to
    c. Greater than
    d. All of the above
    e. None of the above
27. If Doppler shift is 2.6 kHz, no aliasing would result with a pulse repetition frequency of 10 kHz. True or false?
28. If there were a problem in Exercise 27, _____ Doppler ultrasound could be used to avoid it.
29. If red represents a positive Doppler shift and blue represents a negative one, what color is seen for normal flow toward the transducer? What color is seen for aliasing flow toward the transducer? What colors are seen for normal flow away and for aliasing flow away from the transducer?
30. When a pulse is emitted before all the echoes from the previous pulse have been received, which artifact occurs?
31. When a strong reflector is located in the scan plane, which of the following artifacts is likely to occur?
    a. Aliasing
    b. Range ambiguity
    c. Spectrum mirror image
    d. Location mirror image
    e. Speckle
32. Increasing pulse repetition frequency to avoid aliasing can cause the following:
    a. Baseline shift
    b. Range ambiguity
    c. Spectrum mirror image
    d. Location mirror image
    e. Speckle
33. Which of the following decreases the likelihood of range-ambiguity artifact?
    a. Decreasing operating frequency
    b. Decreasing pulse repetition frequency
    c. Decreasing Doppler angle
    d. Baseline shift
    e. Increasing pulser output
34. Range ambiguity produces which error in spectral Doppler studies?
    a. Incorrect spectral peaks
    b. Incorrect gate location
    c. Intensity too high

d. Intensity too low
e. All of the above
35. Range ambiguity produces which error in anatomic imaging?
    a. Range too long
    b. Range too short
    c. Intensity too high
    d. Doppler shift too high
    e. Doppler shift too low
36. If a pulse is emitted 65 μs after the previous one, echoes returning from beyond _____ cm will produce range ambiguity.
    a. 1
    b. 2
    c. 3
    d. 4
    e. 5
37. If the maximum imaging depth is 5 cm, the frequency is 2 MHz, and the Doppler angle is zero, what is the maximum flow speed that will avoid aliasing and range ambiguity?
    a. 100 cm/s
    b. 200 cm/s
    c. 300 cm/s
    d. 400 cm/s
    e. 500 cm/s
38. Does solving aliasing by decreasing operating frequency increase the possibility of range-ambiguity artifact?
39. If operating frequency is increased to decrease the possibility of range ambiguity (by increasing attenuation), does the possibility of aliasing increase?
40. If a pulsed wave Doppler sample volume is located at a depth of 8 cm, the sampled echoes arrive at what time following the emission of the pulse?
    a. 25 μs
    b. 50 μs
    c. 75 μs
    d. 104 μs
    e. 117 μs
41. In Exercise 40, if the pulse repetition frequency is set at 11 kHz, a second gate would be located at what depth?
    a. 1 cm
    b. 2 cm
    c. 3 cm
    d. 4 cm
    e. 5 cm
42. Connect the dots (samples) in Figure 8-41 to determine the Doppler shift frequency. How many cycles are in each example?
    a. _____
    b. _____
    c. _____
    d. _____
    e. _____

43. The frequencies that were sampled in Exercise 42 are shown in Figure 8-42. In which example(s) has aliasing occurred?

44. Which of the following instruments can produce aliasing?

a. Continuous wave Doppler
b. Pulsed wave Doppler
c. Duplex
d. Color flow
e. More than one of the above

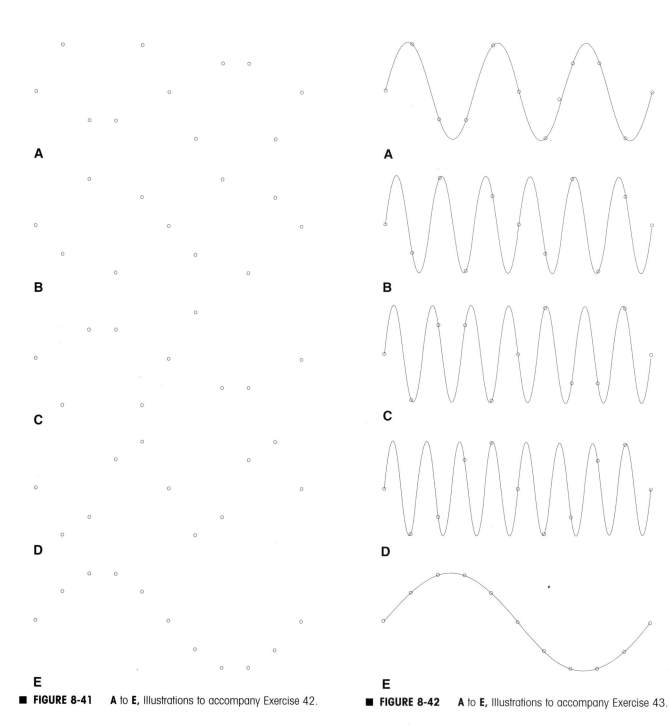

■ FIGURE 8-41 **A** to **E**, Illustrations to accompany Exercise 42.

■ FIGURE 8-42 **A** to **E**, Illustrations to accompany Exercise 43.

45. In Figure 8-43 the solid line shows the Doppler shift and the dots are the samples. The dashed line shows the _____ result. To avoid aliasing in this signal, at least _____ samples would be required.

46. In Figure 8-44 (*R*, red; *B*, blue), assume the color bar shown in *G* and give the direction of blood flow (*R* for from right to the left; *L* for from left to the right) in each case.

47. Figure 8-45 (Color Plate 38) shows five regions of different colors in the flow. Match each of the following with the proper region.

    a. _____   1. 90-degree Doppler angle
    b. _____   2. Unaliased flow toward
    c. _____   3. Unaliased flow away
    d. _____   4. Aliased flow toward
    e. _____   5. Aliased flow away

48. Which part of Figure 8-46 (Color Plates 39 and 40) shows a Doppler-power display?

49. Referring to Figure 8-46, *B*, *C*, and *D* (Color Plates 39 and 40), what is the order of figure parts when they are arranged according to increasing flow speed?

50. What artifact appears in all parts of Figure 8-46 (Color Plates 39 and 40)? What is the additional artifact that appears in Figure 8-46, *D*?

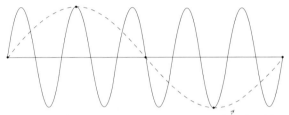

■ **FIGURE 8-43**   Illustration to accompany Exercise 45.

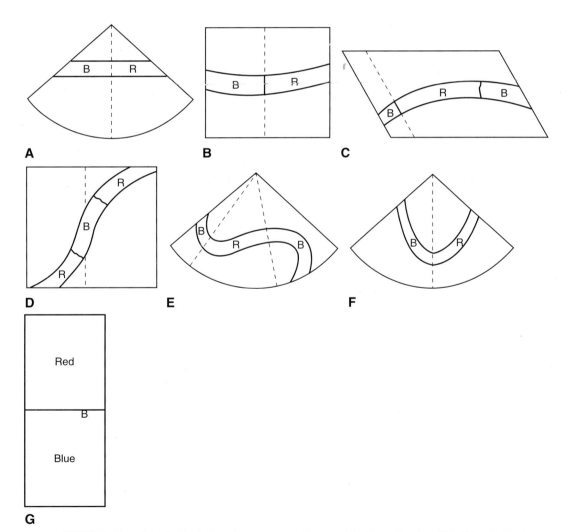

■ **FIGURE 8-44**   **A** to **G**, Illustrations to accompany Exercise 46. (From Kremkau FW: *J Vasc Technol* 18:365-366, 1994.)

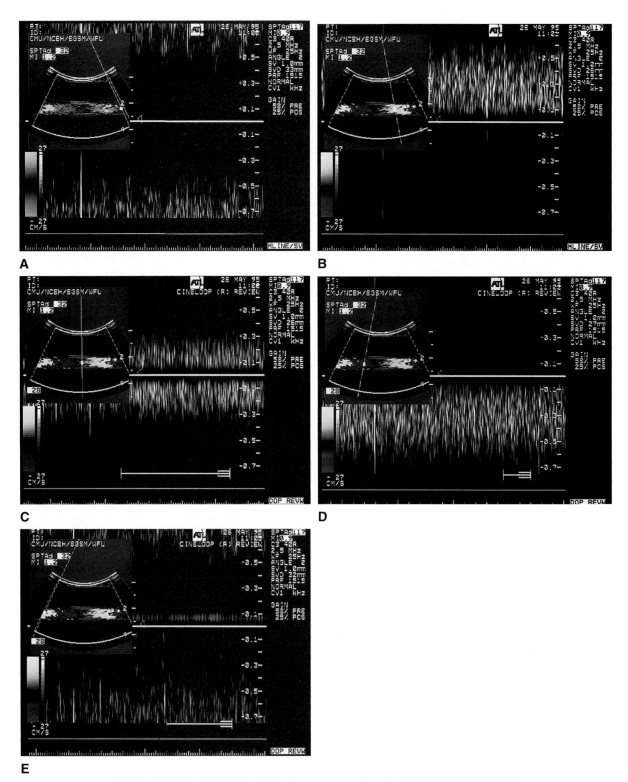

■ **FIGURE 8-45** **A** to **E,** Illustrations to accompany Exercise 47. (See Color Plate 38.)

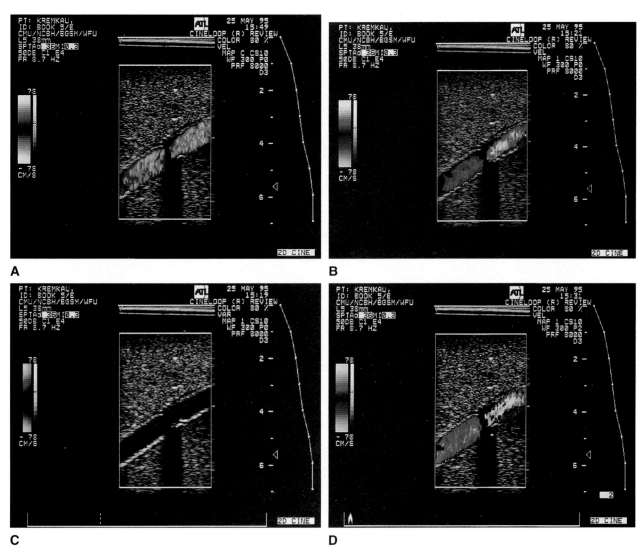

■ **FIGURE 8-46** **A** to **D**, Illustrations to accompany Exercises 48 to 50. (See Color Plates 39 and 40.)

Performance and Safety

LEARNING OBJECTIVES

After reading this chapter, the student should be able to do the following:

- Explain how to determine whether a sonographic or Doppler instrument is working properly.
- List the devices that are available for testing various performance characteristics of instruments.
- Compare a test object and a phantom.
- Describe how instrument output is measured.
- List typical instrument output values.
- Explain what is known about bioeffects in cells, animals, and human beings.
- Describe what is known regarding risk in the use of sonography or Doppler ultrasound.
- Explain how an operator of an ultrasound instrument can implement the ALARA principle by minimizing exposure of the patient to ultrasound during diagnostic scanning.

KEY TERMS

The following terms are introduced in this chapter:

ALARA	Mechanical index	Radiation force
Cavitation	Phantom	Test object
Hydrophone	Polyvinylidene fluoride	Thermal index

Several devices (Figure 9-1) are available for determining whether sonographic and Doppler ultrasound instruments are operating correctly and consistently. These devices are considered in two groups: (1) those that test the operation of the instrument (anatomic imaging and flow evaluation performance) and (2) those that measure the acoustic output of the instrument. Group 1 takes into account the operation of the entire instrument. Group 2 considers only the beam former and the transducer acting together as a source of ultrasound. Imaging and Doppler performance are important for evaluating the instrument as a diagnostic tool. The acoustic output of an instrument is important when considering bioeffects and safety.

Bioeffects are useful in therapeutic applications of ultrasound,[60-64] a subject not considered in this book.

Of interest here is what the known bioeffects of ultrasound suggest about the safety or risk of diagnostic ultrasound. We desire knowledge about the probability of damage or injury and under what conditions this probability is maximized (to avoid those conditions) or minimized (to seek those conditions while obtaining useful diagnostic information).

PERFORMANCE MEASUREMENTS

Imaging performance.[65-67] is determined by measuring primarily the following parameters:

- Detail resolution
- Contrast resolution
- Penetration and dynamic range

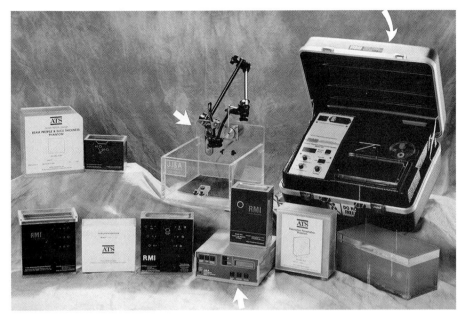

■ **FIGURE 9-1** Several test objects and phantoms. Those intended for Doppler applications are indicated by the arrows. The other devices are used to evaluate sonographic instruments.

■ Time gain compensation operation
■ Accuracy of depth and distance measurement

Several devices are commercially available for testing imaging performance.[68] These devices fall into two categories: tissue-equivalent **phantoms** and **test objects.** Tissue-equivalent phantoms have some characteristics representative of tissues (such as scattering and attenuation properties); test objects do not. Some devices are combinations of the two (e.g., tissue-equivalent phantoms containing resolution targets). Phantoms and test objects can be used not only by service personnel but also by instrument operators. The American College of Radiology Ultrasound Accreditation Program requires that routine quality control testing must occur regularly; a minimum requirement is semiannually. The American Institute of Ultrasound in Medicine (AIUM) Practice Accreditation requires that equipment maintenance and calibration be regularly performed on all ultrasound equipment.

Gray-Scale Test Objects and Tissue-Equivalent Phantoms

Tissue-equivalent phantoms are made of graphite-filled aqueous gels or urethane rubber materials. The graphite particles act as the ultrasound scatterers (echo producers) in the materials. Graphite is the soft carbon that is used in pencils and as a lubricant. Attenuation in these materials is similar to that for soft tissue, and propagation speed is 1.54 mm/μs in the gels and 1.45 mm/μs in the rubber. Compensation for the latter speed error

is accomplished by positioning targets in the rubber material to closer locations. However, errors still can occur because of the speed error. Tissue-equivalent phantoms typically contain echo-free (cystic) regions of various diameters and thin nylon lines (about 0.2 mm in diameter) for measuring detail resolution and distance accuracy.[68] Some phantoms contain cones or cylinders containing material of various scattering strengths (various graphite concentrations) that are hyperechoic or hypoechoic compared with the surrounding material. Figures 9-2 to 9-8 give examples of several phantoms.

Tissue-equivalent phantoms simulate tissue properties, allowing assessment of detail and contrast resolutions, penetration, dynamic range, and time gain compensation operation.

Test objects do not simulate tissue characteristics but do provide some specific measure of instrument performance. The beam-profile slice-thickness test object (Figure 9-9) contains a thin, scattering layer in an echo-free material. The object can be used to show beam width in the scan plane or perpendicular to it (section thickness).

Test objects contain nylon lines and scattering layers to allow evaluation of detail resolution and beam profiles.

Text continued on p. 315.

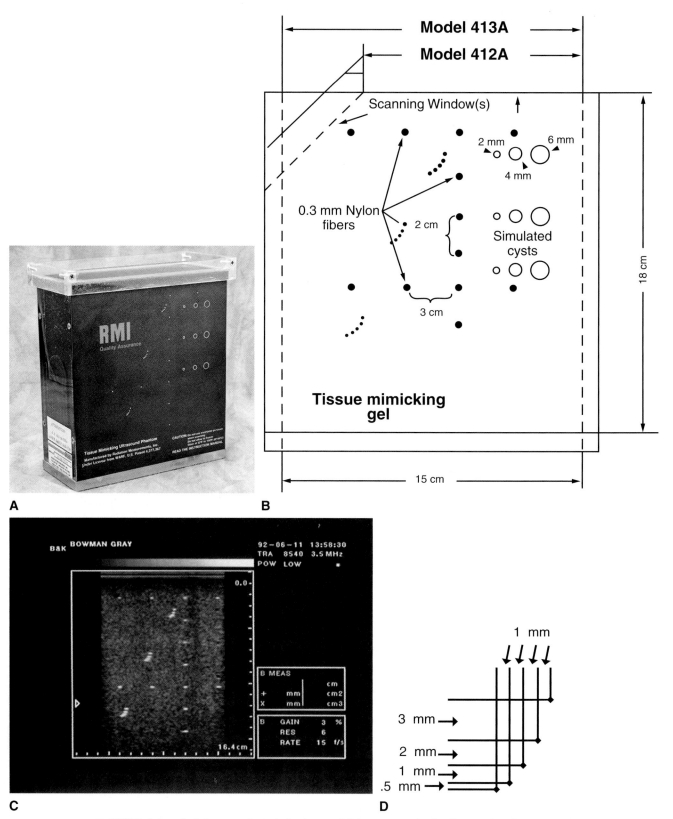

■ FIGURE 9-2 **A,** A tissue-equivalent phantom containing groups of nylon lines and cystic regions of various sizes. **B,** Diagram detailing the construction of such a phantom. **C,** Scan of a phantom. **D,** Arrangement of the axial resolution line set in this phantom and in that pictured in Figure 9-3. This set was used in Figure 3-30, *D* to *F,* to illustrate axial resolution at three frequencies.

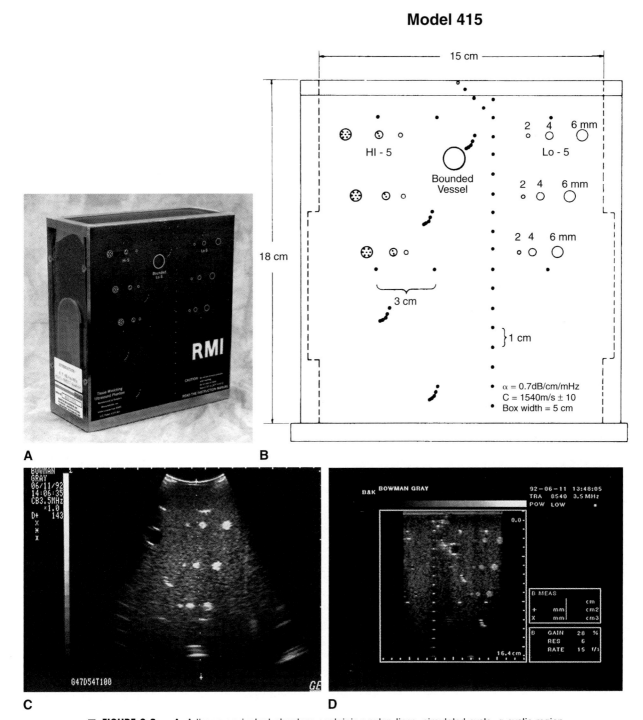

■ **FIGURE 9-3**   **A,** A tissue-equivalent phantom containing nylon lines, simulated cysts, a cystic region with an echogenic rim (simulated bounded vessel), and hyperechoic simulated lesions of various sizes. **B,** Diagram detailing the construction of such a phantom. **C** and **D,** Scans of phantom.

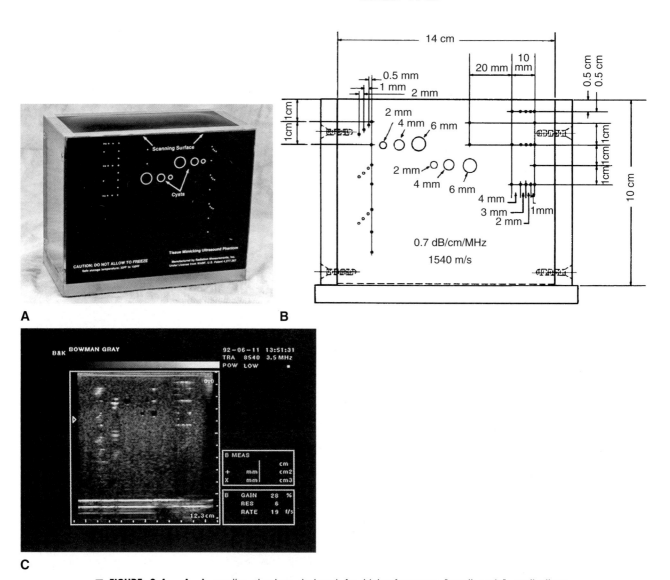

■ **FIGURE 9-4** **A,** A smaller phantom designed for higher-frequency "small parts" applications. **B,** Diagram detailing the construction of such a phantom. **C,** Scan of phantom.

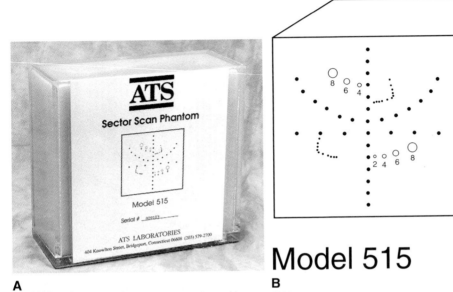

Model 515

A

B

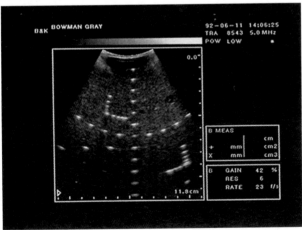

C

■ **FIGURE 9-5** **A,** A phantom designed for sector scan applications. **B,** Diagram detailing the construction of such a phantom. **C,** Scan of phantom.

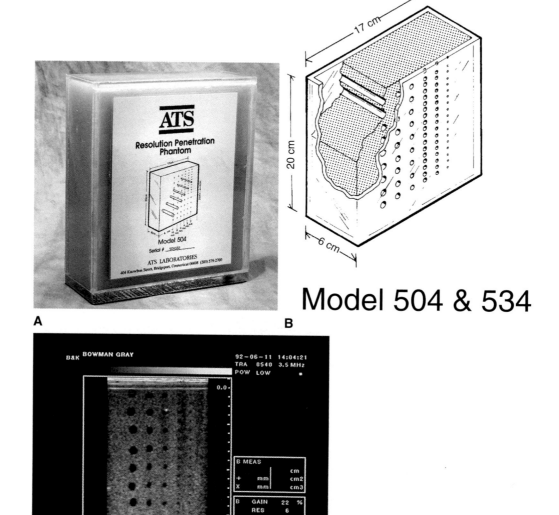

Model 504 & 534

■ **FIGURE 9-6** **A,** A resolution penetration phantom that contains columns of simulated cysts of various sizes. **B,** Diagram detailing the construction of such a phantom. **C,** Scan of phantom. This phantom was used to illustrate resolution and penetration at two frequencies in Figure 3-35.

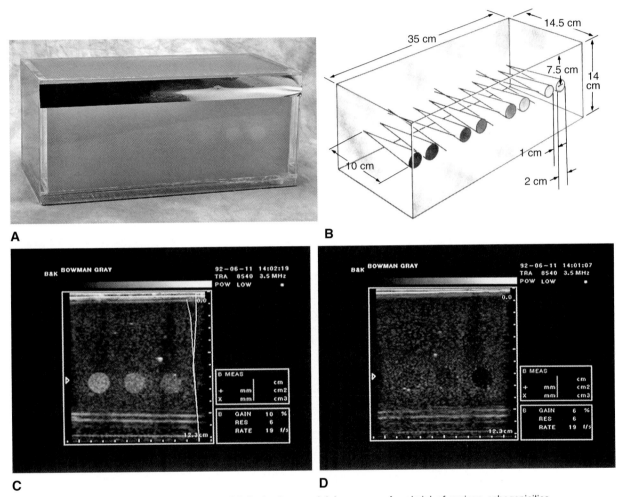

A   **B**

C   **D**

■ **FIGURE 9-7**   **A,** A contrast-detail phantom containing cones of material of various echogenicities.
B, Diagram detailing the construction of such a phantom. **C,** Scan of hyperechoic sections of phantom.
D, Scan of hypoechoic sections of phantom.

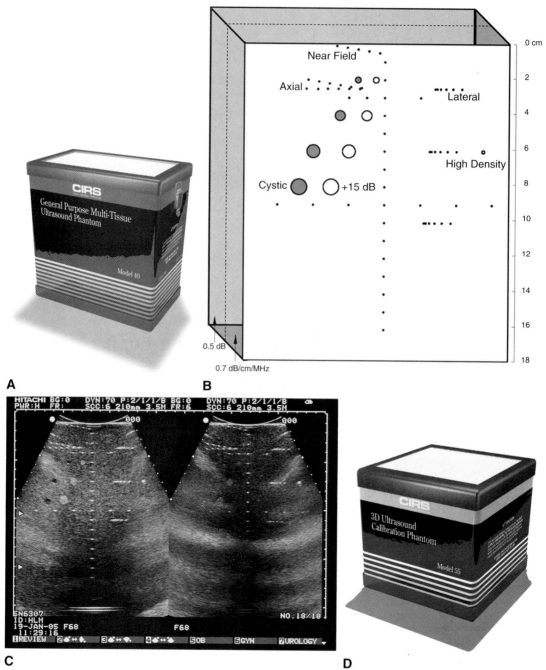

■ FIGURE 9-8   A, General purpose phantom with two background tissue materials (0.5 and 0.7 dB/cm-MHz). **B,** Construction diagram for the phantom in **A. C,** Image scanned with phantom in **A. D,** Three-dimensional calibration phantom for the assessment of volumetric measurement accuracy.

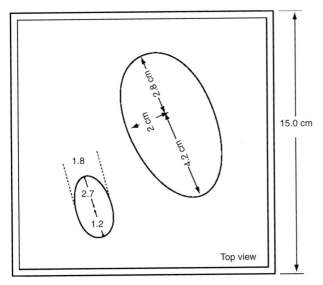

Top scanning window

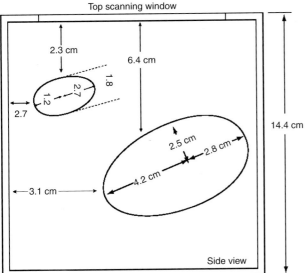

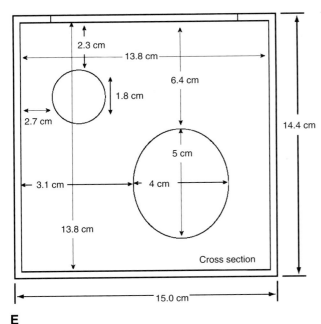

■ FIGURE 9-8, cont'd **E,** Construction diagram for **D.**

Continued.

Doppler Test Objects and Tissue-Equivalent Phantoms

Test objects and tissue- and blood-mimicking phantoms are commercially available for the evaluation of Doppler instruments (Figures 9-10 and 9-11 [Color Plate 29]). These objects are useful for testing the effective penetration of the Doppler beam, the ability to discriminate between different flow directions, the accuracy of sample volume location, and the accuracy of the measured flow speed.[69] Doppler flow phantoms use a flowing blood-mimicking liquid. Doppler test objects use a moving solid object (usually a string) for scattering the ultrasound. They can be calibrated easily and can produce pulsatile and reverse motions.

Phantoms have some disadvantages, such as the presence of bubbles and nonuniform flow, but can simulate clinical conditions easily, such as tissue attenuation (Figure 9-11). These phantoms can be calibrated with an electromagnetic flow meter or by fluid volume collection over time. Figures 7-9, *B,* and 7-9, *C,* illustrate the use of a string test object in the evaluation of Doppler angle correction. Figures 8-30, *A,* and 8-30, *B,* show the use of a string test object in evaluating spectral mirror image. Figure 7-12 illustrates the use of a flow phantom in determining the accuracy of the gate location indicator on the anatomic display. Figure 6-15 shows the use of a flow phantom to illustrate the effect of Doppler angle on Doppler shift. Figure 8-35 illustrates the evaluation of aliasing, Nyquist limit, baseline shifting, and wall filter operation using a flow phantom.

> *Doppler test objects and flow phantoms enable evaluation of spectral calibration and gate location and penetration of spectral and color Doppler instruments.*

OUTPUT MEASUREMENTS

Several devices can measure the acoustic output of ultrasound instruments. These devices normally are used by engineers and physicists rather than by instrument operators. Only the **hydrophone** is discussed here. The hydrophone sometimes is called a microprobe. The hydrophone is used in two forms (Figure 9-12): (1) a small transducer element (with a diameter of 1 mm or less) mounted on the end of a hollow needle, or (2) a large piezoelectric membrane with small metallic electrodes centered on both sides. The membrane is made of **polyvinylidene fluoride** (PVDF). Polyvinylidene fluoride is used in both types of hydrophones because of its wide bandwidth. Various construction approaches are used for hydrophones,[70-74] but these are not considered here. Hydrophones receive sound reasonably

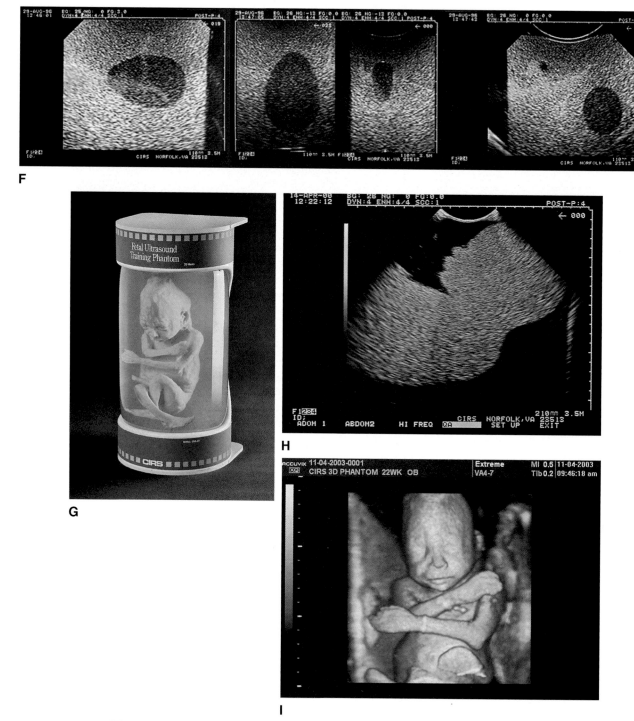

■ **FIGURE 9-8, cont'd**   **F,** Image obtained by scanning **D. G,** Fetal-training phantom. **H,** Two-dimensional image from **G. I,** Three-dimensional image from **G.**

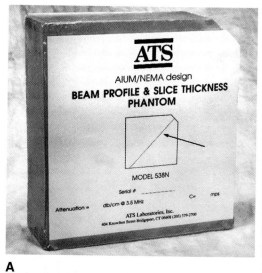

A

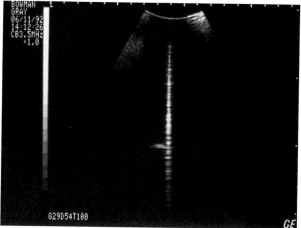

B

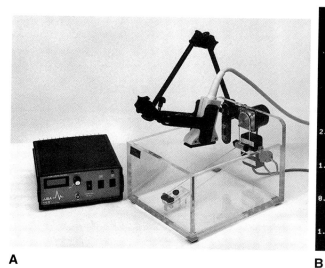

C

■ **FIGURE 9-9** **A,** A beam profile and section thickness test object. It contains a thin, scattering layer *(arrow)* in an anechoic material. **B** and **C,** Scans of beam profiles. Shown in Figure 3-23, *D, E,* and *F* are beam profiles obtained using this test object.

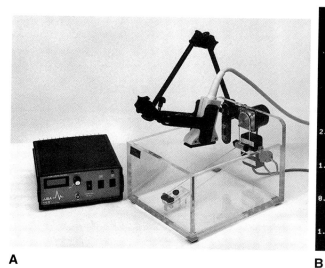

A

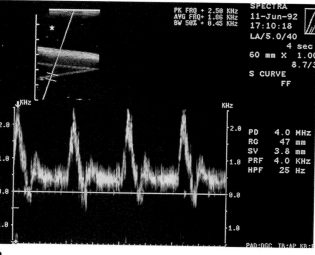

B

■ **FIGURE 9-10** **A,** A moving-string test object and controller. **B,** Spectral display of a moving string (operating in pulsatile mode).

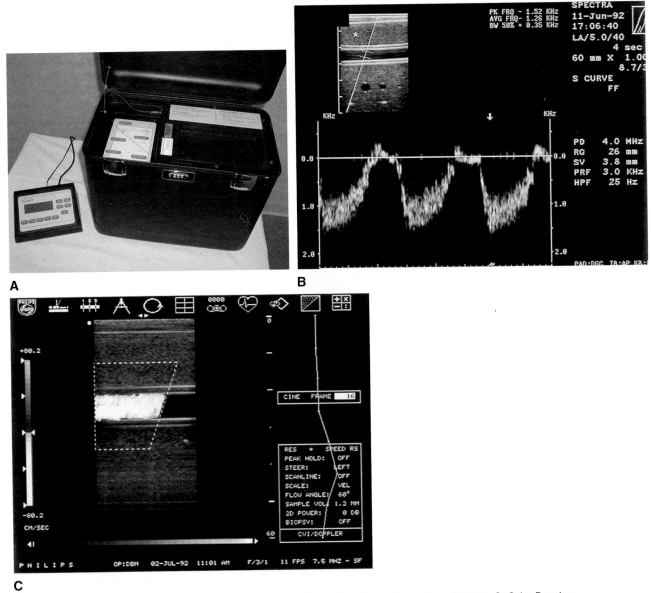

■ **FIGURE 9-11**   **A,** Doppler flow phantom. **B,** Spectral display from a flow phantom. **C,** Color Doppler image from a flow phantom. (See Color Plate 29.)

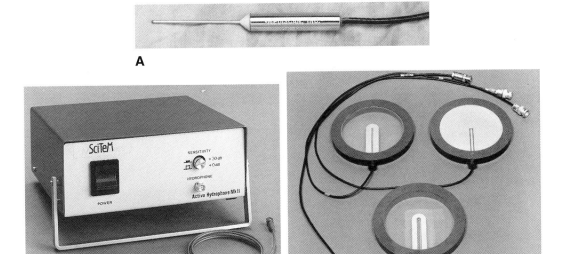

■ **FIGURE 9-12** A hydrophone consists of a small transducer element mounted on the end of a needle (**A** and **B**) or a thin membrane with metal electrodes (**C**). (Courtesy Crown Copyright—The National Physical Laboratory, United Kingdom.)

well from all directions without altering the sound by their presence. In response to the varying pressure of the sound, they produce a varying voltage that can be displayed on an oscilloscope. A picture similar to that in Figure 2-15, *A*, is produced, from which period, pulse repetition period, and pulse duration can be determined. From these quantities, frequency, pulse repetition frequency, and duty factor can be calculated. Using the hydrophone calibration (relationship between the voltage and the acoustic pressure), pressure amplitude also may be determined. In addition, wavelength, spatial pulse length, and intensities also can be calculated. Figure 9-13 shows an array hydrophone system.

Using hydrophones, acoustic pressure output levels have been measured, and intensities and output indexes have been calculated for various diagnostic ultrasound instruments and transducers.[75-78] Figures 9-14 and 9-15 provide summaries of the data from several sources. Generally, sonographic outputs are lowest and pulsed spectral Doppler outputs are highest, with M mode and color Doppler imaging outputs falling between the two. These data will be compared with bioeffects data later in this chapter.

Needle and membrane hydrophones are used to measure pressure amplitude and period, from which several other acoustic pulse parameters can be calculated.

Testing of the functionality of individual transducer elements is possible with an automated probe tester (Figure 9-16).

BIOEFFECTS

The biological effects and safety of diagnostic ultrasound have received considerable attention over the past few years. Several review articles, textbooks, and institutional documents (Figure 9-17) have been published.[79-92] In the remainder of this chapter, we review knowledge regarding bioeffects in cells, plants, and experimental animals, mechanisms of interaction between ultrasound and biological cells and tissues, regulatory activities, epidemiology, risk and safety considerations, and elements of prudent practice.

As with any diagnostic test, there may be some risk, such as some probability of damage or injury with the use of diagnostic ultrasound. This risk, if known, must be weighed against benefit to determine the appropriateness of the diagnostic procedure. Knowledge of how to minimize the risk, even if it is unidentified, is useful to everyone involved in diagnostic ultrasound. Sources of information used in developing policy regarding the use of diagnostic ultrasound are diagrammed in Figure 9-18, *A*. These sources include bioeffects data from experimental systems, output data from diagnostic instruments, and knowledge and experience regarding how the diagnostic information obtained is of benefit

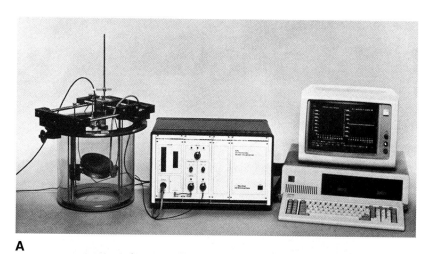

A

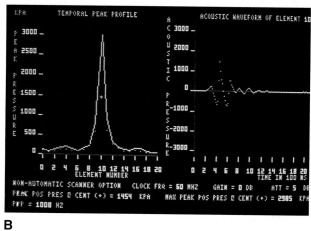

B

■ **FIGURE 9-13**   Linear array membrane hydrophone system **(A)** for measuring pulse waveform and bandwidth **(B)**.

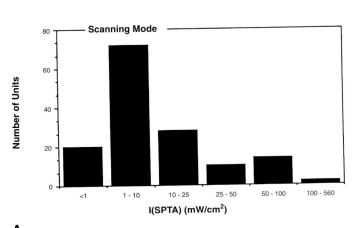

A

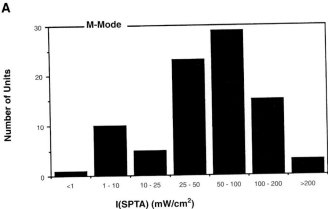

B

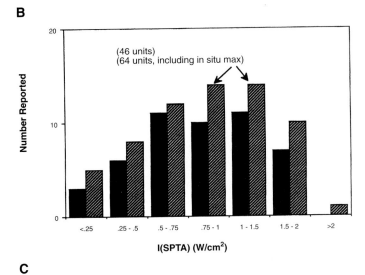

C

■ **FIGURE 9-14** Histograms showing the spatial peak–temporal average (*SPTA*) intensities (*I*) reported by manufacturers participating in the American Institute of Ultrasound in Medicine commendation process for imaging mode **(A)**, M mode **(B)**, and pulsed Doppler **(C)**. (From Ide M, Zagzebski JA, Duck FA: *Ultrasound Med Biol* 15(suppl 1):47-65. Copyright 1989, Pergamon Press, Ltd.)

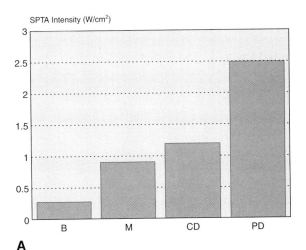

A

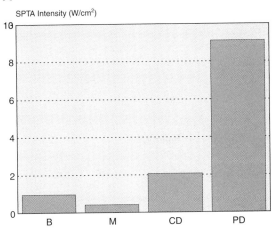

B

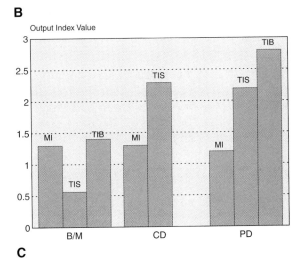

C

■ **FIGURE 9-15** Maximum spatial peak–temporal average (*SPTA*) intensity values found in equipment surveys reported in reference 77 **(A)** and reference 78 **(B).** *B*, B mode; *M*, M mode; *CD*, color Doppler imaging; *PD*, pulsed spectral Doppler. **C,** Maximum mechanical index (*MI*), soft tissue thermal index (*TIS*), and bone thermal index (*TIB*) values found in the equipment survey reported in reference 77. These indexes are discussed later in this chapter. *B*, B mode; *M*, M mode; *CD*, color Doppler imaging; *PD*, pulsed spectral Doppler.

in patient management. Comparison of the first two components allows an assessment of risk, whereas the combination of the latter two components yields an awareness of benefit. It seems reasonable to assume that there is some risk (however small) in the use of diagnostic ultrasound because ultrasound is a form of energy and has at least the potential to produce a biological effect that could constitute risk. Even if this risk is so minimal that it is difficult to identify, prudent practice dictates that routine measures be implemented to minimize the risk while obtaining the necessary information to achieve the diagnostic benefit. This is the **ALARA** (as low as reasonably achievable) principle of prudent scanning.

Our knowledge of bioeffects resulting from ultrasound exposure comes from several sources (Figure 9-18, *B*). These sources include experimental observations in cell suspensions and cultures, plants, and experimental animals; epidemiologic studies in human beings; and studies of interaction mechanisms, such as heating and **cavitation.**

Knowledge of bioeffects is important for the safe and prudent use of sonography.

Cells

Illustrative of end points studied with ultrasound exposure of cells is sister-chromatid exchange (Figure 9-19). Over a 10-year period, about two dozen reports were published on this subject. Most studies yielded negative results; a few reported positive results. Of importance is the fact that there is no independent confirmation of a published positive effect. Attempts to do so have led to the conclusion that the cause for small but statistically significant effects is unknown. It seems clear, however, that the ultrasound exposure does not produce increased exchanges or the effect is not reproducible and is too small to be produced consistently.[93]

Because cells in suspension or in culture are so different from those in the intact patient in a clinical environment, one must exercise restraint in extrapolating in vitro results to clinical significance. Cellular studies are useful in determining mechanisms of interaction and guiding the design of experimental animal studies and epidemiologic studies. The AIUM[92] approved the following statement on in vitro biological effects in 1997:

It is often difficult to evaluate reports of ultrasonically induced in vitro biological effects with respect to their

clinical significance. The predominant physical and biological interactions and mechanisms involved in an in vitro effect may not pertain to the in vivo situation. Nevertheless, an in vitro effect must be regarded as a real biological effect.

Results from in vitro experiments suggest new endpoints and serve as a basis for design of in vivo experiments. In vitro studies provide the capability to control experimental variables and thus offer a means to explore and evaluate specific mechanisms. Although they may have limited applicability to in vivo biological effects, such studies can disclose fundamental intercellular or intracellular interactions.

While it is valid for authors to place their results in context and to suggest further relevant investigations, reports which do more than that should be viewed with caution.

Studies of the effects of ultrasound on cells in culture or suspension are useful for identifying cellular effects and mechanisms of action. They should not be used directly for risk assessment in clinical scanning.

Plants

The primary components of plant tissues—stems, leaves, and roots—contain gas-filled channels between the cell walls. Plants thus have served as useful biological models for studying the effects of cavitation.[94]

Through this mechanism, normal cellular organization and function can be disturbed. Irreversible effects appear to be limited to cell death. Reversible effects include chromosomal abnormalities, mitotic index reductions, and growth-rate reduction. Membrane damage induced by microstreaming shear stress appears to be the cause of cell death in leaves. Intensity thresholds for lysis

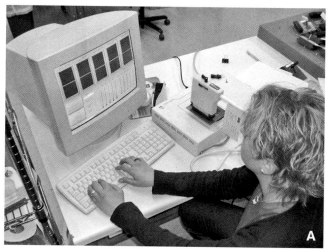

■ **FIGURE 9-16** **A,** System for testing individual elements in a transducer array.

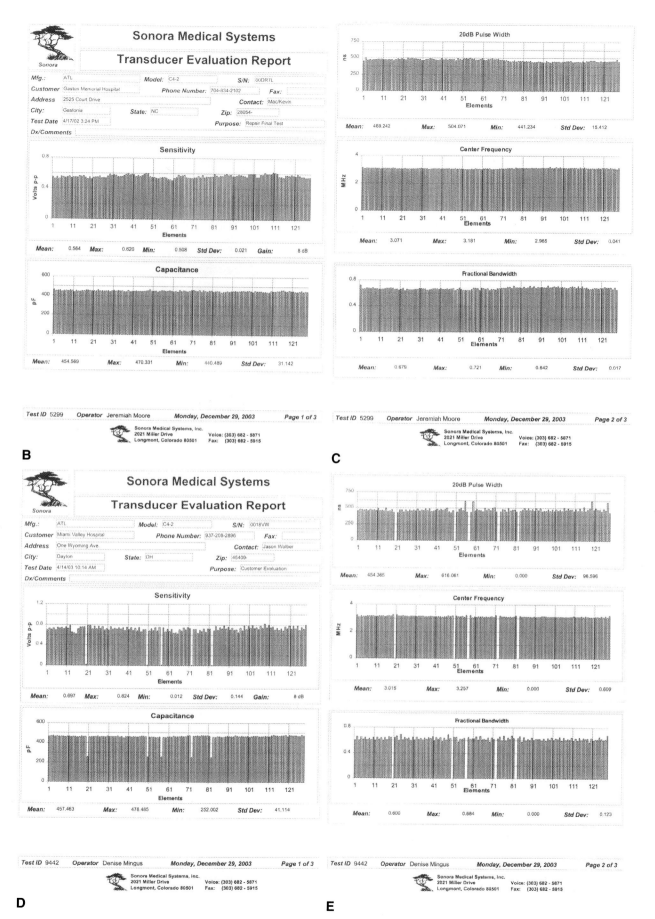

■ **FIGURE 9-16, cont'd** **B** and **C,** Test results for a transducer that is functioning properly. **D** and **E,** Test results for a transducer that has five failed elements.

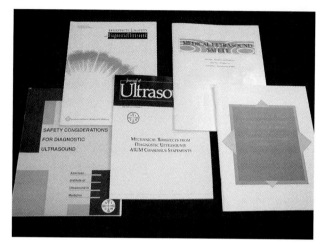

■ **FIGURE 9-17** Publications on safety from the American Institute of Ultrasound in Medicine.[82-85,95]

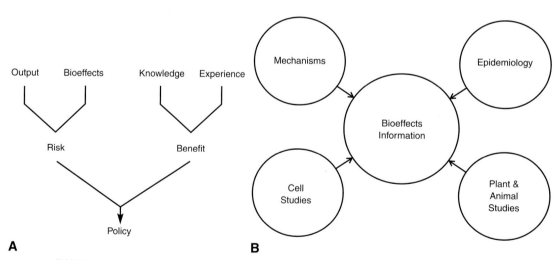

A   **B**

■ **FIGURE 9-18** **A,** Ultrasound risk and benefit information. Risk information comes from experimental bioeffects (including epidemiology) and instrument output data. Benefit information is derived from knowledge and experience in diagnostic ultrasound use and efficacy. Together, they lead to a policy on the prudent use of ultrasound imaging in medicine. **B,** Bioeffects information sources.

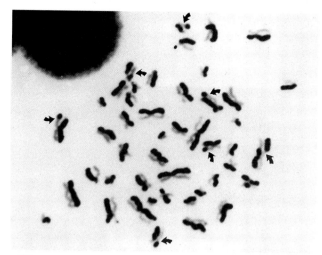

■ **FIGURE 9-19** Sister-chromatid exchange *(arrows)*. Bromodeoxyuridine-substituted, Giemsa-stained human lymphocyte metaphase. (From Kremkau FW: Biologic effects and safety. In Rumack CM, Wilson SR, Charboneau JW, editors: *Diagnostic ultrasound*, St Louis, 1991, Mosby.)

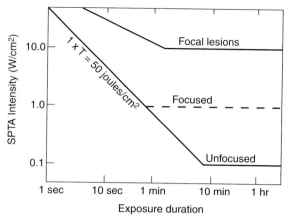

■ **FIGURE 9-20** Comparison of the minimum spatial peak–temporal average *(SPTA)* intensities required for ultrasonic bioeffects specified in the AIUM Statement on Mammalian Bioeffects. The minimum levels required for focal lesions also are shown in the figure for comparison. Note that logarithmic scaling has been used for the axes of this figure, so that the horizontal lines are separated by factors of 10 in intensity. (From American Institute of Ultrasound in Medicine: *Bioeffects and safety of diagnostic ultrasound*, Laurel, Md, 1993, The Institute.)

of leaf cells are much higher with pulsed ultrasound than with continuous wave ultrasound. Apparently, the response of bubbles within the tissues to continuous and pulsed fields is different.

Plant studies are useful primarily for understanding cavitational effects in living tissue.

Animals

With experimental animals, reported in vivo effects include fetal weight reduction, postpartum mortality, fetal abnormalities, tissue lesions, hind limb paralysis, blood flow stasis, wound repair enhancement, and tumor regression.

Many studies on fetal weight reduction in mice and rats have been performed. All rat studies and several mouse studies yielded negative results.

Focal lesion production is a well-documented bioeffect that has been observed over a wide range of intensity and exposure duration conditions (Figure 9-20).

In 1992, the AIUM[92] issued the following statement on mammalian in vivo biological effects:

Information from experiments utilizing laboratory mammals has contributed significantly to our understanding of ultrasonically induced biological effects and the mechanisms that are most likely responsible. The following statement summarizes observations relative to specific ultrasound parameters and indices. The history and rationale for this

statement are provided in *Bioeffects and Safety of Diagnostic Ultrasound*.[84]

In the low megahertz frequency range there have been no independently confirmed adverse biological effects in mammalian tissues exposed in vivo under experimental ultrasound conditions, as follows.

a. When a thermal mechanism is involved, these conditions are unfocused-beam intensities below 100 mW/cm², focused-beam intensities below 1 W/cm², or thermal index values of less than 2. Furthermore, such effects have not been reported for higher values of thermal index when it is less than $6 - \log_{10}t/0.6$ where t is exposure time ranging from 1 to 250 minutes, including off-time for pulsed exposure.

b. When a nonthermal mechanism is involved (for diagnostically relevant ultrasound exposures) in tissues that contain well-defined gas bodies, these conditions are in situ peak rarefactional pressures below approximately 0.3 MPa or mechanical index values of less than approximately 0.3. Furthermore, for other tissues no such effects have been reported.

Figure 9-20 illustrates the intensity and time relations given in part *a* of the statement. Figure 9-21 shows **thermal index** versus exposure time, as given in part *a* of the statement. Figure 9-22 presents pressure versus frequency for a **mechanical index** value of 0.3, as given in part *b* of the statement. These indexes are described in the following discussion on mechanisms.

Studies of bioeffects in experimental animals have allowed the determination of conditions under which thermal and nonthermal bioeffects occur.

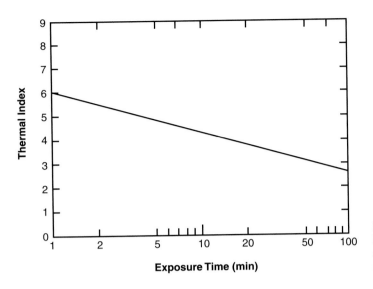

■ **FIGURE 9-21** Thermal index versus exposure time on a log-linear plot, as presented in part 1 of the AIUM statement. (From American Institute of Ultrasound in Medicine: *Bioeffects and safety of diagnostic ultrasound,* Laurel, Md, 1993, The Institute.)

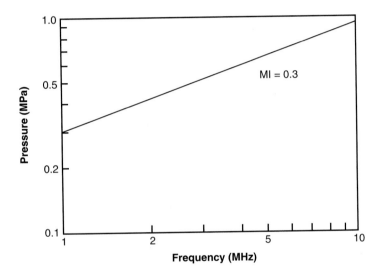

■ **FIGURE 9-22** Peak rarefactional pressure versus frequency on a log-log plot for a mechanical index of 0.3. (From American Institute of Ultrasound in Medicine: *Bioeffects and safety of diagnostic ultrasound,* Laurel, Md, 1993, The Institute.)

Mechanisms

Mechanisms of action by which ultrasound could produce biological effects can be divided into two groups: heating and mechanical. Mechanical is also called nonthermal.

Heat

Recall that attenuation in tissue is primarily due to absorption, that is, conversion of ultrasound to heat. Thus ultrasound produces a temperature rise as it propagates through tissues. The extent of the temperature rise produced depends on the applied intensity and frequency (because the absorption coefficient is approximately proportional to frequency) of sound and on the beam focusing and tissue perfusion. Heating increases as intensity or frequency is increased. For a given transducer output intensity, with increasing tissue depths, heating is decreased at higher frequencies because of the increased attenuation that reduces the intensity arriving at depth. Temperature rises are considered significant if they exceed 2° C. Intensities greater than a few hundred milliwatts per square centimeter can produce such temperature rises. Absorption coefficients are higher in bone than they are in soft tissues. Therefore bone heating, particularly in the fetus, receives special consideration.

Heating has been shown to be an important consideration in some bioeffects reports. Mathematical models have been developed for calculating temperature rises in tissues.[86,87,95] These models have been used to calculate estimated intensities required for a given temperature rise. In 1997 the AIUM[92] approved the following conclusions regarding heat:

1. Excessive temperature increase can result in toxic effects in mammalian systems. The biological effects observed depend on many factors, such as the exposure duration, the type of tissue exposed, its cellular proliferation rate, and its potential for regeneration. Age and stage of development are important factors when considering fetal and neonatal safety. Temperature increases of several degrees Celsius above the normal core range can occur naturally; there have been no significant biologic effects observed resulting from such temperature increases except when they are sustained for extended time periods.

   a. For exposure durations up to 50 hours, there have been no significant, adverse biological effects observed due to temperature increases less than or equal to 2° C above normal.

   b. For temperature increases greater than 2° C above normal, there have been no significant, adverse biological effects observed due to temperature increases less than or equal to $6 - (\log_{10} t/0.6)$ where t is the exposure duration ranging from 1 to 250 minutes. For example, for temperature increases of 4° C and 6° C, the corresponding limits for the exposure duration t are 16 min and 1 min, respectively.

   c. In general, adult tissues are more tolerant of temperature increases than fetal and neonatal tissues. Therefore, higher temperatures and/or longer exposure durations would be required for thermal damage.

2. The temperature increase during exposure of tissues to diagnostic ultrasound fields is dependent upon (a) output characteristics of the acoustic source such as frequency, source dimensions, scan rate, power, pulse repetition frequency, pulse duration, transducer self heating, exposure time and wave shape and (b) tissue properties such as attenuation, absorption, speed of sound, acoustic impedance, perfusion, thermal conductivity, thermal diffusivity, anatomical structure and nonlinearity parameter.

3. For similar exposure conditions, the expected temperature increase in bone is significantly greater than in soft tissues. For this reason, conditions where an acoustic beam impinges on ossifying fetal bone deserve special attention due to its close proximity to other developing tissues.

4. Calculations of the maximum temperature increase resulting from ultrasound exposure in vivo should not be assumed to be exact because of the uncertainties and approximations associated with the thermal, acoustic and structural characteristics of the tissues involved. However, experimental evidence shows that calculations are capable of predicting measured values within a factor of two. Thus, it appears reasonable to use calculations to obtain safety guidelines for clinical exposures where temperature measurements are not feasible. To provide a display of real-time estimates of tissue temperature increases as part of a diagnostic system, simplifying approximations are used to yield values called Thermal Indices. Under most clinically relevant conditions, the soft-tissue thermal index, TIS, and the bone thermal index, TIB, either overestimate or closely approximate the best available estimate of the maximum temperature increase (ΔT_{max}). For example, if TIS is equal to 2, then $\Delta T_{max} \leq 2° C.$*

5. The current FDA regulatory limit for $I_{SPTA.3}$ is 720 mW/cm^2. For this and lesser intensities, the best available estimate of the maximum temperature increase in the conceptus can exceed 2° C.

6. The soft-tissue thermal index, TIS, and the bone thermal index, TIB, are useful for estimating the temperature increase in vivo. For this purpose, these thermal indices are superior to any single ultrasonic field quantity, such as the derated spatial-peak, temporal-average intensity, $I_{SPTA.3}$. That is, TIS and TIB track changes in the maximum temperature increases, ΔT_{max}, thus allowing for implementation of the ALARA principle, whereas $I_{SPTA.3}$ does not. For example,

   a. At a constant value of $I_{SPTA.3}$ TIS increases with increasing frequency and with increasing source diameter.

   b. At a constant value of $I_{SPTA.3}$ TIB increases with increasing focal beam diameter.

*Thermal indices are the nondimensional ratios of the estimated temperature increases to 1° C for specific tissue models.[95]

Experimental measurements have been performed that have shown reasonable confirmation of the mathematical calculations. Bone heating has not been found experimentally to be significantly greater than that calculated for soft tissues. The biological consequences of hyperthermia include fetal absorption or abortion, growth restriction, microphthalmia, cataract production, abdominal wall defects, renal agenesis, palatal defects, reduction in brain waves, microencephaly, anencephaly, spinal cord defects, amyoplasia, forefoot hypoplasia, tibial and fibular deformations, and abnormal tooth genesis. About 80 known biological effects are due to hyperthermia. None have occurred at temperatures of less than 39° C. Above that, the occurrence of a biological effect depends on temperature and exposure time, as shown in Figure 9-23.

Ultrasound is absorbed by tissue producing a temperature rise. If critical time-temperature values are exceeded, tissue damage occurs.

Mechanical

Nonthermal or mechanical mechanisms of interaction include **radiation force**, streaming, and cavitation. Radiation force is the force exerted by a sound beam on an absorber or a reflector. This force can deform or disrupt structures. Radiation force also can cause flow in an absorbing fluid. This flow can cause shear stresses

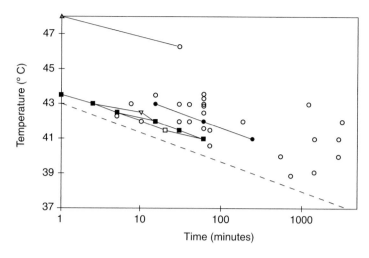

■ **FIGURE 9-23** Thermal bioeffects. A plot of thermally produced biological effects that have been reported in the literature in which the temperature elevation and exposure durations are provided. Each data point represents the lowest temperature reported for any duration or the shortest duration for any temperature reported for a given effect. Solid lines represent multiple data points relating to a single effect. Dashed line represents a lower boundary ($t_{43} = 1$) for observed, thermally induced biological effects. (From Miller MV, Ziskin MC: *Ultrasound Med Biol* 15:707-722, 1989. Copyright 1989 by World Federation of Ultrasound in Medicine and Biology.)

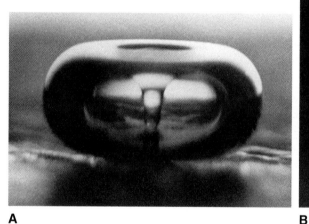
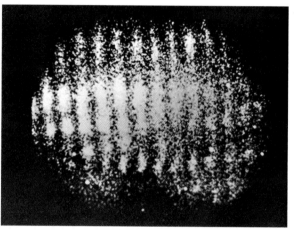

A **B**

■ **FIGURE 9-24** **A,** Photograph of a liquid jet produced by a collapsing cavitation bubble. The width of the bubble is approximately 1 mm. **B,** Photograph taken from the television monitor of an image intensifier system showing light emission from an acoustic standing wave produced in amniotic fluid at 37° C. The vertical bands are separated by approximately 0.75 mm or one half the wavelength for the applied acoustic frequency of 1.0 MHz. The light emission is caused by transient cavitation in the standing wave. (From Kremkau FW: Biologic effects and safety. In Rumack CM, Wilson SR, Charboneau JW, editors: *Diagnostic ultrasound*, St Louis, 1991, Mosby.)

that can deform or disrupt structure. Some bioeffects observed in experimental studies have been attributed to these nonthermal, noncavitational mechanisms of interaction.

Cavitation is the production and behavior of bubbles in a liquid medium. A propagating sound wave is one means by which cavitation can occur. Two types of cavitation are recognized to occur. *Stable cavitation* is the term used to describe bubbles that oscillate in diameter with the passing pressure variations of the sound wave. Streaming of surrounding liquid can occur in this situation, resulting in shear stresses on suspended cells or intracellular organelles. Detection of cavitation in tissues

under continuous wave, high-intensity conditions has been reported. *Transient (collapse) cavitation* occurs when bubble oscillations are so large that the bubble collapses (Figure 9-24, *A*), producing pressure discontinuities (shock waves), localized extremely high temperatures, and light emission in clear liquids (Figure 9-24, *B*). Transient cavitation has the potential for significant destructive effects. Transient cavitation is the means by which laboratory cell disruptors operate. A theory has been developed that predicts that ultrasound could produce transient cavitation under diagnostically relevant conditions in water. A theory also has been developed that incorporates a range of bubble sizes that

yields a predictable dependence of the cavitation threshold on pressure and frequency. Experimental verification of this dependence has been carried out using stabilized microbubbles in water. Thresholds for cavitation in soft tissue and body liquids recently have been determined.

The AIUM[85,92] has summarized information on the cavitation mechanism in its conclusions regarding gas bodies approved in 1993:

1. The temporal peak outputs of some currently available diagnostic ultrasound devices can exceed the threshold for cavitation in vitro and can generate levels that produce extravasation of blood cells in the lungs of laboratory animals.

2. A mechanical index (MI) has been formulated to assist users in evaluating the likelihood of cavitation-related adverse biological effects for diagnostically relevant exposures. The MI is a better indicator than derated spatial peak, pulse average intensity ($I_{SPTA.3}$) or derated peak rarefactional pressure ($p_{r.3}$) for known adverse nonthermal biological effects of ultrasound.*

3. Thresholds for adverse nonthermal effects depend upon tissue characteristics and ultrasound parameters such as pressure amplitude, pulse duration and frequency. Thus far, biologically significant, adverse, nonthermal effects have only been identified with certainty for diagnostically relevant exposures in tissues that have well-defined populations of stabilized gas bodies. For extravasation of blood cells in postnatal mouse lung, the threshold values of MI increase with decreasing pulse duration in the 1-100 μs range, increase with decreasing exposure time and are weakly dependent upon pulse repetition frequency. The threshold value of MI for extravasation of blood cells in mouse lung is approximately 0.3. The implications of these observations for human exposure are yet to be determined.

4. No extravasation of blood cells was found in mouse kidneys exposed to peak pressures in situ corresponding to an MI of 4. Furthermore, for diagnostically relevant exposures, no independently confirmed, biologically significant adverse nonthermal effects have been reported in mammalian tissues that do not contain well-defined gas bodies.

*The MI is equal to the derated peak rarefactional pressure (in MPa) at the point of the maximum pulse intensity integral divided by the square root of the ultrasonic center frequency (in MHz).[95]

Peak rarefactional pressure is illustrated in Figure 9-25. Experimental measurements have been performed that have shown reasonable confirmation of theoretical calculations (Figure 9-26). The only well-documented mammalian biological consequence of gas bodies in an ultrasound beam is blood cell extravasation in inflated lung. It has not occurred at acoustic pressure amplitudes of less than 0.3 MPa. Above that, its occurrence depends on frequency, exposure time, and pulsing conditions.

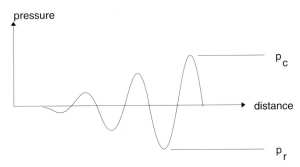

Cavitation can occur in tissues containing gas bubbles with sufficient pressure amplitude and frequency conditions. Damage can result from cavitational activity in tissue.

■ FIGURE 9-25   Pressure versus distance for a three-cycle pulse of ultrasound (p_c, peak compressional pressure; p_r, peak rarefactional pressure).

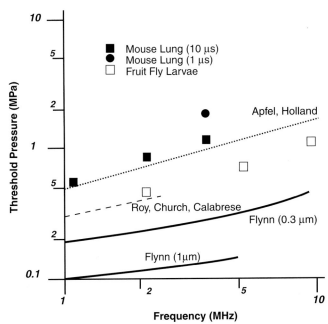

■ FIGURE 9-26   Threshold (in situ) rarefactional pressures for biological effects in vivo of low-temporal-average-intensity, pulsed ultrasound. Pulse durations are shown in parentheses in the legend. In all cases, the tissues contain identifiable, small, stabilized gas bodies. As in diagnostic ultrasound, all exposures consist of repetitive pulses (at 10 μs). Total exposure times were less than 5 minutes. (Adapted from American Institute of Ultrasound in Medicine: *Bioeffects and safety of diagnostic ultrasound,* Laurel, Md, 1993, The Institute.)

The development of contrast agents in diagnostic ultrasound introduces a new consideration regarding cavitation effects. Namely, these agents introduce bubbles (that normally would not be there) into circulation and into tissues. This decreases the acoustic pressure threshold for, and increases the severity of, cavitation bioeffects.[85] Because use of contrast agents is a developing technology, its specific impact on risk and safety has not yet been determined.

SAFETY

Information derived from in vitro and in vivo experimental studies has yielded no known risks in the use of diagnostic ultrasound. Thermal and mechanical mechanisms have been considered but do not appear to be operating significantly at diagnostic intensities. Currently, there is no known risk associated with the use of diagnostic ultrasound. Experimental animal data have helped to define the intensity-exposure time region in which bioeffects can occur. However, differences, physical and biological, between the two situations make it difficult to apply results from one to risk assessment in the other. In the absence of known risk—but recognizing the possibility that bioeffects could be occurring that are subtle, of low incidence, or delayed—a conservative approach to the medical use of ultrasound is recommended. This approach is described in more detail later in this section.

Instrument Outputs

Several reports and compilations of output data have been published. Instrument output may be expressed in many ways. Intensity has been the most popular quantity presented to describe instrument output. Several intensities may be used. Spatial peak–temporal average (SPTA) intensity is used in the AIUM statement on mammalian bioeffects, and it relates reasonably well to a thermal mechanism of interaction. The SPTA is the output intensity most commonly presented. Figures 9-14 and 9-15 give maximum values of SPTA intensities from several sources. Imaging instruments dominate the lower portion of the range, whereas Doppler (especially spectral) instruments dominate the higher portion. In general, spectral Doppler outputs are highest, gray-scale imaging outputs are lowest, and outputs of M mode and color flow fall between the two. Conclusion 5 in "Conclusions Regarding Tissue Models and Equipment Survey," approved by the AIUM in 1997, reads as follows[92]:

> The maximum acoustical output levels of diagnostic ultrasound devices extend over a broad range of values.

a. Historically, maximum MI [mechanical index] values of 1.9 are known to occur for commercially available equipment. Maximum MI values are similar for real-time B-mode, M-mode, pulsed Doppler and color flow imaging.

b. Computed estimates of upper limits to temperature elevations during trans-abdominal scans were obtained in a survey of 1988 and 1990 pulsed Doppler equipment. The vast majority of models yielded upper limits less than 1° C and 4° C for exposures of first-trimester fetal tissue and second-trimester fetal bone, respectively, for dwell times sufficient to achieve steady-state conditions. The largest values obtained were approximately 1.5° C for first-trimester fetal tissue and 7° C for second-trimester fetal bone.

These output intensity measurements usually are made with hydrophones located in the beam in a water bath. Attenuation in water is low compared with that in tissues, so that an intensity at a comparable location within tissue would be considerably less than that in water. Models have been applied to account for the tissue attenuation.[84,86,95]

To compare instrument output intensities with bioeffects knowledge (refer to the AIUM "Statement on Mammalian in Vivo Ultrasonic Biological Effects"[92]), let us assume an average tissue attenuation of 7 dB. This corresponds to an intensity reduction of 80%. Reducing the highest reported value in Figures 9-14 and 9-15 by 80% yields an upper limit of 1.8 W/cm². Because most of the bioeffects studies were done in small animals, such as mice and rats, the attenuation would be negligible and the measured output values can be compared with the AIUM statement value of 1 W/cm² for focused beams because virtually all diagnostic ultrasound uses focused beams. One can see from this comparison that, based on experimental animal studies, clinical bioeffects would not be expected to occur with the output intensities of most current and past diagnostic instrumentation.

Instrument output data are available that allow comparison with conditions necessary for bioeffects to occur.

Food and Drug Administration

Manufacturers are required to submit premarket notifications to the Food and Drug Administration (FDA) before marketing a device for a specific application in the United States. The FDA then reviews this notification to determine whether the device is substantially equivalent, with regard to safety and effectiveness, to instruments on the market before the enactment of the relevant act (1976). If the device is determined to be substantially equivalent, the manufacturer then may market it for that application. Part of the FDA evaluation involves output data for the instrument, which then are compared with maximum values determined for pre-1976 devices. These values are given in the FDA *510(k) Guide for Measuring and Reporting Acoustic Output of Diagnostic Ultrasound Medical Devices* and are presented in Table 9-1. Some of the values have been updated since the 1985 publication of this guide. The current values are shown in the table. To facilitate another path to device approval, a voluntary output display standard was developed by a joint committee involving the AIUM, FDA, National Electrical Manufacturers Association, and several other ultrasound-related professional societies. The goal of this activity was to develop a voluntary standard that would provide a parallel pathway to the current regulatory 510(k) process. The process would allow exemption from the upper limits given in the 510(k) guide (except that an overall upper limit of 720 mW/cm² SPTA still would apply) in exchange for presenting output information on the display. The standard[95,96] includes two indexes that would be displayed: thermal and mechanical. The thermal index (TI) is defined as the transducer acoustic output power divided by the estimated power required to raise tissue temperature by 1°C. The estimated power calculation for the TI involves frequency, aperture, and intensity. Three variations exist on the TI. The TIS (thermal index for soft tissues) applies when the beam travels through soft tissue and does not encounter bone. The TIB (thermal index for bone) applies for bone at or near the beam focus after passing through soft tissue. The TIC (thermal index for cranial tissues) applies when the transducer is close to bone. The mechanical index *(MI)* is equal to the peak rarefactional pressure (Figure 9-25) divided by the square root of the center frequency of the pulse bandwidth,

$$MI = \frac{p \ (MPa)}{[(f)^{1/2} \ (MHz)^{1/2}]}$$

where *p* is pressure amplitude and *f* is frequency.

TABLE 9-1 510(k) Guide to Spatial Peak–Temporal Average in Situ Intensity Upper Limits

Diagnostic Application	I_{SPTA} (mW/cm²)
Cardiac	430
Peripheral vessel	20
Ophthalmic	17
Fetal imaging and other*	94

*Abdominal, intraoperative, pediatric, small organ (breast, thyroid, testes), neonatal cephalic, adult cephalic.

Display of any of these indexes would not be required if the instrument were incapable of exceeding index values of 1. Newer instruments have incorporated this output display standard (Figure 9-27). Maximum values for these indexes, as reported to the FDA,[77] are given in Figure 9-15, *C*. Advice on how to use the indexes in clinical practice is offered in reference 96.

The Food and Drug Administration regulates ultrasound instruments according to application and output intensities and thermal and mechanical indexes.

Epidemiology

A dozen or so studies of an epidemiologic nature have been conducted and published.[97] They indicate that epidemiologic studies and surveys in widespread clinical usage over many years have yielded no evidence of any adverse effect from diagnostic ultrasound. One study included 806 children, approximately half of whom had been exposed to diagnostic ultrasound in utero. The study measured Apgar scores, gestational age, head circumference, birth weight and length, congenital abnormalities, neonatal infection, and congenital infection at birth and also included conductive and nerve measurements of hearing, visual acuity, and color vision, cognitive function and behavioral assessments, and complete and detailed neurologic examinations from the ages of 7 to 12 years. No biologically significant differences between exposed and unexposed children were found. Another study measured the head circumference, height, and weight of 149 sibling pairs of the same sex, one of whom had been exposed to diagnostic ultrasound in utero. No statistically significant differences of head circumference at birth or of height and weight between birth and 6 years of age were found between ultrasound-exposed and unexposed siblings.

Although these studies have limitations and some flaws, they have not revealed any risk associated with the clinical use of diagnostic ultrasound. The AIUM[92] developed and approved in 1995 the following statement regarding epidemiology:

> Based on epidemiologic evidence to date and on current knowledge of interactive mechanisms, there is insufficient justification to warrant a conclusion that there is a causal relationship between diagnostic ultrasound and adverse effects.

The World Federation for Ultrasound in Medicine and Biology[89] approved a similar statement in 1996:

> Epidemiological evidence provides no justification for claiming a causal relationship between diagnostic ultrasound and any adverse effect.

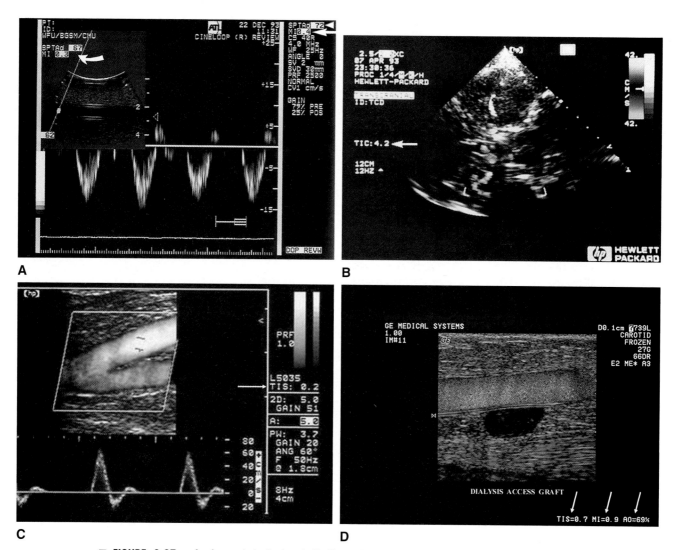

■ **FIGURE 9-27** **A,** A spectral display indicating attenuation-compensated spatial peak–temporal average *(SPTA)* intensity *(arrowhead, upper right)* and mechanical index *(MI; arrow).* The values for the gray-scale image are shown on the inset at upper left *(curved arrow).* **B,** The cranial bone thermal index *(TIC; arrow)* value is indicated on this image of transcranial flow. **C,** The soft-tissue thermal index *(TIS)* is shown *(arrow)* on this vascular image. **D,** The soft tissue thermal index *(TIS),* mechanical index *(MI),* and acoustic output *(AO)* in percent are indicated *(arrows)* on this vascular image.

Epidemiologic studies have yielded no known risk to the use of diagnostic ultrasound.

Prudent Use

Epidemiologic studies have revealed no known risk associated with the use of diagnostic ultrasound. Experimental animal studies have shown bioeffects to occur only at intensities higher than those expected at relevant tissue locations during ultrasound imaging and flow measurements with most equipment. Thus a comparison of instrument output data adjusted for tissue attenuation with experimental bioeffects data does not indicate any risk. We must be open, however, to the possibility that unrecognized, but not zero, risk may exist. Such risk, if it does exist, may have eluded detection up to this point because it is subtle, delayed, or of incidence rates close to normal values. As more sensitive end points are studied over longer periods of time or with larger populations, such risk may be identified. However, future studies might not yield any positive effects, thus strengthening the possibility that medical ultrasound imaging is without detectable risk.

In the meantime, with no known risk and with known benefit to the procedure, a conservative approach to imaging (Figure 9-28) nevertheless should be

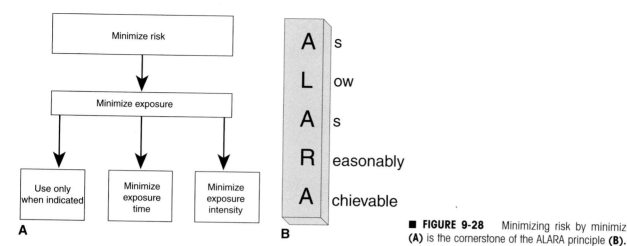

■ **FIGURE 9-28** Minimizing risk by minimizing exposure **(A)** is the cornerstone of the ALARA principle **(B).**

used[82,83]; that is, ultrasound imaging should be used when medically indicated, with minimum exposure of the patient and fetus. Exposure is limited by minimizing instrument output and by minimizing exposure time during a study. Instrument outputs for spectral Doppler studies can be significantly higher than those for other applications (Figures 9-14 and 9-15). It thus seems most likely that the greatest potential for risk in ultrasound diagnosis (although no specific risk has been identified even in this case), is for fetal spectral Doppler studies. These studies combine potentially high-output intensities with stationary geometry and a presumably more sensitive fetus.

The World Health Organization has stated that "the benefits of this imaging modality far outweigh any presumed risks"[90,91] and that

[a]lthough it is difficult to build up a systematic and complete account of all of the possible occurrences and mechanisms that might lead to undesirable consequences of ultrasound exposure, it is possible to make a number of positive statements. Ultrasound has been used in diagnostic medicine for more than 25 years, and in therapeutic applications even longer. Many millions of patients have been exposed to ultrasound during this period, and no verifiable indication has arisen of any adverse effect of the use either of diagnostic procedures or, when properly controlled, of therapy. Nevertheless, because of the general impossibility of fully predicting all the conceivable consequences of human exposure to any given agent, and because of the very large numbers of individuals being exposed, particularly children and fetuses, it is essential to maintain constant vigilance for any evidence of adverse effect.

In this situation, therefore, when risk of injury is at most hypothetical and benefit of some kind is generally expected (though not necessarily always proven) it seems helpful to try to define conditions and working practices that will be "appropriate" to the application being considered....

In using a specific item of equipment to examine a patient, the ALARA principle can be partially implemented by procedures that minimize the examination time. Additionally, if the equipment is provided with means for adjusting the acoustic output, it may be possible further to minimize exposure of the patient. This would be done by reducing the output to the lowest level at which the equipment is diagnostically effective for a specific application.

The AIUM first issued its statement on clinical safety in 1982. The statement was modified in 1997 to the following form[92]:

Diagnostic ultrasound has been in use since the late 1950s. Given its known benefits and recognized efficacy for medical diagnosis, including use during human pregnancy, the American Institute of Ultrasound in Medicine herein addresses the clinical safety of such use:

There are no confirmed biological effects on patients or instrument operators caused by exposures from present diagnostic ultrasound instruments. Although the possibility exists that such biological effects may be identified in the future, current data indicate that the benefits to patients of the prudent use of diagnostic ultrasound outweigh the risks, if any, that may be present.

In 1999 the AIUM issued another statement on prudent use[92]:

The AIUM advocates the responsible use of diagnostic ultrasound. The AIUM strongly discourages the non-medical use of ultrasound for psychosocial or entertainment purposes. The use of either two-dimensional (2D) or three-dimensional (3D) ultrasound to only view the fetus, obtain a picture of the fetus or determine the fetal gender without a medical indication is inappropriate and contrary to responsible medical practice. Although there are no confirmed biological effects on patients caused by exposures from present diagnostic ultrasound instruments, the possibility exists that such biological effects may be identified in the future. Thus ultrasound should be used in a prudent manner to provide medical benefit to the patient.

Prudent practice of sonography involves application of the ALARA principle. By requiring medical indication and by using minimum output and exposure time in diagnostic examinations, exposure and risk are minimized.

In conclusion, extensive mechanistic, in vitro, in vivo, and epidemiologic studies have revealed no known risk devolving with the current ultrasound instrumentation used in medical diagnosis. However, a prudent and conservative approach to ultrasound safety is to assume that there may be unidentified risk, which should be minimized in medically indicated ultrasound studies by minimizing exposure time and output. This is known as the ALARA principle (Figure 9-28).

To make a firm statement about the clinical safety of diagnostic ultrasound is difficult. The experimental and epidemiologic bases for risk assessment are incomplete. However, much work has been done, with no evidence of clinical harm revealed. Patients should be informed that there currently is no basis for concluding that diagnostic ultrasound produces any harmful effects in patients. However, unobserved effects could be occurring. Thus ultrasound should not be used indiscriminately. The AIUM Clinical Safety Statement forms an excellent basis for formulating a response to patient questions and concerns. Prudence in practice is exercised by minimizing exposure time and output. Display of instrument outputs in the form of thermal and mechanical indexes facilitates such prudent use.

In more than 3 decades of use, there has been no report of injury to patients or to operators from medical ultrasound equipment. We in the ultrasound community want to keep that level of safety. In the past, application-specific output limits and the user's knowledge of equipment controls and patient body characteristics were the means of minimizing exposure. Now, more information is available. The mechanical and thermal indexes provide users with information that can be applied specifically to ALARA. Values of mechanical and thermal indexes eliminate some of the guesswork and provide an indication of what actually may be happening within the patient and what occurs when control settings are changed. These values make it possible for the user to obtain the best image possible while following the ALARA principle and thus to maximize the benefit-risk ratio.[96]

REVIEW

The key points presented in this chapter are the following:

- Phantoms and test objects provide means for measuring the detail resolution, distance accuracy, compensation, sensitivity, and dynamic range of diagnostic instruments.

- Hydrophones are used to measure the acoustic output of diagnostic instruments.
- The AIUM has stated that there have been no independently confirmed, significant bioeffects reported to occur in mammalian tissues exposed to focused SPTA intensities of less than 1 W/cm. Furthermore, no risk has been identified with the use of diagnostic ultrasound in human beings.
- Because there is limited specific knowledge, a conservative approach is justified. Such an approach calls for diagnostic ultrasound to be used, with minimum exposure, when medical benefit is expected to be derived from the procedure.

EXERCISES

1. A tissue-equivalent _____ has an attenuation of about 0.5 dB/cm-MHz and a propagation speed of 1.54 mm/µs. A _____ does not mimic tissue but provides a means for measuring some aspect of instrument performance.

2. Match the parameters measured with the items used (answers may be used more than once):

   a. Axial resolution:
   _____, _____
   b. Lateral resolution: _
   _____, _____
   c. Range accuracy:
   _____
   d. Caliper accuracy:
   _____
   e. Contrast resolution:
   _____
   f. Compensation: _____
   g. Sensitivity: _____
   h. Dynamic range: _____
   i. Beam profile: _____
   j. Section thickness: _____

   1. Nylon fibers
   2. Attenuating scattering material
   3. Simulated cysts
   4. Hyperechoic and hypoechoic simulated lesions
   5. Thin scattering layer

3. Match the parameters measured with the correlating types of observation modes (answers may be used more than once):

   a. Axial resolution:
   _____
   b. Lateral resolution:
   _____
   c. Range accuracy:
   _____
   d. Caliper accuracy:
   _____
   e. Compensation:
   _____
   f. Sensitivity: _____
   g. Dynamic range:
   _____,
   _____

   1. Gain settings
   2. Deepest scattering material imaged
   3. Fiber distances from the transducer or from each other on the display
   4. Minimum spacing of separately displayed fibers
   5. Lateral smearing of fibers

4. Test objects and phantoms are available commercially. True or false?

5. Test objects and phantoms can be used by the instrument operator. True or false?

6. A moving _____ test object is useful in checking the accuracy of Doppler spectral displays.

7. A _____ phantom is useful in simulating physiologic _____ conditions for a Doppler instrument.

8. Which of the following is used for Doppler sensitivity measurements?
   a. Cyst phantom
   b. Profile test object
   c. String test object
   d. Contrast phantom
   e. None of the above

9. Tissue-equivalent phantoms attempt to represent some acoustic property of _____.

10. The string test object measures volumetric flow rate. True or false?

11. Using a hydrophone, which of the following can be measured or calculated? (more than one correct answer)
    a. Impedance
    b. Amplitude
    c. Period
    d. Pulse duration
    e. Pulse repetition period

12. All hydrophones consist of a small element mounted on the end of a needle. True or false?

13. A needle hydrophone contains a small _____ element.

14. Because of its small size, a hydrophone can measure spatial details of a sound beam. True or false?

15. A hydrophone
    a. interacts with light.
    b. produces a voltage.
    c. measures intensity directly.
    d. measures total energy.
    e. none of the above.

16. Match the items in column A with those in B and C (answers may be used more than once). (Note: Items in A can be calculated from B if C is known.)
    A
    a. Frequency: _____, _____
    b. Pulse repetition frequency: _____, _____
    c. Duty factor: _____, _____
    d. Wavelength: _____, _____
    e. Spatial pulse length: _____, _____
    f. Energy: _____, _____
    g. Intensity: _____, _____
    B
    1. Wavelength
    2. Period

3. Pulse repetition period
4. Frequency
5. Energy
6. Power
C
7. Number of cycles in the pulse
8. Pulse duration
9. Propagation speed
10. Exposure time
11. Beam area
12. Nothing else

17. The piezoelectric material commonly used in hydrophones is
    a. Quartz
    b. PZT
    c. PVDF
    d. PDQ
    e. PVC

18. The important characteristic of the material used in hydrophones (see Exercise 17) is
    a. impedance.
    b. propagation speed.
    c. efficiency.
    d. density.
    e. bandwidth.

19. Heating depends most directly on
    a. SATA intensity.
    b. SATP intensity.
    c. SPTP intensity.
    d. pressure.

20. Conditions under which cavitation may occur are best described by
    a. SATA intensity.
    b. SATP intensity.
    c. SPTP intensity.
    d. peak rarefactional pressure.

21. Bioeffects have been observed in experimental animals with intensities greater than
    a. 100 mW/cm SPTA.
    b. 1 W/cm SPTA.
    c. 10 W/cm SPTA.
    d. 1 mW/cm SPTP.
    e. 10 mW/cm SPTP.

22. Bioeffects have been observed in experimental animals with focused intensities greater than
    a. 100 mW/cm SPTA.
    b. 1 W/cm SPTA.
    c. 10 W/cm SPTA.
    d. 1 mW/cm SPTP.
    e. 10 mW/cm SPTP.

23. Focal lesions have been observed in experimental animals with intensities greater than
    a. 100 mW/cm SPTA.
    b. 1 W/cm SPTA.
    c. 10 W/cm SPTA.

    d. 1 mW/cm SPTP.

    e. 10 mW/cm SPTP.

24. The available epidemiologic data are sufficient to make a final judgment on the safety of diagnostic ultrasound. True or false?

25. Exposure is minimized by using diagnostic ultrasound

    a. only when indicated.

    b. with minimum intensity.

    c. with minimum time.

    d. all of the above.

    e. none of the above.

26. Which of the following is (are) used currently to indicate output on the display?

    a. Percent

    b. Decibel

    c. SPTA intensity

    d. Mechanical index

    e. All of the above

27. Which of the following affect(s) exposure of a fetus?

    a. Intensity at the transducer

    b. Distance to the fetus

    c. Frequency

    d. Gain

    e. More than one of the above

    f. All of the above

28. There is no possible hazard involved in the use of diagnostic ultrasound. True or false?

29. Ultrasound should not be used as a diagnostic tool because of the bioeffects it can produce. True or false?

30. No independently confirmed, significant bioeffects in mammalian tissues have been reported at intensities below

    a. 10 W/cm^2 SPTP.

    b. 100 mW/cm^2 SPTA.

    c. 10 mW/cm^2 SPTA.

    d. 10 mW/cm^2 SATA.

    e. 1 mW/cm^2 SATP.

31. Is there any known risk with the current use of diagnostic ultrasound?

32. Are there any bioeffects that ultrasound produces in small animals under experimental conditions?

33. Which of the following are mechanisms by which ultrasound can produce bioeffects? (more than one correct answer)

    a. Direction ionization

    b. Absorption

    c. Photoelectric effect

    d. Cavitation

    e. Compton effect

34. Which of the following relates to heating?

    a. Impedance

    b. Sound speed

    c. Absorption

    d. Refraction

    e. Diffraction

35. Which of the following end points is documented well enough in the scientific literature to allow a risk assessment for diagnostic ultrasound to be based on it?

    a. Fetal weight

    b. Sister-chromatid exchange

    c. Fetal abnormalities

    d. Carcinogenesis

    e. None

36. More than one epidemiologic study has shown a statistically significant effect of ultrasound exposure on which of the following end points?

    a. Fetal activity

    b. Birth weight

    c. Fetal abnormalities

    d. Dyslexia

    e. None

37. Which of the following acoustic parameters has (have) been documented in ultrasound epidemiologic studies published thus far?

    a. Frequency

    b. Exposure time

    c. Intensity and pulsing conditions

    d. Scanning patterns

    e. None

38. A device commonly used to measure the output of diagnostic ultrasound instruments is a(n)

    a. Hydrophone

    b. Optical interferometer

    c. Geiger counter

    d. Photoelectric cell

    e. Absorption radiometer

39. A typical output intensity (SPTA) for an ultrasound imaging instrument is

    a. 1540 W.

    b. 13 kW/mm^2.

    c. 3.5 MHz.

    d. 1 mW/cm^2.

    e. 2 dB/cm.

40. Which of the following typically has the highest output intensity?

    a. Fetal monitor Doppler

    b. Duplex pulsed Doppler

    c. Color Doppler shift

    d. Color Doppler-power

    e. Phase array, gray scale

41. As far as we know now, which of the following is the most correct and informative response to a patient's question, "Will this hurt me or my baby?"

    a. No.

    b. Yes.

    c. We don't know.

d. The risks are well understood, but the benefits always outweigh them.

e. There is no known risk with ultrasound imaging as it is applied currently.

42. To minimize whatever risk there may be with ultrasound imaging, which of the following should be done? (more than one correct answer)
    a. Scan for family album pictures
    b. Scan to determine fetal sex
    c. Minimize exposure time
    d. Scan for medical indication(s) only
    e. Minimize exposure intensity

43. Which of the following controls affect instrument output intensity?
    a. Dynamic range, compression
    b. Transmit, output
    c. Near gain, far gain
    d. Overall gain
    e. Slope, time gain compensation

44. Which of the following are correct for a duplex, pulsed wave Doppler instrument? (more than one correct answer)
    a. Tissue anywhere in the Doppler beam is exposed to ultrasound.
    b. Tissue anywhere in the imaging plane is exposed to ultrasound.
    c. Imaging intensities are higher than for conventional gray-scale instruments.
    d. Doppler intensities are higher than for continuous wave fetal monitoring.

45. The tissue of greatest concern regarding bioeffects in an abdominal scan is the
    a. spleen.
    b. pancreas.
    c. liver.
    d. kidney.
    e. fetus.

46. Would it be wise to substitute a duplex, pulsed wave Doppler device for an inoperative fetal monitor for long-term (e.g., 24-hour) monitoring in labor?
    a. Yes
    b. No
    c. Depends on frame rate of image
    d. Depends on frequency of Doppler beam
    e. Depends on gate location

47. Which of the following is (are) likely to be exposed to ultrasound during a diagnostic study?
    a. Patient
    b. Sonographer
    c. Sonologist
    d. Observers in the room
    e. More than one of the above

48. No bioeffects have been observed in nonhuman mammalian tissues at thermal index values of less than
    a. 5.
    b. 4.
    c. 3.
    d. 2.
    e. 1.

49. No bioeffects have been observed in nonhuman mammalian tissues at mechanical index values of less than
    a. 0.5.
    b. 0.4.
    c. 0.3.
    d. 0.2.
    e. 0.1.

50. No bioeffects have been observed in nonhuman mammalian tissues at peak rarefactional pressure values (megapascals) of less than
    a. 0.5.
    b. 0.4.
    c. 0.3.
    d. 0.2.
    e. 0.1.

CHAPTER

10 Review

Diagnostic sonography is medical cross-sectional and three-dimensional anatomic and flow imaging using pulse-echo ultrasound. Pulses of ultrasound are generated by a transducer and are sent into the patient, where they produce echoes at organ boundaries and within tissues. These echoes return to the transducer, where they are detected and then presented on the display of a sonographic instrument. Each pulse produces a series of echoes that is displayed as a scan line. An anatomic image is composed of many scan lines. If flowing blood or moving tissues produce echoes, a frequency change, called a Doppler shift, occurs. Doppler shifts provide motion information that can be presented audibly or as a spectral or two- or three-dimensional color Doppler display.

Ultrasound is sound (a wave of traveling acoustic variables, including pressure, density, and particle motion) having a frequency greater than 20 kHz. Ultrasound is described by frequency, period, wavelength, propagation speed, amplitude, intensity, and attenuation. Pulsed ultrasound is described by additional terms: pulse repetition frequency (PRF), pulse repetition period, pulse duration, duty factor, and spatial pulse length. Propagation speed and impedance are characteristics of the medium that are determined by density and stiffness. Attenuation increases with frequency and path length. Imaging depth decreases with increasing frequency. The soft tissue propagation speed is 1.54 mm/µs, and the attenuation coefficient is 0.5 dB/cm for each megahertz of frequency. When sound encounters boundaries between media with different impedances, part of the sound is reflected (echo) and part is transmitted. With perpendicular incidence, if the two media have the same impedance, there is no reflection. With oblique incidence, the sound is refracted at a boundary between the media where propagation speeds are different. Incidence and reflection angles are always equal. Scattering occurs at rough media boundaries and within

heterogeneous media. The range equation is used to determine distance to reflectors. Pulse-echo round-trip travel time is 13 µs/cm. Using harmonic echoes improves image quality. Contrast media enhance echo generation and detection.

Ultrasound transducers convert electric energy to ultrasound energy and vice versa. They operate on the piezoelectric principle. The preferred operating frequency depends on the element thickness. Axial resolution is equal to one half the spatial pulse length. Pulsed transducers have damping material to shorten the spatial pulse length for acceptable resolution. Transducers produce sound in the form of beams with near and far zones. Lateral resolution is equal to beam width. Beam width is reduced by focusing to improve resolution. Linear and convex are types of array construction. Sequenced, phased, and vector are types of array scanning operation. Phasing also enables electronic control of focus.

Diagnostic ultrasound imaging (sonographic) systems are of the pulse-echo type. They use the strength, direction, and arrival time of received echoes to generate A, B, and M mode displays. Imaging systems consist of a transducer, beam former, signal processor, image processor, and display. Beam formers direct the transmitted beam through the imaged tissue cross section, direct and focus the reception beam, amplify the received echo voltages, compensate for attenuation, and digitize the echo voltages. Signal processors filter, detect, and compress echo signals. Image processors convert scan line signals to image formats, store images in digital form, and perform preprocessing and postprocessing on images. Preprocessing includes persistence, panoramic imaging, spatial compounding, and three-dimensional acquisition. A mode shows echo amplitudes. B and M modes use a brightness display. M mode shows reflector motion in time. B scans show anatomic cross sections in gray scale through the scanning plane. Image memories store echo amplitude information as numbers in memory elements. Contrast resolution improves with increasing bits per pixel (layers of memory). Real-time imaging is the rapid sequential display of ultrasound images resulting in a moving presentation. Such imaging requires automatic, rapid, repeatable, sequential scanning of the sound beam through the tissue. This scanning is accomplished by electronic transducer arrays. Rectangular or sector display formats result from such scanning techniques. Displays are cathode-ray tubes (CRTs) or flat panel liquid-crystal displays (LCDs). Instruments often are connected to peripheral recording devices and to picture archiving and communications systems (PACS).

Fluids (gases and liquids) are substances that flow. Blood is a liquid that flows through the vascular system under the influence of pulsatile pressure provided by the beating heart. Volume flow rate is proportional to pressure difference at the ends of a tube and inversely proportional to the flow resistance. The flow resistance increases with viscosity and tube length and decreases (strongly) with increasing tube diameter. Seven (two temporal and five spatial) flow classifications include steady, pulsatile, plug, laminar, parabolic, disturbed, and turbulent. In a stenosis, flow speeds up, pressure drops (Bernoulli effect), and flow is disturbed. If flow speed exceeds a critical value, as described by the Reynolds number, turbulence occurs. Pulsatile flow is common in the arterial circulation. Diastolic flow or flow reversal or both may occur in some locations within the arterial system. Fluid inertia and vessel compliance are characteristics that are important in determining flow with pulsatile driving pressure.

The Doppler effect is a change in frequency resulting from motion. In most medical ultrasound applications, the motion is that of blood flow in circulation. The change in frequency of the returning echoes with respect to the emitted frequency is called the Doppler shift. For flow toward the transducer, Doppler shift is positive; for flow away, it is negative. The Doppler shift depends on the speed of the scatterers of sound, the angle between their direction and that of the sound propagation, and the operating frequency of the Doppler system. A moving scatterer of sound produces a double Doppler shift. Greater flow speeds and smaller Doppler angles produce larger Doppler shifts but not stronger echoes. Higher operating frequencies produce larger Doppler shifts. Typical ranges of flow speeds (10 to 100 cm/s), Doppler angles (30 to 60 degrees), and operating frequencies (2 to 10 MHz) yield Doppler shifts in the range of 100 Hz to 11 kHz for vascular studies. In Doppler echocardiography, where zero angle and speeds of a few meters per second can be encountered, Doppler shifts can be as high as 30 kHz.

Doppler instruments make use of the Doppler shift to yield information regarding motion and flow. Color Doppler imaging acquires Doppler-shifted echoes from a cross section of tissue scanned by an ultrasound beam. These echoes then are presented in color and are superimposed on the gray-scale anatomic image of nonshifted echoes that were received during the scan. The flow echoes are assigned colors according to the selected color map. Red, orange, yellow, blue, cyan, and white indicate positive or negative Doppler shifts (i.e., approaching or receding flow). Yellow, cyan, or green is used to indicate variance (disturbed or turbulent flow). Several pulses (the number is called the ensemble length) are needed to generate a color scan line. Color controls include gain, color map selection, variance on/off, persistence, ensemble length, color/gray priority, scale (PRF), baseline shift, wall filter, and color window angle, location, and size. Color Doppler instruments are pulsed wave Doppler instruments and are subject to the same limitations—Doppler angle dependence and aliasing—as other Doppler instruments. Doppler-power displays color-encode the strength of the Doppler shifts into a sensitive angle- and aliasing-independent presentation of flow information.

Continuous wave systems provide motion and flow information without depth selection capability. Pulsed wave Doppler systems have the capability of selecting a depth from which Doppler information is received. Spectral analysis provides quantitative information on the distribution of received Doppler-shift frequencies resulting from the distribution of scatterer velocities (speeds and directions) encountered. In addition to audible output, visual presentation of flow spectra is possible in Doppler systems. Combined (duplex) systems using real-time sonography and continuous wave and pulsed wave Doppler are available commercially. The Doppler spectrum is generated by the range of scatterer velocities encountered by the ultrasound beam. The Doppler spectrum is derived electronically using the fast Fourier transform (FFT) and is presented on the display as Doppler shift versus time, with brightness indicating power. Flow conditions at the site of measurement are indicated by the width of the spectrum; spectral broadening indicates disturbed and turbulent flow. Flow conditions downstream, particularly distal flow resistance, are indicated by the relationship between peak systolic and end-diastolic flow speeds. Various indexes for quantitatively presenting this information have been developed.

Axial resolution is determined by spatial pulse length, whereas lateral resolution is determined by beam width. The beam width perpendicular to the scan plane causes section thickness artifacts. Apparent resolution close to the transducer is not related directly to tissue texture but is a result of interference effects from a distribution of scatterers in the tissue (speckle). Reverberation produces a set of equally spaced artifactual echoes distal to the real reflector. Refraction displaces echoes laterally. In the mirror-image artifact, objects that are present on one side of a strong reflector are displayed on the other side as well. Shadowing is caused by high-attenuation objects in the sound path. Enhancement results from low-attenuation objects in the sound path. Propagation speed error and refraction can cause objects to be displayed in improper locations or incorrect sizes or both. Refraction also can cause edge shadowing. Artifacts that can occur with Doppler ultrasound include aliasing, range ambiguity, color Doppler image and Doppler signal mirroring, and spectral trace mirroring. Aliasing is the most common artifact. Aliasing occurs when the Doppler-shift frequency exceeds one half the PRF (the Nyquist limit). Aliasing can be reduced or eliminated by increasing the PRF or Doppler angle, shifting the baseline, reducing operating frequency, or switching to continuous wave operation.

Phantoms and test objects provide means for measuring the detail and contrast resolutions, distance accuracy, compensation, penetration, and dynamic range of diagnostic instruments. Hydrophones are used to measure the acoustic output of diagnostic instruments.

The American Institute of Ultrasound in Medicine has stated that there have been no independently confirmed, significant bioeffects reported to occur in mammalian tissues exposed to focused spatial peak–temporal average intensities of less than 1 W/cm^2. Furthermore, no risk has been identified with the use of diagnostic ultrasound in human beings. Because there is limited specific knowledge, a conservative approach is justified; that is, diagnostic ultrasound should be used, with minimum exposure, when medical benefit is expected to be derived from the procedure.

COMPREHENSIVE EXAMINATION

1. Which of the following frequencies is in the ultrasound range?
   a. 15 Hz
   b. 15 kHz
   c. 15 MHz
   d. 17,000 Hz
   e. 17 km
2. The average propagation speed in soft tissues is
   a. 1.54 mm/μs.
   b. 0.501 m/s.
   c. 1540 dB/cm.
   d. 37.0 km/min.
   e. 1 to 10 MHz.
3. The propagation speed is greatest in
   a. lung
   b. liver
   c. bone
   d. fat
   e. blood
4. Which of the following has a significant dependence on frequency in soft tissues?
   a. Propagation speed
   b. Density
   c. Stiffness
   d. Attenuation
   e. Impedance
5. The frequencies used in diagnostic ultrasound imaging
   a. are much lower than those used in Doppler measurements.
   b. determine imaging depth in tissue.
   c. determine detail resolution.
   d. all of the above.
   e. b and c.
6. An echo from a 5-cm deep reflector arrives at the transducer _____ μs after pulse emission.
   a. 13
   b. 154
   c. 65
   d. 5
   e. 77
7. A small (relative to the wavelength) reflector is said to _____ an incident sound beam.
   a. Focus
   b. Speculate
   c. Scatter
   d. Shatter
   e. Amplify
8. The operating frequency of an ultrasound transducer is determined by which of the following?
   a. Element diameter
   b. Element thickness
   c. Speed of sound in tissue
   d. Element impedance
   e. All of the above
9. The fundamental operating principle of medical ultrasound transducers is
   a. Snell's law.
   b. Doppler law.
   c. magnetostrictive effect.
   d. piezoelectric effect.
   e. impedance effect.
10. The axial resolution of a transducer is primarily determined by
    a. spatial pulse length.
    b. the near-field limit.

c. the transducer diameter.
d. the acoustic impedance of tissue.
e. density.

11. The lateral resolution of a transducer is primarily determined by
    a. spatial pulse length.
    b. the near-field limit.
    c. the aperture.
    d. the acoustic impedance of tissue.
    e. applied voltage.

12. Increasing frequency
    a. improves resolution.
    b. increases penetration.
    c. increases refraction.
    d. a and b.
    e. a and c.

13. Ultrasound bioeffects
    a. do not occur.
    b. do not occur with diagnostic instruments.
    c. are not confirmed below an spatial peak–temporal average intensity of 100 mW/cm^2.
    d. b and c.
    e. none of the above.

14. Diagnostic ultrasound frequency range is
    a. 2 to 10 mHz.
    b. 2 to 10 kHz.
    c. 2 to 15 MHz.
    d. 5 to 15 kHz.
    e. none of the above.

15. What determines the lower and upper limits of frequency range useful in diagnostic ultrasound?
    a. Resolution and penetration
    b. Intensity and resolution
    c. Intensity and propagation speed
    d. Scattering and impedance
    e. Impedance and wavelength

16. Reverberation causes us to think there are reflectors that are too great in
    a. impedance.
    b. attenuation.
    c. range.
    d. size.
    e. number.

17. A flat-panel display is composed of a back-lighted rectangular matrix of thousands of _____ display elements.
    a. Plasma
    b. Television
    c. Fluorescent
    d. Liquid-crystal
    e. Piezo-crystal

18. In an ultrasound imaging instrument, a cathode-ray tube may be used as a
    a. pulser.
    b. digitizer.

c. memory.
d. display.
e. scan converter.

19. The compensation (time gain compensation) control
    a. compensates for machine instability in the warm-up time.
    b. compensates for attenuation.
    c. compensates for transducer aging and the ambient light in the examining area.
    d. decreases patient examination time.
    e. none of the above.

20. A scan converter changes signals from _____ to _____ format.
    a. Gray-scale, color
    b. Radio frequency, video
    c. B mode, M mode
    d. Scan line, image
    e. None of the above

21. Enhancement is caused by a
    a. strongly reflecting structure.
    b. weakly attenuating structure.
    c. strongly attenuating structure.
    d. frequency error.
    e. propagation speed error.

22. Echo intensity is represented in image memory by
    a. positive charge distribution.
    b. a number.
    c. electron density of the scan converter writing beam.
    d. a and c.
    e. all of the above.

23. Which of the following is (are) performed in a signal processor?
    a. Filtering
    b. Detection
    c. Compression
    d. All of the above
    e. None of the above

24. Increasing the pulse repetition frequency
    a. improves detail resolution.
    b. increases maximum unambiguous depth.
    c. decreases maximum unambiguous depth.
    d. both a and b.
    e. both a and c.

25. Attenuation is corrected by
    a. demodulation.
    b. desegregation.
    c. decompression.
    d. compensation.
    e. remuneration.

26. What must be known to calculate distance to a reflector?
    a. Attenuation, speed, density
    b. Attenuation, impedance

c. Attenuation, absorption
d. Travel time, speed
e. Density, speed

27. Which of the following improve(s) sound transmission from the transducer element into the tissue?
    a. Matching layer
    b. Doppler effect
    c. Damping material
    d. Coupling medium
    e. a and d

28. Lateral resolution is improved by
    a. damping.
    b. pulsing.
    c. focusing.
    d. reflecting.
    e. absorbing.

29. Axial resolution is improved by
    a. damping.
    b. pulsing.
    c. focusing.
    d. reflecting.
    e. absorbing.

30. An image memory divides the cross-sectional image into _____.
    a. Frequencies
    b. Bits
    c. Pixels
    d. Binaries
    e. Wavelengths

31. In general, as a reflector approaches a transducer at constant speed, the positive Doppler-shift frequency
    a. increases.
    b. decreases.
    c. remains constant.
    d. b or c.
    e. none of the above.

32. A reduction in vessel diameter produces a(n)
    a. increase in flow resistance.
    b. decrease in area.
    c. increase in flow speed.
    d. decrease in flow speed.
    e. all of the above.

33. Which of the following increases vascular flow resistance?
    a. Decreasing vessel length
    b. Decreasing viscosity
    c. Decreasing vessel diameter
    d. Decreasing pressure
    e. Decreasing flow speed

34. The Doppler effect occurs as
    a. the leukocytes move through the plasma.
    b. the erythrocytes move through the plasma.
    c. the erythrocytes move through the serum.
    d. blood moves relative to the vessel wall.
    e. all of the above.

35. When a reflector is moving toward the transducer,
    a. propagation speed increases.
    b. propagation speed decreases.
    c. Doppler shift is positive (higher frequency).
    d. Doppler shift is negative (lower frequency).
    e. none of the above.

36. Doppler sample volume is determined by
    a. beam width.
    b. pulse length.
    c. frequency.
    d. amplifier gate length.
    e. all of the above.

37. Doppler shift frequencies
    a. are generally in the audible range.
    b. are usually above 1 MHz.
    c. can be applied to a loudspeaker.
    d. a and b.
    e. a and c.

38. The quantitative presentation of frequencies contained in echoes is called
    a. preamplification.
    b. digitizing.
    c. optical encoding.
    d. spectral analysis.
    e. all of the above.

39. The Doppler frequency shift is caused by
    a. relative motion between the transducer and the reflector.
    b. the patient shivering in a cool room.
    c. a high transducer frequency and real-time scanner.
    d. small reflectors in the transducer beam.
    e. changing transducer thickness.

40. The Doppler effect is a change in
    a. intensity.
    b. wavelength.
    c. frequency.
    d. all of the above.
    e. b and c.

41. Doppler shift is zero when the angle between the sound direction and the movement (flow) direction is _____ degrees.
    a. 30
    b. 60
    c. 90
    d. 45
    e. None of the above

42. Duplex Doppler presents
    a. anatomic (structural) data.
    b. physiologic (flow) data.
    c. impedance data.
    d. more than one of the above.
    e. all of the above.

43. Doppler shift frequencies are usually in a relatively narrow range above 20 kHz. True or false?

44. Continuous wave sound is used in
    a. all ultrasound imaging instruments.
    b. only bistable instruments.
    c. all Doppler instruments.
    d. some Doppler instruments.
    e. some M mode instruments.
45. An advantage of continuous wave Doppler over pulsed Doppler is
    a. depth information.
    b. bidirectionality.
    c. no aliasing.
    d. b and c.
    e. all of the above.
46. In color Doppler instruments, hue can represent
    a. sign (+ or −) of Doppler shift.
    b. flow direction.
    c. magnitude of the Doppler shift.
    d. amplitude of the Doppler shift.
    e. all of the above.
47. The Doppler effect for a scatterer moving toward the sound source causes the scattered sound (compared with incident sound) received by the transducer to have
    a. increased intensity.
    b. decreased intensity.
    c. increased impedance.
    d. increased frequency.
    e. decreased impedance.
48. Duplex Doppler instruments include _____.
    a. Pulsed wave Doppler
    b. Continuous wave Doppler
    c. B scan imaging
    d. Dynamic imaging
    e. More than one of the above
49. If the Doppler shifts from normal and stenotic arteries are 4 kHz and 10 kHz, respectively, for which will there be a problem (aliasing) with a pulse repetition frequency of 7 kHz?
    a. Normal artery
    b. Stenotic artery
    c. Both
    d. Neither
50. The signal processor in a Doppler system compares the _____ of the output with the returning echo voltage from the transducer.
    a. Wavelength
    b. Intensity
    c. Impedance
    d. Frequency
    e. All of the above
51. In the Doppler equation that follows, which can normally be ignored?

$$f_D = \frac{2fv}{(c-v)}$$

    a. v in the denominator
    b. v in the numerator
    c. f
    d. f_D
    e. b and c
52. For which of the following is the reflected frequency less than the incident frequency?
    a. Advancing flow
    b. Receding flow
    c. Perpendicular flow
    d. Laminar flow
    e. All of the above
53. Doppler ultrasound can measure flow speed in the
    a. heart.
    b. veins.
    c. arterioles.
    d. capillaries.
    e. a and b.
54. Which of the following are fluids?
    a. Gas
    b. Liquid
    c. Solid
    d. a and b
    e. All of the above
55. The mass per unit volume of a fluid is called its
    a. resistance.
    b. viscosity.
    c. kinematic viscosity.
    d. impedance.
    e. density.
56. The resistance to flow offered by a fluid is called
    a. resistance.
    b. viscosity.
    c. kinematic viscosity.
    d. impedance.
    e. density.
57. Viscosity divided by density is called
    a. resistance.
    b. viscosity.
    c. kinematic viscosity.
    d. impedance.
    e. density.
58. If the following is increased, flow increases.
    a. Pressure difference
    b. Pressure gradient
    c. Resistance
    d. a and b
    e. All of the above
59. Flow resistance depends most strongly on which of the following?
    a. Vessel length
    b. Vessel radius
    c. Blood viscosity
    d. All of the above
    e. None of the above

60. Proximal to, at, and distal to a stenosis, _____ must be constant.
    a. Laminar flow
    b. Disturbed flow
    c. Turbulent flow
    d. Volume flow rate
    e. None of the above
61. Added forward flow and flow reversal in diastole are results of _____ flow.
    a. Volume
    b. Turbulent
    c. Laminar
    d. Disturbed
    e. Pulsatile
62. Turbulence generally occurs when the Reynolds number exceeds
    a. 100.
    b. 200.
    c. 1000.
    d. 2000.
    e. a and b.
63. As diameter at a stenosis decreases, the following pass(es) through a maximum:
    a. Flow speed at the stenosis
    b. Flow speed proximal to the stenosis
    c. Volume flow rate
    d. Doppler shift at the stenosis
    e. a and d
64. The Doppler shift (kilohertz) for 4 MHz, 50 cm/s, and 60 degrees is
    a. 0.5.
    b. 1.0.
    c. 1.3.
    d. 2.6.
    e. 5.0.
65. Physiologic flow speeds can be as much as _____% of the propagation speed in soft tissues.
    a. 0.01
    b. 0.3
    c. 5
    d. 10
    e. 50
66. Which Doppler angle yields the greatest Doppler shift?
    a. −90
    b. −45
    c. 0
    d. 45
    e. 90
67. Doppler shift frequency does not depend on
    a. amplitude.
    b. flow speed.
    c. operating frequency.
    d. Doppler angle.
    e. propagation speed.

68. The Fourier transform technique is not used in color Doppler instruments because it is not _____ enough.
    a. Slow
    b. Fast
    c. Bright
    d. Cheap
    e. None of the above
69. Which of the following on a color Doppler display is (are) presented in real time?
    a. Gray-scale anatomy
    b. Flow direction
    c. Doppler spectrum
    d. a and b
    e. All of the above
70. For a 5-MHz instrument and a 60-degree Doppler angle, a 100-Hz filter eliminates flow speeds below
    a. 1 cm/s.
    b. 2 cm/s.
    c. 3 cm/s.
    d. 4 cm/s.
    e. 5 cm/s.
71. For a 7.5-MHz instrument and a 0-degree Doppler angle, a 100-Hz filter eliminates flow speeds below
    a. 1 cm/s.
    b. 2 cm/s.
    c. 3 cm/s.
    d. 4 cm/s.
    e. 5 cm/s.
72. The functions of a Doppler detector include which of the following?
    a. Amplification
    b. Phase quadrature detection
    c. Demodulation
    d. All of the above
    e. None of the above
73. A later amplifier gate time means a(n) _____ sample volume depth.
    a. Earlier
    b. Shallower
    c. Deeper
    d. Stronger
    e. None of the above
74. The Doppler shift is typically _____ the source frequency.
    a. One thousandth
    b. One hundredth
    c. One tenth
    d. 10 times
    e. 100 times
75. Approximately _____ pulses are required to obtain one line of color Doppler information.
    a. 1
    b. 10
    c. 100

d. 1000

e. 1,000,000

76. There are approximately _____ samples per line on a color Doppler display.
    a. 2
    b. 20
    c. 200
    d. 2000
    e. 2,000,000

77. Which of the following Doppler instruments can produce aliasing?
    a. Continuous wave
    b. Pulsed
    c. Duplex
    d. Color
    e. More than one of the above

78. For normal flow in a large vessel, a _____ range of Doppler shift frequencies is received.
    a. Narrow
    b. Broad
    c. Steady
    d. Disturbed
    e. All of the above

79. Doppler signal power is proportional to
    a. volume flow rate.
    b. flow speed.
    c. Doppler angle.
    d. cell density.
    e. more than one of the above.

80. Stenosis affects
    a. peak systolic flow speed.
    b. end-diastolic flow speed.
    c. spectral broadening.
    d. window.
    e. all of the above.

81. Spectral broadening is a _____ of the spectral trace.
    a. Vertical thickening
    b. Horizontal thickening
    c. Brightening
    d. Darkening
    e. Horizontal shift

82. As stenosis is increased, which of the following increase(s)?
    a. Vessel diameter
    b. Systolic Doppler shift
    c. Diastolic Doppler shift
    d. Spectral broadening
    e. More than one of the above

83. Flow reversal in diastole (normal flow) indicates
    a. stenosis.
    b. aneurysm.
    c. high distal flow resistance.
    d. low distal flow resistance.
    e. more than one of the above.

84. About _____ fast Fourier transforms are performed per second on a spectral display.
    a. 3
    b. 10
    c. 100 to 1000
    d. 700 to 7000
    e. 17,000

85. Each fast Fourier transform appears on a spectral display as a _____.
    a. Dot
    b. Circle
    c. Horizontal line
    d. Vertical line
    e. None of the above

86. Hue is _____.
    a. Color seen
    b. Light frequency
    c. Brightness
    d. Mix with white
    e. More than one of the above

87. A component *not* included in a continuous wave Doppler instrument is a(n) _____.
    a. Loudspeaker
    b. Wall filter
    c. Oscillator
    d. Demodulator
    e. Gate

88. On a spectral display, amplitude is indicated by
    a. brightness.
    b. horizontal position.
    c. vertical position.
    d. b and c.
    e. none of the above.

89. Doppler shift can change because of changes in
    a. velocity.
    b. speed.
    c. direction.
    d. frequency.
    e. all of the above.

90. A gate-open time of 10 μs corresponds to a sample volume length (millimeters) of
    a. 10.
    b. 7.7.
    c. 3.8.
    d. 3.3.
    e. 2.0.

91. Sample volume width is determined by
    a. gate-open time.
    b. pulse duration.
    c. pulse repetition frequency.
    d. pulse repetition period.
    e. beam width.

92. What problem(s) is (are) encountered if pulse repetition frequency is 10 kHz, sample volume is located at 10-cm depth, and the Doppler shift is 4 kHz?

a. Aliasing
b. Mirror image
c. Refraction
d. Range ambiguity
e. More than one of the above

93. What problem(s) is (are) encountered if pulse repetition frequency is 10 kHz, sample volume is located at a 5-cm depth, and the Doppler shift is 6 kHz?
    a. Aliasing
    b. Mirror image
    c. Refraction
    d. Range ambiguity
    e. More than one of the above

94. What problem(s) is (are) encountered if pulse repetition frequency is 10 kHz, sample volume is located at a 10-cm depth, and the Doppler shift is 6 kHz?
    a. Aliasing
    b. Mirror image
    c. Refraction
    d. Range ambiguity
    e. More than one of the above

95. The functions of a color Doppler signal processor include which of the following?
    a. Amplification
    b. Phase quadrature detection
    c. Demodulation
    d. Autocorrelation
    e. All of the above

96. If all cells in a vessel were moving at the same constant speed, the spectral trace would be a _____ line.
    a. Thin horizontal
    b. Thick horizontal
    c. Thin vertical
    d. Thick vertical
    e. None of the above

97. Doppler power displays
    a. are independent of Doppler angle.
    b. are more sensitive than Doppler-shift displays.
    c. are independent of aliasing.
    d. show uniform flow presentations.
    e. all of the above.

98. For a physiologic flow speed, a 5-MHz beam could produce a Doppler shift of about _____.
    a. 5 kHz
    b. 5 MHz
    c. 5 Hz
    d. Depends on the mode (continuous wave or pulsed wave)
    e. None of the above

99. Spectral analysis is performed in a Doppler instrument _____.
    a. Electronically
    b. Mathematically

c. Acoustically
d. Mechanically
e. More than one of the above

100. Doppler shift is proportional to
    a. volume flow rate.
    b. flow speed.
    c. Doppler angle.
    d. cell density.
    e. more than one of the above.

101. Which can be used to evaluate the performance of a Doppler instrument?
    a. Contrast detail phantom
    b. String test object
    c. Flow phantom
    d. b and c
    e. All of the above

102. Place the following instruments in general order of increasing acoustic output: (1) spectral Doppler, (2) sonographic, (3) color Doppler.
    a. 1, 2, 3
    b. 2, 3, 1
    c. 3, 1, 2
    d. 3, 2, 1
    e. 2, 1, 3

103. If operating frequency is 5 MHz, Doppler angle is 60 degrees, pulse repetition frequency is 9 kHz, and Doppler shift is 2 kHz, what problem is encountered if the angle is changed to zero?
    a. Aliasing
    b. Range ambiguity
    c. Mirror image
    d. Refraction
    e. None

104. When angle correction is applied on a color Doppler display, the Nyquist limits (in centimeters per second) on the color map
    a. increase.
    b. decrease.
    c. do not change.
    d. are irrelevant.
    e. are ambiguous.

105. When angle correction is applied on a color Doppler display, the Nyquist limits (in kilohertz) on the color map
    a. increase.
    b. decrease.
    c. do not change.
    d. are irrelevant.
    e. are ambiguous.

106. Flow is _____ if it appears red on a color Doppler display.
    a. Approaching
    b. Receding
    c. Turbulent

d. Disturbed

e. Undetermined (depends on color map)

107. Two different colors in the same vessel indicate
    a. flow reversal.
    b. sector scan.
    c. vessel curvature.
    d. aliasing.
    e. any of the above.

108. The following increase(s) the amount of color appearing in a vessel:
    a. Increased color gain
    b. Increased wall filter
    c. Increased priority
    d. Increased pulse repetition frequency
    e. More than one of the above

109. The following decrease(s) the amount of color appearing in a vessel:
    a. Increased wall filter
    b. Increased pulse repetition frequency
    c. Increased ensemble length
    d. Baseline shift
    e. More than one of the above

110. Which of the following on a color Doppler display is (are) presented as a two-dimensional, cross-sectional display?
    a. Gray-scale anatomy
    b. Flow direction
    c. Doppler spectrum
    d. a and b
    e. All of the above

111. Comparing gray with white is an example of _____.
    a. Hue
    b. Luminance
    c. Saturation
    d. b and c
    e. All of the above

112. Comparing red with green is an example of
    a. Hue
    b. Luminance
    c. Saturation
    d. b and c
    e. All of the above

113. There are about _____ frames per second produced by a color Doppler instrument.
    a. 10
    b. 20
    c. 40
    d. 80
    e. More than one of the above

114. The autocorrelation technique yields
    a. mean Doppler shift.
    b. sign of Doppler shift.
    c. spread around the mean (variance).

d. all of the above.

e. none of the above.

115. Increasing ensemble length _____ color sensitivity and accuracy and _____ frame rate.
    a. Improves, increases
    b. Degrades, increases
    c. Degrades, decreases
    d. Improves, decreases
    e. None of the above

116. Which control can be used to help with clutter?
    a. Wall filter
    b. Gain
    c. Baseline shift
    d. Pulse repetition frequency
    e. Smoothing

117. Doubling the width of a color window produces a(n) _____ frame rate.
    a. Doubled
    b. Quadrupled
    c. Unchanged
    d. Halved
    e. Quartered

118. Steering the color window to the right or left changes the
    a. frame rate.
    b. pulse repetition frequency.
    c. Doppler angle.
    d. Doppler shift.
    e. more than one of the above.

119. Lack of color in a vessel may be due to
    a. low color gain.
    b. low wall filter setting.
    c. small Doppler angle.
    d. low baseline shift.
    e. more than one of the above.

120. Which control(s) can help with aliasing?
    a. Wall filter
    b. Gain
    c. Smoothing
    d. Pulse repetition frequency
    e. More than one of the above

121. Pulse duration is the _____ for a pulse to occur.
    a. Space
    b. Time
    c. Delay
    d. Pressure
    e. Reciprocal

122. Spatial pulse length equals the number of cycles in the pulse multiplied by
    a. period.
    b. impedance.
    c. beam width.
    d. resolution.
    e. wavelength.

123. If pulse duration is 1 μs and the pulse repetition period is 100 μs, duty factor is
    a. 1%
    b. 10%
    c. 50%
    d. 90%
    e. 100%

124. The attenuation of 5-MHz ultrasound in 4 cm of soft tissue is
    a. 5 dB/cm.
    b. 10 dB.
    c. 2.5 MHz/cm.
    d. 2 cm.
    e. 5 dB/MHz.

125. If the maximum value of an acoustic variable in a sound wave is 10 units and the normal (no sound) value is 7 units, the amplitude is _____ units.
    a. 1
    b. 3
    c. 7
    d. 10
    e. 17

126. Impedance equals propagation speed multiplied by
    a. density.
    b. stiffness.
    c. frequency.
    d. attenuation.
    e. path length.

127. Which of the following cannot be determined from the others?
    a. Frequency
    b. Amplitude
    c. Intensity
    d. Power
    e. Beam area

128. For perpendicular incidence, in medium 1, density equals 1 and propagation speed equals 3; in medium 2, density equals 1.5 and propagation speed equals 2. What is the intensity reflection coefficient?
    a. 0
    b. 1
    c. 2
    d. 3
    e. 4

129. For perpendicular incidence, if the intensity transmission coefficient is 96%, what is the intensity reflection coefficient?
    a. 2%
    b. 4%
    c. 6%
    d. 8%
    e. 10%

130. The colors presented on a Doppler-power display represent the _____ of the spectrum.
    a. Mean Doppler shift
    b. Variance
    c. Area
    d. Angle
    e. All of the above

131. For oblique incidence and a medium 2 speed that is equal to twice the speed of medium 1, the transmission angle will be about _____ times the incidence angle.
    a. 0.5
    b. 17
    c. 2
    d. 4
    e. 5

132. The range equation describes the relationship of
    a. reflector distance, propagation time, and sound speed.
    b. distance, propagation time, and reflection coefficient.
    c. number of cows and sheep on a ranch.
    d. propagation time, sound speed, and transducer frequency.
    e. dynamic range and system sensitivity.

133. Axial resolution in a system equals
    a. 4 times the spatial pulse length.
    b. the ratio of reflector size to transducer frequency.
    c. the maximum reflector separation expected to be displayed.
    d. the minimum reflector separation expected to be displayed.
    e. spatial pulse length.

134. In soft tissue, two boundaries that generate reflections are separated in axial distance (depth) by 1 mm. With a two-cycle pulse of ultrasound, the minimum frequency that will axially resolve these boundaries is
    a. 1.0 MHz.
    b. 2.0 MHz.
    c. 3.0 MHz.
    d. 4.0 MHz.
    e. 5.0 MHz.

135. Transducers operating properly in pulse-echo imaging systems have a quality factor of approximately
    a. 1 to 3.
    b. 7 to 10.
    c. 25 to 50.
    d. 100.
    e. 500.

136. Which of the following quantities varies most with distance from the transducer face?
    a. Axial resolution
    b. Lateral resolution
    c. Frequency

d. Wavelength

e. Period

137. The near-zone length for an unfocused, 5-MHz, circular transducer with a 13-mm diameter is greater than that for which of the following 5-MHz transducers with diameters as listed?

a. 19 mm

b. 15 mm

c. 9 mm

d. Depends on impedance

e. None of the above

138. If the near-zone length of an unfocused transducer that is 13 mm in diameter extends (in soft tissue) 6 cm from the transducer face, at which of the following distances from the face can the lateral resolution be improved by focusing the sound from this transducer?

a. 13 cm

b. 8 cm

c. 3 cm

d. 9 cm

e. None of the above

139. The lateral resolution of an ultrasound system depends on

a. the transducer diameter.

b. the transducer frequency.

c. the speed of sound in soft tissue.

d. memory and display.

e. all of the above.

140. Which of the following is a characteristic of a medium through which sound is propagating?

a. Impedance

b. Intensity

c. Amplitude

d. Frequency

e. Period

141. Which of the following cannot be determined from the others?

a. Frequency

b. Period

c. Amplitude

d. Wavelength

e. Propagation speed

142. For perpendicular incidence, if the impedances of two media are the same, there will be no

a. inflation.

b. reflection.

c. refraction.

d. calibration.

e. b and c.

143. What is the transmitted intensity if the incident intensity is 1 and the impedances are 1.00 and 2.64?

a. 0.2

b. 0.4

c. 0.6

d. 0.8

e. 1.0

144. Increasing the intensity produced by the transducer

a. is accomplished by increasing pulser voltage.

b. increases the sensitivity of the system.

c. increases the possibility of biologic effects.

d. all of the above.

e. none of the above.

145. If the propagation speeds of two media are equal, incidence angle equals

a. reflection angle.

b. transmission angle.

c. Doppler angle.

d. a and b.

e. b and c.

146. If no reflection occurs at a boundary, it always means that media impedances are equal in the case of

a. perpendicular incidence.

b. oblique incidence.

c. refraction.

d. a and b.

e. b and c.

147. Increasing spatial pulse length

a. accompanies increased transducer damping.

b. is accompanied by decreased pulse duration.

c. improves axial resolution.

d. all of the above.

e. none of the above.

148. Place the following media in order of increasing sound propagation speed:

a. Gas, solid, liquid

b. Solid, liquid, gas

c. Gas, liquid, solid

d. Liquid, solid, gas

e. Solid, gas, liquid

149. What is the wavelength of 1-MHz ultrasound in tissue with a propagation speed of 1540 m/s?

a. 1×10^6 m

b. 1.54 mm

c. 1540 m

d. 1.54 cm

e. 0.77 cm

150. What is the spatial pulse length for two cycles of ultrasound having a wavelength of 2 mm?

a. 4 cm

b. 4 mm

c. 7 mm

d. 1.5 mm

e. 3 mm

151. Increased damping produces which of the following?

a. Increased bandwidth

b. Shorter pulses

c. Decreased efficiency
d. All of the above
e. None of the above

152. If no refraction occurs as an oblique sound beam passes through the boundary between two materials, what is unchanged as the boundary is crossed?
    a. Impedance
    b. Propagation speed
    c. Intensity
    d. Sound direction
    e. b and d

153. If the spatial average intensity in a beam is 1 W/cm² and the transducer is 5 cm² in area, what is the total acoustic power?
    a. 1 W
    b. 2 W
    c. 3 W
    d. 4 W
    e. 5 W

154. How does the propagation speed in bone compare with that in soft tissue?
    a. Lower
    b. The same
    c. Higher
    d. Cannot say unless soft tissue is specified
    e. b and c

155. Attenuation along a sound path is a decrease in
    a. Frequency
    b. Amplitude
    c. Intensity
    d. b and c
    e. Impedance

156. A focused transducer that is 13 mm in diameter has a lateral resolution at the focus of better than (i.e., smaller than)
    a. 26 mm.
    b. 13 mm.
    c. 6.5 mm.
    d. depends on frequency.
    e. none of the above.

157. An important factor in the selection of a transducer for a specific application is the ultrasonic attenuation of tissue. Because of this attenuation, a 7.5-MHz transducer generally should be used for
    a. imaging deep structures.
    b. imaging superficial structures.
    c. imaging deep and shallow structures.
    d. imaging adult intracranial structures.
    e. all of the above.

158. A real-time scan
    a. consists of many frames produced per second.
    b. depends on how short a time the sonographer takes to make a scan.

c. is made only between 8 AM and 5 PM.
d. yields a gray-scale image, whereas other scans yield only an M mode display.
e. none of the above.

159. Which of the following is determined by the pulser in an instrument?
    a. Amplitude
    b. Pulse repetition frequency
    c. Length of time required for a pulse to reach a specific reflector and return to the instrument
    d. More than one of the above
    e. None of the above

160. If the power at the output of an amplifier is 1000 times the power at the input, the gain is
    a. 60 dB.
    b. 30 dB.
    c. 1000 dB.
    d. 1000 volts.
    e. none of the above.

161. The dynamic range of an ultrasound system is defined as
    a. the speed with which ultrasound examination can be performed.
    b. the range over which the transducer can be manipulated.
    c. the ratio of the maximum to the minimum intensity that can be displayed.
    d. the range of pulser voltages applied to the transducer.
    e. none of the above.

162. The display generally will have a dynamic range _____ than other portions of the ultrasound instrument.
    a. Larger
    b. Smaller

163. The number 30 in the binary system is
    a. 0110.
    b. 1110.
    c. 1001.
    d. 1111.
    e. none of the above.

164. An ultrasound instrument that could represent 64 shades of gray would require an 8-bit memory. True or false?

165. Imaging systems consist of a beam former, display, and _____ and _____ processors.
    a. Beam
    b. Image
    c. Signal
    d. a and b
    e. b and c

166. Phased array systems involve the sequential switching of a small group of elements along the array. True or false?

167. For a two-cycle pulse of 5 MHz in soft tissue, the axial resolution is
    a. 0.1 mm.
    b. 0.3 mm.
    c. 0.5 mm.
    d. 0.7 mm.
    e. 0.9 mm.

168. Postprocessing is the process of assigning numbers to be placed in memory. True or false?

169. The minimum displayed axial dimension of a reflector is approximately equal to
    a. beam diameter.
    b. half the beam diameter.
    c. twice the beam diameter.
    d. spatial pulse length.
    e. half the spatial pulse length.
    f. twice the spatial pulse length.

170. The minimum displayed lateral dimension of a reflector is approximately equal to
    a. beam diameter.
    b. half the beam diameter.
    c. twice the beam diameter.
    d. spatial pulse length.
    e. half the spatial pulse length.
    f. twice the spatial pulse length.

171. M mode recordings have _____ dimension(s).
    a. Two spatial
    b. One spatial and one temporal
    c. One Doppler and one temporal
    d. One Doppler and one spatial
    e. b and c

172. Nonlinear propagation of ultrasound in tissue generates
    a. speckle.
    b. attenuation.
    c. harmonics.
    d. refraction.
    e. reverberations.

173. The operation in the signal processor that reduces noise is
    a. filtering.
    b. time gain compensation.
    c. scan conversion.
    d. compression.
    e. detection.

174. The binary number 01001 is _____ in the decimal system.
    a. 1
    b. 3
    c. 5
    d. 7
    e. 9

175. Reflectors may be added to the display because of
    a. reverberation.
    b. propagation speed error.
    c. enhancement.
    d. oblique reflection.
    e. Doppler shift.

176. If the propagation speed in a soft tissue path is 1.60 mm/µs, a diagnostic instrument assumes a propagation speed too _____ and will show reflectors too _____ the transducer.
    a. High, close to
    b. High, far from
    c. Low, close to
    d. Low, far from
    e. None of the above

177. The reflector information that can be obtained from an M mode display includes
    a. distance and motion pattern.
    b. transducer frequency, reflection coefficient, and distance.
    c. acoustic impedance, attenuation, and motion pattern.
    d. all of the above.
    e. none of the above.

178. Increasing the gain generally produces the same effect as
    a. decreasing the attenuation.
    b. increasing the compression.
    c. increasing the rectification.
    d. both b and c.
    e. all of the above.

179. A gray-scale display shows
    a. gray color on a white background.
    b. reflections with one brightness level.
    c. a white color on a gray background.
    d. a range of reflection amplitudes or intensities.
    e. none of the above.

180. Electric pulses from the pulser are applied through the delays and transmit/receive switch to the
    a. pulser.
    b. transducer.
    c. demodulator.
    d. display.
    e. memory.

181. Peak detection is part of
    a. amplipression.
    b. rejection.
    c. a and b.
    d. compression.
    e. amplitude demodulation.

182. Multiple focus is not used with color Doppler instruments because of
    a. ensemble length.
    b. wall filter.
    c. priority.

d. low frame rate.

e. a and d.

183. If the gain of an amplifier is reduced by 3 dB and input power is unchanged, the output power of the amplifier is _____ what it was before.
    a. equal to.
    b. twice.
    c. one half.
    d. greater than.
    e. none of the above.

184. If gain was 30 dB and output power is reduced by one half, the new gain is _____ dB.
    a. 15
    b. 60
    c. 33
    d. 27
    e. None of the above

185. If four shades of gray are shown on a display, each twice the brightness of the preceding one, the brightest shade is _____ times the brightness of the dimmest shade.
    a. 2
    b. 4
    c. 8
    d. 16
    e. 32

186. The dynamic range displayed in Exercise 185 is _____ dB.
    a. 100
    b. 9
    c. 5
    d. 2
    e. 0

187. Phantoms with nylon lines measure
    a. resolution.
    b. pulse duration.
    c. spatial average–temporal average intensity.
    d. wavelength.
    e. all of the above.

188. The following may be used to measure acoustic output:
    a. Hydrophone
    b. Optical encoder
    c. 100-mm test object
    d. All of the above
    e. None of the above

189. Real-time imaging is made possible by
    a. scan converters.
    b. single-element transducers.
    c. gray-scale display.
    d. transmit/receive switches.
    e. arrays.

190. Gain and attenuation are usually expressed in
    a. decibels.
    b. decibels per centimeter.

c. centimeters.

d. centimeters per decibel.

e. none of the above.

191. Gray-scale display requires
    a. array transducers.
    b. cathode-ray storage tubes.
    c. more than one bit per pixel.
    d. b and c.
    e. all of the above.

192. With which of the following is time represented on one axis?
    a. B mode
    b. B scan
    c. M mode
    d. A la mode
    e. None of the above

193. Analog voltages occur at the output of the
    a. beam former.
    b. transducer.
    c. signal processor.
    d. display.
    e. a and b.

194. Digital signals occur at the output of the
    a. beam former.
    b. transducer.
    c. signal processor.
    d. display.
    e. a and c.

195. Which of the following produce(s) a rectangular image format?
    a. Vector array
    b. Convex array
    c. Phased array
    d. Linear array
    e. All of the above

196. The piezoelectric effect describes how _____ is converted into _____ by a _____.
    a. Electricity, an image, display
    b. Incident sound, reflected sound, boundary
    c. Ultrasound, electricity, transducer
    d. Ultrasound, heat, tissue
    e. None of the above

197. Propagation speed in soft tissues
    a. is directly proportional to frequency.
    b. is inversely proportional to frequency.
    c. is directly proportional to intensity.
    d. is inversely proportional to intensity.
    e. none of the above.

198. Doppler-power imaging indicates (with color) the _____ of flow.
    a. Presence
    b. Direction
    c. Speed
    d. Character
    e. More than one of the above

199. As frequency is increased,
    a. wavelength increases.
    b. a three-cycle ultrasound pulse decreases in length.
    c. imaging depth decreases.
    d. propagation speed decreases.
    e. b and c.

200. Focusing
    a. improves lateral resolution.
    b. improves axial resolution.
    c. increases beam width in the focal region.
    d. shortens pulse length.
    e. increases duty factor.

Glossary

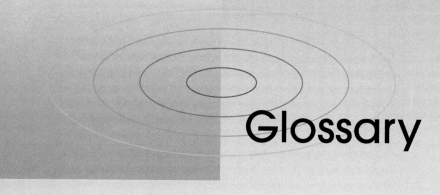

All of the key terms that were listed at the beginning of the individual chapters are compiled and defined here. More detailed and complete compilations of terminology are available.[98,99]

A mode. A display presentation of echo amplitude versus depth (used in ophthalmology).

Absorption. Conversion of sound to heat.

Acoustic. Having to do with sound.

Acoustic variables. Pressure, density, and particle vibration; sound wave quantities that vary in space and time.

ALARA. Acronym for "as low as reasonably achievable"; the principle that it is prudent to obtain diagnostic information with the least amount possible of energy exposure to the patient.

Aliasing. Improper Doppler-shift information from a pulsed wave Doppler or color Doppler instrument when the true Doppler shift exceeds one half the pulse repetition frequency.

Amplification. The process by which small voltages are increased to larger ones.

Amplifier. A device that accomplishes amplification.

Amplitude. Maximum variation of an acoustic variable or voltage.

Analog. Related to a procedure or system in which data are represented by proportional, continuously variable, physical quantities (e.g., electric voltage).

Analog-to-digital converter. A device that converts voltage amplitude to a number. Abbreviated ADC.

Anechoic. Echo-free.

Aperture. Size of a transducer element (for a single-element transducer) or group of elements (for an array).

Apodization. Nonuniform (i.e., involving different voltage amplitudes) driving of elements in an array to reduce grating lobes.

Array. A transducer assembly containing several piezo-electric elements.

Attenuation. Decrease in amplitude and intensity with distance as a wave travels through a medium.

Attenuation coefficient. Attenuation per centimeter of wave travel.

Autocorrelation. A rapid technique, used in most color Doppler instruments, for obtaining mean Doppler-shift frequency.

Axial. In the direction of the transducer axis (sound travel direction).

Axial resolution. The minimum reflector separation along the sound path that is required to produce separate echoes (i.e., to distinguish between two reflectors).

B mode. Mode of operation in which the display presents a spot of appropriate brightness for each echo received by the transducer.

B scan. A B mode image that represents an anatomic cross section through the scanning plane.

Backscatter. Sound scattered back in the direction from which it originally came.

Bandwidth. Range of frequencies contained in an ultrasound pulse; range of frequencies within which a material, device, or system can operate.

Baseline shift. Movement of the zero Doppler-shift frequency or zero flow speed line up or down on a spectral display.

Beam. Region containing continuous wave sound; region through which a sound pulse propagates.

Beam area. Cross-sectional area of a sound beam.

Beam former. The part of an instrument that accomplishes electronic beam scanning, apodization, steering, focusing, and aperture with arrays.

Bernoulli effect. Pressure reduction in a region of high-flow speed.

Bidirectional. Indicating Doppler instruments capable of distinguishing between positive and negative Doppler shifts (forward and reverse flow).

Bistable. Having two possible states (e.g., on or off, white or black).

Bit. Binary digit.

Cathode-ray tube. A display device that produces an image by scanning an electron beam over a phosphor-coated screen. Abbreviated CRT.

Cavitation. Production and dynamics of bubbles in sound.

Channel. A single one- or two-way path for transmitting electric signals, in distinction from other parallel paths; an independent transmission delay line and transducer element path; an independent reception transducer element, amplifier, analog-to-digital converter, and delay line path.

Cine loop. Sequential display of all the frames stored in memory at a controllable frame rate.

Clutter. Noise in the Doppler signal that generally is caused by high-amplitude, Doppler-shifted echoes from the heart or vessel walls.

Coded excitation. A sophisticated form of transmission in which the driving voltage pulses have intrapulse variations in amplitude, frequency, and/or phase.

Color Doppler display. The presentation of two-dimensional, real-time Doppler-shift information superimposed on a real-time, gray-scale, anatomic, cross-sectional image. Flow directions toward and away from the transducer (i.e., positive and negative Doppler shifts) are presented as different colors on the display.

Comet tail. A series of closely spaced reverberation echoes.

Compensation. Equalization of received echo amplitude differences caused by different attenuations for different reflector depths; also called depth gain compensation or time gain compensation.

Compliance. Distensibility; nonrigid stretchability of vessels.

Composite. Combination of a piezoelectric ceramic and a nonpiezoelectric polymer.

Compression. Reduction in differences between small and large amplitudes. Region of high density and pressure in a compressional wave.

Constructive interference. Combination of positive or negative pressures.

Continuous wave. A wave in which cycles repeat indefinitely; not pulsed. Abbreviated CW.

Continuous wave Doppler. A Doppler device or procedure that uses continuous wave ultrasound.

Contrast agent. A suspension of bubbles or particles introduced into circulation to enhance the contrast between anatomic structures, thereby improving their imaging.

Contrast resolution. Ability of a gray-scale display to distinguish between echoes of slightly different intensities.

Convex array. Curved linear array.

Cosine. The cosine of angle A in Figure 5-20, *C,* is the length of side *b* divided by the length of side *c.* Abbreviated cos.

Coupling medium. A gel used to provide a good sound path between a transducer and the skin by eliminating the air between the two.

Critical Reynolds number. The Reynolds number above which turbulence occurs.

Cross-talk. Leakage of strong signals in one direction channel of a Doppler receiver into the other channel; can produce the Doppler mirror-image artifact.

Crystal. Element.

Curie point. Temperature at which an element material loses its piezoelectric properties.

Cycle. One complete variation of an acoustic variable.

Damping. Material attached to the rear face of a transducer element to reduce pulse duration; the process of pulse duration reduction.

Decibel. Unit of power or intensity ratio; the number of decibels is 10 times the logarithm (to the base 10) of the power or intensity ratio. Abbreviated dB.

Demodulation. Detection.

Density. Mass divided by volume.

Depth gain compensation. See *compensation.* Abbreviated DGC.

Destructive interference. Combination of positive and negative pressures.

Detail resolution. The ability to image fine detail and to distinguish closely spaced reflectors. (See *axial resolution* and *lateral resolution.*)

Detection. Conversion of voltage pulses from radio frequency to video form. Also called demodulation, amplitude detection, and envelope detection.

Digital. Related to a procedure or system in which data are represented by numeric digits.

Digital-to-analog converter. A device that converts a number to a proportional voltage amplitude. Abbreviated DAC.

Disk. A thin, flat, circular object.

Display. A device that presents a visual image derived from voltages received from an image processor.

Disturbed flow. Flow that cannot be described by straight, parallel streamlines.

Doppler angle. The angle between the sound beam and the flow direction.

Doppler effect. A change in frequency caused by motion of reflectors.

Doppler equation. The mathematical description of the relationship between Doppler shift, frequency, Doppler angle, propagation speed, and reflector speed.

Doppler-power display. Color Doppler display in which colors are assigned according to the strength (amplitude, power, intensity, energy) of the Doppler-shifted echoes.

Doppler shift. Reflected frequency minus incident frequency; a change in frequency that occurs as a result of motion.

Doppler spectrum. The range of frequencies present in Doppler-shifted echoes.

Duplex instrument. An ultrasound instrument that combines gray-scale sonography with pulsed Doppler and, possibly, continuous wave Doppler.

Duty factor. Fraction of time that pulsed ultrasound is on.

Dynamic aperture. Aperture that increases with increasing focal length (to maintain constant focal width).

Dynamic focusing. Continuously variable reception focusing that follows the increasing depth of the transmitted pulse as it travels.

Dynamic range. Ratio (in decibels) of largest to smallest power that a system can handle; ratio of the largest to smallest intensity of echoes encountered.

Echo. Reflection.

Eddies. Regions of circular flow patterns present in turbulence.

Element. The piezoelectric component of a transducer assembly.

Elevational resolution. The detail resolution in the direction perpendicular to the scan plane. It is equal to the section thickness and is the source of section thickness artifact.

Energy. Capability of doing work.

Enhancement. Increase in echo amplitude from reflectors that lie behind a weakly attenuating structure.

Ensemble length. Number of pulses used to generate one color Doppler image scan line.

f number. Focal length divided by transducer size (aperture).

Far zone. The region of a sound beam in which the beam diameter increases as the distance from the transducer increases; also called far field.

Fast Fourier transform. Digital computer implementation of the Fourier transform.

Filter. An electric circuit that passes frequencies within a certain range.

Flat-panel display. A back-lighted rectangular matrix of thousands of liquid crystal display elements.

Flow. To move in a stream; volume flow rate.

Fluid. A material that flows and conforms to the shape of its container; a gas or liquid.

Focal length. Distance from a focused transducer to the center of a focal region or to the location of the spatial peak intensity.

Focal region. Region of minimum beam diameter and area.

Focal zone. Length of the focal region.

Focus. The concentration of the sound beam into a smaller beam area than would exist otherwise.

Fourier transform. A mathematical technique for obtaining a Doppler frequency spectrum.

Fractional bandwidth. Bandwidth divided by operating frequency.

Frame. A single image produced by one complete scan of the sound beam.

Frame rate. Number of frames of echo information stored each second.

Fraunhofer zone. Far zone.

Freeze-frame. Constant display of one of the frames in memory.

Frequency. Number of cycles per second.

Frequency spectrum. The range of Doppler-shift frequencies present in the returning echoes.

Fresnel zone. Near zone.

Fundamental frequency. The primary frequency in a collection of frequencies that can include odd and even harmonics and subharmonics.

Gain. Ratio (in decibels) of amplifier output to input electric power.

Gate. A device that allows only echoes from a selected depth (arrival time) to pass.

Grating lobes. Additional weaker beams of sound traveling out in directions different from the primary beam as a result of the multielement structure of transducer arrays.

Gray scale. Range of brightnesses between white and black.

Harmonics. Frequencies that are even and odd multiples of another, commonly called the fundamental or operating frequency.

Hertz. Unit of frequency, one cycle per second; unit of pulse repetition frequency, one pulse per second. Abbreviated Hz.

Hue. The color perceived based on the frequency of light.

Hydrophone. A small transducer element mounted on the end of a narrow tube; a piezoelectric membrane with small metallic electrodes.

Hypoechoic. Having relatively weak echoes. Opposite of hyperechoic (having relatively strong echoes).

Image. A reproduction, representation, or imitation of the physical form of a person or thing.

Image memory. The part of the image processor where echo information is stored in image format.

Image processor. An electronic device that manipulates and prepares images for visual presentation.

Impedance. Density multiplied by the sound propagation speed.

Incidence angle. Angle between incident sound direction and a line perpendicular to the boundary of a medium.

Inertia. Resistance to acceleration.

Instrument. An electronic system that electrically drives a transducer, receives returning echoes, and presents them on a visual display as an anatomic image, Doppler spectrum, or color Doppler presentation.

Intensity. Power divided by area.

Intensity reflection coefficient. Reflected intensity divided by incident intensity; the fraction of incident intensity reflected.

Intensity transmission coefficient. Transmitted intensity divided by incident intensity; the fraction of incident intensity transmitted into the second medium.

Interference. Combinations of positive and/or negative pressures.

Kilohertz. One thousand hertz. Abbreviated kHz.

Laminar flow. Flow in which fluid layers slide over each other in a smooth, orderly manner, with no mixing between layers.

Lateral. Perpendicular to the direction of sound travel.

Lateral gain control. Gain controls that enable different gain values to be applied laterally across an image to compensate for differing attenuation values in different anatomic regions.

Lateral resolution. Minimum reflector separation perpendicular to the sound path that is required to produce separate echoes.

Lead zirconate titanate. A ceramic piezoelectric material. Abbreviated PZT.

Lens. A curved material that focuses a sound or light beam.

Linear. Adjectival form of *line*.

Linear array. Array made of rectangular elements arranged in a line.

Linear image. An anatomic image presented in a rectangular format.

Linear phased array. Linear array operated by applying voltage pulses to all elements, but with small time differences (phasing) to direct ultrasound pulses out in various directions.

Linear sequenced array. Linear array operated by applying voltage pulses to groups of elements sequentially.

Longitudinal wave. Wave in which the particle motion is parallel to the direction of wave travel (compressional wave).

Luminance. Brightness of a presented hue and saturation.

M mode. A B mode presentation of changing reflector position (motion) versus time (used in echocardiography).

Mass. Measure of the resistance of an object to acceleration.

Matching layer. Material attached to the front face of a transducer element to reduce the reflections at the transducer surface.

Mechanical index. An indicator of nonthermal mechanism activity; equal to the peak rarefactional pressure divided by the square root of the center frequency of the pulse bandwidth.

Medium. Material through which a wave travels.

Megahertz. One million hertz. Abbreviated MHz.

Mirror image. An artifactual gray-scale, color flow, or Doppler signal appearing on the opposite side (from the real structure or flow) of a strong reflector.

Multiple reflection. Several reflections produced by a pulse encountering a pair of reflectors; reverberation.

Natural focus. The narrowing of a sound beam that occurs with an unfocused flat transducer element.

Near zone. The region of a sound beam in which the beam diameter decreases as the distance from the transducer increases; also called near field.

Nonlinear propagation. Sound propagation in which the propagation speed depends on pressure causing the wave shape to change and harmonics to be generated.

Nyquist limit. The Doppler-shift frequency above which aliasing occurs; one half the pulse repetition frequency.

Oblique incidence. Sound direction that is not perpendicular to media boundaries.

Operating frequency. Preferred (maximum efficiency) frequency of operation of a transducer.

Panoramic imaging. An expansion of the field of view beyond the normal limits of a transducer scan plane.

Parabolic flow. Laminar flow with a profile in the shape of a parabola.

Penetration. Imaging depth.

Period. Time per cycle.

Perpendicular. Geometrically related by 90 degrees.

Perpendicular incidence. Sound direction that is perpendicular to the boundary between media.

Persistence. Averaging sequential frames together.

Phantom. Tissue-equivalent device that has characteristics that are representative of tissues (e.g., scattering, propagation speed, and attenuation).

Phase. A description of progress through a cycle; one full cycle is divided into 360 degrees of phase.

Phase quadrature. Two signals differing by one fourth of a cycle.

Phased array. An array that steers and focuses the beam electronically (with short time delays).

Phased linear array. Linear sequenced array with phased focusing added; linear sequenced array with phased steering of pulses to produce a parallelogram-shaped display.

Picture archiving and communications system. The system provides means for electronically communicating images and associated information to work stations and devices external to the sonographic instrument, the examining room and even the building in which the scanning is done. Abbreviated PACS.

Piezoelectricity. Conversion of pressure to electric voltage.

Pixel. Picture element; the unit into which imaging information is divided for storage and display in a digital instrument.

Plug flow. Flow with all fluid portions traveling with the same flow speed and direction.

Poise. Unit of viscosity.

Poiseuille's equation. The mathematical description of the dependence of volume flow rate on pressure, vessel length and radius, and fluid viscosity.

Polyvinylidene fluoride. A piezoelectric thin-film material.

Postprocessing. Image processing done after memory.

Power. Rate at which work is done; rate at which energy is transferred.

Preprocessing. Signal and image processing accomplished before memory.

Pressure. Force divided by the area in a fluid.

Priority. The gray-scale echo strength below which color Doppler information is shown preferentially on a display.

Probe. Transducer assembly.

Propagation. Progression or travel.

Propagation speed. Speed with which a wave moves through a medium.

Pulsatile flow. Flow that accelerates and decelerates with each cardiac cycle.

Pulsatility index. A description of the relationship between peak systolic and end-diastolic flow speeds or Doppler shifts.

Pulse. A brief excursion of a quantity from its normal value; a few cycles.

Pulse duration. Interval of time from beginning to end of a pulse.

Pulse repetition frequency. Number of pulses per second; sometimes called pulse repetition rate. Abbreviated PRF.

Pulse repetition period. Interval of time from the beginning of one pulse to the beginning of the next.

Pulsed Doppler. A Doppler device or procedure that uses pulsed wave ultrasound.

Pulsed ultrasound. Ultrasound produced in pulsed form by applying electric pulses or voltages of one or a few cycles to the transducer.

Pulse-echo technique. Ultrasound imaging in which pulses are reflected and used to produce a display.

Radiation force. The force exerted by a sound beam on an absorber or a reflector.

Radio frequency. Voltages representing echoes in cyclic form. Abbreviated RF.

Range ambiguity. An artifact produced when echoes are placed too close to the transducer because a second pulse was emitted before they were received.

Range equation. Relationship between round-trip pulse travel time, propagation speed, and distance to a reflector.

Range gating. Selection of the depth from which echoes are accepted based on echo arrival time.

Rarefaction. Region of low density and pressure in a compressional wave.

Rayl. Unit of impedance.

Real time. Imaging with a rapid frame sequence display.

Real-time display. A display that, with a sufficient frame rate, appears to image moving structures or a changing scan plane continuously.

Reflection. Portion of sound returned from a media boundary; echo.

Reflection angle. Angle between the reflected sound direction and a line perpendicular to the media boundary.

Reflector. Media boundary that produces a reflection; reflecting surface.

Refraction. Change of sound direction on passing from one medium to another.

Refresh rate. The number of times each second that information is sent from image memory to the display. The number of times per second that a computer monitor redraws the information found in memory.

Resistance (flow). Pressure difference divided by volume flow rate for steady flow.

Resolution. The ability to distinguish echoes in terms of space, time, or strength (called detail, temporal, and contrast resolutions, respectively).

Resonance. The condition where a driven mechanical vibration is of a frequency similar to a natural vibration frequency of the structure.

Resonance frequency. Operating frequency.

Reverberation. Multiple reflection.

Reynolds number. A number that depends on flow speed and viscosity to predict the onset of turbulence.

Ring-down artifact. An artifact resulting from a continuous stream of sound emanating from an anatomic site.

Sample volume. The anatomic region from which pulsed Doppler echoes are accepted.

Saturation. The amount of hue present in a mix with white.

Scan converter. An electronic device that reformats echo data into an image form for image processing, storage, and display.

Scan line. A line produced on a display that represents ultrasonic echoes returning from the body. A sonographic image is composed of many such lines.

Scanhead. Transducer assembly.

Scanning. The sweeping of a sound beam through anatomy to produce an image.

Scatterer. An object that scatters sound because of its small size or its surface roughness.

Scattering. Diffusion or redirection of sound in several directions upon encountering a particle suspension or a rough surface.

Section thickness. Thickness of the scanned tissue volume perpendicular to the scan plane; also called slice thickness.

Sector. A geometric figure bounded by two radii and the arc of the circle included between them.

Sector image. An anatomic image presented in a pie slice–shaped format.

Sensitivity. Ability of an imaging system to detect weak echoes.

Shadowing. Reduction in echo amplitude from reflectors that lie behind a strongly reflecting or attenuating structure.

Side lobes. Weaker beams of sound traveling out from a single element in directions different from that of the primary beam.

Signal. Information-bearing voltages in an electric circuit; an acoustic, visual, electric, or other conveyance of information. The physical representation of a message or information.

Signal processor. An electronic device that manipulates electric signals in preparation for appropriate presentation of information contained in them.

Sonography. Medical two-dimensional, cross-sectional, and three-dimensional anatomic and flow imaging using ultrasound.

Sound. Traveling wave of acoustic variables.

Sound beam. The region of a medium that contains virtually all of the sound produced by a transducer.

Source. An emitter of ultrasound; transducer.

Spatial compounding. Averaging of frames that view anatomy from different angles.

Spatial pulse length. Length of space over which a pulse occurs.

Speckle. The granular appearance of images and spectral displays that is caused by the interference of echoes from the distribution of scatterers in tissue.

Spectral analysis. Separation of frequencies in a Doppler signal for display as a Doppler spectrum; the application of the Fourier transform to determine the frequency components present in a Doppler signal.

Spectral broadening. The widening of the Doppler-shift spectrum; that is, the increase in the range of Doppler-shift frequencies present that occurs because of a broadened range of flow velocities encountered by the sound beam. This occurs for disturbed and turbulent flow.

Spectral display. The presentation of Doppler information in a quantitative form. Visual display of a Doppler spectrum.

Spectrum analyzer. A device that derives a frequency spectrum from a complex signal.

Specular reflection. Reflection from a large (relative to wavelength), flat, smooth boundary.

Speed error. Propagation speed that is different from the assumed value (1.54 mm/μs).

Stenosis. Narrowing of a vessel.

Stiffness. Property of a medium; applied pressure divided by the fractional volume change produced by the pressure.

Streamline. A line representing the path of motion of a particle of fluid.

Strength. Nonspecific term referring to amplitude or intensity.

Temporal resolution. Ability to distinguish closely spaced events in time; improves with increased frame rate.

Test object. A device without tissuelike properties that is designed to measure some characteristic of an imaging system.

Thermal index. An indicator of thermal mechanism activity (estimated temperature rise); a value equal to transducer acoustic output power divided by the estimated power required to raise tissue temperature by $1°$ C.

Time gain compensation. Equalization of echo amplitude differences caused by different attenuations for different reflector depths; also called depth gain compensation. Abbreviated TGC.

Transducer. A device that converts energy from one form to another.

Transducer assembly. Transducer element(s) with damping and matching materials assembled in a case.

Transmission angle. Angle between the transmitted sound direction and a line perpendicular to the media boundary.

Turbulence. Random, chaotic, multidirectional flow of a fluid with mixing between layers; flow that is not laminar.

Ultrasound. Sound having a frequency greater than what humans can hear, that is, greater than 20 kHz.

Ultrasound transducer. A device that converts electric energy to ultrasound energy and vice versa.

Variance. Square of standard deviation; one of the outputs of the autocorrelation process; a measure of spectral broadening (i.e., spread around the mean).

Vector array. Linear sequenced array that emits pulses from different starting points and (by phasing) in different directions.

Video. Demodulated amplitude voltages representing echoes.

Viscosity. Resistance of a fluid to flow.

Volumetric flow rate. Volume of fluid passing a point per unit of time (i.e., per second or minute).

Wall filter. An electric filter that passes frequencies above a set level and eliminates strong, low-frequency Doppler shifts from pulsating heart or vessel walls.

Wave. Traveling variation of one or more quantities.

Wavelength. Length of space over which a cycle occurs.

Window. An anechoic region appearing beneath echo frequencies presented on a Doppler spectral display.

Work. Force multiplied by displacement.

Zero-crossing detector. An analog detector that yields mean Doppler shift as a function of time.

Answers to Exercises

Chapter 1

1. Pulses, ultrasound, echoes, image
2. Pulse-echo
3. Strength
4. Vertical, parallel
5. Origin
6. Rectangular
7. Slice, pie
8. Pointed, curved
9. Origin
10. Pulse, echo, location, strength, location, brightness
11. Transducer
12. Ultrasound pulses, echoes
13. Two-dimensional
14. Cross sections
15. d
16. Motion
17. d
18. Blood, loudspeakers, display
19. Strip-chart, spectral, color
20. Shift, power
21. a
22. d
23. e
24. c
25. b

Chapter 2

1. Wave variables
2. Acoustic variables
3. 20,000
4. Pressure, density, particle vibration
5. c, d, e
6. a, e
7. Cycles
8. Hertz, Hz
9. Time
10. Frequency
11. Space
12. Wave or cycle
13. Propagation speed, frequency
14. Density, stiffness
15. Stiffness or hardness
16. 1540, 1.54
17. e
18. a, c, b
19. 0.22
20. Decreases
21. 10
22. Higher
23. d (fastest in solids)
24. b
25. Gases
26. Mechanical, longitudinal or compressional
27. Doubled
28. Unchanged (determined by the medium)
29. 1
30. Information
31. c
32. True
33. 6
34. d
35. c
36. e (c and d)
37. Frequencies, even, odd, fundamental, harmonics
38. 1,540,000
39. True
40. True
41. Density, propagation speed
42. 0.1 μs, 10 MHz; b. 0.25 μs, 4 MHz
43. 1.54
44. 0.38
45. Continuous wave
46. Pulses
47. Pulses
48. Period

49. Decreases
50. Time
51. Length, space
52. Duty factor
53. Period
54. Wavelength
55. 1 (100%)
56. 6
57. 0.6 (Soft tissue propagation speed is 1.54 mm/μs; wavelength is 0.3 mm.)
58. 0.4 (Period is 0.2 μs; soft tissue is irrelevant.)
59. 1 (1000 pulses per second; $1/_{1000}$ second from one pulse to the next)
60. 0.0004 (0.04%)
61. d
62. e (50,000)
63. c
64. Less than
65. Variation
66. Power, area
67. W/cm^2 or mW/cm^2
68. Amplitude
69. Doubled
70. Halved
71. Unchanged
72. Quadrupled
73. 5
74. 100
75. Temporal average
76. b
77. 100
78. 2
79. 3, 4
80. Amplitude, intensity
81. Absorption, reflection, scattering
82. Centimeter
83. dB, dB/cm
84. 0.5
85. 1.5 dB/cm
86. Increases
87. Doubled, doubled, quadrupled
88. Unchanged
89. Sound, heat
90. No (Attenuation includes absorption.)
91. Higher
92. 50, 50, 80
93. 5
94. 2.5
95. Frequency
96. Decreases
97. 0.32 (Attenuation is 8 dB and intensity ratio is 0.16.)
98. 0.00000002 (Attenuation is 80 dB, and intensity ratio is 0.00000001.
99. c (0.5 × 7.5 MHz × 0.8 cm = 3 dB)

100. a. 1; b. −1; c. 2; d. −3
101. 6 dB (Intensity ratio is 0.25.)
102. 20, 4
103. 1.9 (Intensity ratio is 0.63.)
104. e
105. Impedances
106. Impedances, intensity
107. Impedances
108. 0.0008, 1.9992
109. 0.0002, 1.9998
110. 0.0008, 1.9992
111. 0.01, 1 (incident intensity not needed)
112. 0.99, 99
113. 20 (intensity ratio of 0.01; use Table 2-3)
114. 0.01
115. 0 (Impedances are equal.)
116. 5, 0 (total reflection)
117. True, for perpendicular incidence
118. False, in general (true for perpendicular incidence if propagation speeds are also equal)
119. False, in general (true for perpendicular incidence if densities are also equal)
120. False
121. 0.9990
122. Air, reflection
123. 0.01
124. 0.43
125. d
126. Direction, propagation speed
127. Larger than, equal to
128. Smaller than, equal to
129. Equal to, equal to
130. 30, 21
131. 30, 30
132. 30, 39
133. Perpendicular incidence, equal media propagation speeds
134. 32
135. Scattering
136. True
137. False
138. a
139. True
140. c
141. e (a, b, and c are correct.)
142. Propagation speed, time
143. 4
144. 7
145. 7.7
146. 1
147. 3 cm
148. 10
149. 65 μs
150. a
151. e

152. a. 4; b. 1; c. 3; d. 5; e. 2
153. 100 μs, 50 μs, 0.5, 10 kHz, 17 μs, 60 kHz
154. d
155. Impedances
156. False
157. 80 (9-dB increase; do not forget round-trip)
158. a. 1; b. 4; c. 2; d. 3
159. d
160. c ($0.5 \times 0.99 \times 0.5 \times 0.01 \times 0.5 \times 0.99 \times 0.5 =$ 0.0006, or 0.06%)
161. a. 0.33 (33%); b. 2.5; c. 3.5
162. e (unitless)
163. Frequencies
164. 9 (yielding the same frequency penetration product, 45 cm-MHz)
165. d (double the fundamental frequency)

Chapter 3

1. Energy
2. Electric, ultrasound
3. Piezoelectric
4. Disks
5. Thickness
6. Element, assembly
7. Element, assembly
8. Pulse, frequency
9. Thickness
10. Decreases
11. Cycles, axial resolution, bandwidth, quality (Q) factor
12. Efficiency, sensitivity
13. Two, three
14. 0.2
15. e
16. Reflection
17. Air
18. False
19. False
20. Back
21. Front
22. Intermediate
23. Rectangles
24. f (a, b, c)
25. Resonance frequency
26. Composites
27. Broad bandwidth
28. No (because these frequencies are outside the bandwidth [4.5 to 5.5 MHz])
29. No (because these frequencies are outside the 2.5-MHz bandwidth [3.75 to 6.25 MHz])
30. Near, far
31. Near zone
32. Aperture
33. Frequency, aperture, distance
34. Aperture, frequency
35. Half
36. Two
37. Decreases
38. Increases
39. Increases
40. c
41. 30
42. 3, 6, 9
43. Longer
44. Shorter
45. False (can focus only in the near zone)
46. c
47. Increases
48. Doubles
49. Increased
50. d (all of the above)
51. False (See Figure 3-15.)
52. Focal length
53. c
54. b (Wavelength is 0.3 mm.)
55. a. 3; b. 2; c. 2; d. 1; e. 1 (See Table 3-3.)
56. Elements
57. Sequencing
58. a. 1; b. 2, 3; c. 2, 3; d. 1, 2, 3; e. 1; f. 3; g. 1, 2, 3
59. One (the lateral dimension in the scan plane)
60. Curved, lens
61. Elements
62. a. 1; b. 2; c. 1
63. b
64. c
65. a, e
66. b, c, d
67. c
68. The same, different
69. Different, origin
70. Convex, vector
71. Sound travel or scan lines, echoes
72. Spatial pulse length
73. True
74. 1.5
75. 1
76. Wavelength, 0.3
77. Halved
78. Doubled
79. False
80. False
81. 2
82. 15 (less than 15 MHz in many applications)
83. Wavelength, spatial pulse length
84. Attenuation
85. Separation, echoes
86. Beam width
87. f
88. True

89. True
90. False, in general (only true near the transducer)
91. b, c, e, f
92. a. 4; b. 3; c. 2; d. 1
93. a, d
94. a. 10; b. 0.15; c. 14; d. 6.5; e. 13; f. 14
95. c
96. Half, near-zone
97. Focal
98. 6.5 (frequency not needed)
99. 0.7 (size not needed)
100. True
101. False
102. Focal
103. True
104. False
105. a. 1, 2, 3; b. 2; c. 2; d. 1
106. e
107. a
108. b, c, d
109. True (axial resolution 0.3 mm)
110. Resolution, penetration
111. 2, 15
112. 1, 1.5
113. 3 mm, 2 mm
114. 4 cm
115. a. 1; b. 4; c. 3; d. 5; e. 2

Chapter 4

1. Pulse
2. Amplitude, intensity
3. a (A minimum echo reception time of 130 μs is required.)
4. Filtering, detection, compression
5. a. 2; b. 4; c. 5; d. 1; e. 3
6. 10, 100, 20
7. 1
8. 10
9. b
10. Depth
11. Times
12. Dynamic, display, vision
13. 2.0
14. Radio frequency, video
15. False
16. c
17. Zero, maximum, values, higher, weakest, strongest
18. 30
19. 50, 75, 87.5
20. 20
21. 10
22. 40
23. 32
24. 45, 32,000

25. −2, 2, 0.63
26. a. 6; b. 9; c. 10; d. 13; e. 14
27. a (43/32)
28. c (45/64)
29. a. 5; b. 3; c. 2; d. 6; e. 1; f. 4
30. e
31. a. 4; b. 5; c. 6; d. 7; e. 8
32. 50,000
33. c
34. e
35. a
36. Two (0 and 1)
37. Bit
38. Two, on, off
39. a. 3; b. 7; c. 8; d. 5; e. 4; f. 2; g. 1; h. 6
40. 25
41. 1101
42. a. 5; b. 10; c. 3; d. 1; e. 9; f. 2; g. 8; h. 7; i. 4; j. 6
43. a. 1 (0); b. 1 (1); c. 3 (101); d. 4 (1010);
    e. 5 (11001); f. 5 (11110); g. 6 (111111);
    h. 7 (1000000); i. 7 (1001011); j. 7 (1100100)
44. a. 3 (111); b. 4 (1111); c. 2 (11); d. 9 (111111111);
    e. 10 (1111111111); f. 6 (111111); g. 8 (11111111);
    h. 1 (1); i. 7 (1111111); j. 5 (11111)
45. a. 1 (0, 1); b. 2 (00, 01, 10, 11); c. 3 (000, 001,
    010, 011, 100, 101, 110, 111); d. 4; e. 4; f. 5; g. 5;
    h. 6; i. 7; j. 7
46. B (brightness), M (motion), A (amplitude), all,
    cardiac, ophthalmologic
47. a. 1, 2, 4; b. 2, 3, 5
48. Cathode, ray, CRT, flat, panel
49. Deflection
50. Brightness
51. M
52. Scan
53. Gray-scale, B mode
54. Image memory
55. c
56. d
57. 33
58. 63
59. a. 1; b. 2; c. 2; d. 2
60. 40
61. 1200
62. True (10 × 1 × 100 × 30 = 30,000, which is less than 77,000)
63. c
64. Transducer, beam former, signal processor, image processor, display
65. a. 4; b. 1; c. 2; d. 5; e. 3
66. a. 1, 2; b. 1, 2; c. 1, 2, 3; d. 3; e. 1; f. 1; g. 1, 2;
    h. 1, 2; i. 1, 2, 3; j. 1, 2, 3; k. 1, 2; l. 1, 2;
    m. 1, 2, 3; n. 1, 2, 3; o. 1, 2; p. 1, 2
67. a
68. b

69. d
70. c
71. Scan converter
72. c
73. b
74. b
75. d
76. 2, 60
77. d
78. Echoes
79. Pulse-echo
80. Brightness
81. Strength, direction, time
82. b
83. Display, voltages
84. Beam former
85. Beam former
86. Signal processor
87. a
88. a
89. Transducer
90. b
91. c
92. d
93. c
94. b
95. a
96. False
97. A, M
98. B
99. Electronic
100. Frame
101. Pulsed
102. Lines, frame
103. Frame rate
104. Increase
105. Improved, decreases, increased
106. $256 \times 512 = 131,072$; $512 \times 512 = 262,144$
107. b; e (a, c, d)
108. $1000/20 = 50$ lines per frame (one scan line for each pulse)
109. d
110. b
111. e (approaching the focus)
112. d
113. b
114. Image processor
115. Contrast

Chapter 5

1. a, c, d, e, g, h
2. Capillaries
3. a, b, f
4. d
5. c
6. Stream
7. Plasma, erythrocytes, water
8. d
9. a
10. e
11. b
12. c
13. Viscosity
14. Density
15. Density
16. 1.05 g/mL, 0.035 poise
17. Force
18. c
19. Difference, gradient
20. a
21. Pump, gravity
22. Difference, distance or separation
23. Pressure, resistance
24. d
25. Decreases
26. d
27. c
28. Vessels
29. e
30. d
31. d
32. b
33. b
34. d
35. e
36. e
37. e
38. c
39. Disturbed
40. Turbulent
41. Reynolds
42. Stenosis
43. d
44. a
45. Decrease
46. Increase
47. e
48. e
49. a
50. e
51. 33 cm/s
52. 16 cm/s, 960; 64 cm/s, 1920; 16 cm/s, 960
53. d
54. e
55. b
56. d
57. e
58. b
59. d

60. e
61. Doppler, flow
62. Frequency
63. Frequency, motion
64. Greater
65. Less
66. Equal to
67. Motion
68. 0.02, 1.02
69. 0.026
70. −0.026
71. Received, emitted
72. Cosine
73. 0.01, 1.01 (The Doppler shift is cut in half.)
74. 0, 1.00 (no Doppler shift at 90 degrees)
75. 110
76. a. 1.62; b. 0; c. 50; d. 2.5; e. 6.49; f. 0; g. 150; h. 5; i. 14.6; j. 2.81; k. 60; l. 90; m. 100; n. 3.25; o. any value; p. 30; q. 5; r. 0
77. c
78. 0.26 kHz
79. 0.44 kHz
80. 1.95 kHz
81. 100 cm/s
82. 50 cm/s
83. Decrease
84. Increase
85. 0.65 kHz
86. −6.5 kHz
87. 4.9935 MHz
88. 3.25 kHz
89. 5.62 kHz
90. False
91. Constant
92. Scatter the ultrasound; that is, produce echoes.
93. b (~5 m/s)
94. c
95. Doppler angle
96. Speed, angle
97. a
98. Doubled
99. Doubled
100. Decreased
101. 649 kHz
102. 4, 10, and 20 MHz
103. 45 degrees
104. 10 MHz, 200 cm/s
105. 5 MHz, 100 cm/s
106. 5, 0.1
107. θ_1, θ_D, θ_3, θ_1, θ_2, 90 degrees
108. b
109. d
110. Low
111. 100
112. 100
113. 2
114. It decreases as the Doppler angle increases.
115. 2, 1

Chapter 6

1. e (a, b, d; strictly speaking, black and white are not colors)
2. e (d because of c)
3. a
4. False (A small Doppler angle causes the large Doppler shift.)
5. e (aliasing at flow speeds exceeding about 64 cm/s)
6. Flow or motion, anatomy
7. d
8. Red, blue, blue, red, red, blue, unknown
9. Autocorrelation
10. Mean, sign, variance, power
11. True (power displays have no angle dependence)
12. c
13. No
14. False
15. b
16. c
17. e (a, b, or c)
18. False
19. False (It also can mean aliasing or changing Doppler angle.)
20. False (Remember the Doppler angle.)
21. Decreases
22. Autocorrelation
23. Decreases
24. d
25. a and c
26. a, b, c
27. d
28. c and d
29. c
30. a
31. c
32. d
33. a
34. b
35. False
36. False
37. 100
38. d
39. c
40. b, c
41. c
42. e (c and d)
43. b
44. e

45. False
46. a. 3; b. 2; c. 1; d. 4; e. 5
47. e (wall filter setting)
48. From right to left
49. b
50. False (nonzero Doppler angle)
51. a. 3; b. 1, 5; c. 2, 5; d. 6; e. 7; f. 1, 4; g. 2, 4
52. Left to right
53. Blue
54. Large variance
55. d
56. b
57. e
58. a
59. e (a, b, c, d)
60. Cannot determine in power display
61. a. 5; b. 4; c. 3 or 2; d. 1
62. Attenuation
63. e (a, b, c)
64. d
65. b

Chapter 7

1. False
2. Direction, bidirectional
3. False (They are undamped dual elements.)
4. Transducer, oscillator (part of beam former), Doppler detector (part of signal processor), loudspeakers, spectrum analyzer (part of signal processor), image processor, display
5. Amplitude, frequency
6. Frequency, time
7. Gray, color
8. Speeds, directions
9. True
10. Pulser, gated amplifier
11. Beam former
12. Depths, arrival times
13. False
14. True
15. True
16. Pulse repetition frequency
17. Fast Fourier transform
18. FFT
19. Pulsed
20. Pulsed
21. 50 seconds
22. 100 seconds
23. Damped, longer, efficient
24. c
25. c
26. e
27. b

28. Continuous wave and pulsed wave
29. Continuous wave
30. Pulsed wave
31. Duplex
32. Pulsed wave
33. Doppler-shift detector
34. a
35. Doppler angle
36. Cathode, ray
37. Wall, wall thump
38. 5, 30, gate, pulse
39. Baseline
40. Beam width
41. Continuous wave
42. False
43. False
44. False
45. c
46. Components or frequencies, order
47. c
48. e (a and b)
49. Shifts
50. Speeds, directions
51. Single
52. a
53. e (More accurately, it is near-plug flow or blunted flow, not true plug flow.)
54. Amplitude, power, time
55. Second
56. Color, gray scale
57. d
58. a
59. c
60. b
61. d
62. True
63. False
64. Laminar undisturbed
65. b
66. e (a, c, or d) (These would each yield a small Doppler shift.)
67. False
68. e
69. a
70. a
71. c
72. False
73. False
74. e (b, c, d)
75. False (Remember the Doppler angle.)
76. b
77. c
78. a
79. a. 2; b. 1; c. 3

80. Narrow
81. Higher
82. False
83. False (See Figure 7-30.)
84. c (high-resistance vascular bed)
85. True
86. Varies, compliant, higher, lower
87. Small Doppler angle
88. Large Doppler angle
89. False (Remember the Doppler angle.)
90. e
91. b
92. c
93. e
94. e
95. a
96. b
97. c
98. e
99. a
100. A, B, C, D
101. D, E, F, G
102. A, G
103. D
104. D
105. A, G
106. All are the same (flow speed constant, approximately 50 cm/s, in the straight tube with constant diameter).
107. All are the same (volume flow rate must be constant throughout the tube).
108. a
109. b
110. d
111. 50
112. Doppler angle
113. 60
114. 2.5
115. c

Chapter 8

1. Range, ambiguity
2. 11, 1
3. c (assumes 1.54 mm/µs, lower than the actual speed)
4. False
5. a
6. e (a, b, d)
7. False (This is the display of the interference pattern [speckle] of scattered sound from the distribution of scatterers within the ultrasound pulse in the tissue.)
8. Section thickness
9. c, d, e, f
10. True (edge shadowing)
11. Figure 8-40, A (Figure 8-40, B, shows a comet tail artifact originating as reverberations within a structure.)
12. a. 1; b. 2, 3; c. 3; d. 4, 5; e. 4, 5
13. Separation
14. Weaker
15. b
16. d
17. True
18. b
19. b
20. b
21. c
22. Refraction (double image)
23. e
24. e (c and d)
25. e
26. a
27. True
28. Continuous wave
29. Red, blue, blue, red
30. Range ambiguity
31. d
32. b
33. b
34. b
35. b
36. e
37. c
38. Yes (less attenuation, greater penetration, later echoes)
39. Yes (Doppler shift increases with increasing frequency.)
40. d
41. a
42. a. 3; b. 4; c. 3; d. 2; e. 1
43. b, c, d
44. e (b, c, d)
45. Aliased, 10
46. a. R (Color changes at a 90-degree angle because scan lines go in different directions; they are heading upstream on the right and downstream on the left.); b. L (Vessel curvature causes flow to be away from the transducer on the left and toward the transducer on the right.); c. R (The blue area at right is aliasing.); d. L (The blue in the center is aliasing.); e. L; f. L (The color changes because the vessel is curved; flow is away from the transducer on the left and toward the transducer on the right.)
47. a. 4; b. 2; c. 1; d. 3; e. 5
48. a
49. c, b, d
50. Shadowing, aliasing

Chapter 9

1. Phantom, test object
2. a. 1, 3; b. 1, 3; c. 1; d. 1; e. 4; f. 2; g. 2; h. 2; i. 5; j. 5
3. a. 4; b. 5; c. 3; d. 3; e. 1; f. 2; g. 1, 2
4. True
5. True
6. String
7. Flow, flow
8. e
9. Tissues
10. False
11. b, c, d, e
12. False
13. Transducer or piezoelectric
14. True
15. b
16. a. 2, 12; b. 3, 12; c. 3, 8; d. 4 or 2; f. 9; e. 1, 7; f. 6, 10; g. 6, 11
17. c
18. e
19. a
20. d
21. a
22. b
23. c
24. False
25. d
26. e
27. e (a, b, c)
28. False
29. False
30. b
31. No
32. Yes
33. b and d
34. c
35. e
36. e
37. e
38. a
39. d
40. b
41. e
42. c, d, e
43. b
44. a, b, d
45. e (pregnancy possibility in fertile female)
46. b
47. a
48. d
49. c
50. c

Chapter 10

Following each answer is the chapter number in which the subject is discussed. Most answers also have explanatory comments.

1. c. Ultrasound is sound of frequency greater than 20 kHz (0.02 MHz). Answer e is not in frequency units. (Chapter 2)
2. a. Propagation speeds in soft tissues are in the range of about 1.4 to 1.6 mm/μs. Answers c and e are not in speed units. (Chapter 2)
3. c. Solid; high stiffness. (Chapter 2)
4. d. Propagation speed and impedance increase only slightly with frequency. (Chapter 2)
5. e. (Chapters 2 and 3)
6. c. Round-trip travel time is 13 μs/cm. (Chapter 2)
7. c. Scattering occurs with rough surfaces and with heterogeneous media (made up of small particles relative to the wavelength). Large, flat, smooth surfaces produce specular reflections. (Chapter 2)
8. b. The operating frequency of a transducer is such that its thickness is equal to one half the wavelength in the transducer element material. (Chapter 3)
9. d. Transducer elements expand and contract when a voltage is applied; conversely, when returning echoes apply pressure to the element, a voltage is generated. (Chapter 3)
10. a. Axial resolution is equal to one half the spatial pulse length. (Chapter 3)
11. c. Lateral resolution is equal to beam width. Beam width depends on the aperture (size of the element or group of elements generating the beam). (Chapter 3)
12. a. Penetration decreases with increasing frequency, and frequency has no effect on refraction. (Chapter 3)
13. c. This is part of the American Institute of Ultrasound in Medicine "Statement on Mammalian in Vivo Ultrasonic Biological Effects." (Chapter 9)
14. c. Frequencies lower than this range do not provide the needed resolution, whereas frequencies greater than this range do not allow for adequate penetration for medical purposes. (Chapters 2 and 3)
15. a. See answer to question 14. (Chapters 2 and 3)
16. e. Reverberation adds additional reflectors on the display that are deeper than the true ones. (Chapter 8)
17. d. (Chapter 4)
18. d. (Chapter 4)
19. b. (Chapter 4)
20. d. (Chapter 4)
21. b. (Chapter 8)

22. b. (Chapter 4)
23. d. (Chapter 4)
24. c. Pulse repetition frequency has no direct effect on detail resolution. (Chapters 4 and 8)
25. d. (Chapter 4)
26. d. Distance equals one half the speed multiplied by the round-trip time. (Chapter 2)
27. e. The matching layer improves sound transmission by reducing the reflection at the transducer-skin boundary. The coupling medium improves it by removing the air layer between the transducer and the skin. (Chapter 3)
28. c. (Chapter 3)
29. a. (Chapter 3)
30. c. (Chapter 4)
31. d. If the transducer is in the path of the reflector, answer c is correct because the Doppler angle is zero. If this is not the case, then b is correct because the Doppler angle will increase (decreasing the Doppler shift) as the reflector approaches. (Chapter 5)
32. e. The diameter referred to can be the entire vessel diameter or the diameter of a small portion of it (stenosis). For the former, d is correct. For the latter, c is correct at the stenosis. In either case, a and b are correct. (Chapter 5)
33. c. Poiseuille's equation shows that resistance increases with increasing vessel length, increasing fluid viscosity, or decreasing vessel diameter. (Chapter 5)
34. d. The blood cells move along with the plasma, not through it. (Chapter 5)
35. c. Propagation speed is determined by the medium, not by motion. (Chapters 2 and 5)
36. e. (Chapter 7)
37. e. (Chapter 5)
38. d. Spectral comes from *spectrum*, referring to color spectrum. A prism is an optical spectrum analyzer that breaks down white light into its component colors. (Chapter 7)
39. a. (Chapter 5)
40. e. If frequency changes, wavelength changes also. (Chapter 5)
41. c. (Chapter 5)
42. d. Answers a and b are correct. Anatomic data are provided by the real-time B scan, and physiologic data are provided by the pulsed Doppler portion of the instrument. (Chapter 7)
43. False. Physiologic Doppler-shift frequencies are usually in the audible frequency range. (Chapter 5)
44. d. All imaging instruments and some Doppler instruments use pulsed ultrasound. (Chapters 4, 6, and 7)
45. c. (Chapters 7 and 8)
46. e. (Chapter 6)

47. d. (Chapter 5)
48. e. They include pulsed Doppler (and sometimes continuous wave Doppler) and dynamic B scan imaging. (Chapter 7)
49. c. Both Doppler shifts exceed one half the pulse repetition frequency. (Chapter 8)
50. d. (Chapters 6 and 7)
51. a. This is because physiologic speeds (*v*) are small compared with the speed of sound (*c*) in tissues. (Chapter 5)
52. b. (Chapter 5)
53. e. Arterioles and capillaries are too small. (Chapter 5)
54. d. (Chapter 5)
55. e. (Chapter 5)
56. b. (Chapter 5)
57. c. (Chapter 5)
58. d. This is Poiseuille's law. Increasing resistance *decreases* flow. (Chapter 5)
59. b. It depends on radius to the fourth power. (Chapter 5)
60. d. This is the continuity rule. (Chapter 5)
61. e. (also results of distensible vessels) (Chapter 5)
62. d. (Chapter 5)
63. e. See Figure 5-11. (Chapter 5)
64. c. (assuming a *reflector* moving at 50 cm/s) (Chapter 5)
65. b. (that is, about 5 m/s) (Chapter 5)
66. c. (smaller angle, larger cosine, larger shift) (Chapter 5)
67. a. (Chapter 5)
68. e. Spectrum is not needed; it cannot be displayed in a pixel. (Chapters 6 and 7)
69. d. The spectrum can be shown *in addition* to the color Doppler display. (Chapter 6)
70. c. (Chapters 5 and 7)

$$v = \frac{77 \times 0.100}{(5 \times 0.5)} = 3.08$$

71. a. (Chapters 5 and 7)

$$v = \frac{77 \times 0.100}{7.5} = 1.03$$

72. d. (Chapter 7)
73. c. (13 μs of delay per centimeter of depth) (Chapter 7)
74. a. This is because flow speeds are typically one thousandth the speed of sound in tissues. (Chapter 5)
75. b. The range is about 4 to 32. (Chapter 6)
76. c. The range is about 40 to 400. (Chapter 6)
77. e. Any pulsed instrument (b, c, d) can. (Chapter 8)
78. a. This is called near-plug flow. (Chapter 5)
79. d. (Chapter 6)

80. e. A stenosis generally increases a, b, and c and decreases d. (Chapters 5 and 7)
81. a. (that is, a widening of the spectrum) (Chapter 7)
82. e. Items b, c, and d are increased; a is decreased. (Chapters 5 and 7)
83. c. The blood flows back out of the high-impedance vascular bed during the low-pressure portion of the cardiac cycle. (Chapter 7)
84. c. (Chapter 7)
85. d. (Chapter 7)
86. e. (a resulting from b) (Chapter 6)
87. e. (Chapter 7)
88. a. (gray level or, sometimes, color) (Chapter 7)
89. e. (a = b + c) (Chapter 5)
90. b. (Chapter 7)
91. e. Items a and b determine sample volume length. (Chapter 7)
92. d. Echoes from the sample volume arrive after another pulse is emitted. (Chapters 7 and 8)
93. a. The shift exceeds the Nyquist limit (5 kHz). (Chapters 7 and 8)
94. e. (a and d) (Chapters 7 and 8)
95. e. (Chapter 6)
96. a. (Chapter 7)
97. e. (Chapter 6)
98. a. Because physiologic flow speeds are about one thousandth the ultrasound propagation speed (1540 m/s), Doppler shifts are about one thousandth the operating frequency. (Chapter 5)
99. e. (a and b) (Chapter 7)
100. b. (also proportional to the *cosine* of the Doppler angle) (Chapter 5)
101. d. Item a is for gray-scale instruments. (Chapter 9)
102. b. (Chapter 9)
103. e. Shift increases to 4 kHz, which is still less than the Nyquist limit (4.5 kHz). (Chapter 8)
104. a. A nonzero Doppler angle increases calculated equivalent flow speed. (Chapters 6 and 8)
105. c. The Nyquist limit is still one half of the pulse repetition frequency. (Chapters 6 and 8)
106. e. (Chapter 6)
107. e. (Chapters 6 and 8)
108. e. (a and c) (Chapter 6)
109. e. (a and b; c increases amount of color) (Chapter 6)
110. d. Item c is not strictly part of the color flow display. Also, it is not a cross-sectional display but rather a frequency-versus-time presentation. (Chapter 6)
111. b. White is brighter than gray. (Chapter 6)
112. a. Red and green are different hues, representing different light wave frequencies. (Chapter 6)
113. e. (a, b, c; about 5 to 50 frames per second are displayed) (Chapter 6)
114. d. (Chapter 6)
115. d. (Chapter 6)
116. a. The wall filter removes the lower-frequency clutter Doppler shifts. (Chapters 6 and 7)
117. d. (twice as many scan lines per frame) (Chapter 6)
118. e. Items c and d change because the scan line (pulse path) orientation changes. (Chapter 6)
119. a. Items b and c increase the amount of color. (Chapter 6)
120. d. Increasing pulse repetition frequency increases the Nyquist limit, reducing aliasing. (Chapter 8)
121. b. (Chapter 2)
122. e. The wavelength is the length of each cycle in a pulse. (Chapter 2)
123. a. Duty factor is pulse duration divided by pulse repetition period. (Chapter 2)
124. b. The attenuation coefficient of 5-MHz ultrasound is approximately 2.5 dB/cm. The attenuation coefficient multiplied by the path length yields the attenuation (in decibels). Only answer b is given in attenuation (decibel) units. (Chapter 2)
125. b. Amplitude is the maximum amount that an acoustic variable varies from the normal value (in this case, 10 − 7 units). (Chapter 2)
126. a. (Chapter 2)
127. a. Amplitude, intensity, power, and beam area are related to one another. If two of these are known, the others can be found. Frequency is independent of these. All four of them can be known, and yet frequency remains undetermined. (Chapter 2)
128. a. Impedance 1 equals 3, which equals impedance 2; thus there is no reflection. (Chapter 2)
129. b. If 96% of the intensity is transmitted, 4% is reflected because what is not reflected is transmitted (i.e., the two must add up to 100%). (Chapter 2)
130. c. (Chapter 6)
131. c. If the second speed is twice the first speed, then the transmission angle is approximately twice the incidence angle. (Chapter 2)
132. a. Reflector distance = $\frac{1}{2}$ × speed × time. (Chapter 2)
133. d. If reflectors are separated by less than the axial resolution, they are not separated on the display. (Chapter 3)
134. b. Axial resolution is equal to one half the spatial pulse length. Spatial pulse length is equal to the number of cycles in the pulse multiplied by wavelength. Wavelength is equal to propagation speed divided by frequency. For 1 MHz, wavelength is 1.54 mm, spatial pulse length is 2 × 1.54, and axial resolution is 1.54 mm, so that

two reflectors separated by 1 mm would not be resolved. For 2 MHz the resolution is 0.77 and the reflectors would be resolved. (Chapter 3)

135. a. For highly damped transducers the quality factor (Q) is approximately equal to the number of cycles in the pulse. (Chapter 3)

136. b. Beam width changes with distance from transducer and thus so does lateral resolution. (Chapter 3)

137. c. Near-zone length increases with transducer diameter so that the only transducer that would have a shorter near-zone length would be a transducer of smaller diameter. (Chapter 3)

138. c. Focusing can be accomplished only in the near zone of a beam. (Chapter 3)

139. e. Answers a, b, and c affect the beam. Resolution of the *system* also is affected by the electronics of the instrument. (Chapter 3)

140. a. All the others are characteristics of the sound. (Chapter 2)

141. c. Frequency, period, wavelength, and propagation speed are related to one another. However, all four of these can be known and yet the amplitude is undetermined. (Chapter 2)

142. e. For perpendicular incidence, there is no refraction. For equal impedances, there is no reflection. (Chapter 2)

143. d. (Chapter 2)

$$IRC = \left(\frac{2.64 - 1.00}{2.64 + 1.00}\right)^2 = \left(\frac{1.64}{3.64}\right)^2 = (0.45)^2 = 0.2$$

For an intensity reflection coefficient *(IRC)* of 0.2 and an incident intensity of 1, the reflected intensity is 0.2 and the transmitted intensity is 0.8. (Chapter 2)

144. d. (Chapters 4 and 9)

145. d. Incidence angle always equals reflection angle. For equal propagation speeds, incidence angle equals transmission angle as well. (Chapter 2)

146. a. For oblique incidence, it is possible to have no reflection, even if the media impedances are unequal. (Chapter 2)

147. e. Increased transducer damping decreases the spatial pulse length. Increasing spatial pulse length is accompanied by increased pulse duration and degraded axial resolution. (Chapters 2 and 3)

148. c. (Chapter 2)

149. b. Wavelength is equal to propagation speed divided by frequency. (Chapter 2)

150. b. Spatial pulse length is equal to wavelength multiplied by the number of cycles in the pulse. (Chapter 2)

151. d. (Chapter 3)

152. e. No refraction means that there is no change in sound direction. This is a result of no change in

propagation speed (i.e., equal propagation speeds on both sides of the boundary). (Chapter 2)

153. e. If there is 1 W in each square centimeter of area, then there are 5 W in 5 cm^2 of area. (Chapter 2)

154. c. Speeds in solids are higher than in liquids. Soft tissue behaves acoustically as a liquid (as it is mostly water). (Chapter 2)

155. d. (Chapter 2)

156. c. An unfocused 13-mm transducer has a beam width of 6.5 mm at the near-zone length. Focusing would reduce the lateral resolution below this value (i.e., improve it). (Chapter 3)

157. b. A 7.5-MHz transducer can image to a depth of only a few centimeters in tissue. (Chapter 2)

158. a. The other answers make little sense. (Chapters 3 and 4)

159. d. (a and b) (Chapter 4)

160. b. For each 10 dB, there is a factor of 10 increase in power. (Chapter 4)

161. c. (Chapter 4)

162. b. (Chapter 4)

163. e. Decimal numbers greater than 15 require at least five bits in a binary number. The number 30 in binary is 11110. (Chapter 4)

164. False. Sixty-four shades require a 6-bit memory. (Chapter 4)

165. e. (Chapter 4)

166. False. This is a description of a linear sequenced array rather than a phased array. (Chapter 3)

167. b. (Chapter 3)

$$AR = \tfrac{1}{2}\, SPL = 0.5 \times n \times c/f = (\tfrac{1}{2})\,(2)\,(1.54/5) = 0.3$$

168. False. Postprocessing is the assignment of display brightness to numbers coming out of memory. (Chapter 4)

169. e. (Chapter 3)

170. a. (Chapter 3)

171. b. In M mode, echo depth is displayed as a function of time. (Chapter 4)

172. c. (Chapter 2)

173. a. (Chapter 4)

174. e. (1 + 8 = 9) (Chapter 4)

175. a. (Chapter 8)

176. c. The instrument assumes a speed of 1.54 mm/μs. Echoes will arrive sooner because of their higher propagation speed and will be placed closer to the transducer than they should be. (Chapters 2 and 8)

177. a. (Chapter 4)

178. a. Increasing gain or decreasing attenuation increases echo intensity. (Chapters 2 and 4)

179. d. (Chapter 4)

180. b. (Chapters 3 and 4)

181. e. (Chapter 4)

182. e. Multiple pulses per scan line (ensemble length) are required for color Doppler imaging.

More pulses per scan line for multiple foci would make the frame rate unacceptably low. (Chapter 6)

183. c. A reduction of 3 dB is a 50% reduction. (Chapter 4)
184. d. See answer to Exercise 183. (Chapter 4)
185. c. (Chapter 4)
186. b. A factor of 8 is three doublings (i.e., 3 + 3 + 3 dB). (Chapter 4)
187. a. (Chapter 9)
188. a. (Chapter 9)
189. e. (Chapter 3)
190. a. (Chapters 2 and 4)
191. c. (Chapter 4)
192. c. (Chapter 4)
193. e. Transmission output side (to the transducer) of a beam former is analog. (Chapters 3 and 4)
194. e. Reception output side of a beam former (to the signal processor) is digital. (Chapter 4)
195. d. (Chapter 3)
196. c. (Chapter 3)
197. e. Propagation speed is independent of frequency and intensity. (Chapter 2)
198. a. (Chapter 6)
199. e. (Chapter 2)
200. a. (Chapter 3)

A Compilation of Key Points

For convenient reference, all the key points listed at the end of each chapter in this book are compiled here.

CHAPTER 1

- Medical imaging with ultrasound is called sonography.
- Sonography is accomplished with a pulse-echo technique.
- Echoes from anatomic structures represent these structures in a sonographic image.
- Sonographic images are composed of many scan lines.
- Sonographic images are presented in linear and sector forms.
- Sonographic images are of 2D and 3D types.
- The Doppler effect is a change in frequency caused by moving objects.
- Doppler information is presented in audible, color display, strip-chart, and spectral display forms.

CHAPTER 2

- Sound is a wave of pressure and density variations and particle vibration.
- Ultrasound is sound having a frequency greater than 20 kHz.
- Frequency denotes the number of cycles occurring in a second.
- Harmonic frequencies are generated as sound travels through tissue.
- Wavelength is the length of a cycle of sound.
- Propagation speed is the speed of sound through a medium.
- The medium determines the propagation speed.
- The average propagation speed of sound through soft tissue is 1.54 mm/μs.
- Pulsed ultrasound is described by pulse repetition frequency, pulse repetition period, pulse duration, duty factor, and spatial pulse length.
- Amplitude and intensity describe the strength of sound.

- Six intensities (SATA, SPTA, SAPA, SPPA, SATP, and SPTP) are used to describe pulsed ultrasound.
- Attenuation is the weakening of sound caused by absorption, reflection, and scattering.
- Attenuation increases with frequency and path length.
- The average attenuation coefficient for soft tissues is 0.5 dB/cm for each megahertz of frequency.
- Imaging depth decreases with increasing frequency.
- Impedance is the density of a medium times its propagation speed.
- When sound encounters boundaries between media with different impedances, part of the sound is reflected and part is transmitted.
- With perpendicular incidence, and if the two media have the same impedance, there is no reflection.
- The greater the difference in the impedances of the media at a boundary, the greater the intensity of the echo that is generated at the boundary.
- With oblique incidence, the sound is refracted at a boundary between media for which propagation speeds are different.
- Incidence and reflection angles at a boundary are always equal.
- Scattering occurs at rough media boundaries and within heterogeneous media.
- Contrast agents are used to enhance echogenicity in sonography and Doppler ultrasound.
- Pulse-echo round-trip travel time is 13 μs/cm. This time is used to determine the distance to a reflector.

CHAPTER 3

- Transducers convert energy from one form to another.
- Ultrasound transducers convert electric energy to ultrasound energy and vice versa.
- Transducers operate on the piezoelectric principle.
- Transducers are operated in pulse-echo mode.
- The operating frequency depends on the element thickness.

- Axial resolution is equal to one half the spatial pulse length.
- Pulsed transducers have damping material to shorten the spatial pulse length for acceptable resolution.
- Transducers produce sound in the form of beams with near and far zones.
- Lateral resolution is equal to beam width.
- Beam width can be reduced by focusing to improve resolution.
- Detail resolution improves with increasing frequency.
- Linear and convex are types of array construction.
- Sequenced, phased, and vector are types of array scanning operations.
- Phasing also enables electronic control of focus.

CHAPTER 4

- Sonographic instruments are of the pulse-echo type.
- These instruments use the strength, direction, and arrival time of received echoes to generate A, B, and M mode displays.
- Sonographic instruments include a beam former, signal processor, image processor, and display, and often are attached to peripheral recording and display devices.
- The beam former is responsible for directing, focusing, and optimizing the ultrasound beam on transmission and reception. The beam former also amplifies the echo voltages, compensates for attenuation using TGC, and digitizes the voltages.
- The signal processor filters, detects, and compresses the echo signal.
- The scan converter converts the echo data in scan line format to image format for storage and display.
- A mode presents an echo versus amplitude display.
- B and M modes use a brightness display echo strength as brightness.
- M mode shows reflector motion in time. M mode is a presentation of echo depth versus time.
- B mode scans show anatomic cross sections through the scanning plane.
- Image memories store echo intensity information as binary numbers in memory elements.
- Contrast resolution improves with increasing bits per pixel.
- Real-time imaging is the rapid sequential display of ultrasound images (frames), resulting in a moving presentation.
- Real-time imaging requires rapid, repeatable, sequential scanning of the sound beam through the tissue. This is accomplished with electronic transducer arrays.
- Increasing frame rate improves temporal resolution.

CHAPTER 5

- Fluids (gases and liquids) are substances that flow.
- Blood is a liquid that flows through the vascular system.
- The heart provides the pulsatile pressure necessary to produce blood flow.

- Volumetric flow rate is proportional to pressure difference at the ends of a tube.
- Volumetric flow rate is inversely proportional to flow resistance.
- Flow resistance increases with viscosity and tube length and decreases greatly with increasing tube diameter.
- Flow classifications include steady, pulsatile, plug, laminar, parabolic, disturbed, and turbulent.
- In a stenosis, flow speeds up, pressure drops (Bernoulli effect), and flow is disturbed.
- If flow speed exceeds a critical value, as described by the Reynolds number, turbulence occurs.
- Pulsatile flow is common in arterial circulation.
- Diastolic flow and/or flow reversal occur in some locations within the arterial system.
- Fluid inertia and vessel compliance are characteristics that are important in determining flow with pulsatile driving pressure.
- The Doppler effect is a change in frequency resulting from motion.
- In medical ultrasound applications, blood flow and tissue motion are the sources of the Doppler effect.
- The change in frequency of the returning echoes with respect to the emitted frequency is called the Doppler shift.
- For flow toward the transducer, the Doppler shift is positive.
- For flow away from the transducer, the Doppler shift is negative.
- The Doppler shift depends on the speed of the scatterers of sound, the Doppler angle, and the operating frequency of the Doppler system.
- Reporting of a Doppler shift frequency without specifying the operating frequency and Doppler angle is incomplete reporting.
- A moving scatterer of sound produces a double Doppler shift.
- Greater flow speeds and smaller Doppler angles produce larger Doppler shifts, but not stronger Doppler-shifted echoes.
- Higher operating frequencies produce larger Doppler shifts.
- Typical ranges of flow speeds (10 to 100 cm/s), Doppler angles (30 to 60 degrees), and operating frequencies (2 to 10 MHz) yield Doppler shifts in the range of 100 Hz to 11 kHz for vascular studies.
- In Doppler echocardiography, in which zero angle and speeds of a few meters per second can be encountered, Doppler shifts can be as high as 30 kHz.

CHAPTER 6

- Color Doppler imaging acquires Doppler-shifted echoes from a two-dimensional cross section of tissue scanned by an ultrasound beam.
- Doppler-shifted echoes are presented in color and are superimposed on the gray-scale anatomic image

of nonshifted echoes that were received during the scan.

■ Flow echoes are assigned colors according to the color map chosen.

■ Several pulses (the number is called the ensemble length) are needed to generate a color scan line.

■ Color controls include gain, map selection, variance on/off, persistence, ensemble length, color/gray priority, scale (PRF), baseline shift, wall filter, and color window angle, location, and size.

■ Doppler shift displays are subject to Doppler angle dependence and aliasing.

■ Doppler-power displays color-encode Doppler-shift strengths into angle-independent, aliasing-independent, more sensitive presentations of flow information.

CHAPTER 7

■ Doppler instruments make use of the Doppler shift to yield information regarding motion and flow.

■ Continuous wave Doppler systems provide motion and flow information without depth selection capability.

■ Pulsed wave Doppler systems provide the ability to select the depth from which Doppler information is received.

■ Spectral analysis provides visual information on the distribution of Doppler-shift frequencies resulting from the distribution of the scatterer speeds and directions encountered.

■ In addition to audible output, Doppler systems provide visual presentation of flow spectra.

■ Duplex systems including gray-scale sonography and CW and PW Doppler are available commercially. Color Doppler capability also can be included.

■ The Doppler spectrum is generated by the range of scatterer velocities encountered by the ultrasound beam.

■ The spectrum is derived electronically using the FFT and is presented on the display as Doppler shift versus time, with brightness indicating power.

■ Flow conditions at the site of measurement are indicated by the width of the spectrum, with spectral broadening and loss of window indicative of disturbed and turbulent flow.

■ Flow conditions downstream, especially distal flow impedance, are indicated by the relationship between peak systolic and end-diastolic flow speeds.

■ Various indexes for quantitatively presenting flow information have been developed.

CHAPTER 8

■ Axial resolution is determined by spatial pulse length.

■ Lateral resolution is determined by beam width.

■ The beam width perpendicular to the scan plane causes section thickness artifacts.

■ Apparent resolution close to the transducer is not related directly to tissue texture but is a result of interference effects from a distribution of scatterers in the tissue (speckle).

■ Reverberation produces a set of equally spaced artifactual echoes distal to the real reflector.

■ In the mirror-image artifact, objects that are present on one side of a strong reflector are displayed on the other side as well.

■ Refraction displaces echoes laterally.

■ Propagation speed error and refraction can cause objects to be displayed in improper locations or incorrect sizes or both.

■ Shadowing is caused by high-attenuation objects in the sound path.

■ Refraction also can cause edge shadowing.

■ Enhancement results from low-attenuation objects in the sound path.

■ Aliasing occurs when the Doppler-shift frequency exceeds one half the PRF.

■ Aliasing can be reduced or eliminated by increasing the PRF or Doppler angle, using baseline shift, reducing operating frequency, or using a continuous wave instrument.

CHAPTER 9

■ Phantoms and test objects provide means for measuring the detail resolution, distance accuracy, compensation, sensitivity, and dynamic range of diagnostic instruments.

■ Hydrophones are used to measure the acoustic output of diagnostic instruments.

■ The AIUM has stated that there have been no independently confirmed, significant bioeffects reported to occur in mammalian tissues exposed to focused SPTA intensities of less than 1 W/cm. Furthermore, no risk has been identified with the use of diagnostic ultrasound in human beings.

■ Because there is limited specific knowledge, a conservative approach is justified. Such an approach calls for diagnostic ultrasound to be used, with minimum exposure, when medical benefit is expected to be derived from the procedure.

APPENDIX

B List of Symbols

LISTED BY SYMBOL

Symbol	Represents
A	area
a	attenuation
a_c	attenuation coefficient
a_p	aperture
AR	axial resolution
c	propagation speed
cos	cosine
c_t	element propagation speed
d	diameter; distance to reflector; distance from transducer
DF	duty factor
d_f	focal beam diameter
F	f number
f	frequency
f_D	Doppler-shift frequency
fl	focal length
f_o	operating frequency
FR	frame rate
f_R	received (echo) frequency
FR_m	maximum frame rate
f_T	transmitted (operating) frequency
I	intensity
I_i	incident intensity
I_r	reflected intensity
IRC	intensity reflection coefficient
I_t	transmitted intensity
ITC	intensity reflection coefficient
L	path length; tube length
LPF	lines per frame
LR	lateral resolution
n	number of cycles per pulse; number of foci; ensemble length
NL	Nyquist limit
P	power
p	pressure amplitude
PD	pulse duration
pen	penetration

Symbol	Represents
PRF	pulse repetition frequency
PRP	pulse repetition period
Q	volumetric flow rate
R	flow resistance
r	radius
R_e	Reynolds number
SPL	spatial pulse length
T	period
th	element thickness
v	flow speed, scatterer speed
v_a	average flow speed
v_r	receiver speed
v_s	source speed
w_b	beam width
z	impedance
ΔP	pressure difference; pressure drop
η	viscosity
θ_D	Doppler angle
θ_i	incidence angle
θ_r	reflection angle
θ_t	transmission angle
λ	wavelength
ρ	density

LISTED BY PARAMETER

Parameter	Represented by
aperture	a_p
area	A
attenuation	a
attenuation coefficient	a_c
average flow speed	v_a
axial resolution	AR
beam width	w_b
cosine	cos
density	ρ
diameter	d
distance from transducer	d
distance to reflector	d
Doppler angle	θ_D

377

Parameter	Represented by
Doppler-shift frequency	f_D
duty factor	DF
element propagation speed	c_t
element thickness	th
ensemble length	n
f number	F
flow resistance	R
flow speed	v
focal beam diameter	d_f
focal length	fl
frame rate	FR
frequency	f
impedance	z
incidence angle	θ_i
incident intensity	I_i
intensity	I
intensity reflection coefficient	IRC
intensity transmission coefficient	ITC
lateral resolution	LR
lines per frame	LPF
maximum frame rate	FR_m
number of cycles per pulse	n
number of foci	n
Nyquist limit	NL
operating frequency	f_o
path length	L
penetration	pen
period	T
power	P
pressure amplitude	p
pressure difference	ΔP
pressure drop	ΔP
propagation speed	c
pulse duration	PD
pulse repetition frequency	PRF
pulse repetition period	PRP
radius	r
received (echo) frequency	f_R
receiver speed	v_r
reflected intensity	I_r
reflection angle	θ_r
Reynolds number	R_e
scatterer speed	v
source speed	v_s
spatial pulse length	SPL
transmission angle	θ_t
transmitted intensity	I_t
transmitted (operating) frequency	f_T
tube length	L
viscosity	η
volumetric flow rate	Q
wavelength	λ

APPENDIX C
Compilation of Equations

For convenient reference, the equations in this book (excepting those in Advanced Concepts sections) are compiled here.

CHAPTER 2

$$T \text{ (μs)} = \frac{1}{f \text{ (MHz)}}$$

$$\lambda \text{ (mm)} = \frac{c \text{ (mm/μs)}}{f \text{ (MHz)}}$$

$$PRP \text{ (ms)} = \frac{1}{PRF \text{ (kHz)}}$$

$$PD \text{ (μs)} = n \times T \text{ (μs)}$$

$$DF = \frac{PD \text{ (μs)}}{PRP \text{ (μs)}} = \frac{PD \text{ (μs)} \times PRF \text{ (kHz)}}{1000}$$

$$SPL \text{ (mm)} = n \times \lambda \text{ (mm)}$$

$$I \text{ (mW/cm}^2\text{)} = \frac{P \text{ (mW)}}{A \text{ (cm}^2\text{)}}$$

$$a \text{ (dB)} = a_c \text{ (dB/cm)} \times L \text{ (cm)}$$

$$a \text{ (dB)} = \frac{1}{2} \text{ (dB/cm-MHz)} \times f \text{ (MHz)} \times L \text{ (cm)}$$

$$z \text{ (rayls)} = \rho \text{ (kg/m}^3\text{)} \times c \text{ (m/s)}$$

$$IRC = \frac{I_r \text{ (W/cm}^2\text{)}}{I_i \text{ (W/cm}^2\text{)}} = \left[\frac{(z_2 - z_1)}{(z_2 + z_1)}\right]^2$$

$$ITC = \frac{I_t \text{ (W/cm}^2\text{)}}{I_i \text{ (W/cm}^2\text{)}} = 1 - IRC$$

$$\theta_i \text{ (degrees)} = \theta_r \text{ (degrees)}$$

$$d \text{ (mm)} = \frac{1}{2} [c \text{ (mm/μs)} \times t \text{ (μs)}]$$

CHAPTER 3

$$f_o \text{ (MHz)} = \left[\frac{c_t \text{ (mm/μs)}}{2 \times th \text{ (mm)}}\right]$$

$$AR \text{ (mm)} = \frac{SPL \text{ (mm)}}{2}$$

$$LR \text{ (mm)} = w_b \text{ (mm)}$$

CHAPTER 4

$$pen \text{ (cm)} \times PRF \text{ (kHz)} \leq 77 \text{ (cm/ms)}$$

$$PRF \text{ (Hz)} = n \times LPF \times FR \text{ (Hz)}$$

$$pen \text{ (cm)} \times n \times LPF \times FR \text{ (Hz)} \leq 77,000 \text{ cm/s}$$

CHAPTER 5

$$Q \text{ (mL/s)} = \frac{\Delta P \text{ (dyne/cm}^2\text{)}}{R \text{ (poise)}}$$

$$R \text{ (g/cm}^4\text{-s)} = 8 \times L \text{ (cm)} \times \frac{\eta \text{ (poise)}}{\pi \times [r^4 \text{ (cm}^4\text{)}]}$$

$$Q \text{ (mL/s)} = \frac{\Delta P \text{ (dyne/cm}^2\text{)} \times \pi \times d^4 \text{ (cm}^4\text{)}}{128 \times L \text{ (cm)} \times \eta \text{ (poise)}}$$

$$R_e = \frac{v_a \text{ (cm/s)} \times d \text{ (cm)} \times \rho \text{ (g/mL)}}{\eta \text{ (poise)}}$$

$$v_a \text{ (cm/s)} = \frac{[\Delta p \text{ (dyne/cm}^2\text{)} \times d^2 \text{ (cm}^2\text{)}]}{[32 \times L \text{ (cm)} \times \eta \text{ (poise)}]}$$

$$f_D \text{ (kHz)} = f_R \text{ (kHz)} - f_T \text{ (kHz)} = f_0 \text{ (kHz)} \times \frac{[2 \times v \text{ (cm/s)}]}{c \text{ (cm/s)}}$$

$$v \text{ (cm/s)} = \frac{77 \text{ (cm/ms)} \times f_D \text{ (kHz)}}{f_0 \text{ (MHz)}}$$

$$f_D \text{ (kHz)} = \frac{[f_0 \text{ (kHz)} \times 2 \times v \text{ (cm/s)} \times (\cos \theta)]}{c \text{ (cm/s)}}$$

$$v \text{ (cm/s)} = \frac{[77 \text{ (cm/ms)} \times f_D \text{ (kHz)}]}{[f_0 \text{ (MHz)} \times \cos \theta]}$$

CHAPTER 6

$$FR_m \text{ (Hz)} = \frac{77,000 \text{ (cm/s)}}{\text{pen (cm)} \times \text{LPF} \times n}$$

CHAPTER 8

$$NL \text{ (kHz)} = \tfrac{1}{2} \times PRF \text{ (kHz)}$$

CHAPTER 9

$$MI = \frac{p \text{ (MPa)}}{[(f)^{1/2} \text{ (MHz)}^{1/2}]}$$

APPENDIX D

Compilation of Boxes and Tables

For convenient reference, all the boxes and tables in this book are compiled here.

TABLE 2-1 Common Ultrasound Periods and Wavelengths in Tissue

Frequency (MHz)	Period (μs)	Wavelength (mm)*
2.0	0.50	0.77
3.5	0.29	0.44
5.0	0.20	0.31
7.5	0.13	0.21
10.0	0.10	0.15
15.0	0.07	0.10

*Assuming a (soft tissue) propagation speed of 1.54 mm/μs (1540 m/s).

TABLE 2-2 Sound Levels

Sound	Level (dB)
Pain threshold	130
Rock concert	115
Chain saw	100
Lawn mower	90
Vacuum cleaner	75
Normal conversation	60
Whisper	30
Hearing threshold	0

TABLE 2-3 Attenuation for Various Intensity Ratios*

Attenuation (dB)	Intensity Ratio	Percent Intensity Ratio
0	1.00	100
1	0.79	79
2	0.63	63
3	0.50	50
4	0.40	40
5	0.32	32
6	0.25	25
7	0.20	20
8	0.16	16
9	0.13	13
10	0.10	10
15	0.032	3.2
20	0.010	1.0
25	0.003	0.3
30	0.001	0.1
35	0.0003	0.03
40	0.0001	0.01
45	0.00003	0.003
50	0.00001	0.001
60	0.000001	0.0001
70	0.0000001	0.00001
80	0.00000001	0.000001
90	0.000000001	0.0000001
100	0.0000000001	0.00000001

*The intensity ratio is the fraction of the original intensity remaining after attenuation.

TABLE 2-4 Average Attenuation Coefficients in Tissue

Frequency (MHz)	Average Attenuation Coefficient for Soft Tissue (dB/cm)	Intensity Reduction in 1-cm Path (%)	Intensity Reduction in 10-cm Path (%)
2.0	1.0	21	90
3.5	1.8	34	98
5.0	2.5	44	99.7
7.5	3.8	58	99.98
10.0	5.0	68	99.999

TABLE 2-5   Common Values for Attenuation Coefficient and Penetration

Frequency (MHz)	Attenuation Coefficient (dB/cm)	Penetration (cm)
2.0	1.0	30
3.5	1.8	17
5.0	2.5	12
7.5	3.8	8
10.0	5.0	6
15.0	7.5	4

TABLE 2-6   Pulse Round-Trip Travel Time for Various Reflector Depths

Depth (cm)	Travel Time (μs)
0.5	6.5
1	13
2	26
3	39
4	52
5	65
10	130
15	195
20	260

TABLE 2-7   Sonographic Parameters in Tissue

Parameter	Symbol or Abbreviation	Range of Common Values
Frequency	f	2-15 MHz
Period	T	0.07-0.5 μs
Wavelength	λ	0.1-0.8 mm
Propagation speed	c	1.44-1.64 mm/μs
Impedance	z	1,300,000-1,700,000 rayls
Pulse repetition frequency	PRF	4-15 kHz
Pulse repetition period	PRP	0.07-0.25 ms
Cycles per pulse	n	1-3
Pulse duration	PD	0.1-1.5 μs
Spatial pulse length	SPL	0.1-2.5 mm
Duty factor	DF	0.1% to 1%
Pressure amplitude	p	0.1-4 MPa
SPTA intensity	I_{SPTA}	0.01-100 mW/cm²
SPPA intensity	I_{SPPA}	0.01-100 W/cm²
Attenuation coefficient	a_c	1-8 dB/cm

TABLE 2-8   Dependence of Various Factors on Increasing (↑) Frequency

Parameter	Symbol or Abbreviation	Dependence (↑ Increase; ↓ Decrease)
Period	T	↓
Wavelength	λ	↓
Pulse duration	PD	↓
Spatial pulse length	SPL	↓
Attenuation	a	↑
Penetration	pen	↓

BOX 3-1   Common Transducer Types

Linear array
Convex array
Phased array
Vector array

BOX 3-2   Array Terminology

(Phased) linear (sequenced) array
(Phased) convex (sequenced) array
(Linear) phased array
(Phased and sequenced) (linear) vector array
The words in parentheses are implied in the abbreviated common terminology.

TABLE 3-1   Transducer Element Thickness* for Various Operating Frequencies

Frequency (MHz)	Thickness (mm)
2.0	1.0
3.5	0.6
5.0	0.4
7.5	0.3
10.0	0.2

*Assuming an element propagation speed of 4 mm/μs.

TABLE 3-2   Near-Zone Length (NZL) for Unfocused Elements

Frequency (MHz)	Width (mm)	NZL (cm)
2.0	19	12
3.5	13	10
3.5	19	20
5.0	6	3
5.0	10	8
5.0	13	14
7.5	6	4
10.0	6	6

TABLE 3-3   f-Number Ranges

Focus	f Number
Weak	>6
Moderate	2-6
Strong	<2

TABLE 3-4   Terms Used to Describe Arrays

Term	Construction	Scanning	Focusing
Array	√		
Linear	√		
Sequenced		√	
Convex	√		
Phased		√	√

TABLE 3-5   Transducer Characteristics

Type	Beam Scanned by Sequencing	Beam Scanned by Phasing	Beam Focused by Phasing
Linear array	√		√
Convex array	√		√
Phased array		√	√
Vector array	√	√	√

TABLE 3-6   Display Formats

Type	Rectangle or Parallelogram	Sector	Flat Top	Curved Top	Pointed Top
Linear array	√		√		
Convex array		√		√	
Phased array		√			√
Vector array		√	√		

TABLE 3-7   Typical Imaging Depth and Axial Resolution (Two-Cycle Pulse) in Tissue

Frequency (MHz)	Imaging Depth (cm)	Axial Resolution (mm)
2.0	30	0.77
3.5	17	0.44
5.0	12	0.31
7.5	8	0.20
10.0	6	0.15
15.0	4	0.10

BOX 4-1   Functions of the Beam Former

Generate voltages that drive the transducer.
Determine pulse repetition frequency, coding, frequency, and intensity.
Scan, focus, and apodize the transmitted beam.
Amplify the returning echo voltages.
Compensate for attenuation.
Digitize the echo voltage stream.
Direct, focus, and apodize the reception beam.

BOX 4-2   Functions of the Signal Processor

Bandpass filtering
Amplitude detection (radio frequency to video)
Compression (dynamic range reduction)

BOX 4-3   Functions of the Image Processor

Scan conversion
Preprocessing
    Persistence
    Panoramic imaging
    Spatial compounding
    Three-dimensional acquisition
Storing image frames
    Cine loop
Postprocessing
    Gray scale
    Color scale
    Three-dimensional presentation
Digital-to-analog conversion

TABLE 4-1   Gain (Expressed in Decibels) and Corresponding Power and Amplitude Ratios*

Gain (dB)	Power Ratio	Amplitude Ratio
0	1.0	1.0
1	1.3	1.1
2	1.6	1.3
3	2.0	1.4
4	2.5	1.6
5	3.2	1.8
6	4.0	2.0
7	5.0	2.2
8	6.3	2.5
9	7.9	2.8
10	10	3.2
15	32	5.6
20	100	10
25	320	18
30	1,000	32
35	3,200	56
40	10,000	100
45	32,000	180
50	100,000	320
60	1,000,000	1,000
70	10,000,000	3,200
80	100,000,000	10,000
90	1,000,000,000	32,000
100	10,000,000,000	100,000

*The power (amplitude) ratio is output power (amplitude) divided by input power (amplitude).

TABLE 4-2   Binary and Decimal Number Equivalents

Decimal	Binary	Decimal	Binary
0	000000	32	100000
1	000001	33	100001
2	000010	34	100010
3	000011	35	100011
4	000100	36	100100
5	000101	37	100101
6	000110	38	100110
7	000111	39	100111
8	001000	40	101000
9	001001	41	101001
10	001010	42	101010
11	001011	43	101011
12	001100	44	101100
13	001101	45	101101
14	001110	46	101110
15	001111	47	101111
16	010000	48	110000
17	010001	49	110001
18	010010	50	110010
19	010011	51	110011
20	010100	52	110100
21	010101	53	110101
22	010110	54	110110
23	010111	55	110111
24	011000	56	111000
25	011001	57	111001
26	011010	58	111010
27	011011	59	111011
28	011100	60	111100
29	011101	61	111101
30	011110	62	111110
31	011111	63	111111

TABLE 4-3 **Characteristics of Digital Memories**

Bits per Pixel	Lowest Number Stored		Highest Number Stored		No. of Shades
	Decimal	Binary	Decimal	Binary	
4	0	0000	15	1111	16
5	0	00000	31	11111	32
6	0	000000	63	111111	64
7	0	0000000	127	1111111	128
8	0	00000000	255	11111111	256

TABLE 4-4 **Bits (Binary Digits or Memory Elements) in Digital Memories with 512 × 512 (262,144) Pixels**

Bits per Pixel	Total Bits	Total Kilobytes*
4	1,048,576	128
5	1,310,720	160
6	1,572,864	192
7	1,835,008	224
8	2,097,152	256

*1 byte = 8 bits; 1 kilobyte = 1024 bytes, or 8192 bits.

TABLE 4-5 **Contrast Resolution of Digital Memories**

Bits per Pixel	40-dB Dynamic Range		60-dB Dynamic Range	
	Decibels per Shade	Intensity Difference (%)*	Decibels per Shade	Intensity Difference (%)*
4	2.5	78	3.8	140
5	1.2	32	1.9	55
6	0.6	15	0.9	23
7	0.3	7	0.5	12
8	0.2	5	0.2	5

*The average difference required between two echoes for the echoes to be assigned different shades.

TABLE 4-6 **Pulse Repetition Frequencies (PRF) and Frame Rates (FR) Permitted for Various Single-Focus Imaging Depths (Penetration) and 100 or 200 Scan Lines per Frame**

Penetration (cm)	PRF (Hz)	FR	
		100 Lines	200 Lines
20	3,850	38	19
15	5,133	51	25
10	7,700	77	38
5	15,400	154	77

TABLE 5-1 Doppler Frequency Shifts for Various Scatterer Speeds toward* the Sound Source at a Zero Doppler Angle

Incident Frequency (MHz)	Scatterer Speed (cm/s)	Reflected Frequency (MHz)	Doppler Shift (kHz)
2	50	2.0013	1.3
5	50	5.0032	3.2
10	50	10.0065	6.5
2	200	2.0052	5.2
5	200	5.013	13.0
10	200	10.026	26.0

*Motion away from the source would yield negative Doppler shifts.

TABLE 5-2 Cosines for Various Angles

Angle A (degrees)	cos A
0	1.00
5	0.996
10	0.98
15	0.97
20	0.94
25	0.91
30	0.87
35	0.82
40	0.77
45	0.71
50	0.64
55	0.57
60	0.50
65	0.42
70	0.34
75	0.26
80	0.17
85	0.09
90	0.00

TABLE 5-3 Doppler Frequency Shifts for Various Angles and Scatterer Speeds toward the Sound Source of Frequency 5 MHz

Scatterer Speed (cm/s)	Angle (degrees)	Doppler Shift (kHz)
100	0	6.5
100	30	5.6
100	60	3.2
100	90	0.0
300	0	19.0
300	30	17.0
300	60	9.7
300	90	0.0

TABLE 5-4 Cosine and Calculated-Speed Errors for Angle Errors of 2 and 5 Degrees

True Angle (degrees)	Cosine Error (%)		Speed Error (%)	
	+2 Degrees	+5 Degrees	+2 Degrees	+5 Degrees
0	−0.1	−0.4	+0.1	+0.4
10	−0.7	−1.9	+0.7	+2.0
20	−1.3	−3.6	+1.3	+3.7
30	−2.1	−5.4	+2.1	+5.7
40	−3.0	−7.7	+3.1	+8.3
50	−4.2	−10.8	+4.4	+12.1
60	−6.1	−15.5	+6.5	+18.3
70	−9.6	−24.3	+10.7	+32.1
80	−19.9	−49.8	+24.8	+99.2

TABLE 5-5 Doppler Shifts (for 4 MHz) at Various Doppler Angles for the Same Flow Yielding a Consistent Calculated Flow Speed

Doppler Shift (kHz)	Angle (degrees)	Calculated Flow Speed (cm/s)
2.25	30	50
1.99	40	50
1.84	45	50
1.67	50	50
1.30	60	50

 TABLE 5-6 Doppler Shifts for Various Frequencies, Angles, and Speeds

Frequency (MHz)	Angle (degrees)	Speed (cm/s)	Shift (kHz)
2	0	10	0.26
2	0	50	1.30
2	0	100	2.60
2	30	10	0.22
2	30	50	1.12
2	30	100	2.25
2	45	10	0.18
2	45	50	0.92
2	45	100	1.84
2	60	10	0.13
2	60	50	0.65
2	60	100	1.30
5	0	10	0.65
5	0	50	3.25
5	0	100	6.49
5	30	10	0.56
5	30	50	2.81
5	30	100	5.62
5	45	10	0.46
5	45	50	2.30
5	45	100	4.59
5	60	10	0.32
5	60	50	1.62
5	60	100	3.25
10	0	10	1.30
10	0	50	6.49
10	0	100	13.0
10	30	10	1.12
10	30	50	5.62
10	30	100	11.2
10	45	10	0.92
10	45	50	4.59
10	45	100	9.18
10	60	10	0.65
10	60	50	3.25
10	60	100	6.49

BOX 6-1 Types of Flow Information Provided by Doppler Ultrasound

Presence of flow
- Yes
- No

Direction of flow
- ←
- →

Speed of flow
- Slow
- Fast

Character of flow
- Laminar
- Turbulent

BOX 6-2 Various Forms of Presentation of Doppler Information

Audible sounds
Strip-chart recording
Spectral display
Color Doppler display

BOX 6-3   Advantages and Disadvantages of Doppler-Power Displays with Respect to Doppler-Shift Displays

ADVANTAGES
Angle independence
No aliasing
Improved sensitivity (deeper penetration, smaller vessels, slower flows)

DISADVANTAGES
No directional information
No flow speed information
No flow character information

TABLE 6-1   Comparison of Doppler-Shift and Doppler-Power Displays

	Doppler-Shift Display	Doppler-Power Display
Quantitative	No	No
Global	Yes	Yes
Perfusion	No	Yes

TABLE 7-1   Echo Arrival Time for Various Reflector Depths (Gate Locations)

Depth (mm)	Time (μs)
10	13
20	26
30	39
40	52
50	65
60	78
70	91
80	104
90	117
100	130
150	195
200	260

TABLE 7-2   Spatial Gate Length for Various Temporal Gate Lengths

Length (mm)	Time (μs)
1	1.3
2	2.6
3	3.9
4	5.2
5	6.5
10	13.0
15	19.5
20	26.0

TABLE 7-3   The Amount Added to Effective Gate Length by Pulse Length for Various Cycles per Pulse and Frequencies

Amount Added (mm)	Cycles	f (MHz)
1.9	5	2
3.8	10	2
7.7	20	2
0.8	5	5
1.5	10	5
3.1	20	5
0.4	5	10
0.8	10	10
1.5	20	10

TABLE 7-4   Spectral Display Indexes

Name	Abbreviation	Expression*
Pulsatility index	PI	$\dfrac{A - B}{mean}$
Resistance index	RI	$\dfrac{A - B}{A}$
RSystolic-to-diastolic ratio	SDR	$\dfrac{A}{B}$
RB/A ratio	BAR	$\dfrac{B}{A}$

*A represents the maximum value at systole, and B represents the minimum value at end-diastole (Figure 7-29).

TABLE 7-5   Comparison of Doppler-Shift, Doppler-Power, and Spectral Displays

	Color Doppler-Shift Display	Color Doppler-Power Display	Spectral Display
Quantitative	No	No	Yes
Global	Yes	Yes	No
Perfusion	No	Yes	No

TABLE 5-5 Doppler Shifts (for 4 MHz) at Various Doppler Angles for the Same Flow Yielding a Consistent Calculated Flow Speed

Doppler Shift (kHz)	Angle (degrees)	Calculated Flow Speed (cm/s)
2.25	30	50
1.99	40	50
1.84	45	50
1.67	50	50
1.30	60	50

TABLE 5-6 Doppler Shifts for Various Frequencies, Angles, and Speeds

Frequency (MHz)	Angle (degrees)	Speed (cm/s)	Shift (kHz)
2	0	10	0.26
2	0	50	1.30
2	0	100	2.60
2	30	10	0.22
2	30	50	1.12
2	30	100	2.25
2	45	10	0.18
2	45	50	0.92
2	45	100	1.84
2	60	10	0.13
2	60	50	0.65
2	60	100	1.30
5	0	10	0.65
5	0	50	3.25
5	0	100	6.49
5	30	10	0.56
5	30	50	2.81
5	30	100	5.62
5	45	10	0.46
5	45	50	2.30
5	45	100	4.59
5	60	10	0.32
5	60	50	1.62
5	60	100	3.25
10	0	10	1.30
10	0	50	6.49
10	0	100	13.0
10	30	10	1.12
10	30	50	5.62
10	30	100	11.2
10	45	10	0.92
10	45	50	4.59
10	45	100	9.18
10	60	10	0.65
10	60	50	3.25
10	60	100	6.49

BOX 6-1 Types of Flow Information Provided by Doppler Ultrasound

Presence of flow
- Yes
- No

Direction of flow
- ←
- →

Speed of flow
- Slow
- Fast

Character of flow
- Laminar
- Turbulent

BOX 6-2 Various Forms of Presentation of Doppler Information

Audible sounds
Strip-chart recording
Spectral display
Color Doppler display

BOX 6-3 **Advantages and Disadvantages of Doppler-Power Displays with Respect to Doppler-Shift Displays**

ADVANTAGES
Angle independence
No aliasing
Improved sensitivity (deeper penetration, smaller vessels, slower flows)

DISADVANTAGES
No directional information
No flow speed information
No flow character information

TABLE 6-1 **Comparison of Doppler-Shift and Doppler-Power Displays**

	Doppler-Shift Display	Doppler-Power Display
Quantitative	No	No
Global	Yes	Yes
Perfusion	No	Yes

TABLE 7-1 **Echo Arrival Time for Various Reflector Depths (Gate Locations)**

Depth (mm)	Time (μs)
10	13
20	26
30	39
40	52
50	65
60	78
70	91
80	104
90	117
100	130
150	195
200	260

TABLE 7-2 **Spatial Gate Length for Various Temporal Gate Lengths**

Length (mm)	Time (μs)
1	1.3
2	2.6
3	3.9
4	5.2
5	6.5
10	13.0
15	19.5
20	26.0

TABLE 7-3 **The Amount Added to Effective Gate Length by Pulse Length for Various Cycles per Pulse and Frequencies**

Amount Added (mm)	Cycles	f (MHz)
1.9	5	2
3.8	10	2
7.7	20	2
0.8	5	5
1.5	10	5
3.1	20	5
0.4	5	10
0.8	10	10
1.5	20	10

TABLE 7-4 **Spectral Display Indexes**

Name	Abbreviation	Expression*
Pulsatility index	PI	$\dfrac{A - B}{mean}$
Resistance index	RI	$\dfrac{A - B}{A}$
RSystolic-to-diastolic ratio	SDR	$\dfrac{A}{B}$
RB/A ratio	BAR	$\dfrac{B}{A}$

*A represents the maximum value at systole, and *B* represents the minimum value at end-diastole (Figure 7-29).

TABLE 7-5 **Comparison of Doppler-Shift, Doppler-Power, and Spectral Displays**

	Color Doppler-Shift Display	Color Doppler-Power Display	Spectral Display
Quantitative	No	No	Yes
Global	Yes	Yes	No
Perfusion	No	Yes	No

BOX 8-1 Sonographic Artifacts

PROPAGATION GROUP
Axial resolution
Comet tail
Grating lobe
Lateral resolution
Mirror image
Range ambiguity
Refraction
Reverberation
Ring-down
Section thickness
Speckle
Speed error

ATTENUATION GROUP
Enhancement
Focal enhancement
Refraction (edge) shadowing
Shadowing

BOX 8-2 Methods of Reducing or Eliminating Aliasing

1. Increase the pulse repetition frequency.
2. Increase the Doppler angle.
3. Shift the baseline.
4. Use a lower operating frequency.
5. Use a continuous wave device.

TABLE 8-1 Aliasing and Range-Ambiguity Artifact Values

Pulse Repetition Frequency (kHz)	Doppler Shift Above Which Aliasing Occurs (kHz)	Range Beyond Which Ambiguity Occurs (cm)
5.0	2.5	15
7.5	3.7	10
10.0	5.0	7
12.5	6.2	6
15.0	7.5	5
17.5	8.7	4
20.0	10.0	3
25.0	12.5	3
30.0	15.0	2

TABLE 8-2 Aliasing and Range-Ambiguity Limits*

Depth (cm)	PRF (kHz)	Nyquist Limit (kHz)	Maximum Flow Speed (cm/s) 0	30	60
1	77.0	38.5	593	685	1186
2	38.5	19.2	296	342	593
4	19.2	9.6	148	171	296
8	9.6	4.8	74	86	148
16	4.8	2.4	37	43	74

*For various depths the maximum pulse repetition frequency (PRF) that avoids range ambiguity and the corresponding maximum Doppler shift frequency (Nyquist limit) that avoids aliasing are listed. Maximum flow speeds corresponding to the maximum Doppler shift also are listed for three Doppler angles (0, 30, and 60 degrees), assuming a 5-MHz operating frequency.

TABLE 8-3   Artifacts and Their Causes

Artifact	Cause
Axial resolution	Pulse length
Comet tail	Reverberation
Grating lobe	Grating lobe
Lateral resolution	Pulse width
Mirror image	Multiple reflection
Refraction	Refraction
Reverberation	Multiple reflection
Ring down	Resonance
Section thickness	Pulse width
Speckle	Interference
Speed error	Speed error
Range ambiguity	High pulse repetition frequency
Shadowing	High attenuation
Edge shadowing	Refraction or interference
Enhancement	Low attenuation
Focal enhancement	Focusing
Aliasing	Low pulse repetition frequency
Spectrum mirror	High Doppler gain

TABLE 9-1   510(k) Guide to Spatial Peak–Temporal Average in Situ Intensity Upper Limits

Diagnostic Application	I_{SPTA} (mW/cm^2)
Cardiac	430
Peripheral vessel	20
Ophthalmic	17
Fetal imaging and other*	94

*Abdominal, intraoperative, pediatric, small organ (breast, thyroid, testes), neonatal cephalic, adult cephalic.

E Mathematics Review

Algebra and trigonometry are used in the discussion of ultrasound and Doppler principles. Logarithms are involved in decibels, and binary numbers are involved in digital electronics. Mathematical concepts that are applicable to the material in this book are reviewed in this appendix. Relevant aspects of algebra, trigonometry, logarithms, scientific notation, binary numbers, units, and statistics are covered.

First, we review some mathematical terminology. In algebraic equations such as

$$x + y = z$$
$$x - y = z$$

x and y are called *terms*. Terms are connected with each other by addition or subtraction. With addition, the result is called the sum. With subtraction the result is called the difference.

In the equations

$$x \times y = z$$
$$\frac{x}{y} = z$$

x and y are called *factors*. Factors are connected with each other by multiplication or division. When multiplied, the result is called the product. When divided, the result is called the quotient.

The inverse or reciprocal of x is $1/x$, sometimes described as "one over" x.

ALGEBRA

Transposition of quantities in algebraic equations is accomplished by performing identical mathematical operations on both sides.

Example E-1

For the equation

$$x + y = z$$

transpose to get x alone (solve for x). To do this, subtract y from both sides:

$$x + y - y = z - y$$

Since $y - y = 0$, the left-hand side of the equation is

$$x + y - y = x + 0 = x$$

so that

$$x = z - y$$

Example E-2

For the equation

$$x - y = z$$

Solve for x. Add y to both sides:

$$x - y + y = z + y$$
$$x + 0 = z + y$$
$$x = z + y$$

Example E-3

For the equation

$$xy = z$$

solve for x. Divide both sides by y:

$$\frac{xy}{y} = \frac{z}{y}$$

Since $y/y = 1$

$$\frac{xy}{y} = x(1) = x$$

and

$$x = \frac{z}{y}$$

391

Example E-4

For the equation

$$\frac{x}{y} = z$$

solve for x. Multiply both sides by y:

$$\left(\frac{x}{y}\right) y = zy$$

$$x(1) = zy$$

$$x = zy$$

Example E-5

Using some numbers, and combining the previous examples, consider the equation

$$\left(\frac{5x + 3}{2}\right) - 3 = 1$$

and solve for x. First, add 3 to both sides:

$$\left(\frac{5x + 3}{2}\right) - 3 + 3 = 1 + 3$$

$$\frac{5x + 3}{2} = 4$$

Multiply by 2:

$$\left(\frac{5x + 3}{2}\right) \times 2 = 4 \times 2$$

$$5x + 3 = 8$$

Subtract 3:

$$5x + 3 - 3 = 8 - 3$$

$$5x = 5$$

Divide by 5:

$$x = 1$$

Substitution of the answer into the original equation shows that the equality is satisfied and the answer is correct:

$$\left[\frac{5(1) + 3}{2}\right] - 3 = 1$$

$$\left(\frac{8}{2}\right) - 3 = 1$$

$$4 - 3 = 1$$

$$1 = 1$$

Example E-6

For the equation

$$c = f \times \lambda$$

solve for wavelength. Divide by frequency:

$$\frac{c}{f} = \frac{f \times \lambda}{f}$$

$$\frac{c}{f} = \lambda$$

Example E-7

If the intensity reflection coefficient (IRC) is 0.1 and the reflected intensity (I_r) is 5 mW/cm^2, find the incident intensity (I_i), given that

$$IRC = \frac{I_r}{I_i}$$

Multiply by incident intensity:

$$IRC \times I_i = \frac{I_r}{I_i} \times I_i$$

Divide by intensity reflection coefficient:

$$\frac{IRC \times I_i}{IRC} = \frac{I_r}{IRC}$$

$$I_i = \frac{I_r}{IRC} = \frac{5 \text{ mW/cm}^2}{0.1} = 50 \text{ mW/cm}^2$$

Example E-8

If the intensity reflection coefficient (IRC) is 0.01 and the impedance for medium 1 (z_1) is 4.5, find the medium 2 impedance (z_2), given that

$$IRC = \left(\frac{z_2 - z_1}{z_2 + z_1}\right)^2$$

Take the square root of each side:

$$IRC^{1/2} = \frac{z_2 - z_1}{z_2 + z_1}$$

Multiply by the sum of z_2 and z_1:

$$IRC^{1/2} \times (z_2 + z_1) = (z_2 - z_1)$$

Add z_1:

$$IRC^{1/2} \times (z_2 + z_1) + z_1 = z_2$$

Subtract $IRC^{1/2} \times z_2$:

$$(IRC^{1/2} \times z_1) + z_1 = z_2 - (IRC^{1/2} \times z_2)$$

$$z_1 (1 + IRC^{1/2}) = z_2 (1 - IRC^{1/2})$$

Divide by $(1 - IRC^{1/2})$ and interchange sides of the equation:

$$z_2 = z_1 \left[\frac{(1 + IRC^{1/2})}{(1 - IRC^{1/2})} \right]$$

$$= 4.5 \left[\frac{1 + (0.01)^{1/2}}{1 - (0.01)^{1/2}} \right]$$

$$= 4.5 \left(\frac{1 + 0.1}{1 - 0.1} \right) = 4.5 \left(\frac{1.1}{0.9} \right) = 4.5 \,(1.22) = 5.5$$

TRIGONOMETRY

If the sides and angles of a right triangle ("right" means one of the angles equals 90 degrees) are labeled as in Figure E-1, the sine of angle A (sin A), the cosine of angle A (cos A), and the tangent of angle A (tan A) are defined as follows:

$$\sin A = \frac{\text{length of side } a}{\text{length of side } c}$$

$$\cos A = \frac{\text{length of side } b}{\text{length of side } c}$$

$$\tan A = \frac{\text{length of side } a}{\text{length of side } b}$$

Example E-9

If the lengths of the sides a, b, and c are 1, $\sqrt{3}$, and 2, respectively, what are sin A and cos A?

$$\sin A = \frac{1}{2} = 0.5$$

$$\cos A = \frac{\sqrt{3}}{2} = 0.87$$

If the sine or cosine is known, angle A may be found using a calculator or a table such as Table E-1.

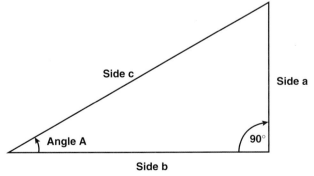

FIGURE E-1 If the sides and angles of a right triangle are labeled as in this figure, the cosine of angle A (cos A) is equal to the length of side b divided by the length of side c. Sine A is equal to the length of side a divided by the length of side c.

TABLE E-1

Angle (°)	Sine	Cosine	Tangent
0	0	1.00	0
30	0.50	0.87	0.58
45	0.71	0.71	1.00
60	0.87	0.50	1.73
90	1.00	0	∞

Note: The symbol ∞ indicates infinity or indeterminate; that is, dividing by zero can be executed an unlimited number of times.

Example E-10

If sin A is 0.5, what is A? From Table E-1, A = 30 degrees.

Example E-11

If cos A is 0.87, what is A? From Table E-1, A = 30 degrees.

If angle A is known, sin A or cos A may be found using a calculator or a table such as Table E-1.

Example E-12

If A = 45 degrees, what are the sin A and cos A? From Table E-1, sin A = 0.71 and cos A = 0.71.

LOGARITHMS

The logarithm to the base 10 (log) of a number is equal to the number of tens that must be multiplied together to result in that number. More generally, the logarithm is the power to which 10 must be raised to give a particular number.

Example E-13

What is the logarithm of 1000? To obtain 1000, three tens must be multiplied together:

$$10 \times 10 \times 10 = 1000$$

Three tens then yield the logarithm (log) of 1000.

$$\log 1000 = 3$$

The logarithm of the reciprocal of a number is equal to the negative of the logarithm of the number.

Example E-14

What is the logarithm of 0.01?

$$0.01 = \frac{1}{100}$$

$$\log 100 = 2$$

$$\log 0.01 = \log \frac{1}{100} = -2$$

Decibels are quantities that result from taking 10 times the logarithm of the ratio of two powers or intensities.

Example E-15

Compare the following two powers in decibels: power 1 = 1 W; power 2 = 10 W.

$$10 \log \left(\frac{\text{power 1}}{\text{power 2}} \right) = 10 \log \left(\frac{1}{10} \right) = 10 \, (-\log 10) = 10 \, (-1) = -10 \text{ dB}$$

Power 1 is 10 dB less than power 2, or power 1 is 10 dB below power 2. Also

$$10 \log \left(\frac{\text{power 2}}{\text{power 1}} \right) = 10 \log \left(\frac{10}{1} \right) = 10 \, (\log 10) = 10 \, (1) = 10 \text{ dB}$$

Power 2 is 10 dB more than power 1, or power 2 is 10 dB above power 1.

Example E-16

An amplifier has a power output of 100 mW when the input power is 0.1 mW. What is the amplifier gain in decibels?

$$\text{amplifier gain (dB)} = 10 \log \left(\frac{\text{power out}}{\text{power in}} \right)$$

$$= 10 \log \left(\frac{100}{0.1} \right) = 10 \log 1000 = 10(3) = 30 \text{ dB}$$

Example E-17

An electric attenuator has a power output of 0.01 mW when the input power is 100 mW. What is the attenuation of the attenuator in decibels?

$$\text{attenuator attenuation (dB)} = -10 \log \left(\frac{\text{power out}}{\text{power in}} \right)$$

$$= -10 \log \left(\frac{0.01}{100} \right) = -10 \log \left(\frac{1}{10,000} \right) = -10(-\log 10,000)$$

$$= -10(-4) = 40 \text{ dB}$$

The first minus sign is used in the equation to give the attenuation as a positive number. If the minus number had not been used, the "gain" of the attenuator would have been calculated, which would have turned out to be −40 dB. A gain of −40 dB is the same as an attenuation of 40 dB.

Example E-18

Compare intensity 2 with intensity 1; intensity 1 = 10 mW/cm^2; intensity 2 = 0.01 mW/cm^2.

$$10 \log \left(\frac{\text{intensity 2}}{\text{intensity 1}} \right) = 10 \log \left(\frac{0.01}{10} \right)$$

$$= 10 \log \left(\frac{1}{1000} \right) = 10(-\log 1000) = 10(-3) = -30 \text{ dB}$$

Intensity 2 is 30 dB less than or below intensity 1.

Example E-19

As sound passes through a medium, its intensity at one point is 1 mW/cm^2 and at a point 10 cm farther along is 0.1 mW/cm^2. What are the attenuation and attenuation coefficient? (See Chapter 2.)

$$\text{attenuation (dB)} = -10 \log \left(\frac{\text{intensity at second point}}{\text{intensity at first point}} \right)$$

$$= -10 \log \left(\frac{0.1}{1} \right) = -10 \log \left(\frac{1}{10} \right) = -10(-\log 10) = -10(-1) = 10 \text{ dB}$$

See Example E-17 for comment on the first minus sign. The attenuation coefficient is the attenuation (dB) divided by the separation between the two points:

$$\text{attenuation coefficient (dB/cm)} = \frac{\text{attenuation (dB)}}{\text{separation (cm)}}$$

$$= \frac{10 \text{ dB}}{10 \text{ cm}} = 1 \text{ dB/cm}$$

Example E-20

Show by example that $\log x^2$ is equal to $2 \log x$.
Let $x = 5$.
Then $\log x = 0.70$ and $2 \log x = 1.40$.
Thus $x = 5^2 = 25$ and $\log 25 = 1.40$.

Example E-21

Power and intensity are proportional to amplitude squared. A power or intensity ratio expressed in decibels is calculated using the definition

$$10 \log \left(\frac{\text{power 1}}{\text{power 2}} \right)$$

This is equivalent to

$$20 \log \left(\frac{\text{amplitude 1}}{\text{amplitude 2}} \right)$$

as seen with the following values:
Amplitude 1 = 4
Amplitude 2 = 3
Power 1 = 4^2 = 16
Power 2 = 3^2 = 9

$$\text{power ratio (dB)} = 10 \log \left(\frac{\text{power 1}}{\text{power 2}} \right)$$

$$= 10 \log \left(\frac{16}{9} \right) = 2.5$$

$$\text{amplitude ratio (dB)} = 20 \log \left(\frac{\text{amplitude 1}}{\text{amplitude 2}} \right)$$

$$= 20 \log \left(\frac{4}{3} \right) = 2.5$$

TABLE E-2 Decibel Values of Attenuation or Gain for Various Values of Power or Intensity Ratio*

Decibel Gain or Attenuation	Attenuation	Gain
1	0.79	1.3
3	0.50	2.0
6	0.25	4.0
10	0.10	10.0
30	0.001	1000
100	0.0000000001	10,000,000,000

*The ratio is output power or intensity divided by input power or intensity.

Table E-2 lists various values of power or intensity ratio with corresponding decibel values of gain or attenuation.

Some authors put output or end-of-path values in the numerator of the equation used for calculating decibels. If the numerator value is less than the denominator value (e.g., attenuation) a negative decibel value is calculated. For example, if the input and output powers for an electrical attenuator were 2 W and 1 W, respectively, −3 dB results; that is, this attenuator has −3 dB of gain. In this book, only positive decibel values are considered with clarification regarding whether attenuation or gain is considered. In this example, the result would be given as 3 dB *of attenuation*.

SCIENTIFIC NOTATION

Scientific notation uses factors of 10, expressed in exponential form, to shorten the expression of very large or very small numbers. For example, 1,540,000 mm/s can be expressed as 1.54×10^6. In the expression x^y, x is called the base and y is called the exponent. When multiplying factors in scientific notation, the exponents are added. When dividing, the exponents are subtracted.

Example E-22

$$\frac{(1.54 \times 10^6 \text{ mm/s}) \times (3.60 \times 10^3 \text{ s/hr})}{(1.61 \times 10^6 \text{ mm/mile})} = 3.44 \times 10^3 \text{ mph}$$

Here, the multiplication result is 5.54×10^9. Then the division by 1.61×10^6 yields 3.44×10^3.

BINARY NUMBERS

The use of digital memories in ultrasound imaging instruments presents a need for understanding the binary numbering system. Digital (computer) memories and data processors use binary numbers in carrying out their functions because they contain electronic components that operate in only two states, off (0) and on (1).

Binary digits (bits) consist of only zeros and ones, represented by the symbols 0 and 1. As in the decimal numbering system, with which we are so familiar, other numbers must be represented by moving these symbols to different positions (columns). In the decimal system, where there are ten symbols (0 through 9), there is no symbol for the number ten (nine is the largest number for which there is a symbol). To represent ten in symbolic form, the symbol for one is used, moving it to the second (from the right) column. A zero is placed in the right column to clarify this so that ten is, symbolically, 10. The symbols for one and zero have been used in such a way that they no longer represent one or zero, but rather ten.

A similar procedure is used in the binary numbering system. The symbol 1 represents the largest number (one) for which there is a symbol in the system. To represent the next number (2), the same thing is done as in the decimal system; that is, the symbol 1 is placed in the next column to represent the number 2. Columns in the two systems represent values as follows:

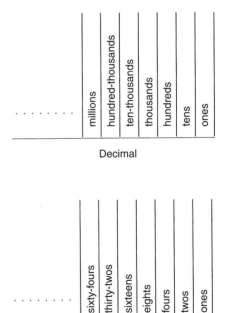

In the decimal system, each column represents 10 times the column to the right. In the binary system each column represents 2 times the column to the right.

The decimal number 1234 represents (reading from right to left) four ones, three tens, two hundreds, and one thousand; that is, 4 + 30 + 200 + 1000 = 1234. Likewise, the decimal number 10,110 represents zero ones, one ten, one hundred, zero thousands, and one ten thousand. The binary number 10110 represents zero ones, one two, one four, zero eights, and one sixteen, or 0 + 2 + 4 + 0 + 16 = 22 in decimal form. This represents a straightforward way of converting a number from the binary system to the decimal system.

Example E-23

Convert the binary number 101010 to decimal form. This number represents 0 + 2 + 0 + 8 + 0 + 32, or 42 in decimal form.

To convert a number from decimal to binary form, one must successively subtract the largest possible multiples of 2, which are the binary column values, in succession from the decimal number.

Example E-24

Convert the decimal number 60 to binary form:
a. Can 64 be subtracted from 60? No. (Enter 0 in the 64 column of the binary number.)
b. Can 32 be subtracted from 60? Yes. (Enter 1 in the 32 column.)
   60 − 32 = 28 (the difference)
c. Can 16 be subtracted from 28? Yes. (Enter 1 in the 16 column.)
   28 − 16 = 12 (the difference)
d. Can 8 be subtracted from 12? Yes. (Enter 1 in the 8 column.)
   12 − 8 = 4 (the difference)
e. Can 4 be subtracted from 4? Yes. (Enter 1 in the 4 column.)
   4 − 4 = 0 (the difference)
f. Can 2 be subtracted from 0? No. (Enter 0 in the 2 column.)
g. Can 1 be subtracted from 0? No. (Enter 0 in the 1 column.)

Therefore the decimal 60 equals 0111100 in the binary system. As in the decimal system, we normally drop leading zeroes, i.e., those to the left of the first nonzero digit. The result is 111100. To check this answer, convert it back to decimal form. This number, 111100, reading from the right, represents 0 + 0 + 4 + 8 + 16 + 32, or 60 in decimal form.

Table E-3 lists the binary forms of the decimal numbers 0 to 63. Numbers 64 to 127 would have one additional digit, and so forth with higher multiples of 2.

 TABLE E-3   Binary and Decimal Number Equivalents

Decimal	Binary	Decimal	Binary
0	000000	32	100000
1	000001	33	100001
2	000010	34	100010
3	000011	35	100011
4	000100	36	100100
5	000101	37	100101
6	000110	38	100110
7	000111	39	100111
8	001000	40	101000
9	001001	41	101001
10	001010	42	101010
11	001011	43	101011
12	001100	44	101100
13	001101	45	101101
14	001110	46	101110
15	001111	47	101111
16	010000	48	110000
17	010001	49	110001
18	010010	50	110010
19	010011	51	110011
20	010100	52	110100
21	010101	53	110101
22	010110	54	110110
23	010111	55	110111
24	011000	56	111000
25	011001	57	111001
26	011010	58	111010
27	011011	59	111011
28	011100	60	111100
29	011101	61	111101
30	011110	62	111110
31	011111	63	111111

UNITS

Units for the physics and acoustics quantities discussed in this book are presented in this section. They are drawn primarily from the international system of units (SI).

Table E-4 lists units for the quantities discussed in this book. Table E-5 gives equivalent units. Table E-6 lists prefixes for units, and Table E-7 gives conversion factors between common units.

In algebraic equations involving these units, the units for the quantity solved for are determined by manipulation of the units for the other quantities in the equation.

TABLE E-4   Units and Unit Symbols for Physics and Acoustic Quantities

Quantity	Unit	Unit Symbol or Abbreviation
Acceleration	meters/second^2	m/s^2
Angle	degrees	°
Area	meters^2	m^2
Attenuation	decibels	dB
Attenuation coefficient	decibels/meter	dB/m
Beam area	meters^2	m^2
Current	amperes	A
Density	kilograms/meter^3	kg/m^3
Displacement	meters	m
Doppler shift	hertz	Hz
Energy	joules	J
Force	newtons	N
Frequency	hertz	Hz
Gain	decibels	dB
Heat	joules	J
Impedance	rayls	—
Intensity	watts/meter^2	W/m^2
Mass	kilograms	kg
Period	seconds	s
Power	watts	W
Pressure	newtons/meter^2	N/m^2
Propagation speed	meters/second	m/s
Pulse duration	seconds	s
Pulse repetition frequency	hertz	Hz
Pulse repetition period	seconds	s
Resistance	ohms	Ω
Spatial pulse length	meters	m
Speed	metes/second	m/s
Stiffness	newtons/meter^2	N/m^2
Temperature	degrees Kelvin	°K
Time	seconds	s
Velocity	meters/second	m/s
Voltage	volts	V
Volume	meters^3	m^3
Wavelength	meters	m
Work	joules	J

TABLE E-5   Equivalent Units for Physics and Acoustics Quantities

Unit Given in Table E-4	Equivalent Unit	Equivalent Unit Abbreviation
Hertz	1/second	1/s
Joules	newton-meters	N-m
Joules	watt-seconds	W-s
Rayls	kilograms/meter^2-second	kg/m^2-s
Newtons	kilogram-meters/second^2	kg-m/s^2
Newtons/meter	pascals	Pa
Watts	joules/second	J/s

TABLE E-6   Unit Prefixes

Prefix	Factor*	Symbol or Abbreviation
mega	1,000,000	M
kilo	1,000	k
centi	0.01	c
milli	0.001	m
micro	0.000001	μ

* *Factor* is the number of unprefixed units in a unit with the prefix. For example, there are 1000 Hz in 1 kHz, and there is 0.001 m in 1 mm.

TABLE E-7   Conversion Factors among Common Units

To Convert	From	To	Multiply by
Area	m^2	cm^2	10,000
	cm^2	m^2	0.0001
Displacement	m	mm	1,000
	m	cm	100
	m	km	0.001
	mm	m	0.001
	mm	km	0.000001
	km	mm	1,000,000
Frequency	Hz	kHz	0.001
	Hz	MHz	0.000001
	kHz	MHz	0.001
	MHz	kHz	1,000
	kHz	Hz	1,000
	MHz	Hz	1,000,000
Intensity	W/cm^2	W/m^2	10,000
	W/cm^2	kW/m^2	10
	W/cm^2	mW/cm^2	1,000
	W/m^2	W/cm^2	0.0001
	W/m^2	mW/cm^2	0.1
	W/m^2	kW/m^2	0.001
Speed	m/s	km/s	0.001
	km/s	m/s	1,000
	km/s	mm/μs	1

Example E-25

Determine the unit for frequency in the equation

$$\text{frequency} = \frac{\text{propagation speed (m/s)}}{\text{wavelength (m)}}$$

The units on the right-hand side of the equation are

$$\frac{m/s}{m} = \frac{1}{s}$$

From Table E-5, it can be found that

$$\frac{1}{s} = \text{Hz}$$

Therefore, the frequency unit is hertz.

Example E-26

Determine the unit for frequency in the equation

$$\text{frequency} = \frac{\text{propagation speed (m/s)}}{\text{wavelength (mm)}}$$

The units on the right-hand side of the equation are

$$\frac{m/s}{mm}$$

From Table E-6, it can be found that 1 mm equals 0.001 m, so that

$$\frac{m/s}{0.001 \text{ m}} = 1000 \text{ 1/s}$$

and from Tables E-5 and E-6,

$$1000 \text{ 1/s} = 1000 \text{ Hz} = 1 \text{ kHz}$$

Therefore, the frequency unit is kilohertz. To convert a frequency given in kilohertz to megahertz, multiply by 0.001. To convert a frequency given in kilohertz to hertz, multiply by 1000.

Example E-27

Determine the unit for intensity in the equation

$$\text{intensity} = \frac{\text{power (W)}}{\text{area (cm}^2)}$$

The units on the right-hand side of the equation are W/cm^2; therefore the intensity unit is watts per centimeter squared.

Example E-28

Determine the unit for impedance in the equation

$$\text{impedance} = \text{density (kg/m}^3) \times \text{propagation speed (km/s)}$$

The units on the right-hand side of the equation are

$$\text{kg/m}^3 \times \text{km/s}$$

From Table E-6,

$$\text{kg/m}^3 \times \text{km/s} = \text{kg/m}^3 \times 1000 \text{ m/s} = 1000 \text{ kg/m}^2 \cdot \text{s}$$

From Table E-5,

$$1000 \text{ kg/m}^2 \cdot \text{s} = 1000 \text{ rayls}$$

From Table E-6,

$$1000 \text{ rayls} = 1 \text{ krayl}$$

Therefore, the impedance unit is kilorayl. Because this is uncommon, it would be better to keep the result in rayls.

STATISTICS

Several concepts are used in evaluating the usefulness of diagnostic tests. These tests can be qualitative, as in the case of interpreting an anatomic image, or they can be quantitative, as with Doppler flow values. Diagnoses are positive and negative; that is, the test indicates the presence or absence of disease. Table E-8 defines the various groups involved in testing for disease.

The sensitivity *(SENS)* of a test is the proportion of those having the disease *(TD)* who test positive *(TPV)*:

$$\text{SENS} = \frac{\text{TPV}}{\text{TD}}$$

The specificity *(SPEC)* of a test is the proportion of those who are disease-free *(TND)* who test negative *(TNV)*:

$$\text{SPEC} = \frac{\text{TNV}}{\text{TND}}$$

The positive predictive value *(PPV)* of a test is the proportion of all positive *(TP)* test results that are correct, that is, the number of true positive results *(TPV)*:

$$\text{PPV} = \frac{\text{TPV}}{\text{TP}}$$

The positive predictive value is the probability that a person who tests positive actually has the disease.

TABLE E-8	Definitions of Numbers in Groups Tested*		
Test Result	**Disease**	**Nondiseased**	**TOTAL**
Positive	TPV	FPV	TP
Negative	FNV	TNV	TN
TOTAL	TD	TND	TOT

*A positive test indicates disease. A negative test indicates disease-free. *TPV* (true-positive value), the number of diseased persons (in the study) testing positive; *FPV* (false-positive value), the number of nondiseased persons who tested positive; *TP*, the total number of persons testing positive; *FNV* (false-negative value), the number of diseased persons testing negative; *TNV* (true-negative value), the number of disease-free persons testing negative; *TN*, the total number of persons testing negative; *TD*, the total number of diseased persons; *TND*, the total number of nondiseased persons; *TOT*, the total number of persons in the study.

The negative predictive value *(NPV)* of a test is the proportion of all negative *(TN)* test results that are correct, that is, the number of true negative results *(TNV)*:

$$NPV = \frac{TNV}{TN}$$

The negative predictive value is the probability that a person who tests negative is actually disease-free.

The accuracy *(ACC)* of a test is the proportion of all tests in the study *(TOT)* that have the correct result

$$ACC = \frac{(TPV + TNV)}{TOT}$$

Example E-29

Given the following table, calculate TD, TND, TP, TN, TOT, SENS, SPEC, PPV, NPV, and ACC.

Test Result	Disease	Nondiseased	TOTAL
Positive	8	2	TP
Negative	5	85	TN
TOTAL	TD	TND	TOT

Test Result	Disease	Nondiseased	TOTAL
Positive	8	2	10
Negative	5	85	90
TOTAL	13	87	100

$$SENS = \frac{8}{13} = 0.62$$

$$SPEC = \frac{85}{87} = 0.98$$

$$PPV = \frac{8}{10} = 0.80$$

$$NPV = \frac{85}{90} = 0.94$$

$$ACC = \frac{(8+85)}{100} = 0.93$$

EXERCISES

1. Solve each of the following for *x*:
   a. $x + y + 2 = z$
   b. $x - y = z - 1$
   c. $2xy = z$
   d. $\frac{x}{y} = 3z$
   e. $\frac{(x + 5)}{4} - 2 = 4$
   f. $\frac{(3x + 3)}{2} - 2 = 4$

2. Solve each of the following for the quantity with the asterisk:
   a. propagation speed = frequency* × wavelength
   b. intensity $= \frac{power}{beam\ area*}$
   c. period $= \frac{1}{frequency*}$

3. The age of an ultrasound instrument is equal to 3 times its age 3 years from now minus 3 times its age 3 years ago. What is its present age?

4. Let
   $$y + x = \tfrac{1}{2}(7y - 3x)$$
   Subtract $2x$ from both sides so that
   $$y - x = \tfrac{1}{2}(7y - 3x) - 2x$$
   Divide both sides by $(y - x)$:
   $$\frac{(y - x)}{(y - x)} = \frac{(7y - 3x)}{2(y - x)} - \frac{2x}{(y - x)}$$
   Combine right side into single fraction:
   $$\frac{(y - x)}{(y - x)} = \frac{(7y - 3x - 4x)}{2(y - x)} = \frac{7(y - x)}{2(y - x)}$$
   Multiply both sides by 2:
   $$2\left[\frac{(y - x)}{(y - x)}\right] = 7\left[\frac{(y - x)}{(y - x)}\right]$$
   Therefore 2 = 7. What went wrong?

5. If side a, b, and c in Figure E-1 have lengths of 3, 4, and 5, respectively, then sin A is _____ and cos A is_____.

6. If angle A is 90 degrees, sin A is _____ and cos A is _____.

7. If sin A is 0.17, angle A is _____ degrees.

8. If cos A is 0.94, angle A is _____ degrees.

9. Give the logarithms of the following numbers:
   a. 10 _____
   b. 0.1 _____
   c. 100 _____
   d. 0.001 _____

10. One watt is _____ dB below 100 W.

11. One watt is _____ dB above 100 mW.

12. If the input power is 1 mW and the output is 10,000 mW, the gain is _____ dB.

13. If the input power is 1 W and the output is 100 mW, the gain is _____ dB. The attenuation is _____ dB.

14. If the intensities of traveling sound are 10 mW/cm^2 and 0.1 mW/cm^2 at two points 5 cm apart, the attenuation between the two points is _____ dB. The attenuation coefficient is _____ dB/cm.

15. If an amplifier has a gain of 33 dB, the ratio of output power to input power is _____. (Use Table E-2.)

16. If an attenuator has an attenuation of 2b dB, the ratio of output power to input power is _____. (Use Table E-2.)
17. If the intensity at the start of a path is 3 mW/cm² and the attenuation over the path is 13 dB, the intensity at the end of the path is _____ mW/cm². (Use Table E-2.)
18. If the output of a 22-dB gain amplifier is connected to the input of a 24-dB gain amplifier, the total gain is _____ dB. The overall power ratio is _____. (Use Table E-2.)
19. If a 17-dB attenuator is connected to a 14-dB amplifier, the net gain is _____ dB. The net attenuation is _____ dB. For a 1-W input, the output is _____ W. (Use Table E-2.)
20. In binary numbers, how many symbols are used? _____
21. The term *binary digit* commonly is shortened into the single word _____.
22. Each binary digit in a binary number is represented in memory by a memory element, which at any time is in one of _____ states.
23. Match the following:
    Column in a binary number hgfedcba:
    a. _____
    b. _____
    c. _____
    d. _____
    e. _____
    f. _____
    g. _____
    h. _____
    Decimal number represented by a 1 in the column:
    1. 64
    2. 32
    3. 1
    4. 16
    5. 8
    6. 128
    7. 2
    8. 4
24. The binary number 10110 represents zero ones, one two, one four, zero eights, and one sixteen, that is, 0 + 2 + 4 + 0 + 16 = 22. What decimal number is represented by the binary number 11001? _____
25. The decimal number 13 is made up of one one, zero twos, one four, and one eight (8 + 4 + 0 + 1 = 13). The decimal number therefore is represented by the binary number _____.
26. Match the following:
    a. 1 _____   1. 0001111
    b. 5 _____   2. 0011001
    c. 10 _____   3. 0001010
    d. 15 _____   4. 0110010
    e. 20 _____   5. 0000001

f. 25 _____   6. 1100100
g. 30 _____   7. 0101000
h. 40 _____   8. 0011110
i. 50 _____   9. 0010100
j. 100 _____   10. 0000101

27. How many binary digits are required in the binary numbers representing the following numbers?
    a. 0 _____
    b. 1 _____
    c. 5 _____
    d. 10 _____
    e. 25 _____
    f. 30 _____
    g. 63 _____
    h. 64 _____
    i. 75 _____
    j. 100 _____
28. Match the following:
    Largest decimal number that can be represented by a binary number with this many bits:
    a. 7 _____   1. 1
    b. 15 _____   2. 2
    c. 3 _____   3. 3
    d. 511 _____   4. 4
    e. 1023 _____   5. 5
    f. 63 _____   6. 6
    g. 255 _____   7. 7
    h. 1 _____   8. 8
    i. 127 _____   9. 9
    j. 31 _____   10. 10
29. How many bits are required to store numbers representing each number of different gray shades?
    a. 2 _____
    b. 4 _____
    c. 8 _____
    d. 15 _____
    e. 16 _____
    f. 25 _____
    g. 32 _____
    h. 64 _____
    i. 65 _____
    j. 128 _____
30. The unit of frequency in the equation

$$\text{frequency} = \frac{\text{propagation speed (km/s)}}{\text{wavelength (mm)}}$$

is _____. To convert frequency in this unit to frequency in kilohertz, multiply by _____.
31. A frequency of 50 kHz is equal to _____ MHz and _____ Hz.
32. A speed of 1.5 mm/µs is equal to _____ km/s, _____ m/s, _____ cm/s, and _____ mm/s.
33. If the frequency is 2 MHz and

$$\text{period} = \frac{1}{\text{frequency}}$$

the period is _____ µs, _____ ms, or _____ s.

34. Mass is given in units of
    a. megahertz.
    b. kilogram.
    c. degrees Kelvin.
    d. watt.
    e. none of the above.
35. Displacement is given in
    a. megahertz.
    b. decibel.
    c. ohm.
    d. meter.
    e. all of the above.
36. Attenuation is given in
    a. decirayl.
    b. deciwatt.
    c. decibel.
    d. decimeter.
    e. decihertz.
37. Given the following table, calculate TD, TND, TP, TN, TOT, SENS, SPEC, PPV, NPV, and ACC.

Test Result	Disease	Nondiseased	TOTAL
Positive	80	20	TP
Negative	50	850	TN
TOTAL	TD	TND	TOT

38. Solve the following for x and y:
    $x + y = 1$ $x - y = 2$

ANSWERS

1. a. $z - y - 2$; b. $y + z - 1$; c. $z/2y$; d. $3yz$; e. 19; f. 3
2. a. $\dfrac{\text{propagation speed}}{\text{wavelength}}$
   b. $\dfrac{\text{power}}{\text{intensity}}$
   c. $\dfrac{1}{\text{period}}$
3. 18
4. Division by zero is what went wrong. Note that

$$y + x = \tfrac{1}{2}(7y - 3x)$$

yields

$$2(y + x) = 7y - 3x$$
$$2y + 2x = 7y - 3x$$
$$5x = 5y$$
$$x = y$$

so that dividing by $(y - x)$ is dividing by zero (not allowed in algebra).
5. 0.6, 0.8
6. 1, 0
7. 10
8. 20
9. a. 1; b. −1; c. 2; d. −3
10. 20
11. 10
12. 40
13. −10, 10
14. 20, 4
15. 2000
16. 0.0025
17. 0.15
18. 46, 40,000
19. −3, 3, 0.50
20. Two (0, 1)
21. Bit
22. Two (off, on)
23. a. 3; b. 7; c. 8; d. 5; e. 4; f. 2; g. 1; h. 6
24. 25
25. 1101
26. a. 5; b. 10; c. 3; d. 1; e. 9; f. 2; g. 8; h. 7; i. 4; j. 6
27. a. 1 (0); b. 1 (1); c. 3 (101); d. 4 (1010); e. 5 (11001); f. 5 (11110); g. 6 (111111); h. 7 (1000000); i. 7 (1001011); j. 7 (1100100)
28. a. 3 (111); b. 4 (1111); c. 2 (11); d. 9 (111111111); e. 10 (1111111111); f. 6 (111111); g. 8 (11111111); h. 1 (1); i. 7 (1111111); j. 5 (11111)
29. a. 1 (0, 1); b. 2 (00, 01, 10, 11); c. 3 (000, 001, 010, 011, 100, 101, 110, 111); d. 4; e. 4; f. 5; g. 5; h. 6; i. 7; j. 7
30. Megahertz, 1000
31. 0.05, 50,000
32. 1.5, 1500, 150,000, 1,500,000
33. 0.5, 0.0005, 0.0000005
34. b
35. d
36. c
37.

Test Result	Disease	Nondiseased	TOTAL
Positive	80	20	100
Negative	50	850	900
TOTAL	130	870	1000

$$\text{SENS} = \frac{80}{130} = 0.62$$

$$\text{SPEC} = \frac{850}{870} = 0.98$$

$$\text{PPV} = \frac{80}{100} = 0.80$$

$$\text{NPV} = \frac{850}{900} = 0.94$$

$$\text{ACC} = \frac{(80+850)}{1000} = 0.93$$

38. $x = 1\tfrac{1}{2}$
    $y = -\tfrac{1}{2}$

APPENDIX

F Physics Review

The terms discussed in this appendix are defined in the Glossary. Their units are given in Appendix E. The definitions are amplified here, and the terms are related to one another.

MECHANICS

If there were no forces, everything would be in a state of rest or steady motion. Forces change the state of rest or motion of matter. When considering sound, the force divided by the area over which the force is applied is a useful quantity. This is called pressure, one of the acoustic variables discussed in Chapter 2. Pressure (*p*) is force *(F)* per unit area *(A)* (the concentration of force).

$$p \ (N/m^2) = \frac{F \ (N)}{A \ (m^2)}$$

A given force applied to an object may produce considerably different results if the pressures at which it is applied are different. If, for example, a small force is applied by a hand to an inflated toy balloon, the balloon simply will move. If the same force is applied by a sharp needle, the balloon will break. The difference is that the needle applies the force over a very small area (a very high pressure), breaking the balloon.

Application of force or pressure changes the state of rest or motion of matter. Motion may be described in many ways.

Displacement is the distance that a body has moved.

Speed is the rate at which position is changing. Speed *(s)* is the distance *(d)* moved divided by the time *(t)* over which the movement occurs.

$$s \ (m/s) = \frac{d \ (m)}{t \ (s)}$$

Velocity *(v)* is the same as speed except that the direction of motion is specified.

Acceleration is the rate at which velocity is changing. Acceleration *(a)* is the change in velocity (change in

speed or direction or both) divided by the time over which the change occurs.

$$a \ (m/s^2) = \frac{\Delta v \ (m/s)}{t \ (s)}$$

Mass is a measure of the resistance of an object to acceleration. Weight is the gravitational force between two bodies attracting each other. Weight depends on the masses of the bodies attracting each other. The mass of a body is the same whether it is on the earth or on the moon, but the weights of the body in the two places are different because the mass of the earth is much greater than that of the moon.

Density *(ρ)* is the concentration of mass. Density is the mass *(m)* divided by the volume *(V)* taken up by the mass (mass per unit volume).

$$\rho \ (kg/m^3) = \frac{m \ (kg)}{V \ (m^3)}$$

Stiffness is a description of the resistance of a material to compression. Stiffness *(M)* is equal to the applied pressure divided by the fractional change in volume *(ΔV_F)* resulting from the pressure.

$$M \ (N/m^2) = \frac{p \ (N/m^2)}{\Delta V_F}$$

The fractional volume change is the difference in volume before and after the pressure is applied, divided by the volume before the pressure is applied.

If a material has high stiffness, little change in volume will occur when pressure is applied. If it has low stiffness, a large change in volume will occur when pressure is applied. Stiffness is also called bulk modulus of elasticity and is the reciprocal of the compressibility of a material.

Newton's second law of motion relates three of the physical phenomena discussed in this appendix. The law states that the force applied to a body is equal to the mass of the body multiplied by the acceleration of the body resulting from the applied force.

$$F \text{ (N)} = m \text{ (kg)} \times a \text{ (m/s}^2)$$

If more than one force is applied, the net force (resulting from combination of the applied forces) is the force used in the equation. The acceleration is in the direction of the net force.

ENERGY

Work is done when a force acts against a resistance to produce motion of a body. Work *(W)* is equal to the applied net force multiplied by the distance the body moves (displacement).

$$W \text{ (J)} = F \text{ (N)} \times d \text{ (m)}$$

If there is no motion, no work is done. If a body is in motion but no force is being applied, no work is done.

Energy *(E)* is the capability of doing work. A body must have energy in order to do work on another body. When a body does work, it loses energy. When a body has work done on it, it gives energy. Work may be thought of as the transfer of energy from one body (the one doing the work) to another (the one having work done on it). The energy transferred is equal to the work done.

Power *(P)* is the rate at which work is done or the rate at which energy is transferred. Power is equal to the work done divided by the time required to do the work. Power is also equal to energy transferred divided by the time required to transfer the energy.

$$P \text{ (W)} = \frac{W \text{ (J)}}{t \text{ (s)}} = \frac{E \text{ (J)}}{t \text{ (s)}}$$

Heat is one type of energy. Heat is the energy resulting from thermal molecular motion.

Temperature is the condition of a body that determines transfer of heat to or from other bodies. No heat flows when two bodies of equal temperatures come in contact with each other. Heat flows from a body of higher temperature to one of lower temperature when they come in contact.

Electricity is another type of energy. Electricity is the energy resulting from the displacement or flow of electrons. Electric voltage is the work done when moving a unit electric charge between two points across which the voltage exists. Voltage is measured in volts. Electric current is the rate of flow of electrons in an electric conductor. This flow is caused by a voltage. Electric current is measured in amperes. The quantity of current is determined not only by the voltage but also by the electric resistance of the conductor. Ohm's law relates voltage *(V)*, current *(I)*, and resistance *(R)*.

$$V \text{ (V)} = I \text{ (A)} \times R \text{ (}\Omega\text{)}$$

Electric power is equal to voltage multiplied by current.

$$P \text{ (W)} = V \text{ (V)} \times I \text{ (A)}$$

Combining Ohm's law and the electric power equation yields:

$$P \text{ (W)} = I^2 \text{ (A}^2) \times R \text{ (}\Omega\text{)} = \frac{V^2 \text{ (V}^2)}{R \text{ (}\Omega\text{)}}$$

EXERCISES

1. To convert speed to velocity, _____ must be specified.
2. Increased mass results in _____ weight.
3. Pressure is the concentration of _____.
4. Density is the concentration of _____.
5. Speed is the rate at which _____ changes.
6. Acceleration is the rate at which _____ changes.
7. Newton's second law of motion states that _____ equals _____ times _____.
8. Stiffness is a description of the resistance of a material to _____.
9. If a force of 50 N acts uniformly over an area of 20 m², the pressure is _____ N/m².
10. If a body moves 50 m uniformly in 5 s, its speed is _____ m/s.
11. If a body accelerates uniformly to the east at 5 m/s², its velocity 5 s after starting from zero speed is _____ m/s east.
12. Five kilograms of matter with a volume of 10 m³ has a density of _____ kg/m³.
13. If a pressure of 5 N/m² changes the volume of a body from 0.5 m³ to 0.4 m³, the fractional volume change is _____.
14. The stiffness of the material of the body in Exercise 13 is _____ N/m².
15. A 5-kg mass subjected to a 15-N force west will have acceleration of _____ m/s² in the _____ direction.
16. Match the following:

    a. Pressure: _____   1. Force × displacement
    b. Speed: ____
    c. Acceleration: _____   2. Displacement/time
    d. Density: _____   3. Mass × acceleration
    e. Force: _____
    f. Stiffness: _____   4. Work/time
    g. Work: _____   5. Force/area
    h. Power: _____   6. Velocity change/time
    i. Electric power: 7. Mass/volume
       _____
    j. Voltage: _____   8. Pressure/fractional volume change

9. Current × resistance
10. Voltage × current

17. Power is the rate at which _____ is done.
18. Energy is the capability of doing _____.
19. Temperature is the condition of a body that determines transfer of _____ to or from other bodies.
20. Heat and electricity are two types of _____.
21. If the current is 2 A and the resistance is 12 Ω, the voltage is _____ V and the power is _____ W.
22. If the current is 25 mA and the resistance is 50 kΩ, the voltage is _____ V and the power is _____ W.
23. If current is doubled (constant resistance), voltage is _____ and power is _____.
24. If resistance is doubled (constant current), voltage is _____ and power is _____.
25. Ohm's law relates _____, _____, and _____.
26. Voltage times current equals electric _____.
27. Electric power equals (three correct answers)
    a. Current × resistance
    b. Current × voltage
    c. Voltage × resistance
    d. Current² × resistance
    e. Voltage²/resistance
28. For 10 volts and 5 A, the power is _____ W.
29. For 10 Ω and 5 A, the voltage is _____ V.
30. If a force of 3 N moves body 4 m, the work done is _____ J.
31. If the movement in Exercise 30 occurs in 6 s, the power is _____ J/s or _____ W.
32. In Exercise 30, the energy transferred is _____ J.

ANSWERS

1. Direction
2. Increased
3. Force
4. Mass
5. Position
6. Velocity
7. Force, mass, acceleration
8. Compression
9. 2.5
10. 10
11. 25
12. 0.5
13. 0.2 (Pressure is not needed for the calculation.)
14. 25
15. 3, west
16. a. 5; b. 2; c. 6; d. 7; e. 3; f. 8; g. 1; h. 4; i. 10; j. 9
17. Work
18. Work
19. Heat
20. Energy
21. 24, 48
22. 1250, 31
23. Doubled, quadrupled
24. Doubled, doubled
25. Voltage, current, resistance
26. Power
27. b, d, e
28. 50
29. 50
30. 12
31. 2, 2
32. 12

G Additional Material for Examination Preparation

The outlines for the UPI (Ultrasound Physics and Instrumentation), CPI (Cardiovascular Principles and Instrumentation Physics), and VPI (Vascular Physical Principles and Instrumentation) examinations administered by the American Registry for Diagnostic Medical Sonography (ARDMS) are listed in this appendix (reproduced with permission of the American Registry for Diagnostic Medical Sonography) along with comments, definitions, and references to relevant text material. Comments, definitions, and references are in italics.

First, here is an explanation of terms included in the ARDMS outlines and examinations that are not included in this book or are described with other terminology.

Spatial resolution is called *detail resolution* in this book.

Wave interference, Huygens' Principle, and *diffraction* are, in the opinion of the author, not helpful concepts for the understanding of diagnostic ultrasound by clinical users. They are thus topics not included in this book.

Annular arrays and other *mechanical transducers* are not discussed in this book, being outmoded technology.

Transducer *crystal* is called *element* in this book.

Transmitter is called *pulser* in this book. The pulser is part of the beam former.

Receiver is an archaic term from the era of analog electronics. The concept is not used in the description of modern digital sonographic instruments in this book. The functions of the receiver now are divided between the beam former and the signal processor.

Rectification and *smoothing* are the outmoded terms that describe the analog approach to amplitude demodulation (detection). They are not discussed in this book. Other techniques are used for demodulation in modern digital signal processing.

Rejection is not implemented in modern digital signal processing and is not described in this book.

Television monitors are no longer used as display devices in sonographic instruments. Cathode-ray-tube computer monitors have replaced them. More recently, flat-panel liquid-crystal displays are replacing cathode-ray tube computer monitors.

ULTRASOUND PHYSICS AND INSTRUMENTATION CONTENT OUTLINE*

I. Elementary Principles (8%-12%) *[Chapter 2]*
   A. Nature of Ultrasound
      1. Definition of sound
         Sound is a traveling wave of acoustic variables; that is, quantities that vary in space and time, including pressure, density, and particle vibration.
         a. Propagation of vibration
            (1) Compression
                Region of high density and pressure in a sound wave.
            (2) Rarefaction
                Region of low density and pressure in a sound wave.
      2. Differentiation between audible sound and ultrasound
         Audible sound can be heard by human beings. Audible sound is in the frequency range 20 to 20,000 Hz.
         Ultrasound is inaudible to human beings because of high frequencies (above 20 kHz).
   B. Frequency, Wavelength, Propagation Speed
      1. Definition of terms
         Frequency. Number of cycles per second.
         Wavelength. Length of space over which a cycle occurs.
         Propagation speed. Speed with which a wave moves through a medium.
      2. Relationships

$$\lambda \ (mm) = \frac{c \ (mm/\mu s)}{f \ (MHz)}$$

where λ is wavelength, c is propagation speed, and f is frequency.

---

*Modified by ARDMS: 2/14/2003.

C. Properties of Ultrasound Waves
   1. Amplitude
      Maximum variation of an acoustic variable away from normal.
   2. Pressure
      Force per unit area in a fluid.
   3. Power
      Rate at which work is done; rate at which energy is transferred.
   4. Intensity
      Power divided by area.
D. Decibels
   1. Definition
      a. Related to intensity
         Unit of power or intensity ratio; the number of decibels is 10 times the logarithm (to the base 10) of the power or intensity ratio.
      b. Related to amplitude
         Unit of amplitude ratio; the number of decibels is 20 times the logarithm (to the base 10) of the amplitude ratio.
   2. Numerical examples
      Intensity ratio in dB = 10 $\log_{10}$ (intensity$_2$/intensity$_1$)
      Amplitude ratio in dB = 20 $\log_{10}$ (amplitude$_2$/amplitude$_1$)
E. Physical Units *[Appendix E]*
   1. Scientific notation
      Using exponents to express factors of 10.
      2,000,000 = 2 $\times$ 10^6
      0.05 = 5 $\times$ 10^{-2}
   2. Metric notation (e.g., micro, mega)
      Prefixes meaning various multiples:
      mega = 1,000,000
      kilo = 1000
      deci = 0.1
      centi = 0.01
      milli = 0.001
      micro = 0.000001
   3. Common units
      mm, cm, Hz, s, W, dB
F. Measurement Dimensions
   1. Distance
      a. Linear
      b. Circumference
   2. Area
   3. Volume
II. Propagation of Ultrasound through Tissues (10%–14%) *[Chapter 2]*
A. Speed of Sound
   1. Average speed of sound in tissues
      1.54 mm/µs, 1540 m/s
   2. Range of propagation speeds in the body
      a. Air
         0.33 mm/µs, 330 m/s
      b. Soft tissue (average)
         1.54 mm/µs, 1540 m/s
      c. Soft tissue: specific tissues (e.g., muscle, fat, parenchyma)
         Muscle, 1.57 mm/µs
         Fat, 1.44 mm/µs
         Parenchyma (liver, kidney), 1.56 mm/µs
         Parenchyma (brain), 1.51 mm/µs
      d. Bone
         3.0 to 4.0 mm/µs
B. Reflection
   1. Characteristic acoustic impedance—definition
      Density multiplied by the sound propagation speed.
   2. Reflection and transmission at specular interfaces
      a. Interface size and contour (smooth or irregular)
         Large compared with wavelength. Smooth surface.
      b. Dependence on angle
         Incidence and reflection angles are equal. Echo received by transducer when incidence angle is near or equal to zero.
      c. Dependence on acoustic impedance mismatch
         Echo strength is proportional to impedance difference at boundary.
   3. Scattering
      a. Definition of scattering
         Diffusion or redirection of sound in several directions upon encountering a particle suspension or a rough surface.
      b. Frequency dependence (Rayleigh scattering)
         Intensity proportional to particle radius^4 for particles small compared with wavelength (the condition for Rayleigh scattering).
      c. Interface contour (smooth or irregular)
         Scattering occurs with irregular (rough) surface.
      d. Contrast media
         A suspension of bubbles or particles introduced into circulation to enhance the contrast between anatomic structures, thereby improving their imaging.
      e. Harmonics
         Frequencies that are even and odd multiples of another, commonly called the fundamental or operating frequency.
C. Refraction
   1. Definition of refraction
      Change of sound direction on passing from one medium to another.
   2. Dependence of angle
      Transmission angle is approximately proportional to the incidence angle.

3. Dependence of velocity mismatch
Transmission angle is proportional to the ratio of the propagation speeds in the media.

4. Numerical example
If the incidence angle is 20 degrees and the propagation speeds in the media are 1.54 and 1.45, the transmission angle is

$$T_t = T_i [c_2/c_1] = 20 [1.45/1.54] = 18.8 \text{ degrees}$$

D. Attenuation
1. Definition and sources of attenuation
Decrease in amplitude and intensity with distance as a wave travels through a medium.
   a. Scattering
   Diffusion or redirection of sound in several directions upon encountering a particle suspension or a rough surface.
   b. Absorption
   Conversion of sound to heat. Dominant mechanism for attenuation in soft tissues.
      (1) Heat
      Energy resulting from thermal molecular motion.
      (2) Measurement
      Temperature rise in tissue can be measured by inserting a thermocouple.
   c. Reflection
   Generation of an echo at a specular surface.
2. Typical values in soft tissue
0.5 dB/cm-MHz
3. Variation with frequency—numerical example
Doubling frequency doubles attenuation coefficient.
1.0 dB/cm at 2 MHz
2.0 dB/cm at 4 MHz
4. Effects on images
Increasing frequency increases attenuation and decreases penetration (imaging depth).

E. Useful Diagnostic Frequency Range
1. Numerical values
2 to 15 MHz for most human applications.
2. Tradeoff: penetration vs. spatial resolution
Increasing frequency decreases penetration but improves spatial (detail) resolution by shortening ultrasound pulses and tightening the focus.

F. Terminology Associated with Image Characteristics
1. Echogenic (e.g., hyperechoic, hypoechoic, anechoic, isoechoic, etc.)
Hyperechoic. Having relatively strong echoes.
Hypoechoic. Having relatively weak echoes.
Anechoic. Echo free.
Isoechoic. Of equal or similar echogenicity.
2. Homogeneity, Heterogeneity, etc.
Homogeneous. Of uniform structure or composition.
Heterogeneous. Of nonuniform structure or composition.
3. Other

III. Ultrasound Transducers (17%-25%) [Chapter 3]
A. The Piezoelectric Effect
1. Definition and concept
Piezoelectricity: Conversion of pressure to electric voltage.
2. Curie point
Temperature at which an element material loses its piezoelectric properties.
3. Piezoelectric materials
Lead zirconate titanate (PZT): The common ceramic piezoelectric material.

B. Transducer Construction and Characteristics
1. Thickness resonance of crystal
The natural (resonance) frequency of a crystal is determined by its thickness. Thinner yields a higher frequency.
2. Operating (resonance) frequency
   a. Crystal thickness
   The natural (resonance) frequency of a crystal is such that its thickness is half the wavelength.
   b. Speed of sound in crystal material
   The speed is relatively high, being in a solid crystal. Speed ranges from 4 to 6 mm/μs.
3. Frequency characteristics (spectrum)
   a. Bandwidth
   Range of frequencies contained in an ultrasound pulse; range of frequencies within which a material, device, or system can operate.
      (1) Quality factor
      Operating frequency divided by bandwidth.
      (2) Effect of damping
      Damping shortens a pulse, broadens its bandwidth, and lowers the quality factor.
   b. Multi-Hertz
   The capability of operating a broadband transducer at more than one operating frequency.
      (1) Harmonics
      Frequencies that are even and odd multiples of another, commonly called the fundamental or operating frequency.
4. Damping
Material attached to the rear face of a transducer element to reduce pulse duration; the process of pulse duration reduction.
5. Matching layer-numerical example
Crystal impedance, 30 Mrayl
Tissue impedance, 1.63 Mrayl
Matching layer, 7.0 Mrayl

C. Sound Beam Formation—Near Field and Far Field (Fresnel and Fraunhofer Zones)
   1. Interference phenomena
      Interference is the combination of positive and/or negative pressure either constructively or destructively.
      a. Huygen's principle
         All points on a wavefront can be considered as point sources for the production of spherical secondary wavelets. Later, the new position of the wavefront is the surface of tangency to these secondary wavelets.
      b. Diffraction (divergence)
         The flaring out of a wave after it passes through a small aperture or past a blocking edge. The flaring is accompanied by a interference pattern of maxima and minima.
      c. Bandwidth
   2. Length of near field (focal distance)
      The distance from the source to the narrowest region of a beam.
   3. Shape of near field and far field
      a. Beam width
         In the near field, the beam narrows with increasing distance from the source.
         In the far field, the beam broadens with increasing distance from the source.
      b. Natural focus
         The narrowing of a beam (in the near field) from an unfocused transducer.
   4. Dependence on frequency and crystal or aperture size
      Near-field length increases with increasing frequency or aperture. Increasing frequency or aperture tightens (narrows) the focus of a focused beam.

D. Axial Resolution
   The minimum reflector separation along the sound path that is required to produce separate echoes (i.e., to distinguish between two reflectors).
   1. Dependence on spatial pulse length/pulse duration
      Shorter pulses have improved axial resolution.
   2. Numerical example
      Axial resolution is equal to half the spatial pulse length. Pulse length 1 mm, axial resolution 0.5 mm.
   3. Effect of damping
      Damping shortens a pulse, improving the axial resolution.
   4. Transducer frequency spectrum-relation to pulse duration
      Shortening a pulse broadens its bandwidth.
   5. Bandwidth
      Superior axial resolution is associated with broad bandwidth.

E. Lateral Resolution
   Minimum reflector separation perpendicular to the sound path that is required to produce separate echoes.
   1. Dependence on beam width
      Lateral resolution is equal to beam width.
   2. Frequency
      Higher frequencies improve lateral resolution by tightening focus.
   3. Transducer size and focal characteristics
      Larger aperture or greater curvature tightens the focus, improving lateral resolution.
   4. Range

F. Slice Thickness Resolution (Elevational Resolution)
   The detail resolution in the direction perpendicular to the scan plane. Detail resolution is equal to the section (slice) thickness and is the source of section thickness artifact.
   1. Dependence on beam width
      Elevational resolution is equal to the beam width perpendicular to the scan plane.
   2. Transducer array and focal characteristics
      Arrays focus with phase delay curvature pattern. More delay curvature moves focus closer to transducer. Less delay curvature moves it away (deeper).
   3. Frequency
      Higher frequencies narrow the slice thickness.
   4. Lateral and axial resolution relationship
      Axial resolution is normally better than lateral or elevational.

G. Focusing
   The concentration of the sound beam into a smaller beam area than would exist otherwise.
   1. Methods of focusing
      a. Mechanical (internal and external)
         Internal focus is the use of curved crystals. External focus is the use of a lens on the front of a flat crystal.
      b. Electronic (transmit and receive)
         Using a curved phase delay pattern on transmission and/or correction of curved pattern on reception to focus electronically.
   2. Focal zone characteristics
      a. Focal distance (length)
         Distance from the source to the focus.
      b. Focal zone region
         The region around the focus, usually defined as the region within which the intensity is greater than 50% of the maximum.
         (1) Maximum intensity
            The greatest value of intensity found in beam, usually at the focus.

H. Transducer Arrays and Image Appearance
An array is a transducer assembly containing several piezoelectric elements (crystals).
1. Mechanical and/or electronic construction
2. Multiple element construction
   a. Linear array
      A straight line of elements.
   b. Curved array
      A curved line of elements (also called a convex or curvilinear array).
   c. Annular array
      An array composed of several concentric ring (annulus) elements.
   d. Multi-dimensional array
      A two-dimensional array with several rows of elements. There can be three rows up to a number of rows equal to the number of elements in each row (a square array).
3. Multiple element operation
   a. Sequenced
      Energizing elements in groups from one end of the array to the other.
   b. Phased
      Energizing groups of elements with short time delays (called phasing). Phasing steers the beam in the desired direction and also focuses it electronically.
   c. Annular
      Phasing focuses the annular array in the scan plane and in the slice thickness dimension.
   d. Vector
      Combined sequencing and phasing of element groups.
   e. Multi-dimensional
      Row-to-row phasing to focus in the slice-thickness dimension.
4. Beam steering
   a. Transmission time delays
      A rapid progression from left to right in the array steers the beam to the right.
   b. Reception time delays
      Correcting the delay pattern of received echoes maximizes reception sensitivity in a specific direction.
5. Beam focusing
   a. Time delays
      A curved delay pattern focuses a beam electronically.
   b. Dynamic reception focus
      Delay correction for focusing on reception. Needed correction decreases as echoes arrive from deeper locations. Thus reception focus is dynamic (i.e., continually changing as echoes return from a transmitted pulse).

   c. Multiple transmission foci
      Transmitting more than one pulse down a given scan line, each with a different focus. This in effect produces a long focus. Frame rate is reduced, degrading temporal resolution.
   d. Apodization
      Nonuniform (i.e., involving different voltage amplitudes) driving of elements in an array to reduce grating lobes.
   e. Subdicing
      Dividing an element into smaller subelements. Subdicing weakens grating lobes and reduces mechanical interelement interaction.
   f. Dynamic aperture
      Automatically varying aperture to adjust reception focal width to be constant at various depths.
I. Transducer Care and Maintenance
IV. Pulse Echo Instruments (6%-10%) [Chapter 4]
   A. Range Equation—General Concepts
      Echo arrival time corresponds to reflector depth. Arrival time rule is 13 μs/cm.
   B. Pulsing Characteristics
      1. Pulse repetition frequency
         Number of pulses per second; sometimes called pulse repetition rate.
      2. Pulse repetition period
         Interval of time from the beginning of one pulse to the beginning of the next.
      3. Pulse duration
         Interval of time from beginning to end of a pulse.
      4. Spatial pulse length
         Length of space over which a pulse occurs.
      5. Duty factor
         Fraction of time that pulsed ultrasound is on.
   C. Transmitter (Output)
      1. Effect of transmitter voltage on penetration
         Increasing driving voltage increases imaging penetration, but not strongly (only about 5% increase in penetration with a doubling of output intensity).
      2. Effect of transmitter voltage on intensity and on patient exposure
         Doubling transmitter voltage quadruples the output intensity, increasing exposure dramatically.
   D. Receiver
      1. Amplification (overall gain)
         The process by which small voltages are increased to larger ones.
      2. Compensation (swept gain—TGC or DGC)
         Equalization of received echo amplitude differences caused by different attenuations for different reflector depths; also called swept gain, depth

gain compensation (DGC), or time gain compensation (TGC).
- a. Attenuation with range
  Attenuation is proportional to distance traveled.
- b. Effects on return signal and display
  Echoes from deeper structures are weaker because of greater attenuation due to longer travel distance.
- c. Dynamic frequency tuning
- d. Harmonic processing
3. Compression
Reduction in differences between small and large amplitudes.
- a. Dynamic range
  - (1) Definition
    Ratio (in decibels) of largest to smallest power that a system can handle; ratio of the largest to smallest intensity of echoes encountered.
  - (2) Dynamic range (receiver)
- a. Compare to other system components
  Display and human vision dynamic ranges are much less than that of the returning echoes.
- b. Numerical values (dB)
  Echo dynamic range can be as much as 170 dB. Displays have dynamic ranges up to 30 dB.
4. Demodulation
Conversion of voltage pulses from radio frequency to video form. Also called demodulation, amplitude detection, and envelope detection.
- a. Rectification
  Conversion from an alternating (reversing) to a direct (one-way) form of voltage.
- b. Smoothing (enveloping)
  Filtering out the higher frequency components of a rectified voltage to yield its amplitude.
5. Rejection
Elimination of small-amplitude voltages.

V. Principles of Pulse Echo Imaging (6%-10%) [Chapter 4]
- A. Principal Display Modes (A mode, B mode, 3-D, M mode)
  1. Definition of each mode
    A mode. A display presentation of echo amplitude versus depth (used in ophthalmology).
    B mode. Mode of operation in which the display presents a spot of appropriate brightness for each echo received by the transducer.
    B scan. B mode image that represents an anatomic cross section through the scanning plane.
    3D. Presentation on a two-dimensional display of a three-dimensional (3D) volume of echo information.
    M mode. A B mode presentation of changing reflector position (motion) versus time (used in echocardiography).
  2. Information displayed on each mode
    A mode. Echo amplitude versus depth.
    B mode. Echo amplitude in brightness on a two-dimensional cross-sectional display.
    3D. Echo amplitude in brightness on a two-dimensional display of three-dimensional echo information.
    M mode. Echo amplitude in brightness on depth versus time display.
  3. Advantages and disadvantages of each mode
    A mode. Quantitative amplitude information; not two-dimensional.
    B mode. Qualitative; two-dimensional.
    3D. Unlimited two-dimensional plane orientations; slower acquisition.
    M mode. Quantitative motion information; not two-dimensional.
- B. Principles of Real-Time, B-Mode Image Formation
  1. Relationship between echo amplitude and B-mode display
    Echo brightness increases with echo amplitude.
  2. Positioning of echoes
    Scan line on display tracks the path of the emitted pulse. Echo depth determined from arrival time using range equation.
  3. Harmonics
    Imaging echoes of second harmonic frequency improves image quality by eliminating artifacts and improving resolution.
- C. Scanning Speed Limitations
  1. Applications of range equation and relationship to pulsing characteristics
    Pulse repetition period is adjusted automatically to allow time for all echoes to return before next pulse is emitted. Thus all echoes have come from the last pulse, and their depths can be calculated using the range equation.
  2. Real-time systems-relationships between
    - a. Pulsing characteristics
    - b. Frame rate and time required to generate one frame
      Frame rate is proportional to the pulse repetition frequency and inversely proportional to the number of lines per frame.
      Time to generate one frame is the reciprocal of the frame rate.
    - c. Number of lines per frame
      Increasing lines per frame reduces frame rate.

d. Number of focal regions
Multiple foci require multiple pulses per scan line, thus reducing frame rate.

e. Field of view (e.g., sector angle)
Increasing sector angle increases the number of scan lines per frame and reduces frame rate.

f. Image depth (penetration)
Greater imaging depth requires a reduction in pulse repetition frequency and thus in frame rate.

3. Temporal resolution, ability to evaluate rapid motion
Temporal resolution depends on frame rate. Thus increasing imaging depth, lines per frame, or number of foci degrades temporal resolution.

VI. Images, Storage, and Display (10%-14%) [Chapter 4]

A. Role of Scan Converter

1. Image storage
The image memory stores echo information in the form of numbers that represent echo amplitudes.

2. Scan conversion
The scan converter reformats echo data into an image form for image processing, storage, and display. It takes serial scan line echo data and enters them into appropriate location in image memory corresponding to anatomic locations of echo-generation sites.

B. Digital Devices

1. Binary system
The binary numbering system uses only zeroes and ones to number values. Each column represents double the value of the column to its right.

a. Terminology (bits, bytes, pixels)
bit = binary digit
byte = 8 bits
pixel = picture element. The unit into which imaging information is divided for storage and display in a digital instrument. In image memory an image is divided into a rectangular matrix of pixels with an echo amplitude value stored in each pixel location.

b. Discrete nature of binary numbers

2. Steps in processing echo information

a. Analog-to-digital converter
A to D conversion is a function of the beam former. This is the process of digitizing the echo stream according to amplitudes.

b. Digital memory
Digital memory (image memory) is where the image is stored; that is, the echo information forming the anatomic gray-scale image to be displayed.

(1) Spatial resolution
Spatial (detail) resolution is determined by the length and width of the ultrasound pulse and the pixel density in image memory. From a practical standpoint, the latter is inconsequential because pixels are small compared with the size of the ultrasound pulse.
(a) Pixels
(b) Matrix
(c) Field of view

(2) Contrast resolution
Ability of a gray-scale display to distinguish between echoes of slightly different intensities.
(a) Size of memory
The number of layers of image memory (bits per pixel) determines the number of gray shades that can be stored in each pixel location. Each layer addition doubles the number of shades handled.

c. Digital-to-analog converter
Typically a few hundred thousand pixels are in an image. The individual amplitude numbers stored in image memory are not shown on the display because that approach to imaging would be nearly useless.

d. Display devices
The cathode-ray tube (CRT) for decades has been the classic display device in sonographic instruments. Recently, flat-panel displays were introduced for sonographic instruments. They are lighter in weight, less bulky, consume less power, and generate less heat compared with cathode-ray tubes.

C. Preprocessing vs. Postprocessing

1. Definition
Preprocessing. Signal and image processing accomplished before memory.
Postprocessing. Image processing done after memory.

2. Preprocessing functions

a. Time (depth) gain compensation
Time gain compensation (TGC) is the equalization of received echo amplitude differences caused by different attenuations for different reflector depths; also called depth gain compensation (DGC) or swept gain.

b. Logarithmic compression
The reduction in differences between small and large amplitudes to reduce dynamic range.

c. Write magnification
Magnifying a portion of an image by rescanning and reformatting the echo information

from the smaller portion into the entire image memory, thus assigning many more pixels to the original image portion.

3. Postprocessing function
   a. Freeze frame
   Constant display of one of the frames in memory.
   b. Black/white inversion
   Switching from white echo on black background to black echo on white background format.
   c. Read magnification
   Magnifying a portion of an image by simply enlarging its pixels to fill the full display size.
   d. Contrast variation
   Selecting different echo amplitude versus displayed brightness assignments for the purpose of improving the detection of subtle contrast differences.

4. Preprocessing or postprocessing functions (equipment manufacturers' discretion)
   a. Persistence
   Averaging sequential frames together.
   b. Frame averaging
   c. Edge enhancement
   A signal image processing function that improves the display of tissue boundaries.
   d. Smoothing
   e. Fill-in interpolation
   Filling in missing pixel information by inserting an average of surrounding pixel values.

D. Display devices
   1. TV monitors
   Cathode-ray tube displays that use the commercial television display format (525 horizontal lines and 30 frames per second).
   2. High resolution monitors
   Computer monitors that use various numbers (for example, 768) of horizontal lines (depending on the monitor standard used) and frame rates (commonly 60 frames per second) to display images. They can be cathode-ray tubes or flat-panel displays.
      a. Lines and spatial resolution
      Horizontal lines used in a display; for example, 480, 600, 768, 1024, or 1200.
      b. Brightness
      c. Contrast
      d. Frame rate
      Number of image frames displayed (i.e., read from image memory) per second; for example, 60 or 75. Also called refresh rate. This may or may not be the same as the frame rate written into memory.

E. Recording and Archiving Techniques
   1. Video format
   These recording and archiving approaches are being phased out in favor of digital approaches.
      a. Display (monitors)
      b. Single or multi-image cameras and laser imagers
         (1) Photographic film
         (2) Emulsion film
      c. Recorders
         (1) Fiber-optic
         (2) Videotape cassette
      d. Printer
         (1) Thermal
         (2) Laser
   2. Digital format
      a. Magneto-optical disc (digital still recorder)
      A drive and removable high-capacity disk that can store many images.
      b. PACS (picture archiving and communication systems)
      Picture archiving and communications systems provide means for electronically communicating images and associated information to work stations and devices external to the sonographic instrument, the examining room, and even the building in which the scanning is done.
   3. Contrast and brightness control adjustments
   Contrast and brightness are sources of variability in video devices requiring periodic adjustment.
   4. Advantages and limitations of each type
   Digital devices do not require the routine maintenance and adjustments that video devices do. Digital devices allow for image transfer to computers and communication with PACS. Video devices are being phased out in favor of digital devices and systems.

VII. Hemodynamic, Doppler, Color Flow, and Color Power Imaging (10%-14%) [Appendix I]
   A. Hemodynamics
      1. Energy gradient
      A gradient is an upslope or downslope over some horizontal distance. An energy gradient is the increase or decrease in energy over some distance divided by that distance.
      2. Effects of viscosity, friction, inertia
      Fluid viscosity causes flow resistance and energy loss. Viscosity is the friction of fluid layers (lamina) sliding over each other. Inertia causes cyclic flow to lag cyclic driving pressure.
      3. Pressure/flow relationships
      Poiseuille's equation describes the proportional relationship between pressure difference (ΔP)

and volumetric flow rate (Q); that is, $Q = \Delta P/R$, where R is flow resistance.

4. Velocity
   Flow velocity varies across a vessel. Mean velocity equals Q/A, where A is cross-sectional area of the vessel.

5. Steady flow vs. pulsatile flow
   Steady flow is constant. Pulsatile flow is time-varying and cyclic, driven by a cyclic pressure.

6. Laminar vs. turbulent flow
   Laminar (layer) flow is in parallel streamlines with increasing flow speeds toward the vessel center. Turbulent flow is random and chaotic.

7. Effects of stenosis on flow characteristics
   A stenosis (vessel narrowing) produces an increased flow speed at the stenosis and, usually, turbulent flow downstream. Q is constant proximal, at, and distal to the stenosis.

8. Venous resistance
   Resistance (R) is proportional to viscosity and vessel length and inversely proportional to vessel diameter to the fourth power.

9. Hydrostatic pressure
   Pressure caused by weight of a column of fluid.

10. Pressure/volume relationship
    Pressure and volume are inversely related, that is, increasing pressure produces decreasing volume. The ratio of pressure change to volume change is the bulk modulus of the fluid. Compressibility is the reciprocal of bulk modulus.

11. Effects of respiration (phasicity)
    Repiration-induced flow rate variations occur in some locations of the circulatory system.

B. Doppler Physical Principles
   1. Doppler effect
      A change in frequency caused by motion of a wave source, receiver, or reflector.
      a. Principle as related to sampling red blood cell movement
         A change in echo frequency caused by motion of reflectors (blood cells in the case of blood flow).
      b. Doppler equation

$$f_D \text{ (kHz)} = f_R \text{ (kHz)} - f_T \text{ (kHz)} = f_0 \text{ (kHz)} \times \left\{ \frac{[2 \times v \text{ (cm/s)}]}{c \text{ (cm/s)}} \right\}$$

   2. Factors influencing the magnitude of the Doppler shift frequency
      a. Range of the Doppler shift frequency
         100 Hz to 11 kHz for vascular studies.
      b. Effects of beam angle, transmitted frequency, flow velocity, and flow direction
         Increasing angle decreases Doppler shift. Increasing frequency or flow velocity increases Doppler shift.

Flow direction toward or away from the transducer produces a positive or negative Doppler shift, respectively.

C. Doppler Instruments
   1. Continuous wave and pulsed wave Doppler
      a. Differences
         Continuous wave is not pulsed, has no range resolution, and detects flow anywhere in the beam.
         Pulsed wave has a sample volume located at a depth down the beam determined by the time that the gate opens.
         The sample volume width is determined by the beam width. The sample volume length is determined by how long the gate is open.
      b. Advantages and disadvantages of each
         Continuous wave is good for searching; for example, the peak flow velocity in a jet from a stenotic valve (for determining the pressure drop across the stenotic valve).
         Pulsed wave is good for localizing to a specific chamber or vessel and to localize further within that chamber or vessel.
         (1) Aliasing (Nyquist criteria)
             With pulsed wave Doppler, if the Doppler shift exceeds half the pulse repetition frequency, aliasing occurs, yielding incorrect flow speed information.
         (2) Range ambiguity
             With pulsed wave Doppler, if the pulse repetition frequency is too high, there is more than one sample volume. Flow information could be from any of the sample volumes.
      c. Instrumentation
         (1) Receiver
             Amplifiers in the beam former.
         (2) Demodulator
             The Doppler-shift detector in the signal processor.
         (3) Wall filter for clutter rejection
             Low-frequency reject filter that eliminates the high-amplitude, low-frequency Doppler shifts caused by tissue motion (usually cardiac wall, cardiac valve, or vessel wall).
         (4) Directional devices
             Having the capability to detect and indicate flow direction using positive and negative Doppler shifts.
   2. Duplex instruments-definition and basic principles
      An ultrasound instrument that combines gray-scale sonography with pulsed Doppler and,

possibly, continuous wave Doppler. With pulsed wave Doppler the sample volume location within imaged anatomy is indicated on the display. With continuous wave Doppler the beam path is indicated on the anatomic display.

3. Spectral analysis

Separation of frequencies in a Doppler signal for display as a Doppler spectrum; the application of the Fourier transform to determine the frequency components present in a Doppler signal. The spectral display is the visual display of a Doppler spectrum in quantitative form. The vertical axis represents Doppler shift (usually converted to flow speed) with the baseline representing zero Doppler shift. The horizontal axis represents time.

a. Purpose
   (1) Direction
       Doppler shifts above and below the baseline are positive and negative, respectively; this assignment can be reversed by the instrument operator.
   (2) Velocity
       With proper angle incorporation, the Doppler equation is solved to present flow velocity in meters per second or centimeters per second on the vertical axis of the spectral display.
   (3) Duration
       The temporal length of the flow cycle (or any portion of it) can be measured on the horizontal axis of the spectral display.
   (4) Character
       Flow character (laminar, disturbed, turbulent) is correlated with spectral broadening of the spectral display.
   (5) Magnitude
       The maximum values of forward and reverse flow velocities.

b. Fast Fourier transform (FFT)
   Digital computer implementation of the Fourier transform, a mathematical technique for obtaining a Doppler frequency spectrum.

c. Diagnostic measurements (indices—i.e., pulsatility, resistive)
   Ratios of peak systolic and end-diastolic flow velocity values, related to proximal and distal flow conditions (impedance and resistance).

D. Color Flow Imaging
   1. Basic principles
      Color Doppler imaging is the extension of conventional gray-scale anatomic imaging to include presentation of Doppler-shifted echoes in color.

a. Sampling methods
b. Display of Doppler information
   (1) Reflector direction
       Different colors are assigned to positive and negative Doppler shifts.
   (2) Average velocity
       Different colors are assigned to mean Doppler-shift values.
   (3) Velocity variance
       Colors are assigned to indicate spread of Doppler shifts (variance) around the mean. Variance is the standard deviation squared.
c. Advantages and limitations
   Global two-dimensional view of flow along with anatomy. Not quantitative. Slower frame rates compared with gray-scale sonography.

2. Instrumentation
   a. Autocorrelation
      A rapid technique, used in most color Doppler instruments, for obtaining mean Doppler-shift frequency.
   b. Time domain processing
      A seldom-used technique for flow detection that uses echo-arrival time-shift detection rather than Doppler-shift detection.
   c. Color field size and frame rate
      (1) Ensemble length (packet size, pulse packet)
          Number of pulses used to generate one color Doppler image scan line. Increasing ensemble length reduces frame rate.
      (2) Line density
          Increasing the number of scan lines per frame decreases the frame rate.
      (3) Maximum depth
          Increasing image depth decreases frame rate.
   d. Color maps, assignment, or coding
      (1) Hue
          The color perceived based on the frequency of light.
      (2) Saturation
          The amount of hue present in a mix with white.
      (3) Luminance (significance, brightness, intensity)
          Brightness of a presented hue and saturation.
   e. Artifacts (see section VIII)

E. Color Power (Energy) Mode
   1. Displayed information
      Assigns colors to the amplitude (power, energy) of the Doppler-shifted echoes.

2. Advantages and limitations

More sensitive detection of Doppler shifts; that is, deep or slow flows or flow in tiny vessels. Presents only existence of flow (not direction, speed, or character of flow).

VIII. Artifacts (6%-10%) [Chapter 8]

A. Definition of Artifacts

An incorrect presentation of structure or motion.

B. Artifact Recognition in Performing and Interpreting Examinations

1. Echoes not representing actual interfaces
2. Missing echoes
3. Misrepresented interface location
4. Misrepresented interface amplitude

C. Artifacts Associated with Resolution and Propagation (Axial Resolution, Lateral Resolution, Section Thickness, Acoustic Speckle)

1. Definitions

Axial resolution is observed as axial smearing of tiny structures.

Lateral resolution is observed as lateral smearing of tiny structures.

Section thickness is observed as echoes from adjacent tissues filling in what should be anechoic regions.

Speckle is the granular appearance of images and spectral displays.

2. Mechanisms of Production

Axial, lateral, and section thickness resolutions are caused by the finite length and width of the ultrasound pulse.

Speckle is caused by the interference of echoes from the distribution of scatterers in tissue.

3. Appearance

D. Artifacts Associated with Propagation (Reverberation, Comet-Tail, Ring-Down, Mirror Image, Multipath, Side Lobes, Grating Lobes, Refraction, Speed Error, and Range Ambiguity)

1. Definitions

Reverberation. Multiple reflection.

Comet tail. A series of closely spaced reverberation echoes.

Ring-down artifact. An artifact resulting from a continuous stream of sound emanating from an anatomic site.

Mirror image. An artifactual gray-scale, color flow, or Doppler signal appearing on the opposite side (from the real structure or flow) of a strong reflector.

Multipath is the misplacement of an echo because it took a triangular path from the source to two reflectors and then returned to the source.

Side lobes. Weaker beams of sound traveling out from a single element in directions different from that of the primary beam.

Grating lobes. Additional weaker beams of sound traveling out in directions different from the primary beam as a result of the multielement structure of transducer arrays.

Refraction. Change of sound direction on passing from one medium to another.

Speed error. Propagation speed that is different from the assumed value (1.54 mm/μs).

Range ambiguity. An artifact produced when echoes are placed too close to the transducer because a second pulse was emitted before they were received.

2. Mechanisms of Production

Artifacts associated with propagation occur when the assumptions (the ultrasound pulse travels at the assumed speed directly to a reflector and directly back; the main beam of the transducer is the only beam) of pulse-echo imaging are violated.

3. Appearance

E. Artifacts Associated with Attenuation (Shadowing, Enhancement, and Focal Enhancement or Focal Banding)

1. Definitions

Shadowing. Reduction in echo amplitude from reflectors that lie behind a strongly reflecting or attenuating structure.

Enhancement. Increase in echo amplitude from reflectors that lie behind a weakly attenuating structure.

Focal enhancement or banding is a brightening of the region of an image caused by the increased intensity in the focal region of the beam.

2. Mechanisms of Production

See foregoing definitions.

3. Appearance

Shadowing is an abnormal darkening of echoes. Enhancement is an abnormal brightening of echoes.

F. Artifacts Associated with Doppler and Color Flow Instrumentation (Aliasing, Slice Thickness, Reverberation, Mirror Imaging, Ghosting or Flash, Registration, Incident Beam Angle, and Clutter)

1. Definitions

Aliasing. Improper Doppler-shift information from a pulsed Doppler or color Doppler instrument when the true Doppler shift exceeds one half the pulse repetition frequency.

Section (slice) thickness is observed as echoes from adjacent tissues filling in what should be anechoic regions.

Reverberation. Multiple reflection.

Mirror image. An artifactual gray-scale, color flow, or Doppler signal appearing on the opposite side (from the real structure or flow) of a strong reflector.

Ghosting is a term sometimes applied to reverberation duplication or to refraction doubling (split-image) artifacts.

Flash is a term sometimes applied to clutter (see the following definition).

Registration refers to proper relationship between Doppler-shifted and non–Doppler-shifted echoes in location on an image.

Incident beam angle: Maximum Doppler shift occurs with zero Doppler angle. Maximum echo strength occurs with a 90-degree angle of incidence for specular reflectors (like vessel intimal surface).

Clutter refers to Doppler-shifted echoes caused by tissue motion.

   2. Mechanisms of Production
Aliasing is caused by insufficient sampling of the Doppler shift.
See 1. for causes of other artifacts.

   3. Appearance
See 1.

G. Other (Electronic Noise, Equipment Malfunction)

   1. Definitions

   2. Mechanisms of production

   3. Appearance

H. Artifact Effects on Measurements (velocity or speed error and range ambiguity)

IX. Quality Assurance of Ultrasound Instruments (4%-8%) [Chapter 9]

A. General Concepts Regarding the Need for and Nature of a Quality Assurance Program
Several devices are available for determining whether sonographic and Doppler ultrasound instruments are operating correctly and consistently. These devices include those that test the operation of the instrument (anatomic imaging and flow evaluation performance) and those that measure the acoustic output of the instrument. The former take into account the operation of the entire instrument. The latter consider only the beam former and the transducer, acting together as a source of ultrasound. Imaging and Doppler performance are important for evaluating the instrument as a diagnostic tool. The acoustic output of an instrument is important when considering bioeffects and safety.

B. Methods for Evaluating Instrument Performance

   1. Test objects
Devices without tissuelike properties that are designed to measure some characteristic of an imaging system.

   2. Phantoms (tissue, Doppler, flow)
Tissue-equivalent devices that have characteristics that are representative of tissues (for example, scattering, propagation speed, and attenuation).

C. Parameters to Be Evaluated

   1. Test object

     a. Dead zone

     b. Axial resolution and lateral resolution (beam width)

     c. Depth calibration accuracy

     d. TGC characteristics

     e. Uniformity

     f. System sensitivity

   2. Tissue equivalent (mimicking) phantom

     a. Dead zone

     b. Depth calibration accuracy

     c. Lateral (horizontal) distance measurement accuracy

     d. Axial, lateral, and section thickness (elevational) resolution

     e. TGC characteristics

     f. System sensitivity

     g. Dynamic range

     h. Contrast resolution

     i. Lesion detection

   3. Doppler flow, string, or belt phantoms

     a. Maximum depth

     b. Pulsed Doppler sample volume alignment (gate position accuracy)

     c. Velocity accuracy

     d. Color flow penetration

     e. Image congruency test

D. Preventive Maintenance

   1. Standard precautions

     a. Equipment

       (1) Cleaning

       (2) Disinfecting

       (3) Sterilization

E. Record Keeping

F. Statistical Indices

   1. Sensitivity/specificity
Sensitivity equals the number of correct positive test results divided by the total number of positive test results.
Specificity equals the number of correct negative test results divided by the total number of negative test results.

   2. Negative/positive predictive value
Negative predictive value equals number of correct negative test results divided by total number of negative test results.
Positive predictive value equals number of correct positive test results divided by total number of positive test results.

   3. Accuracy
Accuracy is the number of correct test results divided by the total number of tests.

X. Bioeffects and Safety (6%-10%) *[Chapter 9]*
   A. Acoustic Output Quantities
      1. Pressure
         a. Units (MPa, mmHg)
         b. Peak pressures (compression, rarefaction)
         c. Methods of determining pressure (miniature hydrophone)
      2. Power
         a. Units (mW)
         b. Methods of determining power (radiation force, hydrophone)
      3. Intensity
         a. Units (mW/cm^2, W/cm^2)
         b. Spatial and temporal considerations
            The sound intensity is not uniform across a beam but usually is highest at the center and decreasing away from the center.
         c. Average and peak intensities
            Spatial and temporal
         d. Methods of determining intensity (hydrophones)
         e. Common intensities
            (1) SATA
               Spatial average, temporal average
            (2) SPTA
               Spatial peak, temporal average
            (3) SPPA
               Spatial peak, pulse average
            (4) SPTP
               Spatial peak, temporal peak
      4. Intensity and power values for different operating modes
         Generally lowest for gray-scale anatomic imaging, highest for pulsed Doppler, and intermediate for M mode and color Doppler.
   B. Acoustic Output Labeling Standard
      1. Thermal index
         a. TIS
            Thermal index for soft tissue
         b. TIB
            Thermal index for bone
         c. TIC
            Thermal index for cranium
      2. Mechanical index
         Mechanical index equals the peak rarefactional pressure amplitude divided by the square root of the operating frequency.
   C. Acoustic Exposure
      1. Definition and concepts of prudent use (ALARA)
         Minimize risk by minimizing exposure; that is, implement the ALARA (as low as reasonably achievable) principle.
      2. Methods of reducing acoustic exposure
         Expose only for medical benefit; minimize exposure time; minimize exposure amplitude or intensity.
   D. Primary Mechanisms of Biological Effect Production
      1. Cavitation mechanisms: relevant acoustic parameters
         Cavitation. Production and dynamics of bubbles in sound.
         Relevant parameters are pressure amplitude and frequency.
      2. Thermal mechanisms: relevant acoustic parameters
         Thermal mechanisms relate to tissue heating. Relevant parameters include power, intensity, frequency, and aperture.
   E. Experimental Biological Effect Studies
      The following are summarized by relevant American Institute of Ultrasound in Medicine statements:
      1. Animal studies
      2. In vitro studies
      3. Epidemiologic studies
         a. Limitations
   F. Guidelines and Regulations
      1. American Institute of Ultrasound in Medicine (AIUM) Statements (e.g., mammalian, epidemiology, in vitro)
      2. National Electrical Manufacturers Association (NEMA)
      3. Food and Drug Administration (FDA)
   G. Electrical and Mechanical Hazards
      1. Patient susceptibility to electrical hazard
      2. Equipment components which could present a hazard

SAMPLE QUESTIONS

Each numbered statement or question is followed by a minimum of four options. Select the ONE that is BEST.

1. If the relative output power of an ultrasound instrument is calibrated in decibels and the operator increases the output by 20 dB, the beam intensity is increased by
   A. five percent.
   B. two times.
   C. twenty times.
   D. one hundred times.
   E. one million times.
2. Assuming a fixed frequency, what happens if the diameter of an unfocused circular transducer is increased?
   A. The distance to the far field is reduced.
   B. The beamwidth in the near field is reduced.
   C. The beamwidth in the far field is reduced.

D. The ultrasonic wavelength is increased.

E. The sensitivity is reduced.

3. Which one of the following sets of properties of a test object or phantom is MOST relevant when assessing depth calibration accuracy?

A. Reflector spacing and reflector reflection coefficient

B. Attenuation in the medium and speed of sound in the medium

C. Reflector spacing and ultrasonic attenuation in the medium

D. Reflector reflection coefficient and ultrasonic attenuation in the medium

E. Reflector spacing and speed of sound in the medium

4. From a safety standpoint, which one of the following methods is BEST?

A. Low transmitter output and high receiver gain

B. High transmitter output and low receiver gain

C. High near gain and low far gain

D. Low near gain and high far gain

E. High reject and high transmitter output

5. Which one of the following instruments is a component that stores digital echo signal information?

A. Demodulator

B. Receiver

C. Video monitor

D. Logarithmic amplifier

E. Scan converter

6. The dynamic range of the receiver of an ultrasound instrument refers to the

A. ability of the receiver to track a rapidly moving structure.

B. range of echo signal frequencies that can be processed without distortion.

C. speed with which the receiver recovers following the excitation pulse to the transducer.

D. depth range in tissue over which moving echoes can be received.

E. range of echo signal amplitudes that can be processed without distortion.

7. Which one of the following statements is TRUE about a single pulse of ultrasound from a transducer?

A. It contains a range of frequencies.

B. It contains sound at the nominal frequency of the transducer only.

C. It contains sound at the center frequency of the transducer only.

D. The shorter the pulse the narrower the bandwidth.

E. Sound energy is continuously transmitted.

8. Increasing the gain of pulse echo instruments results in higher echoes displayed in the A mode. This is due to

A. increased amount of sound emitted by the transducer.

B. increased amount of sound reflected.

C. increased efficiency of transducer conversion of sound into electricity.

D. increased amplification in the receiver.

E. decreased amplification in the receiver.

9. A sound wave leaves its source and travels through air. The speed of sound in air is 330 m/sec. One second later, an echo returns to the source. At what distance from the source is the reflector that produced the echo?

A. 1540 meters

B. 770 meters

C. 660 meters

D. 330 meters

E. 165 meters

ANSWER KEY

1. D *Ten decibels is a factor of 10; 20 dB is a factor of 100.*

2. C *A higher frequency produces less beam spreading in the far field.*

3. E *For reflectors to be shown in proper position on a display, they must be in proper position in the test object and the propagation speed must be 1.54 mm/μs as assumed by the instrument.*

4. A *Transmitter output relates to risk and safety. Lower is better.*

5. E *The term* scan converter *sometimes is used loosely to indicate the image memory.*

6. E *This is the definition of dynamic range.*

7. A *This is called the bandwidth. It is broader for shorter pulses.*

8. D *Gain and amplification are equivalent terms.*

9. E *Distance traveled is speed times time. In this case, it is 330 m/s times 1 second, which equals 330 m. But the sound made a round trip so the distance to the reflector is 165 m.*

CARDIOVASCULAR PRINCIPLES AND INSTRUMENTATION PHYSICS CONTENT OUTLINE*

I. Anatomy of the Heart (Review) (4%-8%)

   A. Chambers and Related Septa

   B. Valves and Related Apparatus

   C. Arterial-Venous System

   D. Conduction System

   E. Layers

   F. Relational Anatomy

II. Basic Embryology (1%-3%)

   A. Primitive Heart Tube

      1. Formation from primitive vascular tube

      2. Sinus venosus

      3. Cardiac loop

      4. Aortic arches

      5. Septation

*Modified by ARDMS: 5/21/2003.

6. Valve formation
B. Comparison of Fetal and Postnatal Circulation
III. Congenital Defects (1%-3%)
A. Abnormalities of Septation
B. Abnormal Vasculature and Resulting Lesions
C. Persistence of Normal Fetal Communication
D. Valvular Anomalies
IV. Cardiac Physiology (5%-15%)
A. Electrophysiology and the Conduction System
1. Propagation of electrical activity
2. Excitation contraction coupling
B. Mechanical Considerations and Events
1. Frank Starling law (length-tension relationship)
2. Force-velocity relationship
3. Interval-strength relationship
4. Valve opening and closure
C. Phases of the Cardiac Cycle (Electromechanical Events)
1. Passive filling phase (ventricular diastole)
2. Atrial systole (p-wave on EKG; late diastole)
3. Isovolumic contraction
4. Ventricular ejection
5. Isovolumic relaxation
D. Left Ventricular Function: Indicators and Normal Values
1. Stroke volume
2. Ejection fraction
3. Cardiac output
E. Pulmonary vs. Systemic Circulation: Differences (e.g., Pressure, Oxygen Content, etc.) and Similarities (e.g., Volumes)
F. Intracardiac Pressures and Principles of Flow
1. Normal values
2. Changes during the cardiac cycle and relation to valve opening/closure
G. Maneuvers Altering Cardiac Physiology (e.g., Position)
H. Normal Heart Sound Generation and Timing
I. Cardiovascular Circulation
1. Normal metabolic needs and their variations
2. Component parts of the circulation
3. Control mechanisms
4. Coronary circulation
5. Properties of blood: composition
V. Cardiac Evaluation Methods (5%-15%)
A. Symptoms of Cardiac Diseases and Common Causes
B. Physical Examination and Signs
1. General physical appearance and patient history
2. Correlation of auscultatory findings
a. Normal heart sounds
b. Abnormal heart sounds and common causes

c. Murmurs, timing, location, intensity, character, grading
C. EKG
1. Basic principles and waveforms
2. Common abnormalities: basic pattern recognition
3. Exercise and pharmacologic stress testing: basic principles
D. Phonocardiography: Basic Principles and Waveforms
E. Cardiac Catheterization
1. Basic concepts of hemodynamic recordings
2. Determination of cardiac output
3. Oximetry
4. Coronary angiography
5. Evaluation and definition of gradients (e.g., peak-to-peak, mean, etc.)
6. Recognition of pressure wave forms in common disease states
F. Other Diagnostic Modalities—Correlation to Echocardiography
1. Chest x-ray
2. Nuclear cardiology
3. Phonocardiography
G. Relation of Cardiac Events as Recorded on ECG, Phonocardiogram, Pressure Tracings, etc.
H. Correlation and Integration of Information Obtained with Echocardiography and Various Methods of Cardiac Evaluation
I. Superimposed Respiratory Tracing
J. Knowledge of CPR Techniques
VI. Principles of Cardiac Hemodynamics (5%-15%)
[Chapter 5]
A. Blood Flow Dynamics
1. Factors affecting blood flow (e.g., viscosity, cell number, etc.)
Poiseuille's equation, the mathematical description of the dependence of volume flow rate, involves pressure difference, vessel length and radius, and fluid viscosity.
2. Laminar Flow: definition, characteristics, and types
Flow in which fluid layers slide over each other in a smooth, orderly manner, with no mixing between layers.
Parabolic flow is a specific type of laminar flow that has a flow profile in the shape of a parabola.
3. Disturbed flow: definition, characteristics (vortices, turbulence, etc.)
Disturbed flow is flow that cannot be described by straight, parallel streamlines.
Turbulent flow is random, chaotic, multidirectional flow of a fluid with mixing between layers. Turbulent flow is nonlaminar flow.

Turbulent flow involves vortices, regions of circular flow also called eddies.

  4. Relationships between pressure and velocity: Bernoulli principles and equations used
  The Bernoulli effect is a pressure reduction in a region of high-flow speed. The simplified Bernoulli equation for cardiac application is $\Delta P = 4(v_2)^2$.

  B. Effects of Abnormal Pressures and Loading, Volume Concepts
   1. Heart failure and shock
   2. Valvular stenosis
   3. Valvular regurgitation
   4. Shunts
   5. Pulmonary disease
   6. Pericardial disease
   7. Cardiomyopathies

VII. Elementary Principles (4%-8%) *[Chapter 2]*
  A. Nature of Ultrasound: Definitions, Propagation, Difference from Audible Sound
  Ultrasound is sound having a frequency greater than what human beings can hear; that is, greater than 20 kHz. Sound is a traveling pressure wave.

  B. Frequency, Wavelength, Propagation Speed: Definitions and relationships
  Frequency. Number of cycles per second.
  Wavelength. Length of space over which a cycle occurs.
  Propagation speed. Speed with which a wave moves through a medium.
  Wavelength equals propagation speed divided by frequency.

  C. Properties of Sound Waves (e.g., Amplitude, Pressure, etc.)
  Amplitude. Maximum variation of an acoustic variable.
  Acoustic variables. Pressure, density, and particle vibration; sound wave quantities that vary in space and time.

  D. Decibels: Definition, Relationships to Amplitude, and Intensity
  Decibel. Unit of power or intensity ratio; the number of decibels is 10 times the logarithm (to the base 10) of the power or intensity ratio. The number of decibels is 20 times the logarithm of the amplitude ratio.

  E. Physical Units
   1. Scientific notation
   Expressing a number as a value with digits after the decimal point times 10 to an exponent representing the power of 10.
   2. Engineering notation (e.g., micro vs. Mega)
   Engineering notation is scientific notation where only exponents that are integral multiples of 3 are used.

Micro-, milli-, centi-, deci-, kilo-, and mega- are metric system prefixes that indicate a factor of one millionth, one thousandth, one hundredth, ten, one thousand, and one million, respectively.
   3. Common units
   Meter (m) for length
   Second (s) for time
   Hertz (Hz) for frequency

VIII. Propagation of Ultrasound Through Tissues (4%-8%) *[Chapter 2]*
  A. Speed of Sound
   1. Average speed of sound in tissue
   1.54 mm/μs or 1540 m/s
   2. Range of propagation speeds in the body
   1.44 to 5.0 mm/μs
   3. Speeds in specific tissues (e.g., muscle, bone, fat)
   Typical values (mm/μs):
   Muscle, 1.57
   Bone, 4.0
   Fat, 1.44

  B. Principles Related to Reflection
   1. Characteristic acoustic impedance: definition
   Density times propagation speed.
   2. Reflection and transmission at specular interfaces
   Specular is from Latin meaning "mirrorlike"; that is, a flat, smooth surface.
   Reflection (echo) amplitude depends on impedance difference at the boundary.
   The incident intensity minus the reflected intensity equals the transmitted (into the second medium) intensity.
   3. Scattering
   Diffusion or redirection of sound in several directions upon encountering a particle suspension or a rough surface.

  C. Principles Related to Refraction
  Change of sound direction on passing from one medium to another.

  D. Principles Related to Attenuation
  Attenuation. Decrease in amplitude and intensity with distance as a wave travels through a medium. Attenuation increases with increasing frequency.

  E. Useful Diagnostic Frequency Range
  2 to 15 MHz

IX. Ultrasound Transducers (5%-10%) *[Chapter 3]*
  A. The Piezoelectric Effect
  Piezoelectricity: Conversion of pressure to electric voltage.

  B. Transducer Construction and Characteristics
  The transducer is composed of many piezoelectric elements (crystals) sandwiched between a damping layer behind and matching layers in front.

C. Sound Beam Formation: Near and Far Fields (Fresnel and Fraunhofer zones)
   The near field (Fresnel zone) is the region of the beam from the transducer surface to the focus. The far field (Fraunhofer zone) is the region beyond the focus.
D. Focusing
   1. Methods of focusing and steering
      Focusing is accomplished with lenses and with electronic phasing of the driving voltages.
   2. Focal zone characteristics
      Larger apertures and higher frequencies allow tighter (narrower) focusing.
E. Beam Width and Lateral Resolution
   Lateral resolution is equal to beam width (narrower is better).
F. Pulse Duration and Axial Resolution
   Axial resolution is equal to half the spatial pulse length (shorter is better).
G. Transducer Types
   1. Multiple elements and their arrangements
      Rectangular elements are lined up in a row like a piano keyboard.
      Two-dimensional arrays have several rows of elements.
   2. Mechanical sector scanners
      Mechanically steer the transducer sector format with electric motor.
   3. Single crystals
      Disk shaped commonly used for continuous wave Doppler.
   4. Rationale for selection (frequency, focal characteristics, etc.)
      Lower frequencies and deeper focus for deep applications (adult cardiac, abdominal, pelvic, obstetric).
      Higher frequencies and shallow focus for superficial applications (breast, thyroid, carotid artery).

X. Pulse Echo Instruments (3%-7%)
   [Chapter 4]
   A. Output Power Control
      Controls output amplitude, intensity, power.
   B. Receiver Overall Gain
      Controls the amplification of echo voltages in the beam former.
   C. Receiver Swept Gain (TGC)
      Compensates for attenuation by automatically increasing gain with echo arrival time.
   D. Reject
      Eliminates weaker voltages.
   E. Dynamic range
      Ratio (in decibels) of largest to smallest power that a system can handle; ratio of the largest to smallest intensity of echoes encountered.

F. Compression
   Reduction in differences between small and large amplitudes.
   [There is no G. in the outline.]
H. Magnification (or zoom)
I. Focal zone(s)
   Controls the number of transmission foci and therefore the effective length of the focus.
J. Filters
   Eliminate part of the frequency spectrum; for example, to reduce electronic and acoustic noise or to eliminate fundamental frequency echoes in harmonic imaging.

XI. Principles of Pulse Echo Imaging (5%-10%)
   [Chapter 4]
   A. Principal Display Modes (A-mode, B-mode)
      A mode diplays echo amplitude versus depth.
   B. Principles of B-mode Image Formation
      B mode image is a two-dimensional echo presentation with brightness corresponding to echo strength.
   C. Identification of Major Types of Imaging Equipment
      Two-dimensional and three-dimensional gray-scale, continuous wave and pulsed wave spectral Doppler, and color and power Doppler.
   D. Scanning Speed Limitations
      1. Applications of range equation and relationship to pulsing characteristics
         Echo arrival time is proportional to reflector depth. Pulse repetition frequency must slow down for deeper imaging to allow greater time for echo reception.
      2. Pulsing characteristics (e.g., PRF)
         Pulse repetition frequency is the number of pulses per second; sometimes called pulse repetition rate.
      3. Frame rate and time needed to generate one frame
         Frame rate is the number of images displayed per second. The inverse of the frame rate is the time needed to generate one frame, which is equal to the pulse repetition period times the number of scan lines per frame times the number of foci in use.
      4. Number of lines per frame
         The number of scan lines included in each frame (image).
      5. Field of view (e.g., sector angle)
         Field of view is the depth and width (angular width for sector image) of the imaging area.
      6. Depth to be imaged
         Increasing depth lowers frame rate.

XII. Images, Storage, and Display (1%-5%) [Chapter 4]
   A. General Role and Use of Scan Converters and Digital Memories
      The scan converter reformats echo data into an image form for image processing, storage, and display. It

takes serial scan-line echo data and enters them into appropriate locations in image memory corresponding to anatomic locations of echo-generation sites. *Digital memory is the image memory that stores echoes according to their amplitudes.*

B. Basic Concepts of Digital Systems
Digital signal and image processing is accomplished with mathematical manipulation of numbers that represent echo amplitudes.

C. Image Storage, Resolution, and Field of View

D. Display Devices and Controls

E. Postprocessing
Postprocessing. Image processing done after memory.

F. Recording Techniques (e.g., Videotape, Stripchart, etc.)

G. Display Contrast and Brightness

XIII. Doppler (10%-20%) [Appendix I]

A. Basic Principles

1. Doppler effect: principle as related to sampling red blood cell movement
Doppler effect. A change in frequency caused by motion of a wave source, receiver, or reflector.

2. Scattering (from red blood cells)

a. Frequency dependence
Echo intensity proportional to frequency⁴ for particles small compared with wavelength (the condition for Rayleigh scattering).

b. Strength of emitted signal vs. returned signal
Because erythrocytes are so small compared with wavelength, their echoes are very weak compared with those from tissue, for example, cardiac wall.

3. Doppler equation

a. Range of Doppler shift frequencies—audible
Up to 30 kHz for cardiac studies.

b. Factors influencing magnitude of Doppler shift and special relationships
Doppler equation:

$$f_D \text{ (kHz)} = f_R \text{ (kHz)} - f_T \text{ (kHz)} = f_0 \text{ (kHz)} \times \left\{ \frac{[2 \times v \text{ (cm/s)} \times \cos(\theta_D)]}{c \text{ (cm/s)}} \right\}$$

(1) Transducer frequency
f_D *is proportional to frequency.*

(2) Angle of beam incidence
f_D *is proportional to cosine Doppler angle.*

(3) Flow velocity
f_D *is proportional to flow velocity.*

B. Spectral Analysis

1. Fast Fourier Transform (FFT)
Digital computer implementation of the Fourier transform, a mathematical technique for obtaining a Doppler frequency spectrum.

2. Spectral display (visual and audio)

a. Axis identification (e.g., frequency and time)
The spectral display is the visual display of a Doppler spectrum in quantitative form. The vertical axis represents Doppler shift (usually converted to flow speed) with the baseline representing zero Doppler shift. The horizontal axis represents time.

b. Assignment of gray shades represented on the spectrum
Gray level represents the strength of each Doppler shift present at each point in time.

c. Components of the spectrum
High frequencies represent fast flows or slower flows at small Doppler angles. Low frequencies represent slow flows or faster flows at large angles.

d. Effect of wall filtering and gains
Overgaining artificially broadens the spectrum. Overly high wall-filter settings artificially remove legitimate lower-frequency Doppler shifts.

3. Spectral broadening

a. Influence of sample volume size
Larger sample volumes broaden the spectrum by including more of the flow profile.

b. Flow disturbances
Spectral broadening occurs in the progression from laminar to disturbed to turbulent flow.

4. Spectral artifacts (aliasing, mirroring, etc.)
Aliasing. Improper Doppler-shift information from a pulsed Doppler or color Doppler instrument when the true Doppler shift exceeds one half the pulse repetition frequency.
Mirroring. An artifactual gray-scale, color flow, or Doppler signal appearing on the opposite side (from the real structure or flow) of a strong reflector.
Clutter refers to Doppler shifted echoes caused by tissue motion.

C. Continuous Wave Doppler

1. Transducer configurations
Separate transmitting and receiving elements in transducer assembly.

2. Lack of range resolution (range ambiguity)
Detects flow anywhere in the overlapping region of the transmitting and receiving beams.

3. High velocity measurement capability
Not limited by aliasing.

D. Pulsed Doppler

1. Transducers
Same element(s) used for transmitting and receiving.

2. Range discrimination
   a. Sample volume(s)
      Pulsed Doppler has a sample volume located at a depth down the beam determined by the time that the gate opens.
      The sample volume width is determined by the beam width. The sample volume length is determined by how long the gate is open.
   b. Resolution compared to imaging resolution
      Axial resolution not as good is for imaging because longer pulses are used and the gate length adds to the resolution.
3. Aliasing
   a. Pulse repetition frequency
      Higher pulse repetition frequency avoids aliasing.
   b. Nyquist frequency limit
      Aliasing occurs when Doppler shift exceeds the Nyquist limit, which is half the pulse repetition frequency.
   c. Maximum depth
      Determined by pulse repetition frequency (lower pulse repetition frequency permits deeper sample volume locations without range ambiguity).
   d. Baseline position
      Baseline shift can be used to eliminate aliasing. In extreme cases, increased pulse repetition frequency and baseline shift may be necessary.
E. Color Flow Imaging
   1. Sampling methods
   2. Fundamental variables
      a. Packet size
         Also called ensemble length: number of pulses used to generate one color Doppler image scan line.
      b. Line density
         Number of scan lines per color frame.
      c. Maximum depth
      d. Frame rate
         Increasing any of the foregoing (a, b, c) decreases frame rate.
      e. Echo vs. color threshold
         The echo strength level (operator adjustable on some instruments) at which the instrument chooses to play a gray-scale or color-coded, Doppler-shifted echo at each pixel location.
   3. Evaluation of frequency content
      a. Methods of separating frequencies (e.g., autocorrelation algorithm)
         (1) Mean frequency
             The average of the frequencies present in the Doppler spectrum.

(2) Variance
    The spread of the spectrum around the mean (square of the standard deviation).
4. Color maps
   Assignment rules for encoding Doppler shifts in various colors on the display (operator selectable).
5. Artifacts (aliasing, ghosting, reverberation, dropout)
   Aliasing. Improper Doppler-shift information from a pulsed Doppler or color Doppler instrument when the true Doppler shift exceeds one half the pulse repetition frequency.
   Ghosting is a term sometimes applied to reverberation duplication or to refraction doubling (split-image) artifacts.
   Reverberation. Multiple reflection.
6. Limitations
   Not quantitative; slower frame rates compared with gray-scale sonography.
F. Roles and Limitations of Each Doppler Modality
   Spectral Doppler is localized to the sample volume; it is quantitative.
   Color Doppler is a global two-dimensional view of flow along with anatomy. Color Doppler is qualitative and has slower frame rates compared with gray-scale sonography.
XIV. Image Features and Artifacts (1%-5%) [Chapter 8]
   A. Artifacts: Definition, Role of Recognition in Performing & Interpreting Exams, Understanding Mechanism, and Appearance
      Artifact. An incorrect presentation of structure or motion.
      Artifacts can lead to improper identification and interpretation. They must be recognized and properly handled when encountered.
   B. Reverberation, Refraction, and Other Artifacts (e.g., Beam Width, Electronic Noise)
      Reverberation. Multiple reflection.
      Comet tail. A series of closely spaced reverberation echoes.
      Ring-down artifact. An artifact resulting from a continuous stream of sound emanating from an anatomic site.
      Mirror image. An artifactual gray-scale, color flow, or Doppler signal appearing on the opposite side (from the real structure or flow) of a strong reflector.
      Multipath is the misplacement of an echo because it took a triangular path from the source to two reflectors and then returned to the source.
      Side lobes. Weaker beams of sound traveling out from a single element in directions different from that of the primary beam.

Grating lobes. Additional weaker beams of sound traveling out in directions different from the primary beam as a result of the multielement structure of transducer arrays.

Refraction. Change of sound direction on passing from one medium to another.

Speed error. Propagation speed that is different from the assumed value (1.54 mm/μs).

Range ambiguity. An artifact produced when echoes are placed too close to the transducer because a second pulse was emitted before they were received.

C. Shadowing and Enhancement

Shadowing. Reduction in echo amplitude from reflectors that lie behind a strongly reflecting or attenuating structure.

Enhancement. Increase in echo amplitude from reflectors that lie behind a weakly attenuating structure.

D. Measurements of Dimensions from Images (e.g., area)

E. Artifacts Affecting Measurement

Refraction and speed error (propagation speed that is different from the assumed value [1.54 mm/μs]).

XV. Quality Assurance of Ultrasound Instruments (1%-3%) [Chapter 9]

A. General Concepts Regarding the Need and Nature of a Quality Assurance Program

Several devices are available for determining whether sonographic and Doppler ultrasound instruments are operating correctly and consistently. These devices include those that test the operation of the instrument (anatomic imaging and flow evaluation performance) and those that measure the acoustic output of the instrument. The former take into account the operation of the entire instrument. The latter consider only the beam former and the transducer, acting together as a source of ultrasound. Imaging and Doppler performance are important for evaluating the instrument as a diagnostic tool. The acoustic output of an instrument is important when considering bioeffects and safety.

B. Quality Assurance Evaluation Parameters and Methods

Parameters:

1. *Test object*
   a. *Dead zone*
   b. *Axial resolution and lateral resolution (beam width)*
   c. *Depth calibration accuracy*
   d. *Time gain compensation characteristics*
   e. *Uniformity*
   f. *System sensitivity*
2. *Tissue equivalent (mimicking) phantom*
   a. *Dead zone*
   b. *Depth calibration accuracy*

c. *Lateral (horizontal) distance measurement accuracy*
d. *Axial, lateral, and section thickness (elevational) resolution*
e. *Time gain compensation characteristics*
f. *System sensitivity*
g. *Dynamic range*
h. *Contrast resolution*
i. *Lesion detection*

3. *Doppler flow, string, or belt phantoms*
   a. *Maximum depth*
   b. *Pulsed Doppler sample volume alignment (gate position accuracy)*
   c. *Velocity accuracy*
   d. *Color flow penetration*
   e. *Image congruency test*

Methods:

Test objects

Devices without tissuelike properties that are designed to measure some characteristic of an imaging system.

Phantoms (tissue, Doppler, flow)

Tissue-equivalent devices that have characteristics that are representative of tissues (e.g., scattering, propagation speed, and attenuation).

C. Preventive Maintenance
1. Cleaning
2. Disinfecting
3. Sterilization

D. Record Keeping

XVI. Bioeffects and Safety (2%-6%) [Chapter 9]

A. Dosimetric Quantities (Units and Definitions)

1. Relationship between pressure, intensity, power, and area

Intensity is power divided by beam area. Intensity is proportional to (pressure amplitude)^2.

2. Typical values for diagnostic equipment used in echocardiography in all modes of operation

1 to 25 mW/cm^2 I_{SPTA} for B mode
25 to 200 mW/cm^2 I_{SPTA} for M mode and color Doppler
0.5 to 2.0 W/cm^2 I_{SPTA} for pulsed wave Doppler mode

B. Acoustic Exposure

1. Definition

Intensity and time.

2. Factors affecting and methods of reducing acoustic exposure

Minimize risk by minimizing exposure (intensity and time); that is, implement the ALARA (as low as reasonably achievable) principle.

3. Primary mechanisms of biological effect production

Thermal (heating by absorption) and nonthermal (mechanical), primarily cavitation.

C. American Institute of Ultrasound in Medicine Statements
See Chapter 9.
D. Electrical and Mechanical Hazards

SAMPLE QUESTIONS

Each numbered statement or question is followed by a minimum of four options. Select the ONE that is BEST.

1. In a patient with a grade IV/VI systolic crescendo-decrescendo murmur, the MOST likely pathology is
   A. mitral stenosis.
   B. mitral regurgitation.
   C. aortic stenosis.
   D. aortic regurgitation.
   E. tricuspid regurgitation.

2. When ultrasound waves travel through a medium that contains many small scatterers (e.g. red blood cells), the amount of sound that is scattered would
   A. increase sharply with increasing frequency.
   B. increase sharply with increasing wavelength.
   C. be independent of frequency.
   D. decrease with increasing beam area.
   E. decrease sharply with increasing frequency.

3. With phased array transducers, the transmitted sound beam is swept by
   A. mechanically oscillating the transducer elements.
   B. mechanically rotating the transducer elements.
   C. varying the timing of pulses to the transducer elements.
   D. varying the voltage of pulses to the transducer elements.
   E. varying the resonant frequency of the transducer elements.

4. In a normal individual, during isovolumetric contraction, the
   A. aortic valve opens allowing blood to be ejected from the left ventricle.
   B. mitral valve is open allowing blood flow into the left ventricle.
   C. pressure in the left ventricle increases; no valves are open.
   D. pressure in the left ventricle decreases; no valves are open.
   E. pressure in the left ventricle is the same as it is in end diastole; no valves are open.

5. Myocardial blood flow is most predominant during which phase of the cardiac cycle?
   A. Isovolumic relaxation phase
   B. Systole
   C. Isovolumic contraction
   D. Diastole

6. Myocardial blood flow in the normal heart returns to the right atrium via the
   A. pulmonary veins.
   B. azygos veins.
   C. superior vena cava.
   D. coronary sinus.

ANSWER KEY

1. C
2. A *This is called Rayleigh scattering. Echo intensity is proportional to scatterer size to the fourth power.*
3. C *Short time delays in voltage application from element to element, which is called phasing.*
4. C
5. D
6. D

VASCULAR PHYSICAL PRINCIPLES AND INSTRUMENTATION CONTENT OUTLINE*

I. Ultrasound Physics (35%-45%)
   A. Definition of Sound (6%-10%) *[Chapter 2]*
      1. Sound vs. ultrasound
         Ultrasound is sound having a frequency greater than what humans can hear; that is, greater than 20 kHz. Sound is a traveling pressure wave.
      2. Propagation velocity
         Speed with which a wave moves through a medium.
      3. Frequency
         Number of cycles per second.
      4. Wavelength
         Number of cycles per second.
      5. Frequency vs. depth
         Imaging depth (penetration) decreases with increasing frequency because of increasing attenuation.
      6. Frequency ranges
         2 to 15 MHz
   B. Propagation of Sound in Tissue (6%-10%) *[Chapter 2]*
      1. Speed of sound through tissue: air, bone, soft tissue
         Air, 0.33 mm/μs
         Bone, 3.0 to 4.0 mm/μs
         Soft tissue average, 1.54 mm/μs (1540 m/s)
      2. Speed of sound through blood
         1.57 mm/μs
      3. Acoustic impedance
         Density times propagation speed.
      4. Reflection
         Portion of sound returned from a media boundary; echo.
      5. Refraction
         Change of sound direction on passing from one medium to another.
      6. Absorption
         Conversion of sound to heat.

*Modified by ARDMS: 4/29/2003.

7. Attenuation
   Decrease in amplitude and intensity with distance as a wave travels through a medium.

C. Transducers: Ultrasound (6%-10%) [Chapter 3]
   1. Piezoelectric effect
      Piezoelectricity. Conversion of pressure to electric voltage.
   2. Transducer characteristics
      The transducer is composed of many piezoelectric elements (crystals) sandwiched between a damping layer behind and matching layers in front.
   3. Sound beam characteristics
      a. Effect of beam diameter on resolution
         Lateral resolution equals beam diameter. Smaller is better.
      b. Effect of transducer frequency on beam characteristics
         Increasing frequency shortens the pulse (improving axial resolution) and focuses the beam more tightly (improving lateral resolution).
      c. Beam focusing
         Focusing improves lateral resolution by narrowing the beam.
      d. Near field
         The region of a sound beam in which the beam diameter decreases as the distance from the transducer increases; also called near zone.
      e. Far field
         The region of a sound beam in which the beam diameter increases as the distance from the transducer increases; also called far zone.
   4. Lateral resolution
      Minimum reflector separation perpendicular to the sound path that is required to produce separate echoes.
   5. Axial resolution
      The minimum reflector separation along the sound path that is required to produce separate echoes (that is, to distinguish between two reflectors).
   6. Mechanical transducers
      Beam scanning by moving element(s) with a motor drive.
   7. Electronic transducers
      Beam scanning and focusing accomplished with electronic sequencing and phasing.

D. Doppler Signal Processing (6%-10%) [Chapters 5 to 7]
   1. Doppler effect
      A change in frequency caused by motion of a wave source, receiver, or reflector.
   2. Doppler frequency shift
      Reflected frequency minus incident frequency; a change in frequency that occurs as a result of motion.

3. Effect of transmitting frequency on Doppler frequency shift
   f_D is proportional to frequency.
4. Effect of insonation angle on Doppler frequency shift
   f_D is proportional to cosine of Doppler angle.
5. Reflector speed (velocity)
   f_D is proportional to flow velocity.
6. Extracting the Doppler signal
   Accomplished with autocorrelation in color Doppler and with phase-quadrature detection in spectral Doppler.
7. Audible Doppler signal analysis
   Doppler shifts are sent to loudspeakers for audible analysis.
8. Analog Doppler waveform generation
   Accomplished with zero-crossing detector, an analog detector that yields mean Doppler shift as a function of time.
9. Spectral display characteristics
   The spectral display is the visual display of a Doppler spectrum in quantitative form. The vertical axis represents Doppler shift (usually converted to flow speed) with the baseline representing zero Doppler shift. The horizontal axis represents time.
10. Sample volume size
    The sample volume width is determined by the beam width. The sample volume length is determined by how long the gate is open.
11. Aliasing
    Improper Doppler-shift information from a pulsed Doppler or color Doppler instrument when the true Doppler shift exceeds one half the pulse repetition frequency.

E. Doppler Instruments (6%-10%) [Chapters 6 and 7]
   1. Continuous wave instruments
      Uses a continuous beam; good for searching (for example, a flow jet); detects flow anywhere in the overlapping transmission and reception beams.
   2. Pulsed wave instruments
      Uses pulsed ultrasound and has a sample volume that localizes the received Doppler shifts from a specific depth along the beam.
   3. Bidirectional Doppler
      Detects and presents flow direction by differentiating positive and negative Doppler shifts.
   4. Unidirectional Doppler
      Does not differentiate between positive and negative Doppler shifts.
   5. Color flow
      An instrument that detects Doppler shifts and presents a two-dimensional, real-time Doppler

shift display superimposed on a real-time, gray-scale, anatomic, cross-sectional image. Flow directions toward and away from the transducer (i.e., positive and negative Doppler) are presented as different colors on the display.

    6. Transcranial
       Detection and presentation of intracranial blood flow information.

II.   Ultrasonic Imaging (15%-25%)
    A. Imaging Principles (10%-14%) [Chapter 4]
       1. A-mode: definition
         A display presentation of echo amplitude versus depth (used in ophthalmology).
       2. B-mode: definition
         Mode of operation in which the display presents a spot of appropriate brightness for each echo received by the transducer.
       3. Real-time: definition
         Imaging with a rapid frame sequence display.
       4. Gray scale display
         Display of echo amplitudes as a range of brightnesses between white and black.
       5. Dynamic range
         Ratio (in decibels) of largest to smallest power that a system can handle; ratio of the largest to smallest intensity of echoes encountered.
       6. Frame rate
         Number of frames of echo information stored and displayed each second.
       7. Scan converter
         An electronic device that reformats echo data into an image form for image processing, storage, and display.
       8. Gain
         Ratio (in decibels) of amplifier output to input electric power.
       9. Time gain compensation
         Equalization of echo amplitude differences caused by different attenuations for different reflector depths; also called TGC and depth gain compensation (DGC).
      10. Recording techniques
        a. Multi-imaging camera
        b. Video tape
        c. Thermal video printer
        d. Digital storage
      11. Duplex instrumentation
        An ultrasound instrument that combines gray-scale sonography with pulsed Doppler and, possibly, continuous wave Doppler.
      12. Image resolution
        Detail resolution. The ability to image fine detail and to distinguish closely spaced reflectors; has axial and lateral aspects.

Contrast resolution. Ability of a gray-scale display to distinguish between echoes of slightly different intensities; depends on number of gray shades.
Temporal resolution. Ability to distinguish closely spaced events in time; improves with increased frame rate.

    B. Imaging Artifacts (6%-10%) [Chapter 8]
       1. Artifact: definition
         In imaging, an artifact is anything that is not properly indicative of the structures or motion imaged. Artifact is caused by some problematic aspect of the imaging technique.
       2. Origin of artifacts: technique
         Resulting from improper settings or procedure; for example, improper gain or time gain compensation or inadequate coupling gel.
       3. Origin of artifacts: instrumentation
         Resulting from violation of one or more of the assumptions in pulse-echo imaging.
       4. Enhancement
         Increase in echo amplitude from reflectors that lie behind a weakly attenuating structure.
       5. Multiple reflections
         Several reflections produced by a pulse encountering a pair of reflectors; reverberation.
       6. Reverberation
         See 5.
       7. Shadowing
         Reduction in echo amplitude from reflectors that lie behind a strongly reflecting or attenuating structure.
       8. Refraction
         Change of sound direction on passing from one medium to another.

III. Physiology & Fluid Dynamic (10%-20%) [Chapter 5]
    A. Arterial Hemodynamics (7%-11%)
       1. Energy gradient
         The reduction in pressure and/or flow energy resulting from viscous loss (conversion to heat).
       2. Effects of viscosity, friction, inertia
         Viscosity is the resistance of a fluid to flow. Viscosity is caused by friction between fluid layers flowing at different speeds.
         Inertia is resistance to acceleration or deceleration. For pulsatile flow, inertia causes cyclic pressure and flow velocity to be out of phase with each other.
       3. Pressure/flow relationships
        a. Poiseuille's law
          The relationship between volume flow rate and flow resistance:

$$Q \text{ (mL/s)} = \frac{\Delta P \text{ (dyne/cm}^2) \times \pi \times d^4 \text{ (cm}^4)}{128 \times L \text{ (cm)} \times \eta \text{ (poise)}}$$

b. Bernoulli's principle
The Bernoulli effect is a pressure reduction in a region of high-flow speed. The simplified Bernoulli equation for cardiac application is $\Delta P = 4\ (v_2)^2$.

4. Velocity
The speeds and directions with which various parts of a fluid are flowing.

5. Steady flow vs. pulsatile flow
Steady flow is temporally constant, whereas pulsatile flow varies with time because the driving pressure difference also varies.

6. Effects of stenosis on flow characteristics
   a. Direction, turbulence, disturbed flow
   The progression as lumen is reduced is from laminar to disturbed to turbulent flow.
   b. Velocity acceleration
   Fluid must accelerate to a higher speed as it enters a stenosis.
   c. Entrance/exit effects
   Acceleration and deceleration, respectively. Flow separation from walls and generation of eddies.
   d. Diameter reduction
   A stenosis, by definition, is a lumen reduction.
   e. Peripheral resistance
   f. Collateral effects
   g. Effects of exercise
   Reduction in distal resistance as arterioles dilate.
   h. Occlusion
   Zero lumen diameter; no flow.

B. Venous Hemodynamics (4%-8%)
1. Venous resistance
2. Hydrostatic pressure
3. Pressure/volume relationship
4. Effects of edema
5. Effects of muscle pump mechanism
   a. At rest
   b. Contraction
   c. Relaxation

C. Other (0%-3%)
1. Arteriovenous fistula (traumatic, congenital, access dialysis)
2. Trauma (pseudoaneurysm)

IV. Physical Principles (15%-25%)
A. General (3%-7%)
1. Energy
Ability to do work.
2. Power
Energy per second (1) converted from one form to another or (2) passing a location.
3. Graphical recording
4. Calibration

5. AC/DC coupling
6. Units of measure

B. Tissue Mechanics/Pressure Transmission (1%-5%)
1. Venous occlusion by limb positioning
2. Superficial venous occlusion by tourniquets
3. Volume changes by blood inflow/outflow
4. Arterial occlusion by cuffs

C. Plethysmography (1%-5%)
1. Displacement (pneumatic cuff)
2. Photoplethysmography
3. Oculoplethysmography-pressure

D. Pressure Measurements (6%-10%)
1. Legs
2. Arms

E. Other (0%-3%)
1. Skin temperature
2. Transcutaneous oximetry

V. Ultrasound Safety & Quality Assurance (3%-7%)
[Chapter 9]
A. Instrument Performance (2%-6%)
1. Evaluation of image quality
Test objects and tissue-equivalent phantoms are used to evaluate various aspects of image quality.
2. Evaluation of Doppler quality
String test objects and flow phantoms are used to evaluate Doppler performance.
3. Preventive maintenance

B. Biological Effects (0%-3%)
1. Minimizing exposure time
Implement the ALARA principle by minimizing exposure time and instrument output (thermal index or mechanical index).
2. Mechanisms of production
Thermal (temperature rise caused by absorption) and nonthermal (mechanical, primarily cavitation).
3. Scientific data
See American Institute of Ultrasound in Medicine statements in Chapter 9.
4. Preventing electrical hazards

SAMPLE QUESTIONS

Each numbered statement or question is followed by a minimum of four options. Select the ONE that is BEST.

1. Which one of the following factors does NOT affect the frequency of the Doppler shift?
   A. Size of the Doppler probe
   B. Angle with which the probe is pointed at the vessel
   C. Velocity of the blood in the vessel
   D. Speed of ultrasound in tissue
   E. Transmitting frequency of the Doppler

2. A blood pressure cuff (wider than the thigh) is applied above the knee. A Doppler probe is then

applied over the posterior tibial artery at the ankle. The cuff is inflated above the systolic pressure and slowly deflated. What does the pressure in the cuff represent at the time that the first pulse is detected by the Doppler?
   A. Systolic pressure at the ankle
   B. Mean pressure at the ankle
   C. Diastolic pressure in the popliteal artery
   D. Systolic pressure in the artery(ies) underlying the cuff
   E. Systolic pressure of the common femoral artery above the cuff
3. Lateral resolution is determined mainly by
   A. reflector size.
   B. beam diameter.
   C. pulse duration.
   D. band width.
   E. the TV monitor.
4. In photoplethysmography, a change in blood volume is detected by light
   A. color.
   B. refraction.
   C. frequency shift.
   D. reflection.
   E. penetration.
5. When a 5 MHz Doppler instrument with a pulse repetition frequency of 15 kHz is used, "aliasing" will begin to occur at which frequency?
   A. 3 kHz
   B. 5 kHz
   C. 8 kHz
   D. 15 kHz
   E. 30 kHz
6. Which one of the following is measured by a venous outflow study?
   A. Rate of venous emptying
   B. Venous vascular incompetence
   C. Calf vein obstruction
   D. Limb perfusion
   E. Perforator incompetence
7. Which one of the following results in an increase in acoustic exposure to the patient?
   A. Application of reject
   B. Increase in the swept gain slope rate
   C. Increase in the television monitor brightness
   D. Increase in the examination time
   E. Increase in the overall gain

ANSWER KEY

1. A *B to E are included in the Doppler equation.*
2. D
3. B *Lateral resolution is equal to beam width (diameter for circular cross section).*
4. D
5. C *Nyquist limit is half the operating frequency (7.5 kHz in this case).*
6. A
7. D *None of the other choices affects the acoustic output from the transducer and therefore patient exposure.*

H Compilation of Advanced Concepts

CHAPTER 2

ADVANCED CONCEPTS

Speed is the rate of change of position of an object. Speed sometimes is called velocity, although, strictly speaking, *velocity* is defined as speed *with* direction of motion specified. An example of wind speed might be 25 miles per hour (mph), but its velocity would be 25 mph out of the northwest.

ADVANCED CONCEPTS

The propagation speed in any medium depends on the density (ρ) and stiffness of the medium. By density, we mean *mass density*, which is the mass per unit volume. The stiffness is the resistance to compression, also called the hardness or the bulk modulus of elasticity *(B)*. The reciprocal of bulk modulus is the compressibility of a medium. Specifically, propagation speed depends on the bulk modulus–density ratio:

$$c \text{ (m/s)} = \left[\frac{B \text{ (N/m}^2)}{\rho \text{ (kg/m}^3)} \right]^{1/2}$$

This relationship predicts that an increase in bulk modulus increases propagation speed and that an increase in density decreases propagation speed. If we compare gases, liquids, and solids, we find that generally more dense materials have *higher* propagation speeds, not lower. The reason is that higher-density materials generally have higher stiffness also, and the stiffness differences between materials are generally greater than the density differences. Thus the stiffness differences dominate the effect on the propagation speed so that, in general, solids have higher propagation speeds than liquids and liquids have higher speeds than gases.

ADVANCED CONCEPTS

Bandwidth is specified by some definition of where in the frequency range it starts and stops. For example, a 6-decibel (dB) bandwidth refers to the range of frequencies that includes those that have half or greater the amplitude (one fourth or greater the power) of the strongest one, which is the operating frequency. A 20-dB bandwidth includes amplitudes that are one tenth or greater of the strongest (one hundredth or greater the power). Clearly, a 20-dB bandwidth is greater that a 6-dB bandwidth.

The reciprocal of fractional bandwidth is called quality factor (Q). The quality factor is operating frequency divided by bandwidth. Shorter pulses (with their broader bandwidths) have lower Q's. This may seem like a contradiction because we stated previously that shorter pulses produce better resolution. So how could this be a lower quality? One does best to forget that Q originally stood for "quality" and simply to think of it as "Q." In the early days of electronics, for example, in radio, narrow bandwidth was good (for example, in radio to tune in one station and, at the same time, to tune out another station that is nearby on the frequency dial). In much of

modern electronics (including, for example, the Internet) broad bandwidth is good, being associated with, for example, high-fidelity sound and video and high information transmission rates. Thus in many cases, including sonography, low Q is good Q.

Shorter pulses have broader bandwidth and lower Q's. For short pulses (those having three cycles or fewer), the Q is approximately equal to the number of cycles in the pulse. Figure 2-10 gives two examples.

Bandwidth is an oft-mentioned term regarding connections to the Internet. Broader bandwidth connections permit faster information transfer and thus cost more. To achieve higher information transmission rates, a higher bit rate is required. Bits (and gaps) must be shorter in temporal length to be transmitted at a higher bit rate. Shorter bits have broader bandwidth just as shorter ultrasound pulses do. Thus higher bit rates require broader bandwidth connections to accomplish.

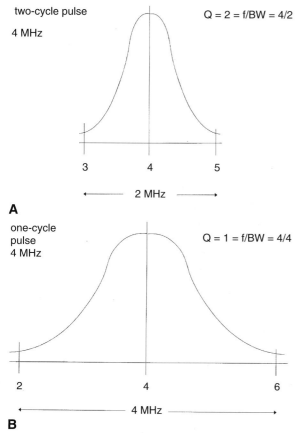

two-cycle pulse

4 MHz

$Q = 2 = f/BW = 4/2$

3   4   5

2 MHz

A

one-cycle pulse 4 MHz

$Q = 1 = f/BW = 4/4$

2   4   6

4 MHz

B

■ **FIGURE 2-10**   **A,** A 4-MHz, two-cycle pulse has a Q factor of approximately 2, and therefore a bandwidth of approximately 2 MHz (from 3 to 5 MHz). **B,** A 4-MHz one-cycle pulse has a Q factor of approximately 1, and therefore a bandwidth of approximately 4 MHz (from 2 to 6 MHz). Shorter pulses have broader bandwidths and lower Q's.

ADVANCED CONCEPTS

Several intensities are encountered in diagnostic ultrasound. Reasons for this are as follows:

1. Like a flashlight beam, intensity is not constant across a sound beam but is usually highest in the center and falls off near the periphery (Figure 2-13).
2. In the case of pulsed ultrasound, intensity varies with time (Figure 2-14); that is, the intensity is some value during each pulse but is zero between pulses.
3. Intensity is not constant within pulses (Figure 2-15) but rather starts out high and then decreases toward the end of the pulse.

For spatial considerations, the spatial peak (SP) and spatial average (SA) values are used. Spatial peak is the greatest intensity found across the beam, usually at the center. Spatial average is the average for all values found across the beam, including the larger values found near the center and the small values near the periphery.

For temporal (time) considerations, temporal average (TA), pulse average (PA), and temporal peak (TP) values are used. Temporal peak is the greatest intensity found in the pulse as it passes by. Pulse average is the average for all values found in a pulse, including the larger values found at its beginning and the small values found near the end. Temporal average includes the "dead" time between pulses where there is zero intensity. Thus temporal average is the lowest value, temporal peak is the highest, and pulse average is in between for a given pulsed beam. Pulse average and temporal average values are related by the duty factor. Temporal average intensity (I_{TA}) is equal to the pulse average intensity (I_{PA}) multiplied by the duty factor.

$$I_{TA} = I_{PA} \times DF$$

Thus if the duty factor is 0.01 (the sound is on 1% of the time), the temporal average intensity will be one hundredth the pulse average intensity. The greater the duty factor, the greater the temporal average intensity will be. If the sound is continuous instead of pulsed, the duty factor is equal to 1, and the pulse average intensity and temporal average intensity are equal to each other.

The pulses shown in Figures 2-7 and 2-14 have constant amplitude and intensity within each pulse. Pulses used in sonography, however, are similar to those shown in Figure 2-15. The peak intensity occurring within each pulse is called the temporal peak intensity. The intensity averaged over the pulse duration is called the pulse average intensity. For constant amplitude pulses, temporal peak intensity and pulse average intensity are equal. Six intensities result from these spatial and temporal considerations:

1. Spatial average–temporal average (I_{SATA})
2. Spatial peak–temporal average (I_{SPTA})

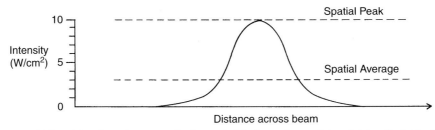

■ **FIGURE 2-13** Intensity varies across the beam. In this figure, the spatial peak intensity (at the beam center) is 10 W/cm^2 and the spatial average is 3 W/cm^2. In addition to varying across the beam, intensity varies along the direction of beam travel because of focusing and attenuation.

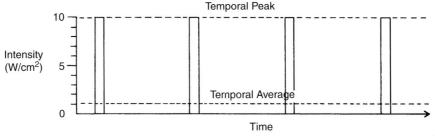

■ **FIGURE 2-14** Intensity versus time for pulsed ultrasound. Temporal peak intensity (10 W/cm^2) is the intensity when the sound is actually on. Temporal average intensity (1 W/cm^2) is the intensity that is averaged over time. In this figure the duty factor is 0.1. This figure assumes constant intensity within pulses. Sonographic pulses are depicted more accurately in Figure 2-9, *B* and *C*, and in Figure 2-15.

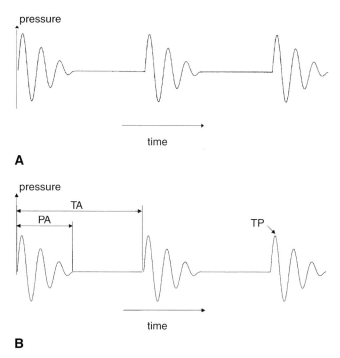

A

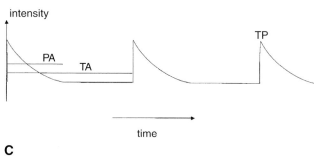

B

C

■ **FIGURE 2-15** **A,** The ultrasound pulses used in sonography have cycles of differing pressure amplitudes within each pulse. They are called damped pulses. **B,** The relevant times for three intensities are shown. Temporal average *(TA)* intensity is averaged over the pulse-repetition period; pulse average *(PA)* intensity is averaged over the pulse duration; and temporal peak *(TP)* intensity is not averaged over time. **C,** Intensity versus time for the pressure waveforms of **A** and **B.** The values for TP, PA, and TA intensities are shown. Temporal peak is the largest value (no averaging). Pulse average is smaller because it is averaged over pulse duration (including the portions with lower intensities). Temporal average is smallest because it is averaged over the pulse repetition period (including the time with no intensity).

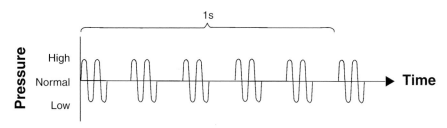

A

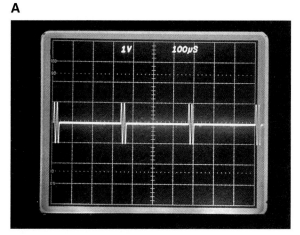

B

■ **FIGURE 2-7** Pulse repetition frequency is the number of pulses occurring in 1 second. **A,** Five pulses (containing two cycles each) occur in 1 second; thus the pulse repetition frequency is 5 Hz. **B,** In this photograph, three pulses occur in 1 millisecond (or one thousandth of a second); thus the pulse repetition frequency is 3 kHz. The total screen width is 1 ms.

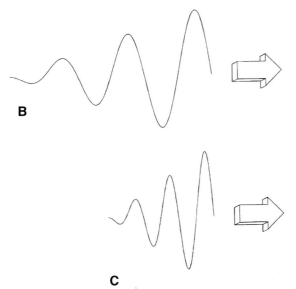

■ **FIGURE 2-9** **B** and **C** show three-cycle damped (decreasing in amplitude) pulses of ultrasound traveling to the right. **B,** Lower-frequency pulse with longer wavelength and spatial pulse length. **C,** Higher-frequency pulse with shorter wavelength and spatial pulse length.

3. Spatial average–pulse average (I_{SAPA})
4. Spatial peak–pulse average (I_{SPPA})
5. Spatial average–temporal peak (I_{SATP})
6. Spatial peak–temporal peak (I_{SPTP})

Spatial average–temporal average averages spatially across the beam and temporally, yielding the lowest value for a given beam. Spatial peak–temporal peak is averaged neither spatially nor temporally, so it is the highest value.

Example 2-1

The spatial peak–pulse average intensity is 500 mW/cm², and the duty factor is 2% (0.02). Calculate spatial peak–temporal average.

$$I_{SPTA} = I_{SPPA} \times DF = 500 \times 0.02 = 10 \text{ mW/cm}^2$$

Example 2-2

The spatial peak–temporal peak and spatial peak–pulse average intensities are 6 and 2 W/cm², respectively. Calculate spatial peak–temporal average if the duty factor is 1%.

$$I_{SPTA} = I_{SPPA} \times DF = 2 \times 0.01 = 0.020 \text{ W/cm}^2 = 20 \text{ mW/cm}^2$$

ADVANCED CONCEPTS

A clarification regarding the distance L (in centimeters) in the equation [a (dB) = ½ (dB/cm-MHz) × f (MHz) × L (cm)] is useful. In this equation, L is the distance (path length) the sound has traveled. For sonographic imaging the sound must make a round trip from the transducer to the reflector and back. Thus the distance that the sound travels to image an object is *twice* the distance to the object. Thus if imaging *depth* is being considered, rather than sound *travel distance*, the attenuation is approximately 1 dB/{[cm (depth)]-MHz} rather than 0.5 dB/{[cm (travel distance)]-MHz}.

ADVANCED CONCEPTS

This impedance ($z = \rho c$) is called the characteristic impedance. The characteristic impedance is the impedance for a propagating plane wave (one for which any acoustic variable has, at any instant of time, the same value anywhere in a plane perpendicular to the direction of propagation). For some acoustic considerations, such as reflection of a plane wave at a boundary, density times propagation speed has greater use as a descriptor of a medium than does either density or propagation speed alone. That is why the name "*characteristic* impedance" is applied.

Impedance in general is the ratio of force amplitude divided by its response amplitude. Impedance was first applied to electrical circuits, where it is the ratio of voltage amplitude to current amplitude. *Acoustic* impedance in general is pressure amplitude divided by particle velocity amplitude. Because pressure is force per unit area, acoustic impedance is impedance per unit area and thus is called specific acoustic impedance, with the term *specific* indicating "per unit amount" (area in this case).

ADVANCED CONCEPTS

Reflection and transmission of ultrasound at a boundary can be expressed in amplitude terms. For a plane wave, pressure amplitude and intensity are related as follows:

$$I = \frac{p^2}{z}$$

That is, intensity depends on pressure amplitude squared. Intensity reflection and transmission coefficients then depend on the square of the amplitude coefficients. Amplitude coefficients are slightly more involved because amplitudes can be positive or negative, whereas intensities are always positive. The amplitude reflection coefficient (ARC) is as follows:

$$ARC = \frac{p_r}{p_i} = \frac{(z_2 - z_1)}{(z_2 + z_1)}$$

where p_r is reflected pressure amplitude and p_i is incident pressure amplitude.

If z_2 equals z_1, there is no reflection (ARC = 0). If z_1 is greater than z_2, p_r is negative. The amplitude transmission coefficient is as follows:

$$ATC = \frac{p_t}{p_i} = \frac{2z_2}{(z_2 + z_1)}$$

where p_t is transmitted pressure amplitude.

If z_2 equals z_1, then ATC equals 1; that is, p_t equals p_i.

If z_1 is greater than z_2, then p_t is less than p_i.

The intensity transmission coefficient in terms of impedances is as follows:

$$ITC = \frac{4z_1 z_2}{(z_2 + z_1)^2}$$

ADVANCED CONCEPTS

The exact relationship between the incidence and transmission angles is known as Snell's law:

$$\left[\frac{\text{sine } (\theta_i)}{\text{sine } (\theta_t)}\right] = \frac{c_1}{c_2}$$

Where c_1 and c_2 are the propagation speeds in media 1 and 2, respectively, in Figure 2-25. This equation can be rearranged to yield the transmission angle:

$$\theta_t = \text{sine}^{-1}\left\{\frac{c_1}{c_2}\left[\text{sine } (\theta_t)\right]\right\}$$

The meaning of "sine^{-1}(S)" is the angle the sine of which is S.

Under the right conditions, there can be an angle at which there is *no* reflection (complete transmission into the second medium).

Because Snell's law involves ratios of sines and speeds, a good approximation allows the use of the ratio of the angles rather than the sines. This is why the angle ratio is approximately equal to the speed ratio as discussed previously. If Snell's law is used in Example 2-9 on p. 38, the calculated incidence angle is 18.8 degrees, confirming validity of using the angles, rather than the sines, as an approximation.

For oblique incidence, the reflection equation involves angles in addition to impedances:

$$\text{ARC} = \frac{(z_2 \cos \theta_i) - (z_1 \cos \theta_t)}{(z_2 \cos \theta_i) + (z_1 \cos \theta_t)}$$

If c_2 is greater than c_1, there is a critical incidence angle (θ_c) beyond which there is *total* reflection (no transmission into the second medium):

$$\theta_c = \text{sine}^{-1}\left(\frac{c_1}{c_2}\right)$$

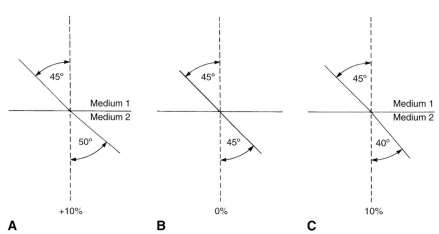

■ **FIGURE 2-25**   Transmission angles for an incidence angle of 45 degrees and propagation speeds through medium 2 that are 10% greater than **(A)**, equal to **(B)**, and 10% less than **(C)** propagation speed through medium 1.

CHAPTER 3

ADVANCED CONCEPTS

When a ceramic crystal is raised beyond the Curie point (about 350° C for lead zirconate titanate ceramics) the molecules in the crystal lattice can reorient with respect to each other. The molecules normally are oriented randomly, yielding no piezoelectric properties. If raised beyond the Curie point while in a strong electric field, the molecules (which are tiny electric dipoles) line up with the electric field. When the crystal is cooled below the Curie point while in the field, the crystal lattice is locked into the molecular structure that piezoelectric crystals naturally have, with the molecular dipoles lined up parallel to each other. Now if a voltage is applied to the front and rear faces of the element, it will get thicker or thinner as the dipoles together rotate toward or away (depending on the polarity of the voltage) from parallelism with the electric field produced by the voltage. If a polarized ceramic element is heated above the Curie point (not in an electric field), the molecules reorient randomly and the element loses its piezoelectric properties.

ADVANCED CONCEPTS

For continuous wave ultrasound, a single matching layer of quarter-wave thickness and impedance that is the geometric mean of the two impedances at the boundary provides the best match at the boundary. The geometric mean is the square root of the product of the two impedances. Because ultrasound pulses are characterized by a bandwidth rather than a single frequency, multiple layers (usually two for practical purposes) of varying impedance values and thicknesses match the impedances better than a single matching layer would. Even so, the matching layers still act as a bandpass filter, limiting the bandwidth of the pulses transmitted from the elements to the tissues.

Under development is a new class of transducer elements called capacitive microfabricated ultrasonic transducers or cMUTs. These elements are composed of thousands of microscopic silicon drums that include thin suspended membranes. Pulse generation is accomplished by applying a voltage to the drum. The voltage creates an electrostatic force on the membrane, causing it to vibrate and emit a pulse of ultrasound. Conversely, echoes arriving at the element cause the membrane to vibrate, producing the corresponding voltage that represents the echo in the electronics. One major advantage of cMUTs is that they have an impedance much lower than ceramic elements, easing the impedance-matching challenge and enabling broader bandwidth (exceeding 100%) pulses to be transmitted into tissues. Another advantage is that with semiconductor-based technology, the elements and electronics are combined in silicon. Thus more of the electronic components can be housed in the probe assembly, allowing more of the signal processing to be accomplished before sending of the electric signals through the probe cable to the instrument. A third advantage is that less energy is lost in the damping material because the pulse is coupled better to the tissues. This makes the transducer more efficient. Finally, the cMUT approach may allow flexible transducers to be fabricated that will conform to the surface of the patient more effectively and will allow a broader area of acoustic coupling to the tissues. In summary, cMUTs will enable more efficient production and coupling of broader-band pulses to the patient.

ADVANCED CONCEPTS

The formation of a beam from an aperture of some size and shape is explained by the Huygens principle and the concept of diffraction. Diffraction is the deviation of the direction of a wave that is *not* attributable to reflection, scattering, or refraction. Diffraction occurs when a wave passes an obstacle or a small (similar to the wavelength) aperture. The Huygens principle states that all points on a wave front or at a source can be considered as point sources for the production of spherical secondary wavelets. As these wavelets propagate, the wave front location and orientation at later times can be constructed by the summation of these wavelets. This principle can be applied to the surface of a transducer to determine the beam profile of the wave that emanates from that surface.

ADVANCED CONCEPTS

The formation of a beam from an aperture of some size and shape is explained by the Huygens principle and the concept of diffraction. Diffraction is the deviation of the direction of a wave that is *not* attributable to reflection, scattering, or refraction. Diffraction occurs when a wave passes an obstacle or a small (similar to the wavelength) aperture. The Huygens principle states that all points on a wave front or at a source can be considered as point sources for the production of spherical secondary wavelets. As these wavelets propagate, the wave front location and orientation at later times can be constructed by the summation of these wavelets. This principle can be applied to the surface of a transducer to determine the beam profile of the wave that emanates from that surface.

The near-zone length is given by

$$NZL = \frac{(a_p)^2}{4\lambda} = \frac{(a_p)^2 f}{4c}$$

where a_p is the disk aperture, i.e., diameter, and c is the propagation speed.

The beam width (w_b) at any location depends on wavelength (λ), aperture (a_p), and distance from the transducer (d).

In the approximation of Figure 3-10, at the end of the near zone, the beam width is equal to one half the transducer width (Figure 3-11). At a distance of 2 times the near-zone length, the beam width is equal to the transducer diameter. Beyond this distance, the beam width increases in proportion to the distance. As a pulse travels through the near zone, its width decreases; as it travels through the far zone, its width increases. In the near zone,

$$w_b = a_p - \frac{2\lambda d}{a_p} = a_p - \frac{2cd}{f\, a_p}$$

where a_p is the diameter for a circular aperture. For a rectangular aperture the expression is more complicated. In the far zone,

$$w_b = \frac{2(\lambda \times d)}{a_p} = \frac{2cd}{f \times a_p}$$

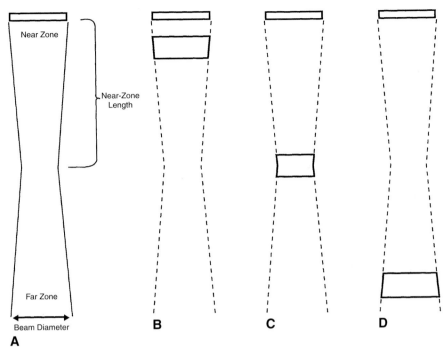

■ **FIGURE 3-10**   **A,** Beam width for a single-element unfocused disk transducer operating in the continuous wave mode. The near zone is the region between the disk and the minimum beam width. The far zone is the region beyond the minimum beam width. Intensity varies within the beam, with intensity variations being greatest in the near zone. This beam approximates the changing pulse diameter as an ultrasound pulse travels away from a transducer. **B,** An ultrasound pulse shortly after leaving the transducer. **C,** Later, the ultrasound pulse is located at the end of the near-zone length, where its width is at a minimum. **D,** Still later, the pulse is in the far zone, where its width is increasing as it travels.

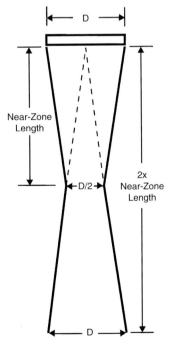

■ **FIGURE 3-11**   Sound beam from a disk transducer. The beam width narrows to half the disk diameter (*D*) at the near-zone length and then widens to the disk diameter at twice the near-zone length.

ADVANCED CONCEPTS

For a rectangular aperture, the minimum beam width (at the focus)—that is, the focal beam diameter (d_f)—can be obtained by multiplying twice the wavelength by the **f number** *(F)*, which is the focal length divided by the aperture.

$$d_f = 2 \times \lambda \times F = \frac{2(\lambda \times fl)}{a_p}$$

As the aperture is increased, the focus narrows, improving the resolution. Also, as frequency is increased, wavelength decreases, again narrowing the focus and improving resolution. Table 3-3 shows f number ranges in use. The best practical focus is with an f number of 2, yielding $d_f = 4\lambda$. Thus the best lateral resolution is about 4 times the best **axial resolution** (which is wavelength for a two-cycle pulse).

TABLE 3-3   f-Number Ranges

Focus	f Number
Weak	>6
Moderate	2-6
Strong	<2

ADVANCED CONCEPTS

As an example of the required delay to steer a beam (and scan line) in a specific direction, let us consider a 40-mm aperture containing 128 elements. We will calculate the case for a beam directed out at a 45-degree angle to the left of the transducer axis. The tangent of 45 degrees is 1; that is, the opposite and adjacent are equal (Figure 3-21, *H*). The hypotenuse is the wave front. The arrow shows the direction of travel that is always perpendicular to the orientation of the wave front.

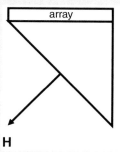

■ FIGURE 3-21   H, Diagram for calculation of phase delay.

The length of the adjacent side of the triangle (also the length of the array aperture) is 40 mm. Thus the length of the opposite side is also 40 mm. Thus the time required for that portion of the pulse to travel from the right-most element to a depth of 40 mm is $t = 40 \div 1.54 = 26$ μs. At this instant in time the left-most element has emitted its contribution to the pulse. Thus the total delay from right to left in energizing the elements is 26 μs. Because the transducer has 128 elements in the 40-mm array, it has a 0.2-μs element-to-element delay $(26 \div 128)$ to achieve a pulse directed at 45 degrees off the array axis.

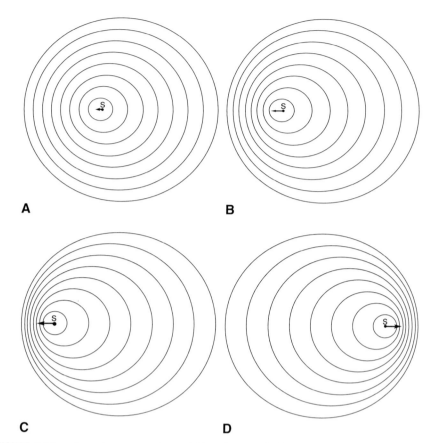

■ **FIGURE 5-14**   A moving source of sound (*s*) produces a shorter wavelength (higher frequency) ahead of it and a longer wavelength (lower frequency) behind it compared with the wavelengths at the sides, which are the same as for a stationary source. **A,** Slow speed. **B,** Medium speed. **C,** High speed. **D,** High-speed movement in the opposite direction.

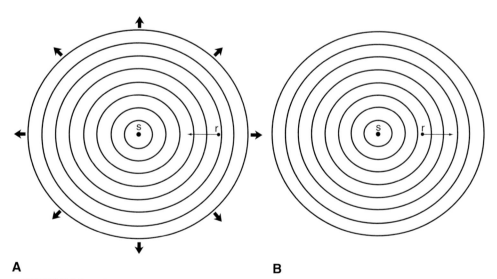

■ **FIGURE 5-13**   **A,** A receiver (*r*) moving toward the source (*s*) experiences a higher frequency (more cycles per second) than a stationary one would. **B,** A receiver moving away from the source experiences a lower frequency than a stationary one would.

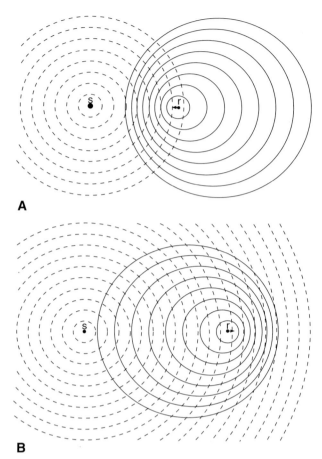

A

B

■ **FIGURE 5-15** A moving reflector (*r*) returns a higher frequency echo if it is approaching the source (*s*) and receiver (*s*) **(A)** and a lower frequency echo if it is moving away from the source and receiver **(B)**.

ADVANCED CONCEPTS

The speed of sound used in the Doppler equation is the average speed of sound in soft tissues: 1540 m/s or 1.54 mm/μs. Use of the speed of sound in blood[22] (1570 to 1575 m/s) is tempting. Strictly speaking, however, this is not appropriate[23-25] because the scatterers (blood cells) are not moving through their medium (blood plasma) but along with it; that is, there is no relative motion between the cells and their suspending medium to produce a Doppler shift. Where then *does* the Doppler shift occur? Doppler shift occurs where the relative motion exists; that is, at the blood-intima boundary for plug flow, in which case the tissue sound speed is relevant. For other types of flow (laminar, disturbed, and turbulent), relative motion occurs between flow layers (laminae), and some (unknown) combination of sound speeds for tissue and blood would be appropriate. Fortunately, this level of accuracy is not required for Doppler techniques to be useful.

CHAPTER 6

ADVANCED CONCEPTS

Autocorrelation is a mathematical process that compares a function with itself, in this case signal phase at different times. Autocorrelation is a measure of similarity (or nonrandomness) of the function at the different times. Autocorrelation is the cross-correlation of the signal with a time-delayed version of itself. Autocorrelation is useful for finding repeating patterns in a signal, such as determining the presence of a periodic signal that has been buried under noise. For our purpose, autocorrelation can determine the phase shift that has occurred over some short time interval. This phase shift is a measure of the Doppler shift and an indicator of the motion of a reflector over the time interval.

ADVANCED CONCEPTS

In Doppler-power displays a cross-correlation calculation yields the integral of power density with respect to time. Noise is less of a problem in Doppler-power displays compared with Doppler-shift displays because noise is spread over all frequencies and thus interferes with all aspects of a Doppler-shift display. However, noise is not spread over all amplitudes but mostly at the weaker levels. Thus the stronger Doppler-shifted echoes are lifted out of the noise and are assigned colors different from the background noise. The result is that Doppler-power displays are more sensitive and can show flow in slower-flow, deeper-vessel, and smaller-vessel situations than Doppler-shift display can. However, directional, speed, and flow character information is not presented. Conventional Doppler-shift displays are still useful for presentation of that information dynamically over cardiac cycle. Because Doppler-power displays show only the presence of flow (and not dynamic changes over cardiac cycle), integration of signal over time also improves signal-to-noise ratio.

CHAPTER 7

ADVANCED CONCEPTS

In the phase quadrature detector, two voltages from the oscillator (one leading by one quarter of a cycle [Figure 7-4], i.e., "quad") are mixed with the returning echo voltages to yield the difference, which is the Doppler shift. The echo voltages contain the Doppler shifts representing flow toward (f_t) and away from (f_a) the transducer. The **filter** outputs of the direct channel and the delayed (quadrature) channel are the Doppler shifts from the echo voltage input. If the Doppler shift is positive, the shift in the direct channel lags behind that in the quadrature channel by one quarter of a cycle (90 degrees). If the Doppler shift is negative, the shift in the quadrature channel lags behind that in the direct channel by one quarter of a cycle. The Doppler shifts in

both of these channels are next shifted by a quarter cycle. A negative Doppler shift in the direct channel at that point leads the one in the quadrature channel (before the additional 90-degree shift) by half a cycle. When added, these two voltages cancel (Figure 7-5), yielding no output. Positive Doppler shifts in these two channels are in **phase** (no lead or lag), yielding output from the direct channel adder. Positive shifts in the quadrature channel lead those in the direct channel by half a cycle, whereas negative shifts in the two channels are in phase. Thus the negative shifts are the output of the quadrature channel adder. The outputs of the two adders are sent to separate loudspeakers so that forward and reverse Doppler shifts can be heard separately. The outputs are also sent to a visual display to show positive and negative Doppler shifts above and below the display baseline, which represents zero Doppler shift.

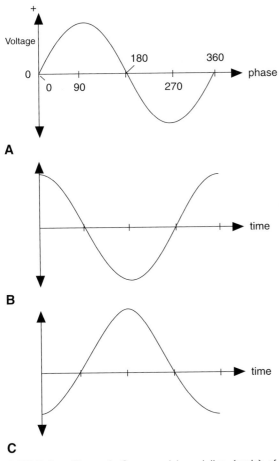

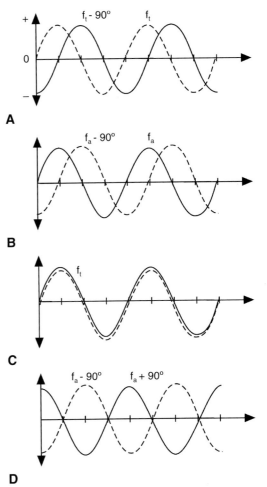

■ **FIGURE 7-4**   Phase. **A,** One complete variation (cycle) of alternating voltage may be thought of as traveling around a 360-degree circle. One quarter of a cycle is 90 degrees of phase angle. Phase is a description of progression through a cycle (analogous to the phase of the moon). One quarter of a cycle is 90 degrees, and one half of a cycle is 180 degrees. The completion of a cycle occurs at 360 degrees, but this is also the 0-degree phase of the next cycle. **B,** This voltage leads that in **A** by 90 degrees (one-quarter cycle). **C,** This voltage lags that in **A** by 90 degrees and lags that in **B** by 180 degrees. If the voltages in **B** and **C** are added together, a zero voltage results. (The two voltages are equal and opposite, so they cancel each other when summed.)

■ **FIGURE 7-5**   The solid curves refer to the direct channel, whereas the dashed curves refer to quadrature. The vertical axis represents voltage and the horizontal one represents time. **A,** Positive Doppler shifts (f_t) at the output of the direct channel filter lag those in the quadrature channel by 90 degrees. **B,** Negative Doppler shifts (f_a) at the output of the quadrature channel lag those in the direct channel by 90 degrees. **C,** Positive Doppler shifts at the input to the direct channel adder are in phase (0-degree phase difference), yielding an f_t output. **D,** Negative Doppler shifts at the input to the direct channel adder are 180 degrees out of phase, yielding a zero f_a output.

ADVANCED CONCEPTS

The **Fourier transform** is defined as follows:

$$F(f) = \int_{\infty}^{\infty} g(t) \, (\cos 2\pi ft - i \sin 2\pi ft) \, dt$$

where f is frequency, $g(t)$ is the function of time to be analyzed, and i is the square root of -1.

The fast Fourier transform is a computation that reduces the number of mathematical operations in the evaluation of the discrete Fourier transform:

$$F(\upsilon) = (1/n) \sum_{\tau=0}^{n-1} g(t) \, (\cos 2\pi\upsilon\tau - i \sin 2\pi\upsilon\tau)$$

where υ is related to frequency and τ is related to the time interval between sample points.

The FFT process includes sampling the complicated, multifrequency Doppler signal at a rate of approximately 25,600 times per second (or higher), which is a 25.6-kHz sampling rate. A 10-ms period of time (yielding 256 samples) is sufficient to provide a useful spectrum. Thus 100 such spectra can be produced per second. Each spectrum can include the amplitudes of 128 frequencies, the lowest of which is equal to the number of FFTs per second (100 Hz in this case) and the highest of which is equal to one half the sampling rate (or 12.8 kHz in this case). This rapid sequence of FFT-generated spectra (100 per second) can be displayed visually in real time. Some current processors can calculate up to 1000 FFTs per second.

ADVANCED CONCEPTS

Spectral broadening also occurs because of the finite size of the sample volume. This sometimes is called geometric spectral broadening. The shorter the gate-open time, the smaller the sample volume and shorter the time the propagating pulse has to interact with the blood flow. This shortens the returning Doppler-shifted echo, broadening its bandwidth. The effective bandwidth of the Doppler-shifted echo is a combination of the various contributions to spectral broadening: the bandwidth of the initial transmitted pulse, the range of flow speeds and angles encountered by the pulse, excessive Doppler gain, beam spreading, and geometric broadening. Effective bandwidth is the broadening resulting from flow character that is of physiologic interest in Doppler analysis.

Doppler Principles (Condensed)

This appendix is a condensed version of the material in Chapters 5 to 7 for those needing less depth and breadth of coverage. Doppler techniques are applied in all areas of diagnostic ultrasound, but in general, those working in cardiac or vascular areas use Doppler techniques more intensely than those in other areas and need a more thorough background in Doppler principles. Additionally, the American Registry for Diagnostic Medical Sonography examinations for the RDMS (Registered Diagnostic Medical Sonographer) and RDCS (Registered Diagnostic Cardiac Sonographer) credentials contains 10% to 20% Doppler questions, whereas the RVT (Registered Vascular Technologist) examination contains 22% to 40%. Thus the RVT examination requires more extensive preparation in Doppler principles than do the RDMS or RDCS examinations.

LEARNING OBJECTIVES

After reading this appendix, the student should be able to do the following:

- List and compare the various kinds of flow encountered in blood circulation.
- Explain how a stenosis affects flow.
- Define and discuss the Doppler effect, the Doppler shift, and the Doppler angle.
- Explain how two-dimensional flow information is color-encoded on a sonographic display.
- Compare Doppler-shift and Doppler-power displays.
- Explain how flow detection is localized to a specific site in tissue using pulsed Doppler techniques.
- Describe spectral analysis.
- Discuss examples of how spectral analysis is applied to evaluate flow conditions at the site of measurement and elsewhere.

KEY TERMS

The following terms are introduced in this chapter:

Autocorrelation	Doppler effect	Flow
Bernoulli effect	Doppler equation	Fluid
Bidirectional	Doppler-power display	Frequency spectrum
Clutter	Doppler shift	Gate
Color Doppler display	Doppler spectrum	Hue
Compliance	Duplex instrument	Inertia
Continuous wave Doppler	Eddies	Laminar flow
Cosine	Ensemble length	Luminance
Disturbed flow	Fast Fourier transform	Parabolic flow
Doppler angle	Filter	Phase quadrature

FLOW

The circulatory system consists of the heart, arteries, arterioles, capillaries, venules, and veins, altogether containing about 5 L of blood. The heart is the pump that produces blood flow through the circulatory system. The heart is a contracting and relaxing muscle (the myocardium) with four chambers: two atria and two ventricles. **Flow** is from the superior and inferior vena cava and pulmonary veins into the right and left atria, respectively, and from there into the ventricles. From the left and right ventricles flow is into the aorta and pulmonary artery, respectively. When the heart contracts, the intended result is forward flow into the aorta and pulmonary artery. Valves are present in the heart to permit forward and prevent reverse flow. Malfunctioning valves can restrict forward flow by not opening sufficiently (stenotic valve) or allow reverse flow by not closing completely (insufficiency or regurgitation). Doppler ultrasound is useful for detecting both of these conditions.

Flow in the heart, arteries, and veins can be detected with Doppler ultrasound. The capillaries are the tiniest vessels, measuring a few micrometers in diameter. The human body has approximately 1 billion capillaries. Across the capillary walls the exchange of gases, nutrients, and waste products with the cells takes place, sustaining their life (this is the reason for the existence of the circulatory system).

The **Doppler effect** is a change in frequency (and wavelength) caused by motion of a sound source, receiver, or reflector. If a reflector is moving toward the source and receiver, the received wave has a higher frequency than would be experienced without the motion. Conversely, if the motion is away (receding), the received wave has a lower frequency. The amount of increase or decrease in the frequency depends on the speed of reflector motion, the angle between the wave propagation direction and the motion direction, and the frequency of the wave emitted by the source.

Fluid

Matter generally is classified into three categories: gas, liquid, and solid. Gases and liquids are fluids; that is, they are substances that flow and conform to the shape of their containers. To flow is to move in a stream, continually changing position and, possibly, direction. Rivers flow downstream. Water flows through a garden hose. Air flows through a fan. Blood flows through the heart, arteries, capillaries, and veins.

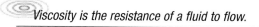
Gases and liquids are materials that flow.

Viscosity is the **resistance** to flow offered by a **fluid** in motion. Viscosity is given in units of **poise** or kilogram per meter-second (kg/m-s). One poise is 1 g/cm-s or 0.1 kg/m-s. Water has a relatively low viscosity compared with molasses, for example, which has a high viscosity. The viscosity of blood plasma is about 50% greater than that of water. The viscosity of normal blood is 0.035 poise at 37° C, approximately 5 times that of water. Blood viscosity can vary from about 0.02 (with anemia) to about 0.10 (with polycythemia). Blood viscosity also varies with flow speed.

Viscosity is the resistance of a fluid to flow.

Pressure, Resistance, and Volumetric Flow Rate

Pressure is the driving force behind fluid flow. Pressure is force per unit area. Pressure is equally distributed throughout a static fluid and exerts its force in all directions (Figure I-1). A pressure *difference* is required for flow to occur. Equal pressures applied at both ends of a liquid-filled tube will result in no flow. If the pressure is greater at one end than at the other, the liquid will flow from the higher-pressure end to the lower-pressure end. This pressure difference can be generated by a pump (e.g., the heart in the circulatory system) or by the force of gravity (i.e., by raising one end of a tube above the other). (Because this is the situation in the lower-extremity veins in a standing person, these vessels have valves in them to prevent reverse flow.) The greater the pressure difference, the greater the flow rate will be. This

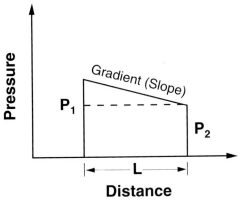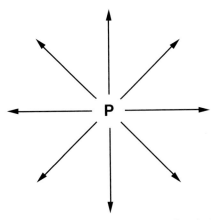

■ **FIGURE I-1** Pressure *(P)* is distributed uniformly throughout a static fluid and exerts its force in all directions.

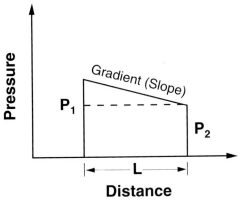

■ **FIGURE I-2** The pressure gradient or slope is the pressure difference *(P₁ – P₂)* divided by the separation *(L)* between the two pressure locations.

pressure difference is sometimes called a pressure gradient, although strictly defined, pressure gradient is the pressure difference *divided by the distance between the two pressure locations*. The term *gradient* comes from the Latin *gradus* and refers to the upward or downward sloping of something. As the pressure drops from one end of the tube to the other, this decrease can be thought of as a slope (i.e., the pressure difference divided by the distance over which the pressure drop occurs; Figure I-2). A constant driving pressure produces steady (unchanging with time) flow. The driving pressure produced by the heart varies with time. This concept is considered later in this section.

Fluid flows in a tube in response to a pressure difference at the ends.

The **volumetric flow rate** *(Q)* (sometimes simply called flow, although that term also is used in other ways) is the volume of blood passing a point per unit of time. Volumetric flow rate usually is expressed in milliliters per minute or per second. The total adult blood flow rate (cardiac output) is about 5000 mL/min (i.e., the total blood volume circulates in about 1 minute). The volumetric flow rate in a long straight tube is determined not only by the pressure difference *(ΔP)* but also by the resistance *(R)* to flow.

$$Q \text{ (mL/s)} = \frac{\Delta P \text{ (dyne/cm}^2)}{R \text{ (poise)}}$$

If pressure difference increases, volumetric flow rate increases.

If flow resistance increases, volumetric flow rate decreases.

The flow resistance in a long, straight tube depends on the fluid viscosity *(η)* and the tube length *(L)* and radius *(r)*, as follows:

$$R \text{ (g/cm}^4\text{-s)} = \frac{8 \times L \text{ (cm)} \times \eta \text{ (poise)}}{\pi \times [r^4 \text{ (cm}^4)]}$$

If tube length increases, flow resistance increases.

If tube radius increases, flow resistance decreases.

If viscosity increases, flow resistance increases.

As expected, an increase in viscosity or tube length increases the resistance, whereas an increase in the radius or diameter of the tube decreases the resistance. The latter effect is particularly strong, with the resistance depending on the radius to the fourth power. Thus doubling the radius of a tube decreases its resistance to one sixteenth its original value. By experience, we know that a longer- or smaller-diameter garden hose reduces water flow rate. And we could guess that if we tried to force molasses through the hose, we would not get nearly the flow rate we get with water.

Poiseuille's Equation

Substituting the equation for flow resistance into the flow rate equation and using tube diameter *(d)* rather than radius yields **Poiseuille's equation** for volumetric flow rate:

$$Q \text{ (mL/s)} = \frac{\Delta P \text{ (dyne/cm}^2) \times \pi \times d^4 \text{(cm}^4)}{128 \times L \text{ (cm)} \times \eta \text{ (poise)}}$$

Recall that this equation is for steady flow in long, straight tubes. Thus the equation serves only as a rough approximation to the conditions in blood circulation. The equation is useful, however, in making qualitative conclusions and predictions, as follows:

If pressure difference increases, flow rate increases.

If diameter increases, flow rate increases.

If length increases, flow rate decreases.

If viscosity increases, flow rate decreases.

The resistance of the arterioles accounts for about half the total resistance in the systemic circulation.[14] The muscular walls of the arterioles can constrict or relax, producing dramatic changes in flow resistance. The walls thus can control blood flow to specific tissues and organs in response to their needs.

The volumetric flow rate in a tube depends on the pressure difference, the length and diameter of the tube, and the viscosity of the fluid.

Types of Flow

Flow can be divided into five spatial categories: plug, laminar, parabolic, disturbed, and turbulent. At the entrance to a tube the speed of the fluid is essentially constant across the tube (Figure I-3). This is called **plug flow** because it is similar to the motion of a solid object (a plug, for example) that does not flow but moves as a unit. As the fluid flows down the tube, laminar (from the Latin term for layer) flow develops. **Laminar flow** is a flow condition in which **streamlines** (which describe the motion of fluid particles) are straight and parallel to each other. Flow speed is maximum at the center of the tube and minimum or zero at the tube walls. A decreasing profile of flow speeds from center to wall exists. Successive layers of fluid slide on each other with relative motion. The pressure difference at each end of

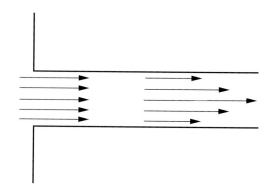

■ **FIGURE I-3**   At the entrance to a tube or vessel, plug flow exists. After some distance, laminar flow is achieved.

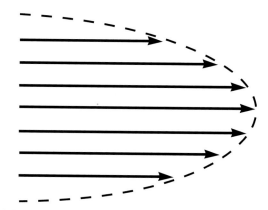

■ **FIGURE I-4**   Parabolic flow profile. The dashed line is a parabola.

the tube overcomes the viscous resistance of the layers sliding over each other, maintaining the laminar flow through the tube. Steady flow in a long, straight tube results in a **parabolic flow** profile (Figure I-4). Parabolic flow is a particular pattern of laminar flow in which varying flow speeds across the tube are described by a parabola (the curved dashed line in Figure I-4). For parabolic flow, the average flow speed across the vessel is equal to one half the maximum flow speed (at the center). Parabolic flow is not commonly seen in blood circulation because the vessels generally are not long and straight. However, nonparabolic laminar flow is commonly seen; indeed, its absence is often an indicator of abnormal flow conditions at a site where there is vascular or cardiac-valvular disease.

Laminar flow is flow where layers of fluid slide over each other.

Various flow profiles are seen in normal flow in various vessels and at different points in the cardiac cycle.[15] For example, a profile approximating a parabolic shape is seen in the common carotid artery at systole (Figure I-5, *A*). A blunted profile approximating plug flow is observed in diastole (Figure I-5, *B*). Even the twisting type of flow called helical is likely to be present in vessels.[16-20]

Disturbed flow occurs when the parallel streamlines describing the flow (Figure I-3) are altered from their straight form (Figure I-6). This occurs, for example, in the region of stenoses or at a bifurcation (the point at which a vessel splits into two). In disturbed flow, particles of fluid still flow in the forward direction. Parabolic and disturbed flows are forms of laminar flow.

In the final category, turbulent flow or **turbulence,** the flow pattern is random and chaotic, with particles moving at different speeds in many directions, even in circles called **eddies,** yet with forward net flow maintained (Figure I-7). As flow speed increases in a tube, turbulent flow eventually will occur (Figure I-7, *A*).

Disturbed flow is a form of laminar flow in which streamlines are not straight. Turbulent flow is nonlaminar flow with random and chaotic speeds and directions.

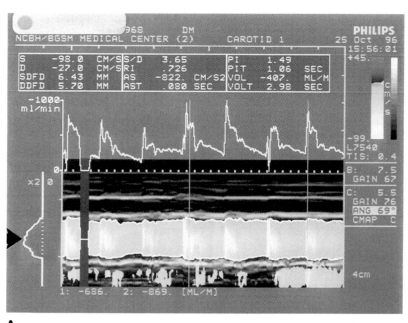

A

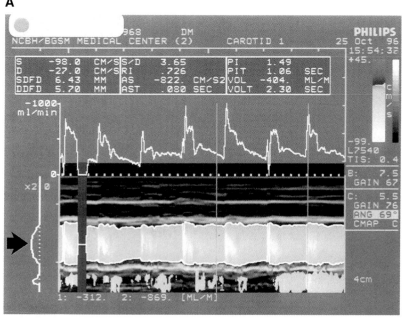

B

■ **FIGURE I-5**   Common carotid flow profiles *(arrows)* are approximately parabolic at systole **(A)** and plug in diastole **(B).**

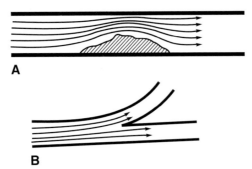

■ FIGURE I-6   Disturbed flow at a stenosis (**A**) and at a bifurcation (**B**).

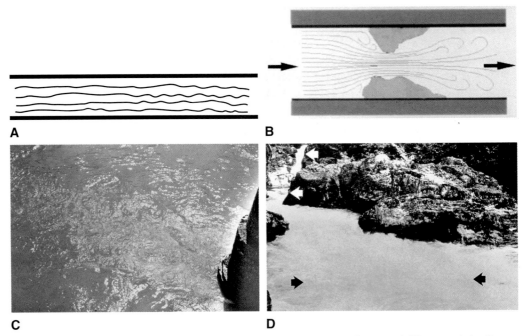

■ FIGURE I-7   Turbulent flow in a vessel may result from too great a flow speed (**A**) or an obstruction (**B**). **C,** Turbulent flow in a river beyond an obstruction (bridge pier). **D,** In a narrow gorge ("stenosis"; *white arrows*), flow speeds are high. Beyond the narrow region *(black arrows)* there is abundant turbulence.

Pulsatile Flow

Thus far we have considered steady flow in which pressures, flow speeds, and flow patterns do not change with time. This is generally the situation on the venous side of the circulatory system, although cardiac pulsations or respiratory cycles can influence venous flow in some locations. However, in the heart and the arterial circulation, flow is pulsatile, directly experiencing the effects of the beating heart with pulsatile variations of increasing and decreasing pressure and flow speed. For steady flow, volumetric flow rate simply is related to pressure difference and flow resistance. With **pulsatile flow,** the relationship between the varying pressure and flow rate depends on the flow impedance, which includes the resistance formerly considered, the **inertia**

of the fluid as it accelerates and decelerates, and the **compliance** (expansion and contraction) of the non-rigid vessel walls. The mathematical analysis is complicated and is not presented here. Two dominant characteristics of interest in this type of flow are the Windkessel effect and flow reversal. When the pressure pulse forces a fluid into a compliant vessel, such as the aorta, the vessel expands and increases the volume within it. (This is why you can feel your pulse on your wrist or neck.) Later in the cycle, when the driving pressure is reduced, the compliant vessel can contract, producing extended flow later in the pressure cycle. This is known as the Windkessel effect. In the aorta the Windkessel effect results in continued flow in the forward direction because aortic valve closure prevents flow back into the heart. In the distal circulation, expan-

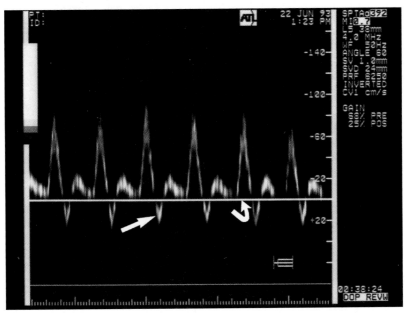

■ **FIGURE I-8**   Flow reversal (*straight arrow*) below the baseline (*curved arrow*) is seen in the superficial femoral artery in diastole.

sion of the distensible vessels results in the reversal of flow in diastole as the pressure decreases and the distended vessels contract. Where there are no valves to prevent it, flow reversal occurs (Figure I-8). This is a normal observation in these locations. Pulsatile flow in compliant vessels thus includes added forward flow and/or flow reversal in diastole, depending on location within arterial circulation. Arterial diastolic flow (absence, presence, direction, quantity) reveals much concerning the state of downstream arterioles, in which flow cannot be measured directly with ultrasound.

> *Pulsatile flow is nonsteady flow, with acceleration and deceleration over the cardiac cycle.*

> *Pulsatile flow in distensible vessels includes added forward flow and/or flow reversal over the cardiac cycle in some locations in circulation.*

Continuity Rule

A narrowing of the lumen of a vessel, or **stenosis,** produces disturbed (Figure I-6, *A*) and possibly turbulent flow (Figure I-7, *B* and *D*). The average flow speed in the stenosis must be greater than that proximal and distal to it, so that the volumetric flow rate is constant throughout the vessel. Examples of increased flow speed at a stenosis and turbulence beyond it are given later

in this appendix. Volumetric flow rate must be constant for the three regions: proximal to, at, and distal to the stenosis because blood is neither created nor destroyed as it flows through the vessel. This is called the continuity rule. Volumetric flow rate is equal to the average flow speed across the vessel multiplied by the cross-sectional area of vessel. Therefore if the stenosis has an area measuring one half that of the proximal and distal vessel, the average flow speed within the stenosis is twice that proximal and distal to it. If a stenosis has a diameter that is one half of that adjacent to it, the area at the stenosis is one fourth that adjacent to it, so the average flow speed in the stenosis must quadruple.

> *Flow speed increases at a stenosis and turbulence can occur distal to it.*

It is sometimes puzzling to students that Poiseuille's law and the continuity rule for a stenosis seem contradictory. One states that flow speed decreases with smaller diameters (Poiseuille's law), whereas the other says that flow speed increases with smaller diameters (continuity rule). How can this be so? The answer is that the two situations are different. Poiseuille's law deals with a long, straight vessel with no stenosis. The diameter in Poiseuille's law is that for the *entire* vessel. By contrast, the diameter in the continuity rule is that for a *short portion* of a vessel (the stenosis). If the diameter of the entire vessel is reduced (as in vasoconstriction), flow speed *is* reduced. If the diameter of only a short segment of a vessel is reduced (stenosis), the flow speed in the vessel is unaffected except at the stenosis, where it is increased. Flow speed increases because the stenosis has little effect on the overall flow resistance of the entire vessel if the stenosis length is small compared with the vessel length and if the lumen in the stenosis is not too small (does not approach occlusion). Figure I-9 illustrates these dependencies[21] of volumetric flow rate and flow speed at the stenosis with increasing stenosis. The maximum normal flow speed in circulation is about 100 cm/s. However, in stenotic regions, flow speeds can increase to a few meters per second. Doppler ultrasound is useful for detecting flow speed increases associated with vascular disease.

The increased flow speed within a stenosis can cause turbulence distal to it. Sounds produced by turbulence, which can be heard with a stethoscope, are called bruits. The ultimate stenosis is called an occlusion, where the vessel is blocked and there is no flow. Using our garden hose analogy again, we can compress the hose (not near the nozzle) and see little effect on the flow at the nozzle until the hose is compressed to near occlusion. At that point turbulence may occur and vibration can be felt at the surface of the hose.

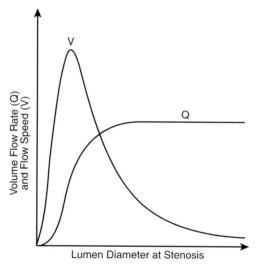

■ **FIGURE I-9** As the diameter of the stenosis is reduced (moving to the left on the horizontal axis; tighter stenosis), volumetric flow rate (Q) is unaffected initially because the stenosis does not contribute substantially to the total vessel resistance. As the diameter continues to decrease, however, the vessel resistance increases, reducing the volumetric flow rate (eventually to zero at occlusion). Volume rate and thus distal pressure begin to drop significantly beyond a diameter reduction of about 50% (area reduction of 75%). As the diameter of the stenosis decreases, flow speed increases (because of the flow continuity requirement), reaches a maximum, and then decreases to zero as the increasing flow resistance effect dominates. (Modified from Spencer MP, Reid JM: *Stroke* 10:326-330, 1979. Reprinted with permission. Copyright 1979 American Heart Association.)

Bernoulli Effect

ADVANCED CONCEPTS

At the stenosis the pressure is less than it is proximal and distal to the stenotic area (Figure I-10). This pressure difference is necessary to allow the fluid to accelerate into the stenosis and decelerate out of it and also to maintain energy balance. (Pressure energy is converted to flow energy upon entry and then vice versa upon exit.) This decreased pressure in regions of high flow speed is known as the **Bernoulli effect** and is described by Bernoulli's equation, a description of the constant energy of the fluid flow through a stenosis, ignoring viscous loss. As flow energy increases, pressure energy decreases. The magnitude of the decrease in pressure (ΔP) that results from the increasing flow speed (v) at the stenosis can be found from Bernoulli's equation. In a simplified form of the equation the flow speed proximal to the stenosis is assumed to be small enough, compared with the flow speed in the stenosis, to be ignored. Pressure drop from a stenotic heart valve can reduce cardiac output. For calculating pressure drop across a stenotic valve, the following form of the equation is used in Doppler echocardiography:

$$\Delta P = 4(v_2)^2$$

In this equation, v_2 is the flow speed (meters/second) in the jet and ΔP (millimeters of mercury) is the pressure drop across the valve. For example, if the flow speed in the jet is 5 m/s, the pressure drop is 100 mm Hg. Thus pressure drop can be calculated from a measurement of flow speed at the stenotic valve using Doppler ultrasound.

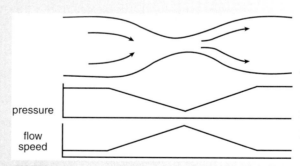

■ **FIGURE I-10** To maintain flow continuity, flow speed must increase through a stenosis. In conjunction with this, the pressure drops (the Bernoulli effect) in the stenosis. (From Kremkau FW: *J Vasc Technol* 17:153-154, 1993. Reprinted with permission.)

The Bernoulli effect is a drop in pressure associated with high flow speed at a stenosis.

If flow speed increases, the magnitude of the pressure drop increases.

DOPPLER EFFECT

The Doppler effect is a change in frequency caused by motion of a sound source, receiver, or reflector. A quantitative description of the Doppler effect is provided by the **Doppler equation**. The Doppler equation can deal with three situations: moving source, receiver, or reflector. Only the moving reflector result will be given because it is the relevant situation of interest for diagnostic Doppler ultrasound.

A moving reflector (Figure I-11) or scatterer of a wave is a combination of a moving receiver and source. For a moving reflector approaching a stationary source, more cycles of a wave will be encountered in 1 second than would be if the reflector were stationary *and* the reflected cycles were compressed in front of the reflector as it moved into its own reflected wave. Both effects increase the frequency of the reflected wave.

Doppler Shift

The *change* in frequency caused by motion is called the Doppler shift frequency or, more commonly, just the **Doppler shift** (f_D). The Doppler shift is equal to the received frequency (f_R) minus the source frequency (f_T). For an approaching reflector (scatterer), Doppler shift is positive; that is, the received frequency is greater than the source frequency. For a receding reflector, Doppler

shift is negative; that is, the received frequency is smaller than the source frequency. The relationship between the Doppler shift and the reflector speed (v) is given by the Doppler equation:

$$f_D \text{ (kHz)} = f_R \text{ (kHz)} - f_T \text{ (kHz)} = f_0 \text{ (kHz)} \times \frac{[2 \times v \text{ (cm/s)}]}{c \text{ (cm/s)}}$$

 If scatterer speed increases, Doppler shift increases. If source frequency increases, Doppler shift increases.

The Doppler shift is the difference between the emitted frequency and the echo frequency returning from moving scatterers.

Take, for example, a source frequency of 5 MHz, a scatterer speed of 50 cm/s (0.5 m/s), and a propagation (sound) speed of 1540 m/s. The scatterer is approaching the source, so the received frequency is greater than the source frequency, with a positive Doppler shift of 0.0032 MHz or 3.2 kHz. For a scatterer moving away from a receiver, the Doppler shift is −3.2 kHz. Other examples using various source frequencies and scatterer speeds are given in Table I-1.

The Doppler shift is what the instruments described in this appendix detect. However, we are interested in the speed of tissue motion or blood flow, not the Doppler shift itself. To facilitate this, the Doppler equation is rearranged to place the speed of motion alone on the left side of the equation. Substituting the speed of sound in tissues (154,000 cm/s) and using units as indicated for the various quantities yields the equation in the following form:

$$v \text{ (cm/s)} = \frac{[77 \text{ (cm/ms)} \times f_D \text{ (kHz)}]}{f_0 \text{ (MHz)}}$$

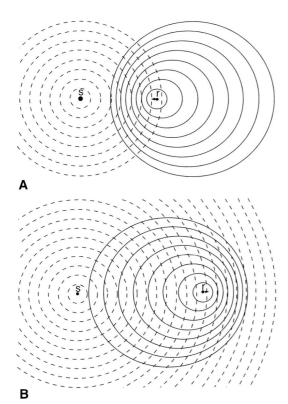

A

B

■ **FIGURE I-11** A moving reflector (*r*) returns a higher frequency echo if it is approaching the source (*s*) and receiver (*s*) **(A)** and a lower frequency echo if it is moving away from the source and receiver **(B).**

TABLE I-1   Doppler Frequency Shifts for Various Scatterer Speeds toward* the Sound Source at a Zero Doppler Angle

Incident Frequency (MHz)	Scatterer Speed (cm/s)	Reflected Frequency (MHz)	Doppler Shift (kHz)
2	50	2.0013	1.3
5	50	5.0032	3.2
10	50	10.0065	6.5
2	200	2.0052	5.2
5	200	5.013	13.0
10	200	10.026	26.0

*Motion away from the source would yield negative Doppler shifts.

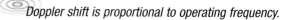*The Doppler equation relates the Doppler shift to the flow speed and the frequency.*

The fact that the Doppler shift is proportional to the blood flow speed explains why the Doppler effect is so useful in medical diagnosis. Doppler instruments measure the Doppler shift. The blood flow is what interests us. The measured shifts are proportional to flow speed, which is the information we seek.

Doppler Ultrasound

With diagnostic medical ultrasound, stationary transducers are used to emit and receive the ultrasound. The Doppler effect is a result of the motion of blood, the flow of which we wish to measure, or the motion of tissue that we wish to evaluate. Physiologic flow speeds, even in highly stenotic jets, do not exceed a few meters per second. Table I-1 gives Doppler shifts resulting from typical physiologic flow speeds. The minimum detectable blood flow speed with Doppler ultrasound is a few millimeters per second. The maximum is determined by aliasing (discussed in Chapter 8).

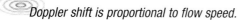*Doppler shift is proportional to flow speed.*

Operating Frequency

For a given flow in a vessel, the Doppler shift measured by an instrument is proportional to the operating frequency of the instrument (Figure I-12 and Table I-1). Thus measurement of Doppler shifts from flow in the same vessel using two transducers operating at 2 MHz and 4 MHz will yield two Doppler shifts. The higher-frequency transducer will have a Doppler shift that is twice that of the lower-frequency transducer. When comparing Doppler shifts, therefore, one must consider the frequency of the devices.[28] The operating frequency is incorporated into the calculation of flow speed. Thus comparisons of flow speeds between different instruments have taken this variable into account.

Doppler shift is proportional to operating frequency.

Doppler frequencies used in vascular studies are slightly less than those used for anatomic imaging because echoes from blood are weaker than those from soft tissues.

Doppler Angle

If the direction of sound propagation is exactly opposite the flow direction, the maximum positive Doppler shift is obtained. If the flow speed and propagation speed directions are the same (parallel), the maximum negative Doppler shift is obtained. If the angle between these two directions (Figure I-13) is nonzero, lesser Doppler shifts will occur. The Doppler shift depends on the **cosine** of the **Doppler angle**.

$$f_D \text{ (kHz)} = \frac{[f_0 \text{ (kHz)} \times 2 \times v \text{ (cm/s)} \times (\cos \theta)]}{c \text{ (cm/s)}}$$

$$v \text{ (cm/s)} = \frac{[77 \text{ (cm/ms)} \times f_D \text{ (kHz)}]}{[f_0 \text{ (MHz)} \times \cos \theta]}$$

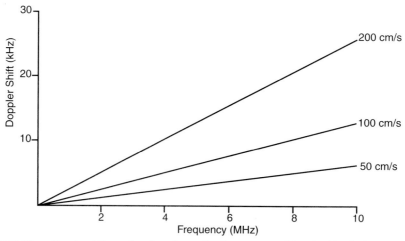

■ **FIGURE I-12** Doppler shift as a function of operating frequency, as determined by the Doppler equation for various flow speeds (at a zero Doppler angle).

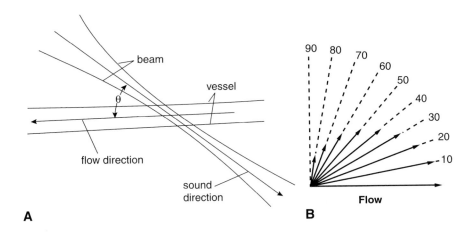

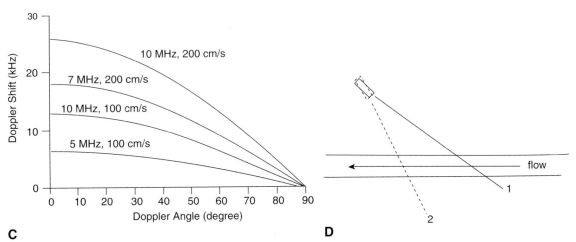

■ **FIGURE I-13** **A,** Doppler angle θ is the angle between the direction of flow and the sound propagation direction. **B,** With constant flow, as the Doppler angle increases, echo Doppler shift frequency decreases. The direction of the arrows indicates the beam direction. The length of the arrows indicates the magnitude of the Doppler shift. **C,** Doppler shift as a function of angle, as determined by the Doppler equation for various incident frequencies and scatterer speeds. **D,** The same flow in a vessel, viewed at different angles, yields different Doppler shifts.

Table I-2 gives cosine values for various angles. Only the portion of the motion direction that is parallel to the sound beam contributes to the Doppler effect. The cosine gives the component of the flow velocity vector that is parallel to the sound beam (Figure I-14). For a given flow, the larger the Doppler angle, the less the Doppler shift (Figure I-13, *B* and *C*). Table I-3 lists examples of Doppler shifts for various angles.

> If Doppler shift increases, calculated scatterer speed increases.
> If source frequency increases, calculated scatterer speed decreases.
> If cosine increases, calculated scatterer speed decreases.
> If Doppler angle increases, calculated scatterer speed increases.

TABLE I-2   Cosines for Various Angles

Angle A (degrees)	cos A
0	1.00
5	0.996
10	0.98
15	0.97
20	0.94
25	0.91
30	0.87
35	0.82
40	0.77
45	0.71
50	0.64
55	0.57
60	0.50
65	0.42
70	0.34
75	0.26
80	0.17
85	0.09
90	0.00

TABLE I-3   Doppler Frequency Shifts for Various Angles and Scatterer Speeds toward the Sound Source of Frequency 5 MHz

Scatterer Speed (cm/s)	Angle (degrees)	Doppler Shift (kHz)
100	0	6.5
100	30	5.6
100	60	3.2
100	90	0.0
300	0	19.0
300	30	17.0
300	60	9.7
300	90	0.0

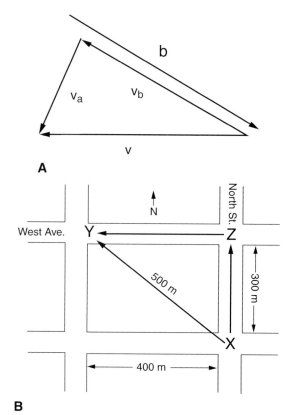

■ **FIGURE I-14**   **A,** The flow velocity vector (*v*) can be broken into two components: one (*v*ᵦ) that is parallel to the sound beam (*b*) direction and one (*v*ₐ) that is perpendicular to the sound beam direction. Only the component parallel to the beam contributes to the Doppler effect. **B,** A city block can be used as an analogy to the vector components in **A.** To get from point X to point Y, one could walk diagonally across the block, a distance of 500 m. However, if buildings blocked that path, an alternate route would be 300 m north on North Street and then 400 m west on West Avenue. The 500-m northwest vector from X to Y is equivalent to a 300-m north vector plus a 400-m west vector (i.e., the result is the same: depart from X and arrive at Y). In this example, the component of the XY vector parallel to North Street is the XZ vector and the component parallel to West Avenue is the ZY vector.

ANGLE ACCURACY

Flow speed calculations based on Doppler shift measurements can be accomplished correctly only with proper Doppler angle incorporation. The calculations therefore are only as good as the accuracy of the measurement, estimate, or guess of that angle. Estimation of the angle normally is done by orienting an indicator line on the anatomic display so that it is parallel to the presumed direction of flow (e.g., parallel to the vessel wall for a straight vessel with no flow obstruction). This is a subjective operation performed by the instrument operator. Error in this estimation of the Doppler angle is more critical at large angles than at small ones because the cosine changes rapidly at large angles. Table I-4 gives error values for various angles. For example, if the correct Doppler angle is 60 degrees but the estimation is 5 degrees in error (the angle estimate is 55 or 65 degrees), the error in the cosine value is about 15%, yielding a calculated speed that is in error by about 18%. Figure I-15 shows how the error in calculated flow speed increases with angle. For this reason, and because Doppler shift frequencies become very small at large angles, thereby reducing the system sensitivity, Doppler measurements (and particularly calculated flow speeds) are not reliably achieved at Doppler angles greater than about 60 degrees. In principle, if angle is incorporated correctly, the calculated flow speed in the vessel should be the same, regardless of what the Doppler angle is. That is, the actual flow speed is certainly not altered by the Doppler angle used in detecting it (Table I-5). Not surprisingly, however, inaccuracies in angle estimation

are experienced. Flow also is often not parallel to vessel walls, even in unobstructed vessels.[15-20]

At Doppler angles less than about 30 degrees, the sound no longer enters the blood at all but is reflected totally at the wall-blood boundary.[29] One generally achieves success, then, at angles greater than this. However, in Doppler echocardiography, Doppler angles of nearly zero *are* useful, and zero commonly is assumed (i.e., angle correction is not incorporated in this application like it is in vascular work). The angle between the beam and the heart wall is large, thereby avoiding the total reflection problem (Figure I-16).

We have considered in this discussion the Doppler angle in the scan plane only. One must remember that the flow may not be parallel to the imaging scan plane,

TABLE I-4   Cosine and Calculated-Speed Errors for Angle Errors of 2 and 5 Degrees

True Angle (degrees)	Cosine Error (%)		Speed Error (%)	
	+2 Degrees	+5 Degrees	+2 Degrees	+5 Degrees
0	−0.1	−0.4	+0.1	+0.4
10	−0.7	−1.9	+0.7	+2.0
20	−1.3	−3.6	+1.3	+3.7
30	−2.1	−5.4	+2.1	+5.7
40	−3.0	−7.7	+3.1	+8.3
50	−4.2	−10.8	+4.4	+12.1
60	−6.1	−15.5	+6.5	+18.3
70	−9.6	−24.3	+10.7	+32.1
80	−19.9	−49.8	+24.8	+99.2

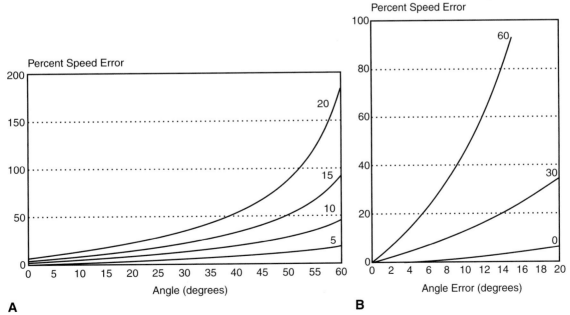

■ **FIGURE I-15   A,** Percent calculated speed error versus correct Doppler angle for 5-, 10-, 15-, and 20-degree angle errors. **B,** Percent calculated speed error versus angle error for three values (0, 30, and 60 degrees) of the correct Doppler angle.

TABLE I-5   Doppler Shifts (for 4 MHz) at Various Doppler Angles for the Same Flow Yielding a Consistent Calculated Flow Speed

Doppler Shift (kHz)	Angle (degrees)	Calculated Flow Speed (cm/s)
2.25	30	50
1.99	40	50
1.84	45	50
1.67	50	50
1.30	60	50

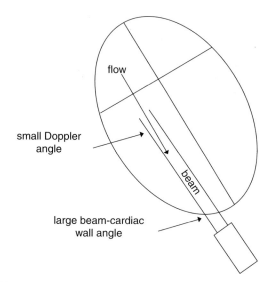

■ **FIGURE I-16**   In cardiac Doppler work, Doppler angles are usually small, whereas the angle between the beam and the cardiac wall is usually large.

which includes the Doppler beam, so that there may be a component of Doppler angle between the flow direction and the scan plane. Thus one must keep in mind the three-dimensional character of the components involved in the process (vessel anatomy, flow, and ultrasound image scan plane).

COLOR DOPPLER INSTRUMENTS

Doppler instruments present information on the presence, direction, speed, and character of blood flow (Box I-1) and on the presence, direction, and speed of tissue motion. This information is present in audible, color Doppler, and spectral Doppler forms (Box I-2). Color Doppler imaging[30-39] presents two-dimensional, cross-sectional, real-time blood flow or tissue motion information along with two-dimensional, cross-sectional, gray-scale anatomic imaging. Two-dimensional real-time presentations of flow information allow the observer readily to locate regions of abnormal flow for further evaluation using **spectral analysis.** The direction of flow

BOX I-1   Types of Flow Information Provided by Doppler Ultrasound

Presence of flow
- Yes
- No

Direction of flow
- ←
- →

Speed of flow
- Slow
- Fast

Character of flow
- Laminar
- Turbulent

BOX I-2   Various Forms of Presentation of Doppler Information

Audible sounds
Strip-chart recording
Spectral display
Color Doppler display

is appreciated readily, and disturbed or turbulent flow is presented dramatically in two-dimensional form. Color Doppler instruments present anatomic information in the conventional gray-scale form but also rapidly detect Doppler-shift frequencies at several locations along each scan line, presenting them in color at appropriate locations in the cross-sectional image.

Color Doppler Principle

Color Doppler imaging (sometimes called color flow imaging) extends the use of the pulse-echo imaging principle to include Doppler-shifted echoes that indicate blood flow or tissue motion. Echoes returning from stationary tissues are detected and presented in gray scale in appropriate locations along scan lines. Depth is determined by echo arrival time, and brightness is determined by echo intensity. If a returning echo has a different frequency than what was emitted, a Doppler shift has occurred because the echo-generating object was moving. Depending on whether the motion is toward or away from the transducer, the Doppler shift is positive or negative. At locations along scan lines where Doppler shifts are detected, appropriate colors are assigned to the display pixels.

Color Doppler imaging is an extension of conventional gray-scale sonography that shows regions of blood flow or tissue motion in color.

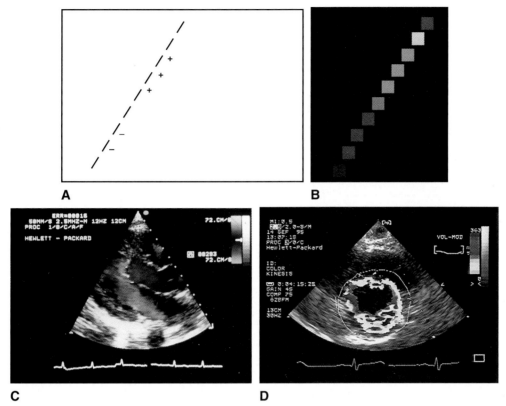

C   D

■ **FIGURE I-17** **A,** Ten echoes are received as a pulse travels through tissues. Three *(red)* have positive Doppler shifts and two *(blue)* have negative shifts. **B,** These echoes are shown as red and blue pixels, respectively, on the color Doppler display. As in gray-scale sonography, a two-dimensional cross-sectional image is made up of many scan lines. **C,** A parasternal long-axis image of normal mitral valve blood flow. **D,** A parasternal short-axis view of myocardial tissue motion (color kinesis). (See Color Plate 4.)

Doppler-shifted echoes can be recorded and presented in color at many locations along each scan line (Figure I-17, *A* and *B* [Color Plate 4, Figure 6-1, *A* and *B* in color insert]). As in all sonography, many such scan lines make up one cross-sectional image (Figure I-17, *C* and *D*). Several of these images (frames) are presented each second, yielding real-time color Doppler sonography.

Linear array presentation of color Doppler information is sometimes inadequate when the vessel runs parallel to the skin surface because the pulses (and scan lines) run perpendicular to the transducer surface (and therefore to the skin surface), resulting in a 90-degree Doppler angle where the pulses intersect the flow in the vessel. If the flow is parallel to the vessel walls, the 90-degree Doppler angle would yield no Doppler shift, and hence no color within the vessel. To solve this problem, phasing is used to steer each emitted pulse from the array in a given direction (e.g., 20 degrees away from perpendicular). All the color pulses and color scan lines are steered at the same angle, resulting in a parallelogram presentation of color Doppler information on the display (Figure I-18 [Color Plate 5, Figure 6-2 in color insert]).

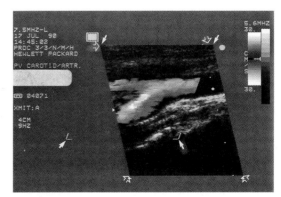

■ **FIGURE I-18** A perpendicular Doppler angle is avoided in this image by electronically steering the color-producing Doppler pulses to the left of vertical. The corners of the resulting parallelogram in which color can be displayed are shown by the solid arrows. Note that on this instrument, the gray-scale anatomic imaging pulses also can be steered (in this case, to the right of vertical). The corners of the resulting gray-scale parallelogram are shown by the open arrows. (See Color Plate 5.) (From Kremkau FW: Principles and pitfalls of real-time color-flow imaging. In Bernstein EF, editor: *Vascular diagnosis*, ed 4, St Louis, 1993, Mosby.)

Instruments

The color Doppler instrument has the same block diagram as the gray-scale sonographic instrument (Figure 4-1, *A*). The beam former, signal processor, image processor, and display perform the same functions as they do in the sonographic instrument. In addition, the signal processor must include the ability to detect Doppler shifts, and the display must be capable of presenting echoes in color.

> *Color Doppler instruments are conventional sonographic instruments that have the ability to detect Doppler shifts and present them on the display in color.*

Doppler-Shift Detection

The signal processor receives the digitized voltages from the beam former that represent the echoes returning from tissue. Non–Doppler-shifted echoes are processed conventionally, as in any sonographic instrument. Doppler-shifted echoes commonly are detected in the signal processor using a mathematical technique called **autocorrelation** that rapidly determines the mean and **variance** of the Doppler-shift signal (Figure I-19) at each location along the scan line (at each selected echo arrival time during pulse travel). The autocorrelation technique[40] is a mathematical process that yields the Doppler-shift information for each sample time (and corresponding depth down the scan line) following pulse emission. The sign, mean, and variance of the

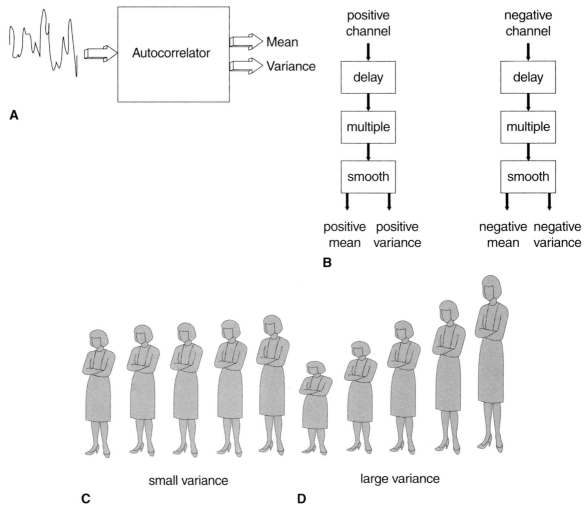

■ **FIGURE I-19** **A,** The autocorrelator rapidly performs Doppler demodulation on the complicated echo signal *(entering at left)*. The outputs of the autocorrelator yield the magnitude of the mean and the variance of the Doppler shifts at each location in the scanned cross section. These items of information are stored in each pixel location in the memory. Color assignments are selected appropriately to indicate these items of information two-dimensionally on the display. **B,** After division of the Doppler signal into positive and negative Doppler-shift channels, each signal is multiplied by a version of itself delayed by one pulse repetition period. High-frequency variations are filtered out (smoothed) to yield the mean and variance of the Doppler shifts. Variance is a measure of data spread around a mean. Variance is equal to the standard deviation squared. **C** and **D,** Two groups of women with equal mean heights but unequal variances.

Doppler signal are stored at appropriate locations in the memory corresponding to anatomic sites where the Doppler shifts have been found. Typically 100 to 400 Doppler samples (locations) per scan line are shown on a **color Doppler display.** Depending on the depth and width of the color presentation, typically 5 to 50 frames per second can be shown. Recall that for gray-scale sonography, a single pulse produces one scan line. For multiple foci, multiple pulses per scan line are required. In color Doppler instruments, multiple pulses are involved in all images because they are required in the autocorrelation process. A three-pulse minimum is required for one speed estimate. More pulses are required for improved accuracy of the estimates, for variance determinations, or to improve detection of lower-frequency mean Doppler shifts (slower flows).

Autocorrelation is the mathematical process commonly used to detect Doppler shifts in color Doppler instruments.

Color Controls

Color controls (Figure I-20) include color **window** location, width and depth, gain, steering angle, color inversion, **wall filter, priority,** baseline shift, velocity range (pulse repetition frequency [PRF]), color map selection, variance, smoothing, and **ensemble length.** Steering angle control permits avoidance of 90-degree angles (Figure I-21 [Color Plates 6 to 8, Figure 6-6 in color insert]). Color inversion alternates the color assignments on either side of the baseline on the color map (Figure I-21, *D* and *E* [Color Plate 7, Figure 6-6]). The wall filter allows elimination of **clutter** caused by tissue

and wall motion (Figure I-22 [Color Plates 9 and 10, Figure 6-7]). However, one must take care not to set the wall filter too high, or slower blood flow signals will be removed (Figure I-22, *C* [Color Plate 9, Figure 6-7]). The operator of a gray-scale sonographic instrument does not have direct control of the PRF. But in Doppler instruments the operator does control the PRF with the scale control. This control sets the PRF and the limit at the color bar extremes. Decreasing the value permits observation of slower flows (smaller Doppler shifts) but increases the probability of aliasing for faster flows (aliasing is described in Chapter 8). Priority selects the gray-scale echo strength below which color will be shown instead of gray level at each pixel location (Figure I-23 [Color Plate 11, Figure 6-8]). Baseline control allows shifting the baseline up or down to eliminate aliasing. Smoothing (also called persistence) provides frame-to-frame averaging to reduce noise (Figure I-24 [Color Plates 12 and 13, Figure 6-9]). Ensemble length is the number of pulses used for each color scan line. The minimum is 3, with 10 to 20 being common. Greater ensemble lengths provide more accurate estimates of mean Doppler shift, improved detection of slow flows, and complete representation of flow within a vessel (Figure I-24 [Color Plates 12 and 13, Figure 6-9]) but at the expense of longer time per frame and therefore lower frame rates (see Figure 6-9 [Color Plates 12 and 13]). Wider color windows (viewing areas) also reduce frame rates because more scan lines are required for each frame (Figure I-25 [Color Plate 14, Figure 6-10]).

Autocorrelation requires several pulses per scan line for Doppler detection. The number of pulses per scan line is called ensemble length.

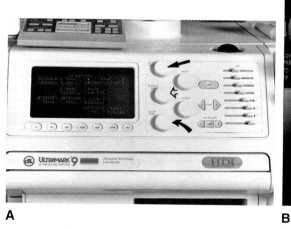
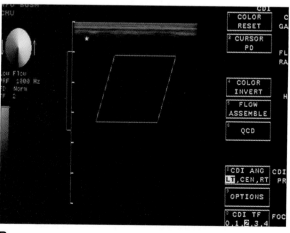

A   **B**

■ **FIGURE I-20**   **A,** Color Doppler gain control *(curved arrow).* The gray-scale *(straight arrow)* and spectral Doppler *(open arrow)* gain controls also are indicated. **B,** Software panel controls for color Doppler functions.

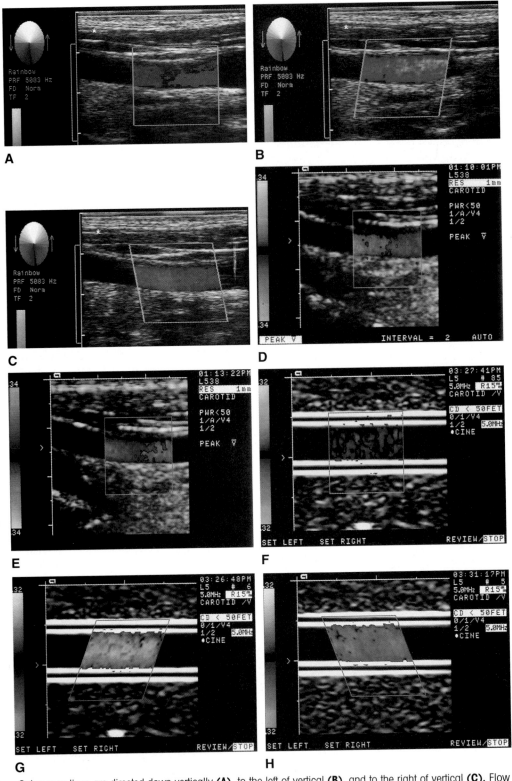

■ **FIGURE I-21**   Color scan lines are directed down vertically **(A),** to the left of vertical **(B),** and to the right of vertical **(C).** Flow is from left to right, producing positive or negative Doppler shifts, depending on the relationship between scan lines and flow. **D,** In this hue map, red and blue are assigned to positive and negative Doppler shifts, respectively, progressing to yellow and cyan (by the addition of green) at the Nyquist limits. **E,** In this map the color assignments are reversed from those presented in **D** (i.e., blue and red are assigned to positive and negative Doppler shifts, respectively). Note the color change occurring within each color window. This is caused by vessel curvature. **F,** With flow in a straight tube, positive and negative Doppler shifts are distributed equally throughout the color window with a Doppler angle of 90 degrees. **G,** Uniform positive Doppler shifts are observed with the color window steered 20 degrees to the left (70-degree Doppler angle). **H,** Uniform negative Doppler shifts are observed with the color window steered to the right. (See Color Plates 6 to 8.) (**A** to **C** from Kremkau FW: *Semin Roentgenol* 27:6-16, 1992; **D** and **E** from Kremkau FW: Principles and pitfalls of real-time color-flow imaging. In Bernstein EF, editor: *Vascular diagnosis,* ed 4, St Louis, 1993, Mosby.)

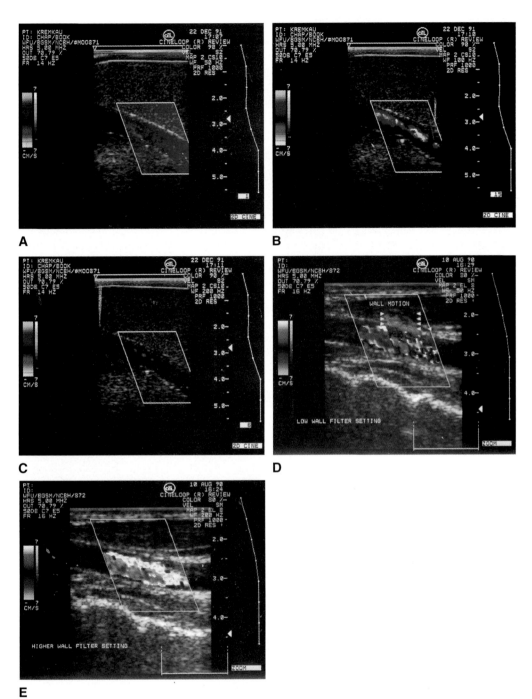

■ **FIGURE I-22**   **A,** Tissue motion causes clutter, obscuring the flow in the vessel and clouding the gray-scale tissue with color Doppler information. **B,** Wall filter has been increased to 100 Hz, thereby eliminating the color clutter. **C,** Wall filter has been increased (too much) to 200 Hz, eliminating virtually all the color Doppler information derived from the vessel. **D,** With a low wall filter setting (50 Hz), wall motion appears in color on the image. **E,** With a higher wall filter setting (200 Hz), this motion no longer appears in color. (See Color Plates 9 and 10.) (**A** to **C** from Kremkau FW: Principles and pitfalls of real-time color-flow imaging. In Bernstein EF, editor: *Vascular diagnosis,* ed 4, St Louis, 1993, Mosby; **D** and **E** from Kremkau FW: Principles and instrumentation. In Merritt CRB, editor: *Doppler color imaging,* New York, 1992, Churchill Livingstone.)

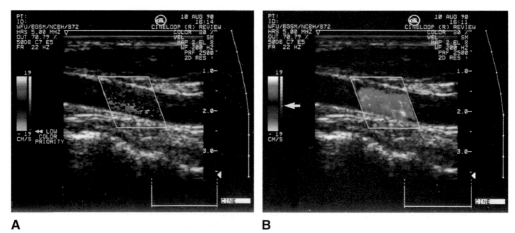

A **B**

■ **FIGURE I-23** **A,** With the color priority set low (at the bottom of the gray bar), weak, non–Doppler-shifted reverberation and off-axis echoes within the vessel take precedence over the Doppler-shifted echoes, and little color is displayed. **B,** With a higher color priority setting (halfway up the gray bar *(arrow)*), the Doppler-shifted echoes *(color)* take precedence over the weaker gray-scale echoes. (See Color Plate 11.) (From Kremkau FW: Principles and instrumentation. In Merritt CRB, editor: *Doppler color imaging,* New York, 1992, Churchill Livingstone.)

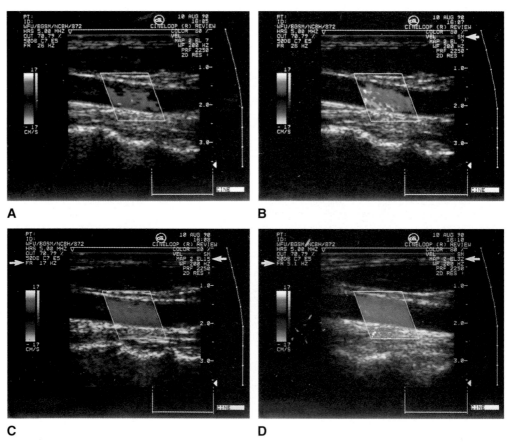

■ **FIGURE I-24** **A,** With no smoothing (persistence), only the Doppler-shifted echoes received from the pulses generating an individual frame are shown. **B,** With smoothing, consecutive frames are averaged, filling gaps in the presentation and presenting a smoother but less detailed representation of flow. **C** and **D,** More accurate and complete detection of flow information is obtained with increasing ensemble lengths. The ensemble lengths shown are 7 **(B),** 15 **(C),** and 32 **(D).** Note the decrease in frame rate from 26 to 17 to 5.1 frames per second. (See Color Plates 12 and 13.) (From Kremkau FW: Principles and instrumentation. In Merritt CRB, editor: *Doppler color imaging,* New York, 1992, Churchill Livingstone.)

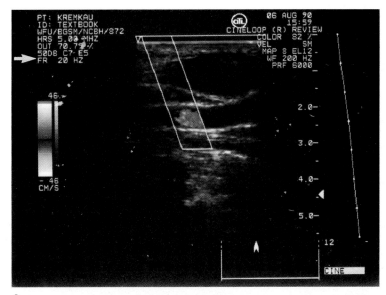

A

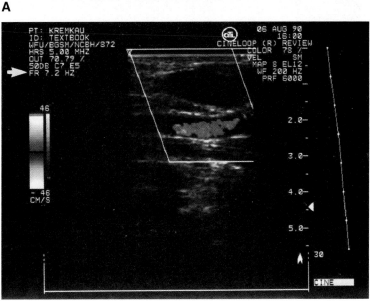

B

■ **FIGURE I-25**   Tripling the color window width decreases the frame rate from 20 Hz **(A)** to 7.2 Hz **(B).** (See Color Plate 14.) (From Kremkau FW: Principles and instrumentation. In Merritt CRB, editor: *Doppler color imaging,* New York, 1992, Churchill Livingstone.)

Color Doppler Limitations

Several aspects of color Doppler imaging are, by their nature, limiting. These aspects include angle dependence, lower frame rates, and lack of detailed spectral information. Spectral Doppler presents the entire range of Doppler-shift frequencies received as they change over the cardiac cycle. Color Doppler displays present only a statistical representation of the complete spectrum at each pixel location on the display. The sign, mean value, and, if chosen, the power or the variance of the spectrum are color-coded into combinations of **hue, satura-**tion, and **luminance** that are presented at each display pixel location. Some Doppler instruments have the capability of reading the quantitative digital values for mean Doppler shift (sometimes converted to angle-corrected equivalent flow speed) at chosen pixel locations (Figure I-26 [Color Plate 15, Figure 6-11]). One must realize that these are mean values that must be compared carefully with the peak systolic values that are used commonly to evaluate spectral displays. Because color Doppler techniques require several pulses per scan line (as opposed to one pulse per scan line for single-focus, gray-scale anatomic imaging), frame rates are

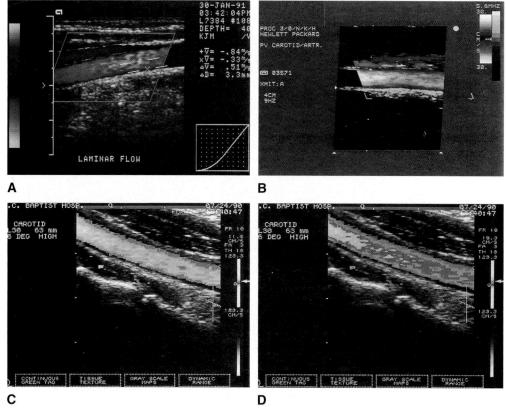

■ FIGURE I-26 **A,** Digital readout of stored mean Doppler shift (converted to mean flow speed) at specific pixel locations. Conversion to speed requires angle correction, just as in spectral Doppler techniques. The value at the vessel center (84 cm/s) is greater than at the edge (33 cm/s), as expected for laminar flow. **B,** Laminar flow. The color bar used in this scan progresses from dark red and dark blue to bright white (indicating decreasing saturation and increasing luminance). The regions near the vessel wall are dark, with progressive brightening and decreasing saturation to white at the center left. This corresponds to the low flow speeds at the vessel wall and high flow speeds at the vessel center that are characteristic of laminar flow. **C,** The green tag is set at a specific level (11.6; *arrow*) on an angle-corrected, calibrated color bar. The green region on the display, therefore, indicates areas where that specific flow speed exists. **D,** The green tag is set at 19.3. As the set flow speed value increases, the indicated region (*green*) moves to the center, where higher speeds are expected. (See Color Plate 15.) (**A** from Kremkau FW: *Semin Roentgenol* 27:6-16, 1992; **B** to **D** from Kremkau FW: Principles and instrumentation. In Merritt CRB, editor: *Doppler color imaging*, New York, 1992, Churchill Livingstone.)

lower than those for gray-scale anatomic imaging. Therefore multiple foci are not used in color Doppler. The relationship between penetration *(pen)*, line density, and frame rate is the same as presented in Chapter 4 except that ensemble length *(n)* replaces number of foci. The maximum permissible frame rate *(FR$_m$)* is as follows:

$$FR_m \text{ (Hz)} = \frac{77,000 \text{ (cm/s)}}{[\text{pen (cm)} \times \text{LPF} \times n]}$$

where *LPF* is lines per frame.

If ensemble length increases, frame rate decreases.

Doppler-Shift Displays

Where Doppler-shifted echoes have been stored, hue, saturation, and luminance appropriate to the shift information are presented according to a choice of schemes, the one selected being presented on the display as a color map (Figure I-27 [Color Plates 17 and 18, Figure 6-13]). The map allows the observer to interpret what the hue, saturation, and luminance mean at each location in terms of sign, magnitude, and variance of the Doppler shifts. Hue indicates Doppler shift sign. Changes in hue, saturation, or luminance up or down the map from the center indicate increasing Doppler-shift magnitude. When selected, variance is shown as a change in hue from left to right across the map.

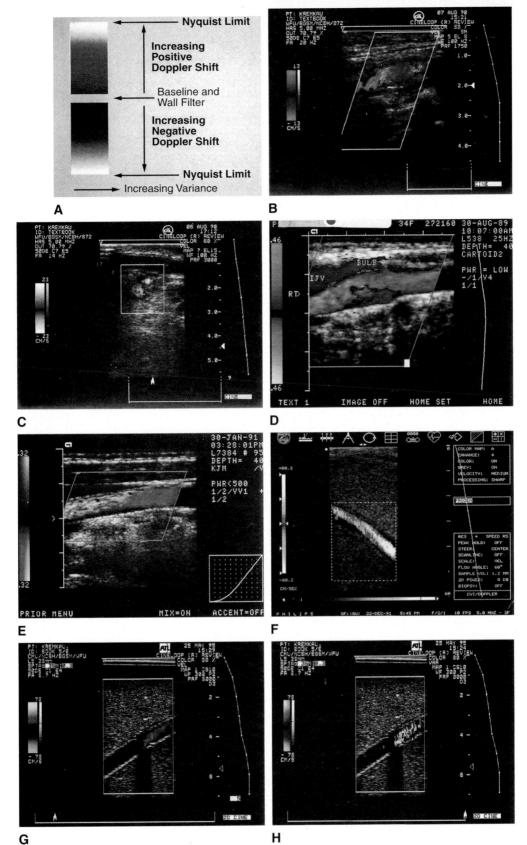

■ **FIGURE I-27** Color map information. **A,** Diagram describing the information contained in a color map or color bar. The color wheel type of map is shown in Figure I-23, *A*, and has the baseline at the bottom and the Nyquist limits joined at the top. **B,** A luminance map. Increasing luminance of red or blue indicates, respectively, increasing positive or negative mean Doppler shifts. **C,** A saturation map is used to show flow transversely in two vessels. Flow in the upper vessel is toward the transducer, yielding positive Doppler shifts *(red).* Flow in the lower vessel is away from the transducer, yielding negative Doppler shifts *(blue).* On this color map, red and blue progress to white (decreasing saturation, increasing luminance) with increasing positive and negative Doppler shift means, respectively. **D,** A hue map showing flow in the carotid artery (with reversal in the bulb) and jugular vein. Increasingly positive Doppler shifts progress from dark blue to bright cyan (blue plus green). Increasingly negative Doppler shifts progress from dark red to bright yellow (red plus green). **E,** A luminance (dark blue and red to bright blue and red) map with variance included. Increasing variance adds green to red or blue (producing yellow or cyan), progressing from left to right across the map. **F,** A saturation map. Red and blue progress toward white. **G,** A stenosis in a tube *(located at the shadow)* increases the flow speed. Proximal to *(left of)* the stenosis, flow speed is too slow to be detected, whereas distal to *(right of)* the stenosis, positive Doppler shifts are seen. **H,** The variance map shows spectral broadening *(green)* in the turbulent flow region distal to the stenosis. (See Color Plates 17 and 18.) (**A** from Kremkau FW: Principles and instrumentation. In Merritt CRB, editor: *Doppler color imaging,* New York, 1992, Churchill Livingstone; **B** to **F** from Kremkau FW: *J Vasc Technol* 15:104-111, 1991.)

⊚ *The color map, always shown on the display, is the key to understanding how the image colors are related to the Doppler characteristics.*

Angle

As with any Doppler technique, angle is important. Figure I-28 (Color Plates 19 and 20, Figure 6-14) shows convex array and linear array views of vascular flow. Note that the images are similar in appearance, with red on the left and blue on the right. But note that the relative position of the color bars is inverted. How is this inconsistency explained? In fact, why does the color change at all, considering that there is no reason not to expect unidirectional flow in these vessels? The color changes in the vessel in *A* because, with the sector image format, pulses and scan lines travel in different directions away from the transducer. They thus have different Doppler angles with the flow in a straight vessel. Some pulses view the flow upstream and some downstream. At the 90-degree Doppler angle point, the color changes because the situation changes from upstream to downstream. However, in *C* this is not the case. All the pulses travel in the same direction (straight down) from this linear array transducer. If the color change is not due to changing scan line directions, then it must be due to changing flow direction. Careful inspection of *C* reveals that the vessel is not perfectly straight but curves up. Flow is from right to left in the vessel, so that flow is away from the transducer on the right (negative Doppler shift is blue on this map) and toward the transducer on the left (positive Doppler shift is red; Figure I-28, *D*). A view further to the left reveals a second color change caused by the curve downward (Figure I-28, *E*). Figure I-28, *F*, shows an example of lack of color in a vessel. This lack of Doppler shift could be caused by lack of flow or flow viewed with a 90-degree Doppler angle. With an acceptable angle (Figure I-28, *G*), flow is revealed.

⊚ *Changing Doppler angle in an image produces various colors in different locations.*

Figure I-29, *A* (Color Plate 21, Figure 6-15, *A*), shows various Doppler shifts as Doppler angle changes across the display in the sector format. Yellow corresponds to a large positive shift, red to a small positive shift, black to a zero shift, blue to a small negative shift, and cyan to a large negative shift. Flow is from left to right. Figure I-29, *B* to *F*, confirms all this by spectral displays, which are discussed later in this appendix.

In Figure I-30 (Color Plate 22, Figure 6-16, *A, C,* and *D*), some interesting questions arise. First, in *A*, what is the blood flow direction? According to the color map in the upper left-hand corner of the figure, negative Doppler shifts are coded in red and yellow, whereas positive Doppler shifts are coded in blue and cyan. The color scan lines (and pulses) are steered to the left, and negative Doppler shifts (red and yellow) are received from the blood flowing within the vessel in the upper and lower portions of the figure. If we are looking to the left and seeing blood flowing away from us (negative Doppler shifts), the blood must be flowing from right to left in the upper and lower horizontal portions of the vessel. What about the central portion of the vessel? Clearly, the blood would have to be flowing from left to right there, but why are negative Doppler shifts also seen in this portion? The answer is that this portion of the vessel is not horizontal but is angled down, so that even though the blood is flowing from left to right, it is also flowing away from the transducer because of the downward direction (more precisely, it is flowing from upper left to lower right). Thus negative Doppler shifts are found throughout the vessel in this scan. Another way to say this is that the flow direction gets close to but never crosses the perpendicular to the scan lines (Figure I-30, *B*).

Another intriguing question arises with respect to Figure I-30, *A*: Does the yellow region in the bend at the upper left indicate where the blood flows fastest? According to the color map, this region is where the highest negative Doppler shifts are generated. Does that mean, however, that this is where the highest flow speeds are encountered? The answer in this case is no. The highest negative Doppler shifts are found in this region because the smallest Doppler angles are encountered there, not because high flow speeds are found there. In this region the flow is approximately parallel to the scan lines (Figure I-30, *B*), yielding Doppler angles of around zero. No evidence of vessel narrowing is present to explain increased flow speed. The increased Doppler shift can be explained purely on grounds of angle.

In Figure I-30, *C*, the region shown in cyan (aqua or blue-green) indicates positive Doppler shifts according to the color map, whereas the blood flow in the rest of the vessel is generating negative Doppler shifts (red and yellow). Again, the scan lines are steered to the left, so that negative Doppler shifts indicate that we are looking downstream, seeing flow away from the transducer. Therefore blood flow is from right to left in this carotid artery, with the head oriented to the left as usual. How then can we explain the positive Doppler shifts found in the upper left-hand portion of the vessel? Possibilities include turbulent flow, flow reversal, and flow speed exceeding 32 cm/s in this region, producing aliasing.

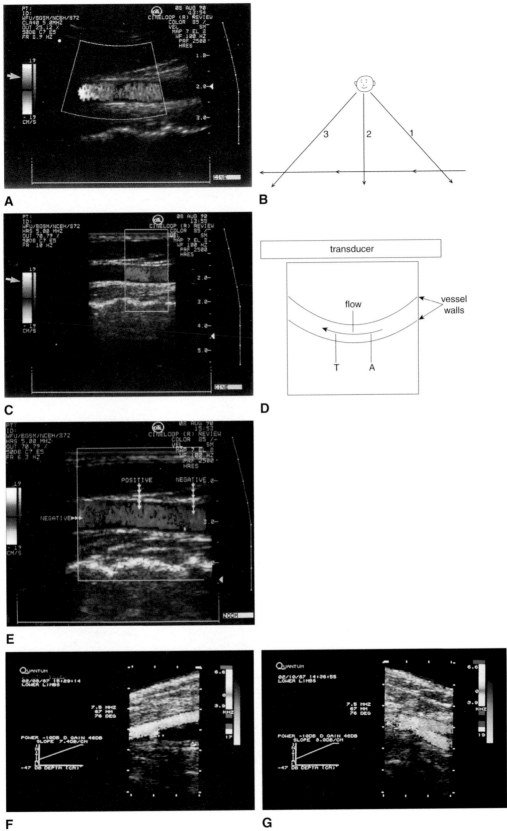

■ FIGURE I-28   **A,** In this saturation map, blue and red are assigned to positive and negative Doppler shifts, respectively, progressing to white at the extremes. **B,** With flow moving from right to left, an observer looking to the right *(1)* is looking upstream; when looking to the left *(3)*, the observer has a downstream view. The perpendicular view *(2)* is neither upstream nor downstream. **C,** In this map the color assignments are reversed from those in **A** (i.e., red and blue are assigned to positive and negative Doppler shifts, respectively). **D,** Exaggerated representation of the image in **C** in which point A represents flow away from the transducer and point T represents flow toward the transducer. **E,** Extension to the left of the color box in **C** reveals another color change caused by vessel curvature (concave-down). **F,** The profunda branch off the femoral artery appears to have no flow (no color within it). **G,** This view of the profunda shows color within it. The 90-degree Doppler angle in **F** causes no Doppler shift, and therefore color is lacking. (See Color Plates 19 and 20.) (**A** and **C** from Kremkau FW: *J Vasc Technol* 15:104-111, 1991; **E** from Kremkau FW: *CJ Vasc Technol* 15:265-266, 1991.)

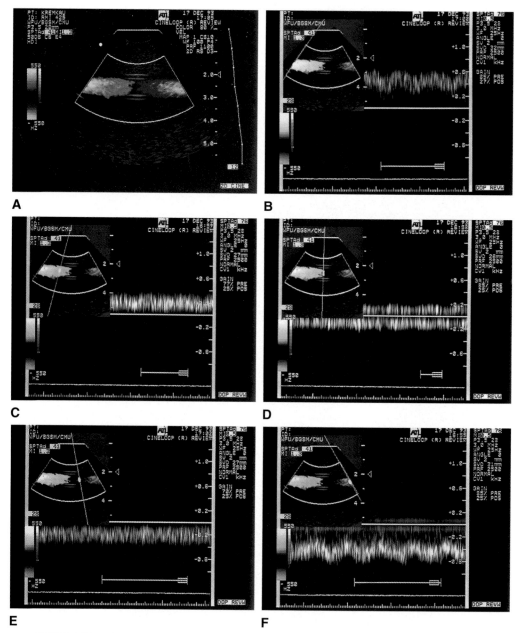

■ **FIGURE I-29** Sector format, color Doppler presentation of flow from left to right in a straight tube. **A,** Approximate Doppler shifts (from the color map) are yellow (500 Hz), red (200 Hz), black (0 Hz), blue (−200 Hz), and cyan (−500 Hz). (See Color Plate 21.) Spectra from these five regions, shown in **B** to **F,** confirm these estimates. Doppler shifts decrease as Doppler angles increase toward the center of the color window.

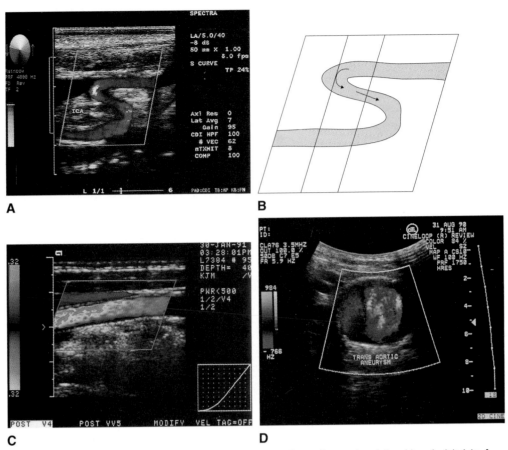

■ **FIGURE I-30** **A,** A tortuous artery. **B,** This drawing shows the angle relationships depicted in **A.** **C,** A (nearly) straight artery. **D,** Circular flow in an aneurysm. The black area between the red and blue areas indicates true flow reversal. (See Color Plate 22.) (**A** and **C** from Kremkau FW: *J Vasc Technol* 16:215-216, 1992.)

Flow reversal and turbulent flow can be eliminated because the region between the negative (red and yellow) and positive (cyan) Doppler shift regions contains no dark or black region (baseline indicating flow reversal). One easily can distinguish between true flow reversal (which involves dark regions, as shown around the baseline of the color bar) (Figure I-30, *D*) and aliasing (which involves bright colors, as indicated at the bar extremes). Thus the aqua region is a region of flow away from the transducer that has exceeded the negative aliasing limit of 32 cm/s and has become an aliased positive Doppler shift (cyan).

Does this mean that the flow speed in the aliased aqua region exceeds 32 cm/s? In this case the answer is no. The aliasing limit, which is one half the PRF, has been exceeded. This aliasing limit has been converted, using the Doppler equation, to an equivalent flow speed of 32 cm/s, as indicated at the map extremes. However, because there is no angle correction in this scan, an angle of zero was assumed in the conversion from Doppler shift to flow speed. Therefore aliased flow

exceeds 32 cm/s only when it is parallel to the scan lines. Because the Doppler angle in this example is approximately 60 degrees, the Doppler shifts are only about one half what they would be at 0 degrees. Therefore the flow in the aliased region has exceeded approximately 64 cm/s. One must exercise care in estimating flow speeds with tagging (Figure I-26, *C* and *D*) or aliasing limits that are converted to flow speed units without correcting for angle.

Proper understanding of the effects of angle on Doppler shift and of how color is related to Doppler shift is necessary to interpret complicated images properly.

Doppler-Power Displays

Doppler-shift displays encode mean Doppler *shifts* in a two-dimensional matrix according to the color map selected. Doppler-power displays present two-dimensional Doppler information by color-encoding the strength of the Doppler shifts. This approach is free of aliasing and angle dependence and is more sensitive to slow flow and flow in small or deep vessels. Names applied to this technique include color power Doppler, ultrasound angio, color Doppler energy, and color power angio. Rather than assigning various hue, saturation, and luminance values to mean Doppler-shift frequency values, as in Doppler-shift displays, this technique assigns these values to Doppler-shift power values. The power of the Doppler shifts is determined by the concentration of moving scatterers producing the Doppler shifts and is independent of Doppler-shift frequency (and thus independent of Doppler angle). In addition to the colors already encountered, magenta (a combination of red and blue) is used on some Doppler-power maps.

Doppler-power displays color-encoded Doppler-shift power values on the display.

Advantages and Disadvantages

The Doppler detector in color Doppler imaging instruments yields the sign, mean, variance, and amplitude and power of the **Doppler spectrum** (Figure I-31, *A*) at each of hundreds of **sample volume** locations in an anatomic cross section. Traditionally, in color Doppler imaging, sign and mean Doppler shift, and sometimes variance (usually in cardiac applications), are color-encoded and displayed. These parameters depend on Doppler angle and are subject to aliasing (Figure I-32, *A* [Color Plate 25, Figure 6-20, *A*]). Power Doppler integrates the area under the spectrum (Figure I-31, *B*). This area is independent of angle and aliasing, displaying the effects of neither (Figure I-32, *B* [Color Plate 25, Figure 6-20, *B*]). Thus an advantage of **Doppler-power display** is the uniform (angle-independent and alias-free) presentation of flow information, although this is accomplished with a loss in direction, speed, and flow character information. This extends even through

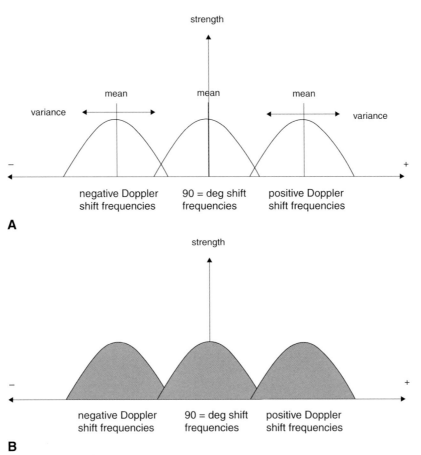

■ **FIGURE I-31** **A,** Spectra for flow toward *(positive)* and away from *(negative)* the transducer and perpendicular (90 degrees) to the sound beam. Conventional color Doppler imaging determines and displays, in color-coded form, the sign and mean (and sometimes the variance) of the Doppler-shift frequency spectrum. **B,** Power Doppler determines and displays, in color-coded form, the size of the area under the spectral curve. The axes of the spectral graph represent strength (amplitude, power, energy, or intensity) versus frequency.

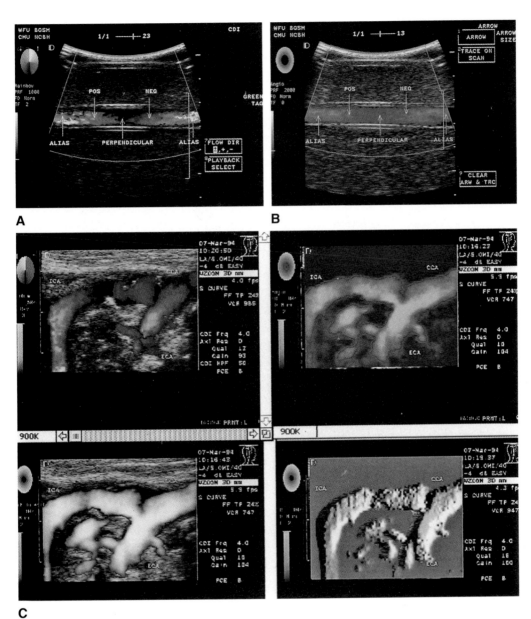

■ FIGURE I-32   A, A color Doppler-shift image of flow in a straight tube, acquired in sector format. The varying Doppler angle from left to right yields aliasing and positive, negative, and zero Doppler-shift regions. **B,** A Doppler-power presentation of the situation shown in **A** yields a uniform image, free of angle dependence and aliasing. However, it contains no directional, speed, or dynamic information. **C,** Angle independence is seen in the Doppler-power images of the carotid artery; compare them to the Doppler-shift display *(upper left)*. Doppler-power imaging is shown in color, topographic, and gray-scale forms *(clockwise from upper right)*. (See also Figure 1-13, *B,* and Color Plates 1 and 25.)

TABLE I-6 **Comparison of Doppler-Shift and Doppler-Power Displays**

	Doppler-Shift Display	Doppler-Power Display
Quantitative	No	No
Global	Yes	Yes
Perfusion	No	Yes

regions of 90-degree Doppler angle (Figure I-32, *B* and *C* [Color Plate 25, Figures 6-20, *B* and *C*]) because the Doppler shift spectrum there has a nonzero area (Figure I-31, *B*), even though its mean is zero, yielding a black region in color Doppler imaging displays (Figure I-32, *A* and *C* [Color Plate 25], Figures 6-20, *A* and *C*). Power Doppler is also essentially free of variations in flow speed (as in the cardiac cycle) and thus can be frame-averaged to improve the signal-to-noise ratio and sensitivity substantially (Figure I-33 [Color Plates 26 and 27, Figure 6-21]). Because aliasing is not a problem in power Doppler, lower PRFs can be used to detect slow flows. Box I-3 lists the advantages and disadvantages of Doppler-power displays. In general, Doppler ultrasound can determine the presence or absence of flow, the direction and speed of flow, and the character of flow. Power Doppler is superior in terms of the first, but at the expense of the other three. Table I-6 compares color Doppler displays.

Doppler-power displays do not have direction, speed, or flow character information included and are insensitive to angle effects and aliasing. they are more sensitive than Doppler-shift displays in that they can present slower flows and flow in deeper or tinier vessels.

SPECTRAL DOPPLER INSTRUMENTS

In addition to color Doppler instruments, two types of spectral Doppler instruments are used for Doppler detection of flow in the heart and blood vessels: continuous wave (CW) and pulsed wave. All three often are combined into one multipurpose instrument (Figure I-34). The CW instrument detects Doppler-shifted echoes in the region of overlap between the beams of the transmitting and receiving transducer elements. A difference between other transducers and those designed exclusively for CW Doppler use is that the latter are not damped. The pulsed wave Doppler instrument emits ultrasound pulses and receives echoes using a single element transducer or an array. Because of the required Doppler frequency shift detection, the pulses are longer than those used in imaging. Through **range gating**, pulsed wave Doppler has the ability to select information from a particular depth along the beam. To use pulsed wave Doppler effectively, it commonly is combined with gray-scale sonography in one instrument. Such instruments are called duplex scanners because of their dual functions (anatomic imaging *and* flow measurement). Continuous wave and pulsed wave instruments present Doppler-shift information in audible form and as a visual display.

Continuous Wave Instruments

Spectral Doppler instruments provide continuous or pulsed voltages to the transducer and convert echo voltages received from the transducer to audible and visual information corresponding to scatterer motion. If an instrument distinguishes between positive and negative Doppler shifts, it is called **bidirectional**. **Continuous wave Doppler** instruments include a CW oscillator and a Doppler detector that detects the changes in frequency (Doppler shifts) resulting from scatterer motion for presentation as audible sounds and as a visual presentation corresponding to the motion.

Components of a Continuous Wave Doppler System

A diagram of the components of a CW Doppler system is presented in Figure I-35, *A*. The oscillator produces a continuously alternating voltage with a 2- to 10-MHz frequency, which is applied to the source transducer element. The ultrasound frequency is determined by the oscillator and is set to equal the operating frequency of the transducer. In the transducer assembly is a separate receiving transducer element that produces voltages with frequencies equal to the frequencies of the returning echoes. If there is scatterer motion, the reflected ultrasound and the ultrasound produced by the source transducer will have different frequencies. The Doppler detector detects the difference between these two

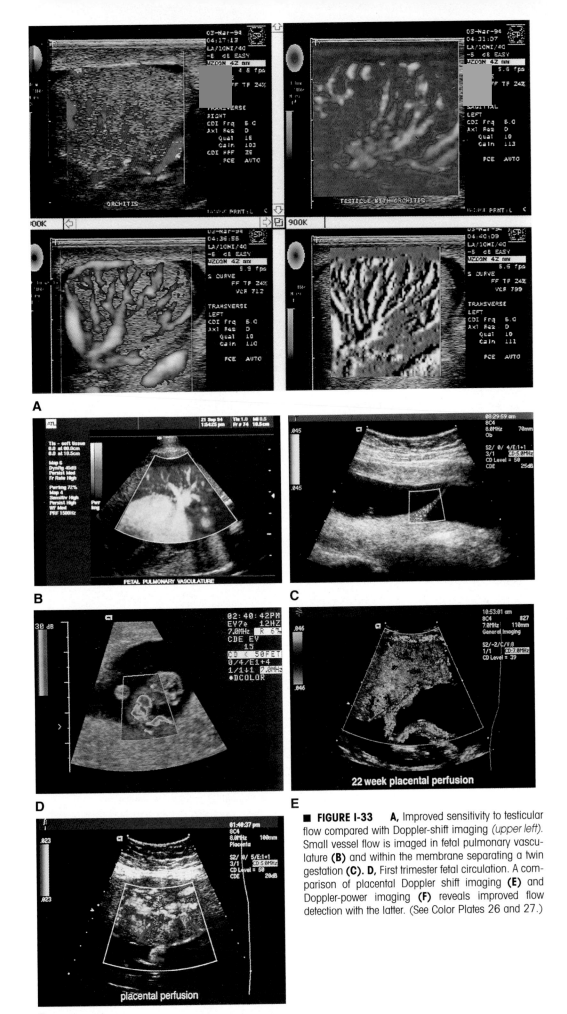

■ **FIGURE I-33** **A,** Improved sensitivity to testicular flow compared with Doppler-shift imaging *(upper left).* Small vessel flow is imaged in fetal pulmonary vasculature **(B)** and within the membrane separating a twin gestation **(C). D,** First trimester fetal circulation. A comparison of placental Doppler shift imaging **(E)** and Doppler-power imaging **(F)** reveals improved flow detection with the latter. (See Color Plates 26 and 27.)

frequencies, which is the Doppler shift, and drives a loudspeaker at this frequency. Doppler shifts are typically one thousandth of the operating frequency, which puts them in the audible range. The Doppler shifts also commonly are sent through a **spectrum analyzer** to a **spectral display** for visual observation and evaluation.

The detector (Figure I-35, *B*) amplifies the echo voltages it receives from the receiving element, detects the Doppler-shift information in the returning echoes, and usually determines motion direction from the

sign of the Doppler shift. Doppler shifts are determined by mixing the returning voltages with the CW voltage from the oscillator. This produces the sum and difference of the oscillator and echo frequencies (Figure I-35, *B*). The difference is the desired Doppler shift. The sum is a much higher frequency (approximately double the operating frequency) and is filtered out easily. The difference is zero for echoes returning from stationary structures. For echoes from moving structures or flowing blood, this difference is the Doppler shift, which provides information about motion and flow.

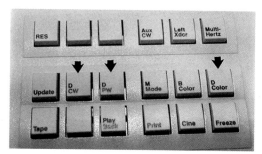

■ **FIGURE I-34** Continuous wave (CW), pulsed wave (PW), and color Doppler instruments can be combined in one device, with each mode selectable from the control panel (*arrows*).

The Doppler detector detects Doppler shifts and determines their sign.

Positive and negative shifts indicate motion toward and away from the transducer, respectively. The detector shown in Figure I-35, *B*, does not provide this directional information. Determining direction and separating Doppler-shift voltages into separate forward and reverse channels is accomplished by the **phase quadrature** detector (Figure I-36).

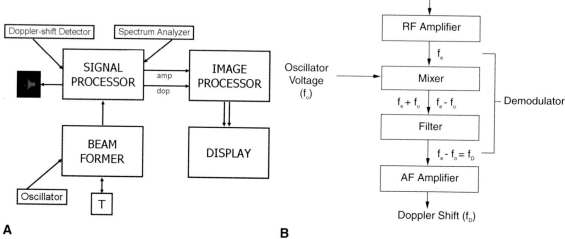

A **B**

■ **FIGURE I-35** **A,** Block diagram of a sonographic instrument functioning as a continuous wave Doppler instrument. The oscillator (part of the beam former) produces a continuously alternating voltage that drives the source transducer element (*T*). The receiving transducer element (*T*) produces a continuous voltage in response to echoes it continuously is receiving. The signal processor includes a Doppler-shift detector that detects differences in frequency between the voltages produced by the oscillator and by the receiving element. The Doppler shifts produce voltages that drive loudspeakers and a visual display. The frequency of the audible sound is equal to the Doppler shift and is proportional to the reflector speed and to the cosine of the angle between the sound propagation direction and the boundary motion. **B,** Block diagram of a continuous wave Doppler detector. The radio frequency (*RF*) amplifier increases the echo voltage amplitude. The frequency of the echo voltage is f_e. In the mixer, this frequency is combined with the oscillator voltage, the frequency of which is f_o. The mixer yields the sum and difference of these two frequency inputs ($f_e + f_o$ and $f_e - f_o$). The low-pass (high-frequency rejection) filter removes $f_e + f_o$, leaving $f_e - f_o$, which is the Doppler-shift frequency (f_D). This frequency then is strengthened in the audio frequency (*AF*) amplifier. The mixer and filter together constitute the Doppler demodulator.

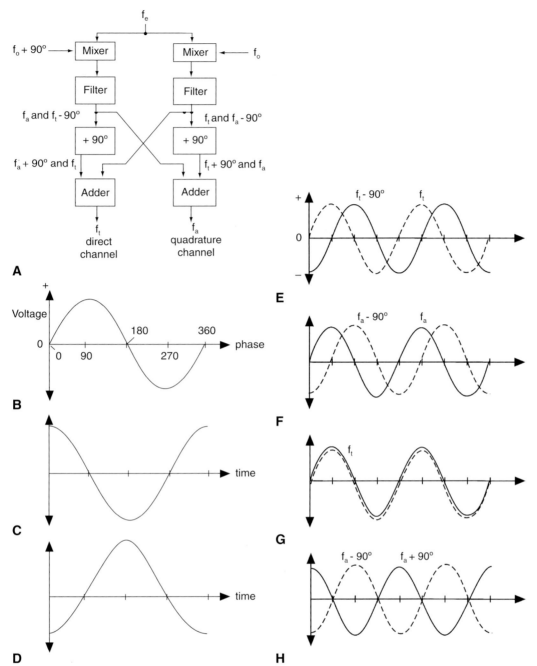

■ FIGURE I-36   A, The phase quadrature detector detects the positive (f_t) and negative (f_a) Doppler shifts contained in the incoming echo voltage (f_e) and separates them into separate channels for delivery to loudspeakers and visual display. These channels are designated as direct and quadrature *(on the left and right,* respectively). Detection proceeds as described in the following. The echo voltage is mixed with the oscillator voltage (f_o) in two mixers. The oscillator voltage in the direct channel leads that in the quadrature channel by one-quarter cycle (90 degrees). This is illustrated in **C,** which leads **B** by 90 degrees (one-quarter cycle). **B** illustrates one complete variation (cycle) of alternating voltage that may be thought of as traveling around a 360-degree circle. One quarter of a cycle is 90 degrees of phase angle. Phase is a description of progression through a cycle (analogous to the phase of the moon). One quarter of a cycle is 90 degrees, and one half of a cycle is 180 degrees. The completion of a cycle occurs at 360 degrees, but this is also the zero-degree phase of the next cycle. **D** lags **B** by 90 degrees. If the voltages in **C** and **D** are added together, a zero voltage results. (The two voltages are equal and opposite, so they cancel each other when summed.) Returning to **A,** the frequency sum $(f_e + f_o)$ is filtered out, as in Figure I-35, *B,* yielding the Doppler shift f_D, which is $f_e - f_o$. The Doppler shift may be positive $(f_t,$ for flow toward the transducer) or negative $(f_a,$ for flow away from the transducer). Because of the oscillator-voltage phase difference ($f_o + 90$ degrees versus f_o), the two filter outputs are different. Positive shifts in the direct channel lag those in the quadrature channel by 90 degrees. This is illustrated in **E.** In **E** to **H,** the solid curves refer to the direct channel, whereas the dashed curves refer to quadrature. The vertical and horizontal axes represent voltage and time, respectively. In **E,** positive Doppler shifts (f_t) at the output of the direct channel filter lag those in the quadrature channel by 90 degrees. **F,** Negative Doppler shifts (f_a) at the output of the quadrature channel lag those in the direct channel by 90 degrees. **G,** Positive Doppler shifts at the input to the direct channel adder are in phase (zero-degree phase difference), yielding an f_t output. **H,** Negative Doppler shifts at the input to the direct channel adder are 180 degrees out of phase, yielding a zero f_a output. Returning to **A,** negative shifts in the quadrature channel lag those in the direct channel by 90 degrees **(F).** Next, another 90-degree phase shift results in the separation of the positive and negative shifts into separate channels—direct and quadrature, respectively—as follows. The phase-shifted positive Doppler shifts in the direct channel are now in phase with the unshifted ones in the quadrature channel **(G),** whereas the negative shifts are 180 degrees out of phase **(H).** When added together, the negative shifts will cancel **(C** and **D),** yielding positive shifts as the output voltage in the direct channel. A similar process in the quadrature channel yields the negative shifts as output.

The forward and reverse channel signals are sent to separate loudspeakers so that forward and reverse Doppler shifts can be heard separately. The signals also are sent to a visual display to show positive and negative Doppler shifts above and below the display baseline, which represents zero Doppler shift (Figure I-37).

Continuous Wave Sample Volume

A CW instrument detects flow that occurs anywhere within the intersection of the transmitting and receiving beams of the dual-transducer assembly (Figure I-38, D). The sample volume is the region from which Doppler-shifted echoes return and are presented audibly or visually. In this case, the sample volume is the overlapping region of the transmitting and receiving beams. Because the sample volume is large, CW Doppler systems can give complicated and confusing presentations if two or more different motions or flows are included in the sample volume (e.g., two blood vessels being viewed simultaneously). **Pulsed Doppler** systems solve this problem by detecting motion or flow at a selected depth with a relatively small sample volume. However, the large sample volume of a CW system is helpful when searching for a Doppler maximum associated with a vascular or valvular stenosis.

Because a distribution of flow velocities is encountered by the beam as it traverses a vessel, a distribution of many Doppler-shifted frequencies returns to the transducer and the instrument. In arterial circulation or in the heart, these Doppler shifts are changing continually over the cardiac cycle and are displayed as a function of time with appropriate real-time frequency-spectrum processing (Figure I-39). These displays provide quantitative data for evaluating Doppler-shifted echoes. The display device is again the cathode-ray tube or flat-panel display. The displayed Doppler information is stored in digital memory before display so that it can be frozen and backed up over the last few seconds of information before freezing.

Angle Incorporation or Correction

To convert a display correctly from Doppler shift versus time to flow speed versus time, the Doppler angle must be incorporated accurately into the calculation process (Figure I-40). This incorporation commonly is called "angle correction." Either term is appropriate because lack of angle incorporation leaves the instrument to assume the Doppler angle is zero, which is incorrect unless the angle is in fact zero. Figure I-40, B and C, illustrates the importance of accurate angle correction. Figure I-40, C to F, shows errors encountered when the Doppler angle is handled incorrectly. Recall that as angle increases, Doppler shift decreases. Thus when the angle indicator on the instrument is set at 60 degrees, the instrument responds by doubling the calculated

flow speed from what is would have been at a Doppler angle of zero. Another way to say this is that the Doppler equation, arranged to have calculated flow speed alone on one side of the equal sign, has cosine Doppler angle in the denominator on the other side. As the angle indicator is increased, the cosine decreases, increasing the calculated speed value. This compensates for the reduction in Doppler shift caused by the Doppler angle actually involved in the ultrasound beam and flow intersection. For example, if the actual Doppler angle is 60 degrees, the Doppler shift is half what it would have been at 0 degrees. If the angle is set properly on the instrument at 60, the cosine in the denominator of the Doppler equation is set at 0.5. This doubles the calculated flow speed to the correct value.

The Doppler sample volume of a continuous wave Doppler instrument is relatively large, being the overlapping region of the transmission and reception beams.

Wall Filter

In vascular studies, to eliminate the high-intensity, low-frequency Doppler-shift echoes called clutter caused by heart or vessel wall or cardiac valve motion with pulsatile flow, a wall filter that rejects frequencies below an adjustable value is used (Figure I-41). Sometimes called a wall-thump filter, the **filter** rejects these strong echoes that otherwise would overwhelm the weaker echoes from the blood. These strong echoes have low Doppler-shift frequencies because the tissue structures do not move as fast as the blood does. The upper limit of the filter is adjustable over a range of about 25 to 3200 Hz. The filter, however, erroneously can alter conclusions regarding diastolic flow and distal flow resistance if not properly used.

Wall filters remove clutter (low-frequency Doppler shifts from moving tissue).

Pulsed Wave Instruments

A diagram of the components of a pulsed Doppler instrument is given in Figure I-42, A. The pulser (in the beam former) is similar to that in the sonographic instrument, except that it generates pulses of several cycles of voltage that drive the transducer where ultrasound pulses are produced. Recall that imaging pulses are two or three cycles long. Pulses used in Doppler

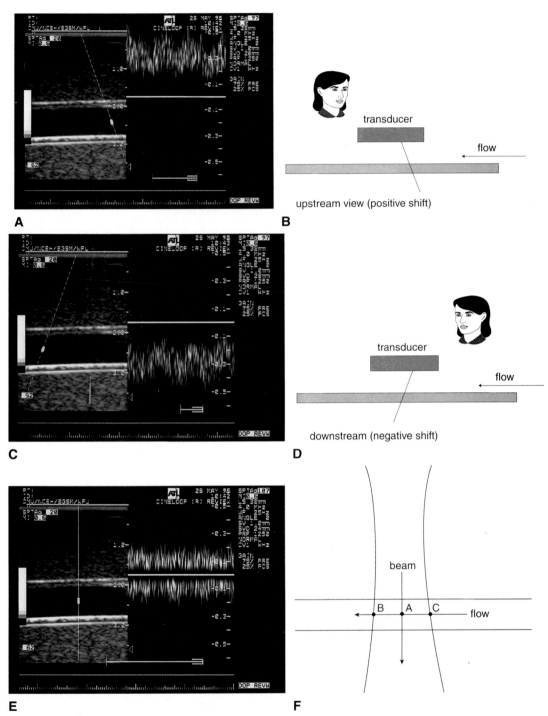

■ FIGURE I-37   The beam is steered to the right and positive Doppler shifts are received **(A).** Thus this is an upstream view **(B),** and flow is from right to left. Therefore steering the beam to the left **(C)** would provide a downstream view **(D)** with negative Doppler shifts. With the beam perpendicular to the flow **(E),** Doppler shifts *are* received, positive and negative, because of beam spreading **(F)**; that is, a portion of the beam views upstream while a portion views downstream. The beam axis portion (90-degree angle) yields a zero Doppler shift.

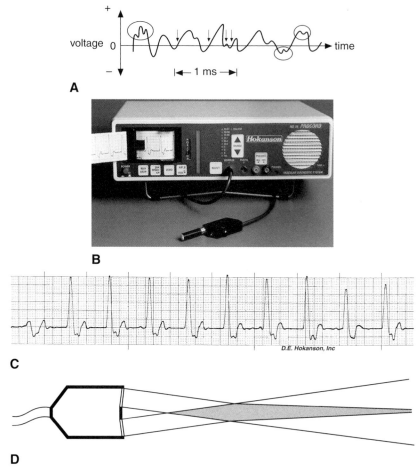

■ **FIGURE I-38** **A,** A zero-crossing detector counts the number of zero crossings per second in the positive or negative direction. In the 1-ms period shown, four zero crossings (negative to positive) occurred *(arrows)*, corresponding to a mean frequency of 4 kHz. Higher frequencies that are missed by the zero-crossing technique are circled. **B,** A zero-crossing continuous wave Doppler instrument. **C,** Chart output from a zero-crossing instrument shows an average Doppler shift. **D,** Continuous wave Doppler systems have dual-element transducer assemblies, one for transmitting and one for receiving. The region over which Doppler information can be acquired (Doppler sample volume) is the region of overlap between the transmitting and receiving beams *(shaded region)*.

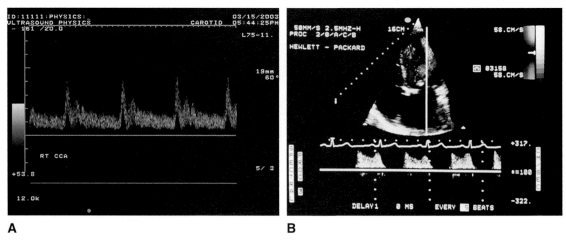

■ **FIGURE I-39** **A,** A display of Doppler-shift frequencies as a function of time. This is a pulsed Doppler spectral display. **B,** A cardiac continuous wave Doppler spectral display.

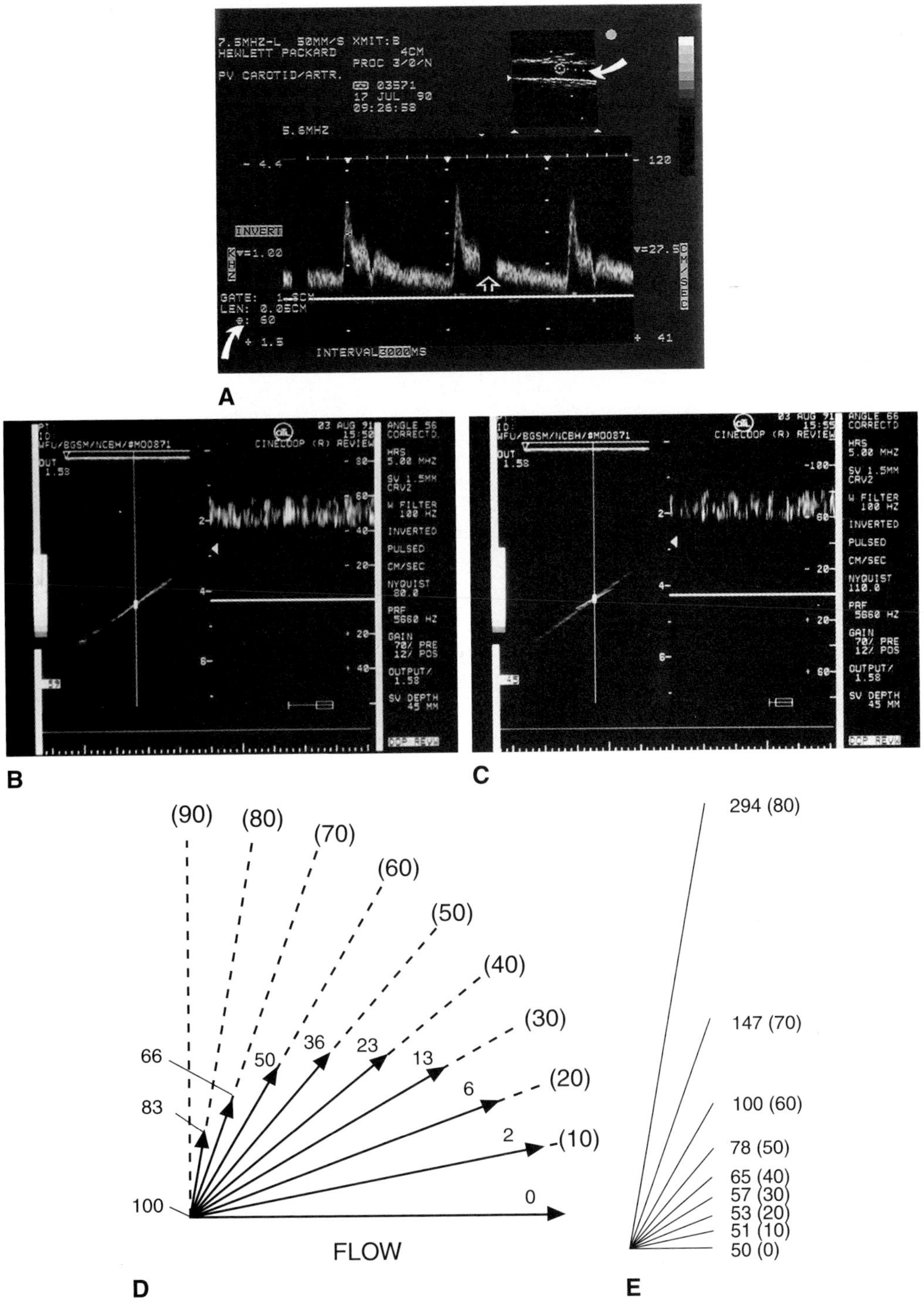

■ **FIGURE I-40** **A,** A spectral display with Doppler-shift (kilohertz) calibration of the vertical axis on the left and flow speed (centimeters per second) calibration on the right. Conversion from the former to the latter requires angle incorporation *(curved arrows)*. The Doppler angle in this example is 60 degrees. The gap in Doppler information *(open arrow)* occurs when the instrument takes time to generate a frame of the anatomic image *(upper right)*. **B** and **C,** A moving-string test object is imaged, resulting in the Doppler spectral display shown. With proper angle incorporation (56 degrees) the 50 cm/s string speed is shown correctly **(B).** With improper angle incorporation (66 degrees), an incorrect string speed of 70 cm/s is shown **(C).** This is a 40% error. **D,** If a zero Doppler angle is assumed correctly, there is zero error in the calculated flow speed. However, if the angle is actually nonzero, error results. The error in flow speed increases as the angle error *(in parentheses)* increases. For example, if the Doppler angle is 10 degrees but is assumed to be zero, the calculated flow speed will be 2% less than the correct value. At 60 and 80 degrees, the errors are 50% and 83%, respectively. At 90 degrees, there is zero Doppler shift. The calculated flow speed is zero (100% error). **E,** If the Doppler angle is zero but is assumed to be some other value, the calculated flow speeds are too large. Here the correct value is 50 cm/s. The error increases with angle *(in parentheses)*. For example, at 60 and 80 degrees, the calculated values are 100 and 294 cm/s, respectively.

Continued.

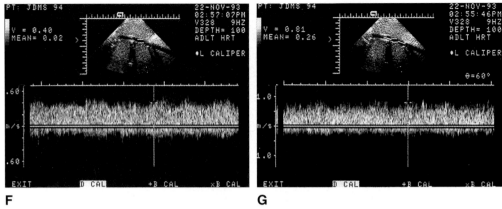

F   **G**

■ **FIGURE I-40, cont'd**   **F,** No angle correction is used in this display. The instrument assumes a Doppler angle of zero and calculates flow speed *(v)* at 40 cm/s. However, the Doppler angle is actually 60 degrees, yielding half the Doppler shift that a 0-degree angle would. **G,** When the cosine of 60 degrees (0.5) is incorporated into the Doppler equation, the result is 81 cm/s. (**B** and **C** from Kremkau FW: *Semin Roentgenol* 27:6-16, 1992; **F** and **G** from Kremkau FW: *J Diagn Med Sonogr* 10:337-338, 1994. Reprinted by permission of Sage Publications, Inc.)

instruments, however, have pulse lengths of about 5 to 30 cycles. This is necessary to determine the Doppler shifts of returning echoes accurately. Echo voltages from the transducer are processed in the detector. In the detector, echo voltages are amplified, their frequency is compared with the pulser frequency, and the Doppler shifts are determined. The Doppler shifts are sent to loudspeakers for audible output and to the display for visual observation. Based on their arrival time (recall the 13 μs/cm rule), echoes coming from reflectors at a given depth may be selected by the amplifier **gate.** Thus motion information may be obtained from a specific depth. This is called range gating. The operator controls the gate length and location.

Range gating enables depth selectivity and a small Doppler sample volume.

A pulsed Doppler instrument does not detect the complete Doppler shift as a CW instrument does but rather obtains samples of it because the pulsed instrument is a sampling system, with each pulse yielding a *sample* of the Doppler shift signal. The Doppler shifts are determined as described previously, except that the mixer does not receive a continuous input echo voltage but rather a sampled one. Echoes arrive from the sample volume depth in pulsed form at a rate equal to the pulse repetition frequency. Each of these returning echoes yields a sample of the Doppler shift from the Doppler detector. These samples are connected and smoothed (filtered) to yield the sampled waveform (Figure I-42, *B* to *E*).

A pulsed wave Doppler system is a sampling system.

Range Gate

The gate selects the sample volume location from which returning Doppler-shifted echoes are accepted (Table I-7 and Figures I-43 to I-45). The width of the sample volume is equal to the beam width. The gate has some length over which it permits reception (Table I-8). For example (applying the 13 μs/cm rule), a gate that passes echoes arriving from 13 to 15 μs after pulse generation is listening over a depth range of 10.0 to 11.5 mm. In this case, the gate is located at a depth of 10.8 mm with a length (depth range) of ±0.8 mm. Longer gate lengths

TABLE I-7   Echo Arrival Time for Various Reflector Depths (Gate Locations)

Depth (mm)	Time (μs)
10	13
20	26
30	39
40	52
50	65
60	78
70	91
80	104
90	117
100	130
150	195
200	260

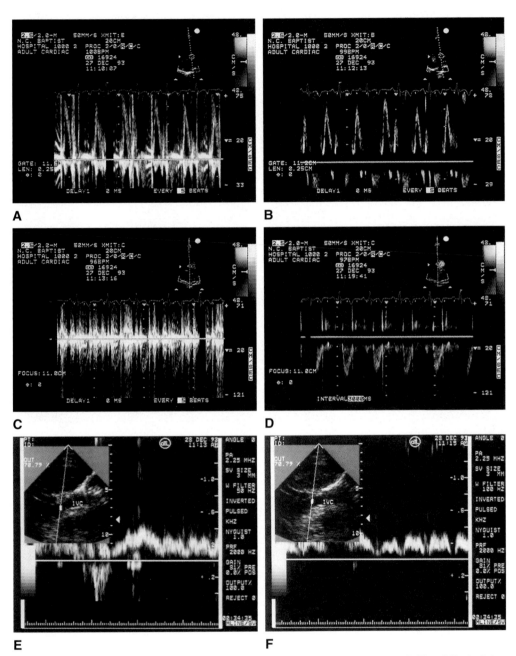

■ **FIGURE I-41**   **A,** Clutter in the spectrum of inflow at the mitral valve is shown. **B,** The clutter in **A** is removed by increasing the wall filter setting. **C,** Clutter in the spectrum of the left ventricular outflow tract. **D,** The clutter in **C** is removed with an increase in the wall filter setting. **E,** Clutter in the display of inferior vena caval flow. **F,** The clutter shown in **E** is removed by adjusting the wall filter.

Continued.

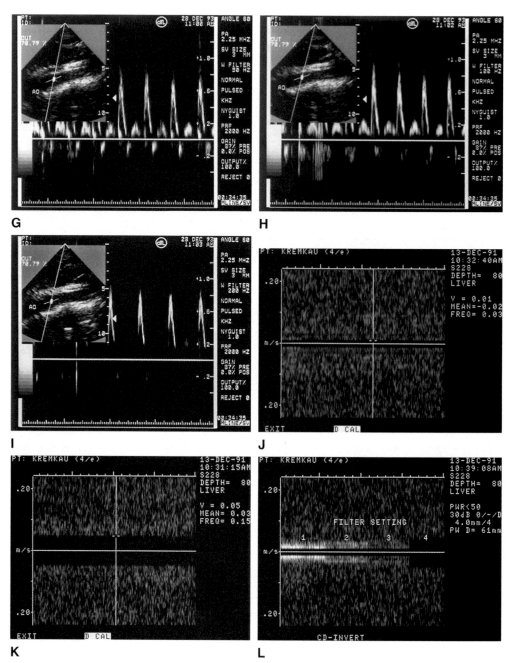

■ **FIGURE I-41, cont'd** **G,** Clutter in the display of aortic flow. **H,** The clutter shown in **G** is removed by adjusting the wall filter. **I,** The wall filter is set too high (200 Hz), eliminating all but the peak systolic portion of the spectrum. **J,** Using electronic noise on the spectrum (with high Doppler gain), a low wall filter setting eliminates Doppler shifts corresponding to flow speeds of less than 1 cm/s. **K,** A higher setting eliminates speeds of less than 5 cm/s. **L,** Four wall filter settings reduce or eliminate frequencies as shown.

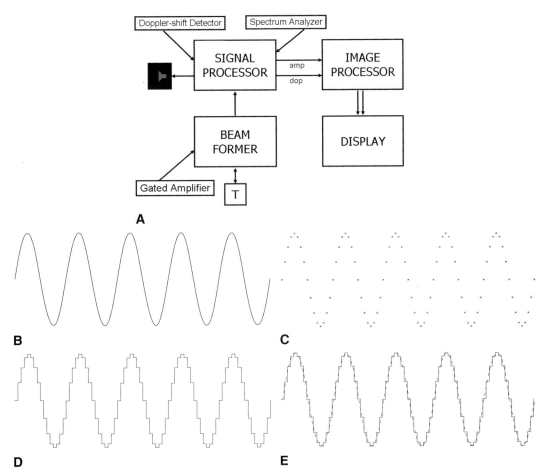

■ FIGURE I-42   A, Block diagram of a sonographic instrument functioning as a pulsed wave Doppler instrument. The beam former produces voltage pulses of several cycles each, which drive the transducer *(T)*. The signal processor includes a Doppler-shift detector, where shift frequencies are compared with the frequency of the outgoing pulses. The difference (Doppler shift) is sent to loudspeakers and, through the spectrum analyzer and image processor, to the display. The beam former also contains a gate that selects echoes from a given depth according to arrival time and thus gives motion information from a selected depth. **B,** Five cycles of a 500-Hz Doppler shift frequency occurring in 10 ms of time. **C,** In a pulsed wave Doppler instrument, each pulse yields echoes from the sample volume. These echoes, after Doppler detection, yield samples (×) of the Doppler shift from the sample volume. In this example, 80 samples are determined in a 10-ms time period. Therefore the pulse repetition frequency of the instrument is 8 kHz (with each pulse yielding one sample of the Doppler shift). **D,** The pulsed wave Doppler gate also is called a sample-and-hold amplifier. It samples the returning stream of echoes (resulting from one emitted pulse of ultrasound) at the appropriate time for the desired depth (Table I-1) and holds the value until the next pulse and sample are accomplished. **E,** Low-pass filtering (which removes higher frequencies) smooths the sampled result *(solid line),* yielding the desired Doppler shift waveform *(dashed line)* comparable to that shown in **B.**

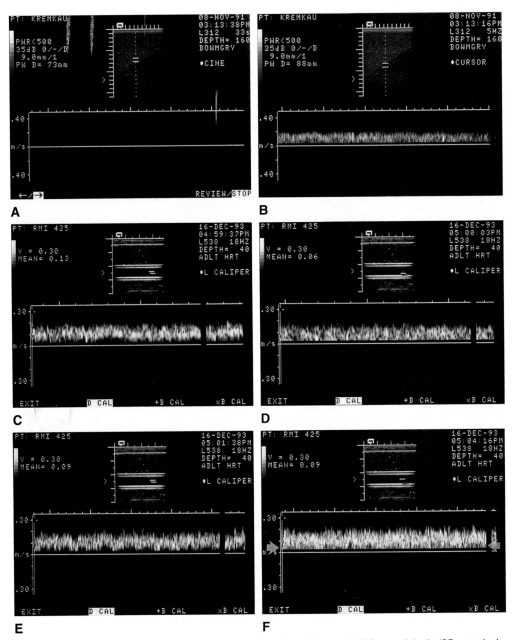

■ FIGURE I-43 **A,** The pulsed wave Doppler sample volume is located at 73 mm of depth (95 μs arrival time). No Doppler shift is seen on the lower display because the Doppler-shifted echoes from within the tube arrive at about 114 μs. **B,** When the gate is open later (corresponding to a depth of 88 mm), the Doppler shifts are received and displayed (indicating a constant flow rate in the tube). **C,** The gate is located in the center of the tube. **D,** The gate is located near the tube wall. Mean flow speed is 6 cm/s compared with 13 cm/s in **C.** This is the expected result with laminar flow. **E,** The gate is again located at the center of the tube. **F,** The gate length is extended to include the flow from the center, out to the tube wall. Note the strengthening of the lower flow speeds (Doppler shifts) *(arrows)* compared with **E,** where the slower flow is not included in the sample volume.

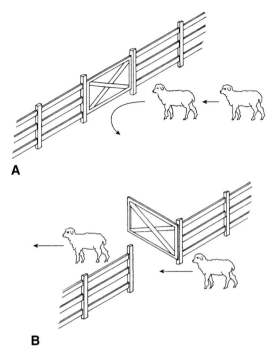

A

B

■ **FIGURE I-44**   **A,** Two sheep arrive at a closed gate and are not received into the pen. **B,** Two sheep arrive later at the gate, when it is open, and are received into the pen. In a Doppler detector the gate accepts and rejects echoes in a similar manner.

TABLE I-9   The Amount Added to Effective Gate Length by Pulse Length for Various Cycles per Pulse and Frequencies

Amount Added (mm)	Cycles	f (MHz)
1.9	5	2
3.8	10	2
7.7	20	2
0.8	5	5
1.5	10	5
3.1	20	5
0.4	5	10
0.8	10	10
1.5	20	10

Volume flow rate (milliliters per second) can be calculated from spatial-mean flow speed multiplied by vessel cross-sectional area. To do this correctly, however, one must average properly the various Doppler shifts representing the cells moving at various speeds, must account properly for the angle to convert mean Doppler shift to mean speed, and must determine the vessel cross-sectional area correctly. Much can go wrong in this complicated process, yielding faulty results.[41-43]

Duplex Instrument

Including pulsed wave Doppler capability in a gray-scale sonographic instrument yields what commonly is called a **duplex instrument** (Figure I-45, G). The duplex instrument has the capacity to image anatomic structures and to analyze motion and flow at a known point in the anatomic field. Imaging allows intelligent positioning of the gate and angle correction in a pulsed wave Doppler system.

Duplex systems must be time-shared. That is, imaging and Doppler flow measurements cannot be done simultaneously. Electronic scanning with arrays permits rapid switching between imaging and Doppler functions (several times per second), allowing what can appear to be simultaneous acquisition of real-time image and Doppler flow information. Imaging frame rates are slowed to allow for acquisition of Doppler information between frames. Likewise, time out is taken from the spectral display to present a sonographic frame (Figure I-40, A, open arrow).

Duplex instruments enable intelligent use of the Doppler sample volume by showing its location in the gray-scale anatomic display.

TABLE I-8   Spatial Gate Length for Various Temporal Gate Lengths

Length (mm)	Time (µs)
1	1.3
2	2.6
3	3.9
4	5.2
5	6.5
10	13.0
15	19.5
20	26.0

are used when searching for the desired vessel and flow location and shorter gate lengths are used for spectral analysis and evaluation. The shorter gate length improves the quality of the spectral display.

The Doppler sample volume is determined by the beam width, the gate length, and the emitted pulse length. One half the pulse length (the same as axial resolution in sonography) is added to the gate length to yield the effective sample volume length (Table I-9). Thus the pulse length must shorten as gate length is reduced. The sample volume width is equal to the beam width at the sample volume depth.

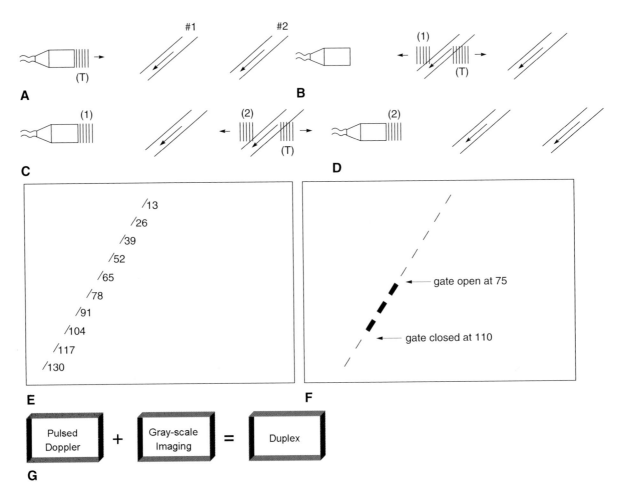

■ **FIGURE I-45** **A,** A pulse *(T)* leaves the transducer. **B,** An echo *(1)* is generated in vessel number 1. **C,** Echo 1 arrives at the transducer. At the same time, another echo *(2)* is generated at vessel number 2. **D,** Echo 2 arrives at the transducer after echo 1. These echoes will be processed by the instrument if the gate is open when they arrive. **E,** Echoes from 1-, 2-, 3-, 4-, 5-, 6-, 7-, 8-, 9-, and 10-cm depths arrive at the times (microseconds) indicated. **F,** If the gate is open from 75 to 110 μs after pulse emission, only the echoes in **E,** arriving at 78, 91, and 104 μs, will be accepted. The others will be rejected. **G,** A duplex instrument is a sonographic instrument with pulsed wave Doppler capability incorporated.

Spectral Analysis

The Doppler-shift voltage from the detector does not go directly to the display but undergoes further processing because it otherwise would look like Figure I-46, *A*. This is the visual picture of what a listener hears from the loudspeaker. Spectral analysis (Figure I-46, *B*) provides a more meaningful and useful way to present the Doppler information visually. The presentation is in the form of a Doppler **frequency spectrum.**

Frequency Spectrum

The term *spectral* means relating to a spectrum. A spectrum is an array of the components of a wave, separated and arranged in order of increasing wavelength or frequency. The term *analysis* comes from a Greek word meaning to break up or to take apart. Thus spectral analysis is the breaking up of the frequency components of a complex wave or signal and spreading them out in order of increasing frequency.

Spectral analysis presents Doppler-shift frequencies in frequency order.

The human auditory system analyzes sound. The ear and brain break down the complex sounds we receive into the component frequencies contained in the sounds. Thus we can listen to a Doppler signal and recognize normal and abnormal flow sounds. Visual presentation of these sounds provides additional capability for recognition of flow characteristics and diagnosis of disease.

Various kinds of flow occur in blood vessels. Changes in vessel size, turns, and abnormalities, such as the presence of plaque or stenoses, can alter the flow character. We have seen that flow can be characterized as plug, laminar, parabolic, disturbed, and turbulent. Portions of the blood flowing within a vessel are moving at different speeds (even for normal flow) and sometimes in different directions. Thus as the ultrasound beam intersects this flow and produces echoes, many different Doppler shifts are received from the vessel by the system, even from a small sample volume. These Doppler shifts are called the Doppler frequency spectrum. The extent of the range of generated Doppler-shift frequencies depends on the character of the flow. For near-plug flow, a narrow range of Doppler-shift frequencies is received. In disturbed and turbulent flow, broader and much broader ranges of Doppler-shift frequencies, respectively, can be received.

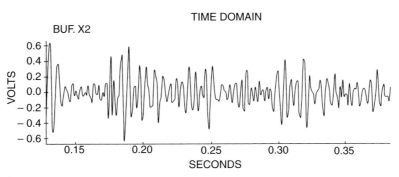

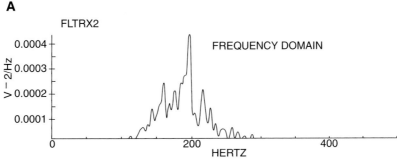

■ **FIGURE I-46** **A,** Demodulated Doppler shift signal for microspheres flowing at nearly uniform speed. When applied to a loudspeaker, a mix of many frequencies is heard. Approximately 10 cycles occur over the time period of 0.20 to 0.25 second. Thus the fundamental period of this signal is about 50 ms, yielding a fundamental frequency of 200 Hz. **B,** After the Fourier transform is applied, a frequency spectrum is obtained. The center frequency is approximately 200 Hz. This is what was predicted in **A.** (From Burns PN: *J Clin Ultrasound* 15:567-590, 1987. Reprinted by permission of John Wiley & Sons, Inc.)

Different flow conditions produce various spectral presentations.

The fast Fourier transform is used to generate Doppler-shift spectral displays.

Fast Fourier Transform

The **fast Fourier transform** is the mathematical technique[44-46] the instrument uses to derive the Doppler spectrum from the returning echoes of various frequencies (Figure I-47). Fast Fourier transform displays can show **spectral broadening**, which is widening of the Doppler-shift spectrum (i.e., an increase in the range of Doppler-shift frequencies present) caused by a broader range of flow speeds and directions encountered by the sound beam with disturbed or turbulent flow.

Spectral Displays

The received Doppler signal is a combination of many Doppler-shift frequencies, yielding a complicated wave-form (Figures I-46, *A*, and I-47, *B*). Using the fast Fourier transform, these frequencies are separated into a spectrum that is presented on a two-dimensional display as Doppler-shift frequency on the horizontal axis and power or amplitude of each frequency component on the vertical axis (Figures I-46, *B*, and I-47, *A* and *C*). Depending on the speed of the processor, about 100 to

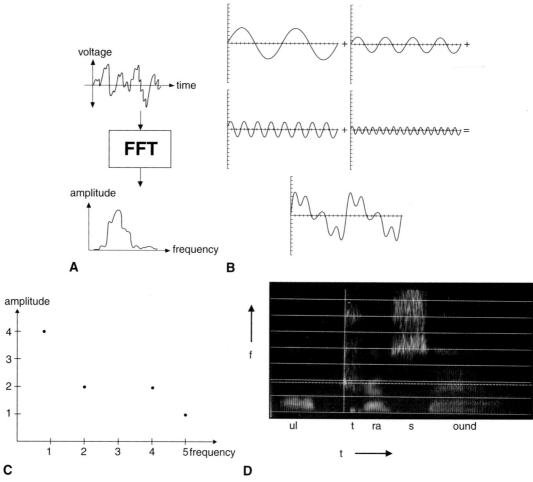

■ **FIGURE I-47**   Fast Fourier transform *(FFT)*. **A,** The Doppler shift signal (containing many frequencies) is transformed by the FFT into a spectrum. (See Figure I-46 for an example of the Doppler signal before **[A]** and after **[B]** FFT processing.) **B,** Four voltages of different frequencies are combined to give the complicated result. **C,** The FFT analysis of this combined voltage yields this spectrum of four frequency components (a frequency of 1 with amplitude 4, two frequencies [2 and 4] with amplitude 2, and one frequency of 5 with amplitude 1). **D,** Spectral analysis of the word *ultrasound*. Time progresses to the right as the word is uttered, and about 100 FFTs are performed. The vertical axis represents frequency. The low frequencies of the *ul, ra,* and *ound* syllables are seen, along with the high frequencies of the *t* and *s* sounds.

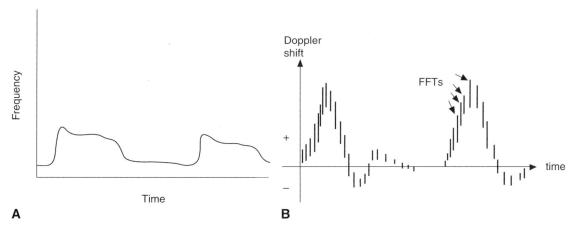

A   B

■ **FIGURE I-48**   **A,** A display of Doppler shift as a function of time for pure plug flow. Doppler-shift frequency is represented on the vertical axis. The amplitude of the Doppler-shift frequency at each instant of time is represented by gray level or color. In this example, there is only a single shift frequency at each instant of time (i.e., no spectrum). **B,** A spectral display for nonplug flow is composed of several (about 100 per second) fast Fourier transform *(FFT)* spectra arranged vertically next to each other across the time (horizontal) axis.

1000 spectra can be generated per second. For venous flow, such a spectral display usually would be rather constant. However, for the pulsatile flow in arterial circulation, such a presentation is changing continually, shifting to the right in systole as the blood accelerates and Doppler shifts increase, shifting to the left in diastole, and changing in amplitude distribution over the cardiac cycle. The interpretation of this changing presentation is difficult, and indeed, the character of the changes over the cardiac cycle could be important. Therefore presentation of this changing spectrum as a function of time is valuable and useful. Such a trace is shown in Figures I-48 and I-49. In these presentations the vertical axis represents Doppler-shift frequency and the horizontal represents time (Figure I-50). The amplitude or power of each Doppler-shift frequency component at any instant now is presented as brightness (gray scale; Figure I-39, *A*) or color (Figure 1-14, *B* [Color Plate 2]). Doppler signal power is proportional to blood cell concentration (number of cells per unit volume). A bright spot on a spectral display means that a strong Doppler-shift frequency component at that instant of time was received (Figure I-39). A dark spot means that a Doppler-shift frequency component at that point in time was weak or nonexistent. Intermediate values of gray shade or brightness indicate intermediate amplitudes or powers of frequency components at the given times. A strong signal at a particular frequency and time means that there are many scattering blood cells moving at speeds and directions corresponding to that Doppler shift. A

weak frequency means that few cells are traveling at speeds and directions corresponding to that Doppler shift at that point in time.

The spectral display is a presentation of Doppler spectra versus time.

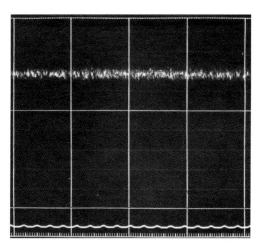

■ **FIGURE I-49**   A spectral display of the signal shown in Figure I-46. The flow is constant, yielding Doppler shift frequencies of approximately 200 Hz. (The horizontal markers represent 100 Hz.) (From Burns PN: *J Clin Ultrasound* 15:567-590, 1987. Reprinted by permission of John Wiley & Sons, Inc.)

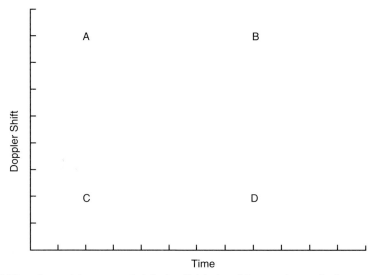

■ **FIGURE I-50** Four points on a spectral display. Points A and C occur at an earlier time, compared with points B and D, which occur later. Points A and B represent higher Doppler-shift frequencies than points C and D.

Spectral Broadening

Spectral trace presentations provide information about flow that can be used to discern conditions at the site of measurement and distal to it.[47,48] Peak flow speeds and spectral broadening are indicative of the degree of stenosis. Spectral broadening means a vertical thickening of the spectral trace (Figure I-51). If all the cells were moving at the same speed, the spectral trace would be a thin line (Figure I-48, A). As stated previously, though, this is not the case in practice. However, narrow spectra can be observed, particularly in large vessels (Figure I-52, A). The apparent narrowing of the spectrum as the blood accelerates in systole can be misinterpreted. A spectrum of consistent width appears to be thinner in a steep-rise portion of a curve (Figure I-53). As flow is disturbed or becomes turbulent, greater variation in velocities of various portions of the flowing blood produce a greater range of Doppler-shift frequencies. This results in a broadened spectrum presented on the spectral display (Figure I-51, A to D). Thus spectral broadening is indicative of disturbed or turbulent flow and can be related to a pathologic condition. However, spectral broadening also can be produced artificially by excessive Doppler gain (Figure I-51, E and F), and some broadening is produced by beam spreading (Figure I-37, F), particularly with wide-aperture arrays.[49,50]

Disturbed or turbulent flow conditions produce spectral broadening.

Downstream Conditions

Doppler flow measurements can yield information regarding downstream (distal) conditions. Flow reversal in early diastole and lack of flow in late diastole (Figures I-8 and I-52, A) indicate high resistance to flow downstream (e.g., because of vasoconstriction of arterioles).[14] If flow resistance is reduced because of vasodilation, impressive differences in the spectral display are observed (Figure I-54). A comparison between low-resistance and high-resistance flow spectra is given in Figure I-55.

High- and low-impedance conditions downstream give rise to different spectral displays.

Normal vessels can be occluded in diastole when pressure drops below the critical value for flow.[14] When this happens, no diastolic Doppler shift is detected.

Table I-10 compares the three types of Doppler displays: color Doppler shift, color Doppler-power, and spectral. Figure I-56 illustrates the Doppler controls discussed in this chapter.

TABLE I-10 Comparison of Doppler-Shift, Doppler-Power, and Spectral Displays

	Color Doppler-Shift Display	Color Doppler-Power Display	Spectral Display
Quantitative	No	No	Yes
Global	Yes	Yes	No
Perfusion	No	Yes	No

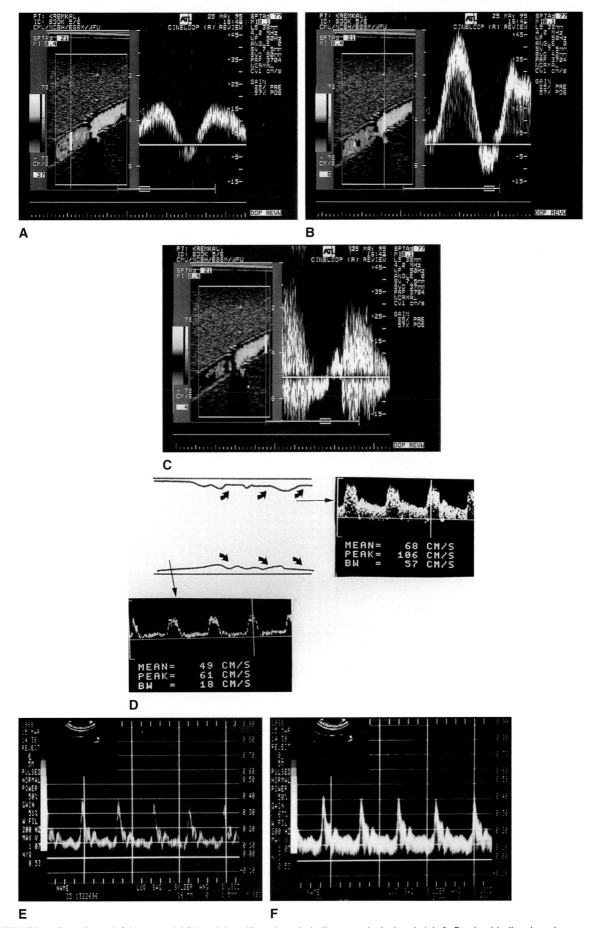

■ **FIGURE I-51** Flow *(lower left to upper right)* in a tube with a stenosis in tissue-equivalent material. **A,** Proximal to the stenosis, a narrow spectrum is observed (indicating approximately plug [i.e., blunted] flow). **B,** At the stenosis a reasonably narrow spectrum still is seen, but the Doppler shifts have tripled because of the high flow speed through the stenosis. **C,** Distal to the stenosis a broad spectrum is observed, along with negative Doppler shifts, both of which are caused by turbulent flow. Compare these observations with the flow conditions in and beyond a narrow gorge (see Figure I-7, *D*). **D,** Spectral broadening produced by atheroma. **E,** Display produced at a correct Doppler gain setting. **F,** Apparent spectral broadening caused by excessive gain. (**D** to **F** from Taylor KJW, Holland S: *Radiology* 174:297-307, 1990.)

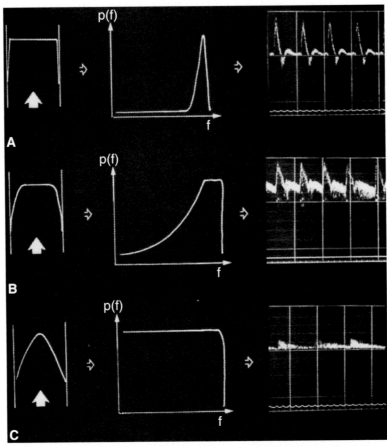

■ **FIGURE I-52** Flow speed profiles *(left),* Doppler spectra (power versus frequency; *center),* and spectral displays *(right)* are shown for nearly plug flow in the aorta **(A),** blunted parabolic flow in the celiac trunk **(B),** and parabolic flow in the ovarian artery **(C).** (From Burns PN: *J Clin Ultrasound* 15:567-590, 1987. Reprinted by permission of John Wiley & Sons, Inc.)

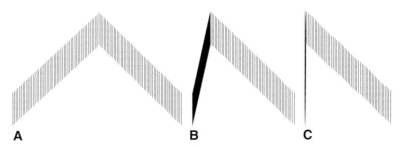

■ **FIGURE I-53**   Apparent spectral narrowing in rapidly accelerating flow. **A,** Slowly accelerating and decelerating flow shows that the spectral widths (bandwidths) are all equal. **B** and **C,** As the acceleration phase becomes steeper, the bandwidths appear to narrow. However, the vertical lines representing bandwidth in all cases are the same.

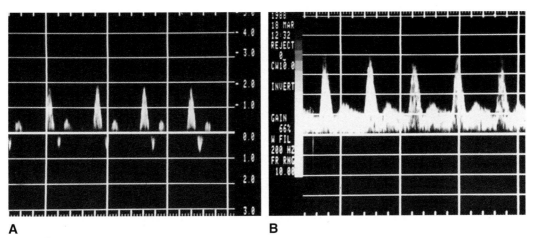

■ **FIGURE I-54**   **A,** High distal resistance flow in the popliteal artery with the patient's leg at rest. **B,** Low distal resistance flow is observed after exercise. (From Taylor KJW, Holland S: *Radiology* 174:297-307, 1990.)

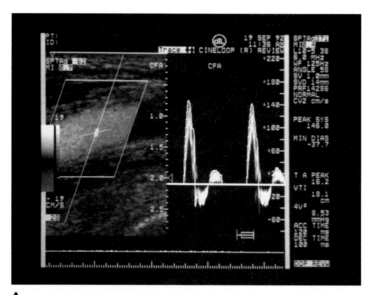

A

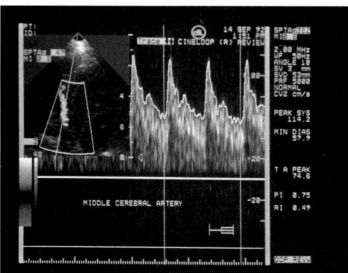

B

■ **FIGURE I-55** **A,** High distal resistance flow is seen in the common femoral artery of the resting lower limb. **B,** Low distal resistance flow is seen in the middle cerebral artery. Although these spectral displays are very different, they are both normal for the locations and conditions given.

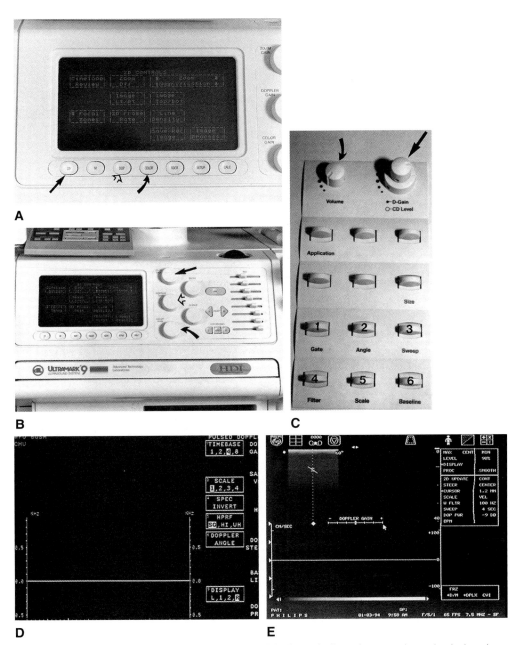

■ **FIGURE I-56** **A,** This instrument provides push-button selection of gray-scale anatomic imaging *(straight arrow)*, spectral Doppler *(open arrow)*, color Doppler imaging *(curved arrow)*, or combinations of these operating modes. **B,** Gray-scale gain *(straight arrow)*, spectral Doppler gain *(open arrow)*, and color Doppler gain controls *(curved arrow)* are shown. **C,** Doppler controls include gain *(straight arrow)*, loud-speaker volume *(curved arrow)*, gate length *(1)*, Doppler angle adjustment *(2)*, spectral display time (horizontal) axis sweep speed *(3)*, wall filter setting *(4)*, spectral display (vertical) axis scale setting (Nyquist limit and pulse repetition frequency control) *(5)*, and baseline shift control *(6)*. **D** and **E,** Software panel controls for Doppler functions.

REVIEW

The key points presented in this appendix are the following:

- The heart provides the pulsatile pressure necessary to produce blood flow.
- Volumetric flow rate is proportional to pressure difference at the ends of a tube.
- Volumetric flow rate is inversely proportional to flow resistance.
- Flow resistance increases with viscosity and tube length and decreases strongly with increasing tube diameter.
- Flow classifications include steady, pulsatile, plug, laminar, parabolic, disturbed, and turbulent.
- In a stenosis, flow speeds up, pressure drops (Bernoulli effect), and flow is disturbed.
- Pulsatile flow is common in arterial circulation.
- Diastolic flow and/or flow reversal occur in some locations within the arterial system.
- The Doppler effect is a change in frequency resulting from motion.
- In medical ultrasound applications, blood flow and tissue motion are the sources of the Doppler effect.
- The change in frequency of the returning echoes with respect to the emitted frequency is called the Doppler shift.
- For flow toward the transducer, the Doppler shift is positive.
- For flow away from the transducer, the Doppler shift is negative.
- The Doppler shift depends on the speed of the scatterers of sound, the Doppler angle, and the operating frequency of the Doppler system.
- Greater flow speeds and smaller Doppler angles produce larger Doppler shifts but not stronger Doppler-shifted echoes.
- Higher operating frequencies produce larger Doppler shifts.
- Typical ranges of flow speeds (10 to 100 cm/s), Doppler angles (30 to 60 degrees), and operating frequencies (2 to 10 MHz) yield Doppler shifts in the range of 100 Hz to 11 kHz for vascular studies.
- In Doppler echocardiography, in which zero angle and speeds of a few meters per second can be encountered, Doppler shifts can be as high as 30 kHz.
- Color Doppler imaging acquires Doppler-shifted echoes from a two-dimensional cross section of tissue scanned by an ultrasound beam.
- Doppler-shifted echoes are presented in color and superimposed on the gray-scale anatomic image of nonshifted echoes that were received during the scan.
- Flow echoes are assigned colors according to the color map chosen.
- Several pulses (the number is called the ensemble length) are needed to generate a color scan line.
- Color controls include gain, map selection, variance on/off, persistence, ensemble length, color/gray priority, scale (PRF), baseline shift, wall filter, and color window angle, location, and size.
- Doppler shift displays are subject to Doppler angle dependence and aliasing.
- Doppler-power displays color-encoded Doppler-shift strengths into angle-independent, aliasing-independent, more sensitive presentations of flow information.
- Continuous wave Doppler systems provide motion and flow information without depth selection capability.
- Pulsed wave Doppler systems provide the ability to select the depth from which Doppler information is received.
- Spectral analysis provides visual information on the distribution of Doppler-shift frequencies resulting from the distribution of the scatterer speeds and directions encountered.
- The Doppler spectrum is generated by the range of scatterer velocities encountered by the ultrasound beam.
- The spectrum is derived electronically using the fast Fourier transform and is presented on the display as Doppler shift versus time, with brightness indicating power.
- Flow conditions at the site of measurement are indicated by the width of the spectrum, with spectral broadening indicative of disturbed and turbulent flow.
- Flow conditions downstream, especially distal flow impedance, are indicated by the relationship between peak systolic and end-diastolic flow speeds.

EXERCISES

1. Which of the following are parts of the circulatory system? (more than one correct answer)
   a. Heart
   b. Cerebral ventricle
   c. Artery
   d. Arteriole
   e. Capillary
   f. Bile duct
   g. Venule
   h. Vein
2. The _____ are the tiniest vessels in the circulatory system.
3. Doppler ultrasound can detect flow in which of the following? (more than one correct answer)
   a. The heart
   b. Arteries
   c. Arterioles
   d. Capillaries
   e. Venules
   f. Veins
4. To flow is to move in a _____.

5. The characteristic of a fluid that offers resistance to flow is called
   a. resistance.
   b. viscosity.
   c. inertia.
   d. impedance.
   e. density.
6. Poise is a unit of _____.
7. Pressure is _____ per unit area.
8. Pressure is
   a. nondirectional.
   b. unidirectional.
   c. omnidirectional.
   d. all of the above.
   e. none of the above.
9. Flow is a response to pressure _____ or _____.
10. If the pressure is greater at one end of a liquid-filled tube or vessel than it is at the other, the liquid will flow from the _____-pressure end to the _____-pressure end.
    a. Higher, lower
    b. Lower, higher
    c. Depends on the liquid
    d. All of the above
    e. None of the above
11. The volumetric flow rate in a tube is determined by _____ difference and _____.
12. If the following is increased, flow increases.
    a. Pressure difference
    b. Pressure gradient
    c. Resistance
    d. a and b
    e. All of the above
13. As flow resistance increases, volumetric flow rate _____.
14. If pressure difference is doubled, volumetric flow rate is
    a. unchanged.
    b. quartered.
    c. halved.
    d. doubled.
    e. quadrupled.
15. If flow resistance is doubled, volumetric flow rate is
    a. unchanged.
    b. quartered.
    c. halved.
    d. doubled.
    e. quadrupled.
16. Flow resistance in a vessel depends on
    a. vessel length.
    b. vessel radius.
    c. blood viscosity.
    d. all of the above.
    e. none of the above.

17. Flow resistance decreases with an increase in which of the following?
    a. Vessel length
    b. Vessel radius
    c. Blood viscosity
    d. All of the above
    e. None of the above
18. Flow resistance depends most strongly on which of the following?
    a. Vessel length
    b. Vessel radius
    c. Blood viscosity
    d. All of the above
    e. None of the above
19. Volumetric flow rate decreases with an increase in which of the following?
    a. Pressure difference
    b. Vessel radius
    c. Vessel length
    d. Blood viscosity
    e. c and d
20. When the speed of a fluid is constant across a vessel, the flow is called _____ flow.
    a. Volume
    b. Parabolic
    c. Laminar
    d. Viscous
    e. Plug
21. The type of flow (approximately) seen in Figure I-57, A, is _____.

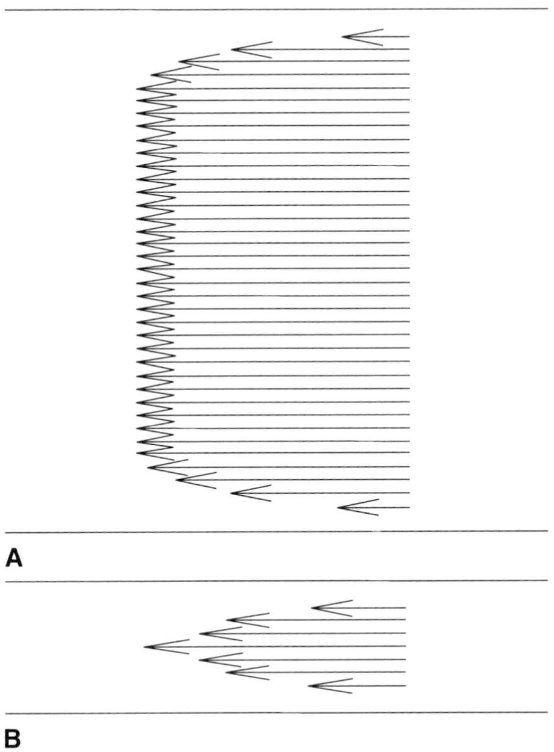

A

B

■ **FIGURE I-57**   Two types of flow patterns (illustration to accompany Exercises 21 and 22).

a. Volume
b. Steady
c. Parabolic
d. Viscous
e. Plug

22. The type of flow seen in Figure I-57, *B*, is _____.
    a. Volume
    b. Steady
    c. Parabolic
    d. Viscous
    e. Plug

23. _____ flow occurs when straight parallel streamlines describing the flow are altered.

24. _____ flow involves random and chaotic flow patterns, with particles flowing in all directions.

25. Turbulent flow is more likely proximal or distal to a stenosis?

26. A narrowing of the lumen of a tube is called a _____.

27. Proximal to, at, and distal to a stenosis, _____ must be constant.
    a. Laminar flow
    b. Disturbed flow
    c. Turbulent flow
    d. Volumetric flow rate
    e. None of the above

28. For the answer to Exercise 27 to be true, flow speed at the stenosis must be _____ that proximal and distal to it.
    a. Greater than
    b. Less than
    c. Less turbulent than
    d. Less disturbed than
    e. None of the above

29. Poiseuille's equation predicts a(n) _____ in flow speed with a decrease in vessel radius.

30. The continuity rule predicts a(n) _____ in flow speed with a localized decrease (stenosis) in vessel diameter.

31. In a stenosis, the pressure is _____ the proximal and distal values.
    a. Less than
    b. Equal to
    c. Greater than
    d. Depends on the fluid
    e. None of the above

32. Added forward flow and flow reversal in diastole can occur with _____ flow.
    a. Volume
    b. Turbulent
    c. Laminar
    d. Disturbed
    e. Pulsatile

33. As stenosis diameter decreases, the following pass(es) through a maximum.
    a. Flow speed at the stenosis
    b. Flow speed proximal to the stenosis
    c. Volumetric flow rate
    d. Doppler shift at the stenosis
    e. a and d

34. In Figure I-58, at which point is pressure lowest?
    a. P
    b. S
    c. D
    d. P and D
    e. None of the above

35. In Figure I-58, at which point is flow speed the lowest?
    a. P
    b. S
    c. D
    d. P and D
    e. None of the above

36. In Figure I-58, at which point is volumetric flow rate the lowest?
    a. P
    b. S
    c. D
    d. P and D
    e. None of the above

37. In Figure I-58, at which point is pressure energy the greatest?
    a. P
    b. S
    c. D
    d. P and D
    e. None of the above

38. The _____ effect is used to detect and measure _____ in vessels.

39. Motion of an echo-generating structure causes an echo to have a different _____ than the emitted pulse.

40. The Doppler effect is a change in reflected _____ caused by reflector _____.

41. If the reflector is moving toward the source, the reflected frequency is _____ than the incident frequency.

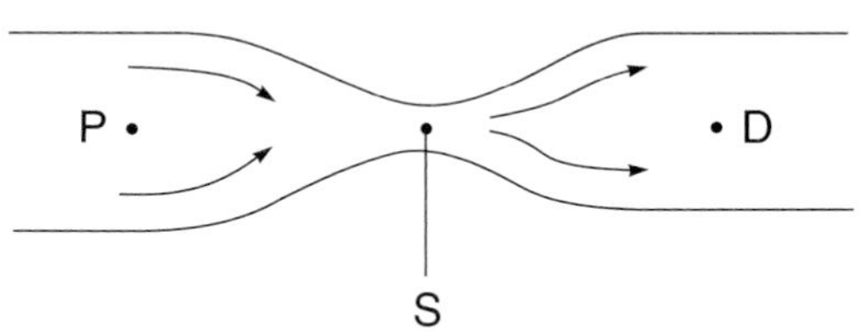

■ **FIGURE I-58** Proximal to *(P)*, at *(S)*, and distal to *(D)* a stenosis (illustration to accompany Exercises 34 to 37). (From Kremkau FW: *J Vasc Technol* 17:153-154, 1993. Reproduced with permission.)

42. If the reflector is moving away from the source, the reflected frequency is _____ than the incident frequency.
43. If the reflector is stationary with respect to the source, the reflected frequency is _____ the incident frequency.
44. Measurement of Doppler shift yields information about reflector _____.
45. If the incident frequency is 1 MHz, the propagation speed is 1600 m/s, and the reflector speed is 16 m/s toward the source, the Doppler shift is _____ MHz, and the reflected frequency is _____ MHz.
46. If 2-MHz ultrasound is reflected from a soft tissue boundary moving at 10 m/s toward the source, the Doppler shift is _____ MHz.
47. If 2-MHz ultrasound is reflected from a soft tissue boundary moving at 10 m/s away from the source, the Doppler shift is _____ MHz.
48. Doppler shift is the difference between _____ and _____ frequencies.
49. When incident sound direction and reflector motion are not parallel, calculation of the reflected frequency involves the _____ of the angle between these directions.
50. If the angle between incident sound direction and reflector motion is 60 degrees, the Doppler shift and reflected frequency in Exercise 45 are _____ MHz and _____ MHz.
51. If the angle between incident sound direction and reflector motion is 90 degrees, the cosine of the angle is _____, and the reflected frequency in Exercise 45 is _____ MHz.
52. For an operating frequency of 2 MHz, a flow speed of 10 cm/s, and a Doppler angle of 0 degrees, calculate the Doppler shift.
53. For an operating frequency of 6 MHz, a flow speed of 50 cm/s, and a Doppler angle of 60 degrees, calculate the Doppler shift.
54. For blood flowing in a vessel with a plug flow profile, the Doppler shift is _____ across the vessel.
55. Which Doppler angle yields the greatest Doppler shift?
    a. −90
    b. −45
    c. 0
    d. 45
    e. 90
56. To proceed from a measurement of Doppler-shift frequency to a calculation of flow speed, _____ _____ must be known or assumed.
57. If operating frequency is doubled, Doppler shift is _____.
58. If flow speed is doubled, Doppler shift is _____.
59. If Doppler angle is doubled, Doppler shift is _____.
60. In Figure I-59, which angle is the incidence angle? Which angle is the Doppler angle? Which angle is the transmission angle? If there is no refraction, which angle is equal to the transmission angle?

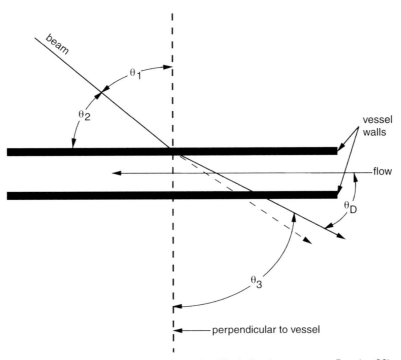

■ **FIGURE I-59**   Diagram of various angles (illustration to accompany Exercise 60).

With no refraction, which angle is equal to the Doppler angle? Incidence angle plus Doppler angle (no refraction) equals what?

61. In Figure I-30, A, (Color Plate 22), red and yellow indicate negative Doppler shifts. Therefore flow in this vessel is
    a. from upper right to lower left.
    b. from lower left to upper right.

62. In the bend at the upper left of Figure I-30, A (Color Plate 22), there is a yellow region in the center of the vessel. This indicates the region in the image where blood flow speed is the greatest. True or false?

63. In Figure I-30, C (Color Plate 22), the region shown in cyan (aqua or blue-green) indicates
    a. turbulent flow.
    b. flow reversal.
    c. flow speed exceeding 32 cm/s.
    d. all of the above.
    e. none of the above.

64. Color Doppler instruments present two-dimensional, color-coded images representing _____ that are superimposed on gray-scale images representing _____.

65. Which of the following on a color Doppler display is (are) presented in real time?
    a. Gray-scale anatomy
    b. Flow direction
    c. Doppler spectrum
    d. a and b
    e. All of the above

66. Color Doppler instruments use an _____ technique to yield Doppler information in real time.

67. The information in Exercise 66 includes _____ Doppler shift, _____, _____, and _____.

68. The angle dependencies of Doppler-shift and Doppler-power displays are different. True or false?

69. Do the different colors appearing in Figure I-28, A and C (Color Plate 19), indicate that flow is going in two different directions in the vessel?

70. In color Doppler instruments, color is used only to represent flow direction. True or false?

71. In practice, approximately _____ pulses are required to obtain one line of color Doppler information.
    a. 1
    b. 10
    c. 100
    d. 1000
    e. 1,000,000

72. About _____ frames per second are produced by a color Doppler instrument.
    a. 10
    b. 20

c. 40
d. 80
e. More than one of the above

73. Doppler-shift displays are not dependent on Doppler angle. True or false?

74. If two colors are shown in the same vessel using a color Doppler instrument, it always means flow is occurring in opposite directions in the vessel. True or false?

75. A region of bright color on a Doppler-shift display always indicates the highest flow speeds. True or false?

76. Increasing the ensemble length _____ the frame rate.

77. The _____ technique commonly is used to detect echo Doppler shifts in color Doppler instruments.

78. Which of the following reduce the frame rate of a color Doppler image? (more than one correct answer)
    a. Wider color window
    b. Longer color window
    c. Increased ensemble length
    d. Higher transducer frequency
    e. Higher priority setting

79. Lack of color in a vessel containing blood flow may be attributable to (more than one correct answer)
    a. low color gain.
    b. a high wall filter setting.
    c. a low priority setting.
    d. baseline shift.
    e. aliasing.

80. Increasing ensemble length _____ color sensitivity and accuracy and _____ frame rate.
    a. Improves, increases
    b. Degrades, increases
    c. Degrades, decreases
    d. Improves, decreases
    e. None of the above

81. Which control can be used to help with clutter?
    a. Wall filter
    b. Gain
    c. Baseline shift
    d. Pulse repetition frequency
    e. Smoothing

82. Color map baselines are always represented by
    a. white.
    b. black.
    c. red.
    d. blue.
    e. cyan.

83. Doubling the width of a color window produces a(n) _____ frame rate.
    a. Doubled
    b. Quadrupled

c. Unchanged
d. Halved
e. Quartered

84. Steering the color window to the right or left produces a(n) _____ frame rate.
    a. Doubled
    b. Quadrupled
    c. Unchanged
    d. Halved
    e. Quartered

85. Autocorrelation produces (more than one correct answer)
    a. the color of Doppler shift.
    b. the mean value of Doppler shift.
    c. variance.
    d. spectrum.
    e. peak Doppler shift.

86. Steering the color window to the right or left changes
    a. frame rate.
    b. pulse repetition frequency.
    c. Doppler angle.
    d. Doppler shift.
    e. more than one of the above.

87. Color Doppler frame rates are _____ gray-scale rates.
    a. Equal to
    b. Less than
    c. More than
    d. Depends on color map
    e. Depends on priority

88. In a single frame, color can change in a vessel because of
    a. vessel curvature.
    b. sector format.
    c. helical flow.
    d. diastolic flow reversal.
    e. all of the above.

89. Angle is not important in transverse color Doppler views through vessels. True or false?

90. Compared with Doppler-shift imaging, Doppler-power imaging is
    a. more sensitive.
    b. angle-independent.
    c. aliasing-independent.
    d. speed-independent.
    e. all of the above.

91. Doppler-power imaging indicates (with color) the _____ of flow.
    a. Presence
    b. Direction
    c. Speed
    d. Character
    e. More than one of the above

92. Doppler-shift imaging indicates (with color) the _____ of flow.
    a. Presence
    b. Direction
    c. Speed
    d. Character
    e. More than one of the above

93. Instruments that distinguish between positive and negative Doppler shifts yield motion _____ information and are called _____.

94. To display the pattern of time change of a Doppler spectrum, a display of Doppler shift _____ versus _____ can be used.

95. In Exercise 94, the amplitude of each frequency component is represented by _____ level or _____.

96. The received frequency spectrum (rather than a single frequency) exists because of the distribution of flow _____ and _____ encountered by the beam.

97. In a duplex instrument the gated detector is part of the _____ _____.

98. The purpose of the gate is to allow selection of Doppler-shifted echoes from specific _____ according to _____.

99. An increased gate-open time increases the length of the sample volume. True or false?

100. A later gate corresponds to a deeper gate location. True or false?

101. Pulsed wave Doppler systems are sampling systems. The sampling rate is the same as the _____.

102. Pulsed wave Doppler instruments use the _____ _____ _____ technique to present Doppler-shift spectra as a function of time.

103. The abbreviation for the technique referred to in Exercise 102 is _____.

104. The functions of a Doppler detector include which of the following?
    a. Amplification
    b. Phase quadrature detection
    c. Doppler-shift detection
    d. Sign determination
    e. All of the above

105. An earlier gate time means a _____ sample volume depth.
    a. Later
    b. Shallower
    c. Deeper
    d. Stronger
    e. None of the above

106. Name the Doppler instrument the sample volume of which is the region of transmitting and receiving transducer beam overlap.

107. Name the instrument the sample volume of which is determined by the detector gate.
108. Name the instrument that combines pulsed wave Doppler with imaging.
109. The _____ detects the difference between the frequencies of the emitted and received ultrasound.
110. To convert a spectral display correctly from Doppler shift to flow speed, the _____ must be incorporated properly.
111. The zero Doppler-shift point on a spectral display is called the _____.
112. Which type of Doppler instrument is most likely to be used in measuring extremely high flow rates?
113. Spectral analysis is the breaking up of the _____ of a complex wave or signal and spreading them out in _____.
114. A Doppler spectrum is produced because many different Doppler _____ are received from the flow.
115. The statement in Exercise 114 is true because portions of the flowing fluid within the heart or a vessel are moving at different _____ and sometimes in different _____.
116. Doppler shift versus time presentations indicate the amplitude or power of each frequency component by _____ or _____.
117. Doppler signal power is proportional to
    a. volume flow rate.
    b. flow speed.
    c. Doppler angle.
    d. cell concentration.
    e. more than one of the above.
118. Doppler ultrasound provides information about flow conditions only at the site of measurement. True or false?
119. Stenosis affects
    a. peak systolic flow speed.
    b. end-diastolic flow speed.
    c. spectral broadening.
    d. window.
    e. all of the above.
120. Spectral broadening is a _____ of the spectral trace.
    a. Vertical thickening
    b. Horizontal thickening
    c. Brightening
    d. Darkening
    e. Horizontal shift
121. If all cells in a vessel were moving at the same constant speed, the spectral trace would be a _____ line.
    a. Thin horizontal
    b. Thin vertical
    c. Thick horizontal

    d. Thick vertical
    e. None of the above
122. Disturbed flow produces a narrower spectrum. True or false?
123. Turbulent flow produces a narrower spectrum. True or false?
124. As stenosis progresses, which of the following increase(s)?
    a. Lumen diameter
    b. Systolic Doppler shift
    c. Diastolic Doppler shift
    d. Spectral broadening
    e. More than one of the above
125. Higher flow speed always produces a higher Doppler shift on a spectral display. True or false?
126. Flow reversal in diastole indicates
    a. stenosis.
    b. aneurysm.
    c. high distal resistance.
    d. low distal resistance.
    e. more than one of the above.
127. Decreased distal resistance normally causes end-diastolic flow to
    a. increase.
    b. decrease.
    c. be disturbed.
    d. become turbulent.
    e. more than one of the above.
128. Under what condition can a relatively low Doppler shift come from a relatively rapidly moving flow?
129. When the spectral trace is calibrated in flow speed (centimeters per second), the highest flow speed shown always represents the fastest cells in the vessel. True or false?
130. If angle correction is set at 60 degrees but should be 0 degrees, the display indicates a flow speed of 100 cm/s. The correct flow speed is _____ cm/s.
    a. 25
    b. 50
    c. 100
    d. 200
    e. 400
131. If angle correction is set at 0 degrees but should be 60 degrees, the display indicates a flow speed of 100 cm/s. The correct flow speed is _____ cm/s.
    a. 25
    b. 50
    c. 100
    d. 200
    e. 400
132. If a 5-kHz Doppler shift corresponds to 100 cm/s, then a 2.5-kHz shift corresponds to _____ cm/s.
133. Which of the following is increased if Doppler angle is increased?

Appendixes   **509**

a. Aliasing
b. Doppler shift
c. Effect of angle error
d. b and c
e. None of the above

ANSWERS TO EXERCISES

1. a, c, d, e, g, h
2. Capillaries
3. a, b, f
4. Stream
5. b
6. Viscosity
7. Force
8. c
9. Difference, gradient
10. a
11. Pressure, resistance
12. d
13. Decreases
14. d
15. c
16. d
17. b
18. b
19. e
20. e
21. e
22. c
23. Disturbed
24. Turbulent
25. Distal
26. Stenosis
27. d
28. a
29. Decrease
30. Increase
31. a
32. e
33. e
34. b
35. d
36. e
37. d
38. Doppler, flow
39. Frequency
40. Frequency, motion
41. Greater
42. Less
43. Equal to
44. Motion
45. 0.02, 1.02
46. 0.026
47. −0.026

48. Received, emitted
49. Cosine
50. 0.01, 1.01 (The Doppler shift is cut in half.)
51. 0, 1.00 (no Doppler shift at 90 degrees)
52. 0.26 kHz
53. 1.95 kHz
54. Constant
55. c
56. Doppler angle
57. Doubled
58. Doubled
59. Decreased
60. θ_1, θ_D, θ_3, θ_1, θ_2, 90 degrees
61. a
62. False (A small Doppler angle causes the large Doppler shift.)
63. e (aliasing at flow speeds exceeding about 64 cm/s)
64. Flow or motion, anatomy
65. d
66. Autocorrelation
67. Mean, sign, variance, power
68. True (Power displays have no angle dependence.)
69. No
70. False
71. b
72. e (a, b, or c)
73. False
74. False (It also can mean aliasing or changing Doppler angle.)
75. False (Remember the Doppler angle.)
76. Decreases
77. Autocorrelation
78. a and c
79. a, b, c
80. d
81. a
82. b
83. d
84. c
85. b, c
86. e (c and d)
87. b
88. e
89. False
90. e
91. a
92. e (a, b, c, d)
93. Direction, bidirectional
94. Frequency, time
95. Gray, color
96. Speeds, directions
97. Signal processor
98. Depths, arrival times
99. True
100. True

101. Pulse repetition frequency
102. Fast Fourier transform
103. FFT
104. e
105. b
106. Continuous wave
107. Pulsed wave
108. Duplex
109. Doppler-shift detector
110. Doppler angle
111. Baseline
112. Continuous wave
113. Components or frequencies, order
114. Shifts
115. Speeds, directions
116. Color, gray scale
117. d

118. False
119. e
120. a
121. a
122. False
123. False
124. e (b, c, d)
125. False (Remember the Doppler angle.)
126. c
127. a
128. Large Doppler angle
129. False (Remember the Doppler angle.)
130. b
131. d
132. 50
133. c

REFERENCES

Preface

1. Szabo TL: *Diagnostic ultrasound imaging: inside out*, New York, 2004, Elsevier/Academic Press.
2. Hill CR, Bamber JC, ter Haar GR, editors: *Physical principles of medical ultrasonics*, ed 2, Hoboken, NJ, 2004, John Wiley & Sons.
3. Edler I, Lindstrom K: The history of echocardiography, *Ultrasound Med Biol* 30:1565-1644, 2004.
4. Goldberg BB: Obstetric US imaging: the past 40 years, *Radiology* 215:622-629, 2000.

Introduction (Chapter 1)

5. Eden A: *The search for Christian Doppler*, New York, 1992, Springer-Verlag.

Ultrasound (Chapter 2)

6. Duck FA: Acoustic properties of tissue at ultrasonic frequencies. In *Physical properties of tissue*, New York, 1990, Academic Press.
7. Goldberg BB, Raichlen JS: *Ultrasound contrast agents*, London, 2001, Marin Dunitz.
8. Burns PN: Microbubble contrast for ultrasound imaging: where, how, and why? In Rumack CM et al, editors: *Diagnostic ultrasound*, ed 3, St Louis, 2005, Elsevier/Mosby.

Transducers (Chapter 3)

9. Ballato A: Piezoelectricity: old effect, new thrusts, *IEEE Trans Ultrason Ferroelectr Freq Control* 42:916-926, 1995.
10. Zemanek J: Beam behavior within the nearfield of a vibrating piston, *J Acoust Soc Am* 49:181-191, 1971.

Imaging Instruments (Chapter 4)

11. Kremkau FW: Clinical benefit of higher acoustic output levels, *Ultrasound Med Biol* 15(suppl 1):69-70, 1989.
12. Hossack J, ed: Coded waveforms in ultrasonic imaging, *IEEE Trans Ultrason Ferroelectr Freq Control (Special Issue)* 52:158-288, 2005.
13. National Electrical Manufacturers Association: *Digital Imaging and Communications in Medicine (DICOM) Set*, Standards PS 3.1-3.16, Rosslyn, Va, 2003, The Association.

Doppler Effect (Chapter 5)

Flow

14. Guyton AC, Hall JE: *Textbook of medical physiology*, ed 10, Philadelphia, 2000, WB Saunders.
15. Milnor WR: *Hemodynamics*, ed 2, Baltimore, 1989, Williams & Wilkins.
16. Nichols WW, O'Rourke MF: *McDonald's blood flow in arteries*, Philadelphia, 1990, Lea & Febiger.
17. Beach KW et al: The systolic velocity criterion for diagnosing significant internal carotid artery stenoses, *J Vasc Technol* 13:65-68, 1989.
18. Ku DN et al: Hemodynamics of the normal human carotid bifurcation: in vitro and in vivo studies, *Ultrasound Med Biol* 11:13-26, 1985.
19. Phillips DJ et al: Should results of ultrasound Doppler studies be reported in units of frequency or velocity? *Ultrasound Med Biol* 15:205-212, 1989.
20. Rosenthal SJ et al: Doppler US of helical flow in the portal vein, *Radiographics* 15:1103-1111, 1995.
21. Spencer MP, Reid JM: Quantitation of carotid stenosis with continuous wave (CW) Doppler ultrasound, *Stroke* 10:326-330, 1979.

Doppler Effect

22. Bradley EL, Sacerio J: The velocity of ultrasound in human blood under varying physiologic parameters, *J Surg Res* 12:290-297, 1972.
23. Wells PNT et al: A second order approximation in the Doppler equation, *Ultrasound Med Biol* 15:73-74, 1989; 16:423, 1990.
24. Kremkau FW: Source of Doppler shift in blood flow, *Ultrasound Med Biol* 16:421-422, 1990; 17:98, 1991.
25. Thorne GC et al: Blood flow measurement by Doppler ultrasound: a question of angles, *Phys Med Biol* 38:1637-1645, 1993.
26. Fuss EL: The technology of burglar alarm systems, *Am Sci* 72:334-337, 1984.
27. Luckman NP et al: Backscattered power in Doppler signals, *Ultrasound Med Biol* 13:669-670, 1987.
28. Kremkau FW: Doppler shift frequency data, *J Ultrasound Med* 6:167, 1987.
29. Kremkau FW: Doppler angle error due to refraction, *Ultrasound Med Biol* 16:523-524, 1990; 17:97, 1991.

Color Doppler Instruments (Chapter 6)

30. Merritt CRB, editor: *Doppler color imaging*, St Louis, 1992, Harcourt Health Sciences.
31. Kremkau FW: Doppler principles, *Semin Roentgenol* 27:6-16, 1992.
32. Kremkau FW: Principles of color flow imaging, *J Vasc Technol* 15:104-111, 1991.
33. Kremkau FW: Color-flow color assignments: I, *J Vasc Technol* 15:265-266, 1991.
34. Kremkau FW: Color-flow color assignments: II, *J Vasc Technol* 15:325-326, 1991.
35. Kremkau FW: Color interpretation: I, *J Vasc Technol* 16:105, 1992.
36. Kremkau FW: Color interpretation: II, *J Vasc Technol* 16:215-216, 1992.
37. Kremkau FW: Color interpretation: III, *J Vasc Technol* 16:309-310, 1992.
38. Kremkau FW: Principles and instrumentation. In Merritt CRB, editor: *Doppler color imaging*, New York, 1992, Churchill Livingstone.
39. Kremkau FW: Principles and pitfalls of real-time color-flow imaging. In Bernstein EF, editor: *Vascular diagnosis*, ed 4, St Louis, 1993, Mosby-Year Book.
40. Kasai C et al: Real-time two-dimensional blood flow imaging using an autocorrelation technique, *IEEE Trans Sonics Ultrason* SU-32:458-464, 1985.

Spectral Doppler Instruments (Chapter 7)

41. Burns PN: Measuring volume flow with Doppler ultrasound: an old nut, *Ultrasound Obstet Gynecol* 2:238-241, 1992.

42. Gill RW: Measurement of blood flow by ultrasound: accuracy and sources of error, *Ultrasound Med Biol* 11: 625-641, 1985.
43. Holland CK, Clancy MJ, Taylor KJW: Volumetric flow estimation in vivo and in vitro using pulsed-Doppler ultrasound, *Ultrasound Med Biol* 22:591-603, 1996.
44. Bracewell RN: The Fourier transform, *Sci Am* 260:86-95, 1989.
45. Bracewell RN: Numerical transforms, *Science* 248:697-704, 1990.
46. Walker JS: *Fast Fourier transforms*, Boca Raton, Fla, 1992, CRC Press.
47. Burns PN: The physical principles of Doppler and spectral analysis, *J Clin Ultrasound* 15:567-590, 1987.
48. Taylor KJW, Holland S: State-of-the-art Doppler ultrasound: I. Basic principles, instrumentation and pitfalls, *Radiology* 174:297-307, 1990.
49. Daigle RJ, Stavros TA, Lee RM: Overestimation of velocity and frequency values by multielement linear array Dopplers, *J Vasc Technol* 14:206-213, 1990.
50. Winkler AJ, Wu J: Correction of intrinsic spectral broadening errors in Doppler peak velocity measurements made with phased sector and linear array transducers, *Ultrasound Med Biol* 21:1029-1035, 1995.

Artifacts (Chapter 8)

51. Waldroup LD, Kremkau FW: Artifacts in ultrasound imaging. In Goldberg BB, editor: *Textbook of abdominal ultrasound*, Baltimore, 1993, Williams & Wilkins.
52. Sanders RC: *Atlas of ultrasonographic artifacts and variants*, ed 2, St Louis, 1992, Mosby-Year Book.
53. Pozniak MA, Zagzebski JA, Seanlan KA: Spectral and color Doppler artifacts, *Radiographics* 12:25-44, 1992.
54. Gill RW et al: New class of pulsed Doppler US ambiguity at short ranges, *Radiology* 173:272-275, 1989.
55. Dickerson KS et al: Comparison of conventional transverse Doppler sonograms, *J Ultrasound Med* 12:497-506, 1993.
56. Hoskins PR, Loupas T, McDicken WN: A comparison of three different filters for speckle reduction of Doppler spectra, *Ultrasound Med Biol* 16:375-389, 1990.
57. Mitchell DG, Burns P, Needleman L: Color Doppler artifact in anechoic regions, *J Ultrasound Med* 9:255-260, 1990.
58. Rahmouni A et al: Color-Doppler twinkling artifact in hyperechoic regions, *Radiology* 199:269-271, 1996.
59. Nelson TR et al: Sources and impact of artifacts on clinical three-dimensional ultrasound imaging, *Ultrasound Obstet Gynecol* 16:374-383, 2000.

Performance and Safety (Chapter 9)

Therapy

60. Baker KG, Robertson VJ, Duck FA: A review of therapeutic ultrasound: effectiveness studies, *Phys Ther* 81:1339-1350, 2001.
61. Baker KG, Robertson VJ, Duck FA: A review of therapeutic ultrasound: biophysical effects, *Phys Ther* 81:1351-1358, 2001.
62. Peter Haar G: Therapeutic ultrasound, *Eur J Ultrasound* 9: 3-9, 1999.
63. Vaezy S et al: Image-guided acoustic therapy, *Ann Rev Biomed Eng* 3:375-390, 2001.
64. Bailey MR et al: Physical mechanisms of the therapeutic effect of ultrasound (a review), *Acoust Phys* 49:369-388, 2003.

Performance

65. American Institute of Ultrasound in Medicine: *Standard methods for measuring performance of pulse-echo ultrasound imaging equipment*, Laurel, Md, 1998, The Institute.
66. American Institute of Ultrasound in Medicine: *Methods for measuring performance of pulse-echo ultrasound imaging equipment. Part II. Digital methods*, Laurel, Md, 1998, The Institute.
67. American Institute of Ultrasound in Medicine: *Quality assurance manual for gray-scale ultrasound scanners*, Laurel, Md, 1998, The Institute.
68. American Institute of Ultrasound in Medicine: *Specifications of available imaging phantoms*, ed 2, Laurel, Md, 1996, The Institute.
69. American Institute of Ultrasound in Medicine: *Performance criteria and measurements for Doppler ultrasound devices*, Laurel, Md, 1998, The Institute.

Output

70. Ziskin MC, Lewin PA, editors: *Ultrasonic exposimetry*, Boca Raton, Fla, 1993, CRC Press.
71. Harris GR: Progress in medical ultrasound exposimetry, *IEEE Trans Ultrason Ferroelectr Freq Control* 52:717-736, 2005.
72. Preston RC: *Output measurement for medical ultrasound*, New York, 1991, Springer-Verlag.
73. American Institute of Ultrasound in Medicine: *Acoustic output labeling standard for diagnostic ultrasound equipment*, Laurel, Md, 2001, The Institute.
74. American Institute of Ultrasound in Medicine: *Acoustic output measurement standard for diagnostic ultrasound equipment*, Laurel, Md, 2004, The Institute.
75. Ide M, Zagzebski JA, Duck FA: Acoustic output of diagnostic equipment, *Ultrasound Med Biol* 15(suppl 1):47-65, 1989.
76. Duck FA, Martin K: Trends in diagnostic ultrasound exposure, *Phys Med Biol* 36:1423-1432, 1991.
77. Patton CA, Harris GR, Phillips RA: Output levels and bioeffects indices from diagnostic ultrasound exposure data reported to the FDA, *IEEE Trans Ultrason Ferroelectr Freq Control* 41:353-359, 1994.
78. Henderson J et al: A survey of the acoustic outputs of diagnostic ultrasound equipment in current clinical use, *Ultrasound Med Biol* 21:699-705, 1995.

Bioeffects and Safety

79. Barnett SB et al: The sensitivity of biological tissue to ultrasound, *Ultrasound Med Biol* 23:805-812, 1997.
80. Barnett SB et al: International recommendations and guidelines for the safe use of diagnostic ultrasound in medicine, *Ultrasound Med Biol* 26:355-366, 2000.
81. Barnett SB, Kossoff G: *Safety of diagnostic ultrasound*, New York, Parthenon, 1998.
82. American Institute of Ultrasound in Medicine: *Safety considerations for diagnostic ultrasound*, Laurel, Md, 1991, The Institute.
83. American Institute of Ultrasound in Medicine: *Medical ultrasound safety*, Laurel, Md, 1994, The Institute.
84. American Institute of Ultrasound in Medicine: *Bioeffects and safety of diagnostic ultrasound*, Laurel, Md, 1993, The Institute.
85. American Institute of Ultrasound in Medicine: Mechanical bioeffects from diagnostic ultrasound: AIUM consensus statements, *J Ultrasound Med* 19:68-168, 2000.

86. National Council on Radiation Protection: *Exposure criteria for medical diagnostic ultrasound. I. Criteria based on thermal mechanisms*, Bethesda, Md, 1992, The Council.

87. National Council on Radiation Protection: *Exposure criteria for medical diagnostic ultrasound: II. Criteria based on all known mechanisms*, Bethesda, Md, 2202, The Council.

88. British Institute of Radiology: *The safe use of ultrasound in medical diagnosis*, London, 2000, The Institute.

89. WFUMB symposium on safety of ultrasound in medicine, *Ultrasound Med Biol* 24(suppl 1):S1-S55, 1998.

90. World Health Organization: *Environmental health criteria 22: ultrasound*, Geneva, 1982, The Organization.

91. World Health Organization: Ultrasound. In *Nonionizing radiation protection*, ed 2, Geneva, 1989, The Organization.

92. American Institute of Ultrasound in Medicine: *Official statements and reports*, Laurel, Md, 2000, The Institute (www.aium.org).

93. Miller MW: Does ultrasound induce sister-chromatid exchanges? *Ultrasound Med Biol* 11:561-570, 1985.

94. Miller DL: The botanical effects of ultrasound: a review, *Environ Exp Bot* 23:1-27, 1983.

95. American Institute of Ultrasound in Medicine: *Standard for real-time display of thermal and mechanical acoustic output indices on diagnostic ultrasound equipment, revision 1*, Laurel, Md, 1998, The Institute.

96. American Institute of Ultrasound in Medicine: How to interpret the ultrasound output display standard for higher acoustic output diagnostic ultrasound devices (version 2), *J Ultrasound Med* 23:723-726, 2004.

97. Salvesen KA, Eik-Nes SH: Is ultrasound unsound? A review of epidemiological studies of human exposure to ultrasound, *Ultrasound Obstet Gynecol* 6:293-298, 1995.

Glossary

98. Institute of Electrical and Electronics Engineers: *The authoritative dictionary of IEEE standard terms*, ed 7, New York, 2000, The Institute.

99. American Institute of Ultrasound in Medicine: *Recommended ultrasound terminology*, ed 2, Laurel, Md, 2002, The Institute.

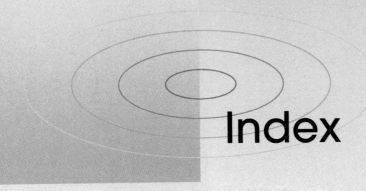

Index

A

A mode, 143, 144f, 145f, 338
Abdomen, scans of, 4, 9, 41f, 100f
Acoustic variables, 17
AIUM. *See* American Institute of Ultrasound in Medicine (AIUM).
ALARA principle, 322, 333f, 334
Aliasing
  causes of, 286f, 287f
  in Doppler echocardiography, 284f
  and Doppler flower, 282f
  and Nyquist limit, 285f, 294f, 296f
  occurring with Doppler ultrasound, 340
  and pulse repetition frequency, 284f
  and range-ambiguity limits, 290t
  and range-ambiguity artifacts, 283t
  reducing of, 285b
  in spectral Doppler displays, 277, 281
American College of Radiology Ultrasound Accreditation Program, 307
American Institute of Ultrasound in Medicine (AIUM)
  performance requirements of, 307
  publications of, 324f
  statement on animals, 340
  statement on cavitation, 329
  statement on heat, 327
  statement on in vitro bioeffects, 322
  statement on instrument output, 330
  statement on prudent ultrasound use, 333-334
  statements on bioeffects, 325
Amplifier(s), and gain, 94, 99-101
Amplitude
  comparisons of, 97f
  definition of, 27, 28f
  and echoes, 42f
  produced by pulser, 92
Analog-to-digital converters (digitizers), 101, 103, 104f, 138f
Aneurysm, scans of, 205f
Angles, in oblique incidence, 37-39
Animals, bioeffects on, 325
Aperture
  dynamic, 74
  and near-zone length, 64
  variable, 72, 73f
Archiving, 145-148

Array
  convex (curved), 67, 68f, 117f, 338
  grating lobes in, 72-73
  (linear) phased, 68-70, 71f, 73f
  linear (sequenced), 66-67, 68f, 117f, 338
    pulsing sequence in, 67
  phased, 338
  terms used for, 75t
  vector, 73-74, 338
Artifact(s)
  attenuation group of
    enhancement, 277, 279f, 340
    focal enhancement (banding), 277, 281f
    refraction, 265, 270f, 271f, 272f
    shadowing, 267, 277, 278f, 279f, 280f, 340
  causes of, 298t
  in harmonic imaging, 105
  interference from electronics, 281f
  occurrence of, 261, 340
  propagation group of
    comet tail, 263, 266f
    grating lobes, 265, 267, 273f, 274f
    mirror image, 265, 268f, 269f, 288, 291f, 292f, 293f, 340
    range ambiguity, 94f, 267, 276f, 283t, 288, 289f, 290f, 340
    refraction, 265, 270f, 271f, 272f, 340
    reverberation, 263, 264f, 265f, 276f, 340
    ring-down, 265, 267f
    section thickness, 79, 262
    speckle, 263
    speed errors, 267
  in spectral Doppler displays
    aliasing, 277, 281, 283f, 288, 297
  types of, 262b
Attenuation
  amplitude and, 27, 28f
  coefficient of, 32-33
  and decibels, 30-32
  definition of, 30
  effects on imaging, 30
  increase of, 338
  intensity and, 27-30
  intensity ratio, determining, 33
  and time gain compensation, 100-101
Autocorrelation, in Doppler shift detection, 188, 190f, 191
Axial resolution. *See* Resolution, detail, axial.

Page numbers followed by f indicate figures; t, tables; b, boxes.